BIODENTAL ENGINEERING V

PROCEEDINGS OF THE 5TH INTERNATIONAL CONFERENCE ON BIODENTAL ENGINEERING, PORTO, PORTUGAL, 22–23 JUNE 2018

Biodental Engineering V

Editors

J. Belinha
Instituto Politécnico do Porto, Porto, Portugal

R.M. Natal Jorge, J.C. Reis Campos, Mário A.P. Vaz &
João Manuel R.S. Tavares
Universidade do Porto, Porto, Portugal

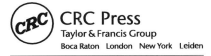

CRC Press is an imprint of the
Taylor & Francis Group, an **informa** business

A BALKEMA BOOK

CRC Press/Balkema is an imprint of the Taylor & Francis Group, an informa business

© 2019 Taylor & Francis Group, London, UK

Typeset by V Publishing Solutions Pvt Ltd., Chennai, India

All rights reserved. No part of this publication or the information contained herein may be reproduced, stored in a retrieval system, or transmitted in any form or by any means, electronic, mechanical, by photocopying, recording or otherwise, without written prior permission from the publisher.

Although all care is taken to ensure integrity and the quality of this publication and the information herein, no responsibility is assumed by the publishers nor the author for any damage to the property or persons as a result of operation or use of this publication and/or the information contained herein.

Library of Congress Cataloging-in-Publication Data

Names: International Conference on Biodental Engineering (5th: 2018: Porto, Portugal), author. | Belinha, Jorge, editor. | Jorge, Renato M. Natal editor. | Campos, J.C. Reis, editor. | Vaz, Mario A.P., editor. | Tavares, Joao Manuel R.S., editor.
Title: Biodental engineering V: proceedings of the 5th International Conference on Biodental Engineering, Porto, Portugal, 22–23 June 2018 / editors, J. Belinha, R.M. Natal Jorge, J.C. Reis Campos, Mario A.P. Vaz & Joao Manuel R.S. Tavares.
Description: London, UK; Boca Raton, FL: Taylor & Francis Group, [2019] | Includes bibliographical references and index.
Identifiers: LCCN 2019000506 (print) | LCCN 2019001080 (ebook) | ISBN 9780429265297 (ebook) | ISBN 9780367210878 (hardcover: alk. paper)
Subjects: | MESH: Dental Materials | Biocompatible Materials | Dental Implants | Biomedical Technology | Medical Informatics | Tissue Engineering | Congress
Classification: LCC RK652.5 (ebook) | LCC RK652.5 (print) | NLM WU 190 | DDC 617.6/95--dc23
LC record available at https://lccn.loc.gov/2019000506

Published by: CRC Press/Balkema
             Schipholweg 107C, 2316 XC Leiden, The Netherlands
             e-mail: Pub.NL@taylorandfrancis.com
             www.crcpress.com – www.taylorandfrancis.com

ISBN: 978-0-367-21087-8 (Hbk)
ISBN: 978-0-429-26529-7 (eBook)

Biodental Engineering V – Belinha et al. (Eds)
© 2019 Taylor & Francis Group, London, ISBN 978-0-367-21087-8

Table of contents

Preface	ix
Acknowledgement	xi
Scientific committee	xiii

Numerical analysis of titanium hybrid-plates in atrophic maxilla 1
M. Prados-Privado, H. Diederich, S.A. Gehrke & J.C. Prados-Frutos

Effects of introducing gap constraints in the masticatory system: A finite element study 5
S.E. Martinez Choy, J. Lenz, K. Schweizerhof & H.J. Schindler

Influence of temperature on the dimensional stability of an addition silicone 11
C.F. Almeida, F. Dantas, A. Portela, M. Vasconcelos & J.C. Reis Campos

Computational analysis for stress intensity factor (KI) measuring in metal-ceramic interface 15
E.M.M. Fonseca, J.F. Piloto, M.G. Fernandes & R.M. Natal Jorge

Thermal stimulation of dentinal tubules 19
P.A.G. Piloto & J.F. Piloto

Analysis tool of skills' acquisition in fine motor skill 25
R.D. Lopes, S. Castro, M.J. Ponces, N. Ramos & M. Vaz

A new approach in 3D finite element analysis in restorative dentistry 27
C. Özcan, C. Muraille, P. Lestriez & Y. Josset

Biological behavior of titanium, zirconia or PEEK dental implant-abutments 31
*M.B. Sordi, S.N.D. Sarwer-Foner, F.H. Schünemann, K. Apaza-Bedoya,
G.M.P. Juanito, B. Henriques, R.S. Magini & C.A.M. Benfatti*

Dental implants fatigue life: A probabilistic fatigue study 43
M. Prados-Privado, S.A. Gehrke, R. Rojo & J.C. Prados-Frutos

Micromorphology, microstructure and micro-Raman spectroscopy of a case
of amelogenesis imperfecta 47
S. Arroyo Bote, A. Villa-Vigil, M.C. Manzanares Céspedes & E. Brau-Aguadé

Influence of resin composite cement on the final color of fixed rehabilitation 53
J.F. Piloto, C.A.M. Volpato, P. Rocha, P.J. Almeida, C. Silva & P. Vaz

Clinical determination of chewing side 57
I. Fediv, A. Carvalho, A. Correia & P. Fonseca

Finishing and polishing of acrylic resins used in provisional restorations 61
S. Matos, F. Araujo, A. Correia & S. Oliveira

3D analysis of the clinical results of VISTA technique combined with connective
tissue graft 65
D.S. Martins, L. Azevedo, N. Santos, T. Marques, C. Alves & A. Correia

3D analysis of rest seats in clinical environment 75
M. Pimenta, F. Araujo, T. Marques, P. Fonseca & A. Correia

Hyaluronic acid vs chlorhexidine in mandibular molar extractions 79
A.A. Martins, B. Leitão, T. Borges, M. Pereira, A. Correia & R. Figueiredo

Research of oral health information by patients of a University dental clinic 83
H. Costa, B. Oliveira, A. Oliveira & A. Correia

Effect of bleaching on microleakage of class V composite resin restorations – in vitro study 89
T. Pereira, A. Azevedo, M. Vasconcelos, P. Mesquita, M.T. Carvalho & C.F. Almeida

Influence of the Er,Cr:YSGG laser and radial firing tips on the push-out bond strength
of glass fiber posts 95
A.I. Araújo, M. Martins, J.C. Reis Campos, A. Barros, A. Azevedo & T. Oliveira

Trigeminal nerve – interdisciplinarity between the areas of dentistry and audiology 101
F. Gentil, J.C. Reis Campos, M. Parente, C.F. Santos, B. Areias & R.M. Natal Jorge

Facial nerve—a clinical and anatomical review 105
F. Gentil, J.C. Reis Campos, M. Parente, C.F. Santos, B. Areias & R.M. Natal Jorge

Prenatal ultrasound features in a case of Arnold Chiari malformation 109
B. Fernandes, I. Côrte-Real, P. Vaz, R. Nogueira, F. Valente & A.C. Braga

Relevance of facial features in ultrasound diagnosis of Holoprosencephaly 111
B. Fernandes, I. Côrte-Real, P. Mesquita, M.H. Figueiral, P. Vaz & F. Valente

Orthodontic stainless steel wire and nickel release 113
S. Castro, M.J. Ponces, J.D. Lopes, M. Vasconcelos, J.C. Reis Campos & C. Pollmann

Influence of thermocycling and colorants in the color of a bis-acryl composite
resin—in vitro study 115
M.G.F. de Macedo, C.A.M. Volpato, B.A.P.C. Henriques, P.C. Vaz,
F.S. Silva & C.F.C.L. Silva

Flexible prosthesis in polyamide: Literature revision 119
R.F.A. da Costa, M.H. Figueiral, M. Sampaio-Fernandes,
S. Oliveira & J.C. Reis Campos

Application of chitosan in dentistry—a review 123
J.M.S. Gomes, J. Belinha & R.M. Natal Jorge

Computational simulation of the vestibular system using a meshless particle method 129
C.F. Santos, M. Parente, J. Belinha, R.M. Natal Jorge & F. Gentil

Using meshless methods to simulate the free vibrations of the cupula under
pathological conditions 135
C.F. Santos, M. Parente, J. Belinha, R.M. Natal Jorge & F. Gentil

Development of an image processing based algorithm to define trabecular bone
mechanical properties using the fabric tensor concept 141
M. Marques, J. Belinha, R.M. Natal Jorge & A.F. Oliveira

A homogenization multiscale procedure for trabecular bone tissue using meshless methods 147
M. Marques, J. Belinha, R.M. Natal Jorge & A.F. Oliveira

Bone remodeling mathematical models using advanced discretization techniques: A review 155
M.M.A. Peyroteo, J. Belinha, L.M.J.S. Dinis & R.M. Natal Jorge

Predicting the trabecular architecture in the vicinity of natural teeth: A comparison
between finite elements and meshless methods 161
M.M.A. Peyroteo, J. Belinha, L.M.J.S. Dinis & R.M. Natal Jorge

Comparing the stress distribution between atrophic maxillary rehabilitation techniques
using FEM 167
K.F. Vargas, G.A.R. Caldas, J. Belinha, R.M. Natal Jorge, P.A.G. Hernandez,
A. Ozkomur, R. Smidt, M.M. Naconecy & L.E. Schneider

The numerical analysis of 4-On-Pillars technique using meshless methods 171
K.F. Vargas, G.A.R. Caldas, J. Belinha, R.M. Natal Jorge, P.A.G. Hernandez,
A. Ozkomur, R. Smidt, M.M. Naconecy & L.E. Schneider

Numerical analysis of support structures on an adhesive dental bridge 177
G.A.R. Caldas, J. Belinha & R.M. Natal Jorge

Predicting in-silico structural response of dental restorations using meshless methods 183
G.A.R. Caldas, J. Belinha & R.M. Natal Jorge

Using meshless methods to analyse bone remodelling after the insertion
of a femoral implant 189
A.T.A. Castro, M.M.A. Peyroteo, J. Belinha & R.M. Natal Jorge

Using meshless methods to predict *in-silico* the stress distribution around
bone sarcoma 195
A.T.A. Castro, J. Belinha, E.M.M. Fonseca, R.M. Natal Jorge,
V.C.C. Oliveira & A.F. Oliveira

Using meshless methods to predict the biomechanical behaviour of red blood cells 201
S.D. Ferreira, J. Belinha & R.M. Natal Jorge

The computational mechanical simulation of healthy and pathological red blood cells
with meshless methods 207
S.D. Ferreira, J. Belinha & R.M. Natal Jorge

Predicting the stress distribution in the mandible bone due to the insertion of implants:
A meshless method study 213
H.I.G. Gomes, J. Belinha & R.M. Natal Jorge

Studying the mandible bone tissue remodelling in the vicinity of implants using
a meshless method computational framework 219
H.I.G. Gomes, J. Belinha & R.M. Natal Jorge

Computational structural analysis of dental implants using radial point interpolation
meshless methods 225
C.C.C. Coelho, J. Belinha & R.M. Natal Jorge

The biomechanical simulation of a zygomatic bar implant using meshless methods 231
C.C.C. Coelho, J. Belinha & R.M. Natal Jorge

Wound healing angiogenesis: An overview on mathematical models 237
A.C. Guerra, J. Belinha & R.M. Natal Jorge

The influence of a blood clot in hemodynamics: A meshless method study 245
M.I.A. Barbosa, J. Belinha & R.M. Natal Jorge

Miscellaneous

Masticatory muscles assessment with infrared imaging in oral rehabilitation—a case report 253
A. Moreira, R. Batista, J. Mendes, S. Oliveira, J.C. Reis Campos & M.H. Figueiral

Tips on implant screws tightening – an overview 259
A. Moreira, R. Batista, S. Oliveira, P. Ferrás, F. Góis & J.C. Reis Campos

Immediate loading in every dental implant protocol – is it safe? 263
D. Soares, J.S. Marques, J.C. Reis Campos, M. Sampaio-Fernandes, C. Silva &
J.C. Sampaio-Fernandes

Immediate loading of dental implants – planning and provisional restauration: A case report 267
J.S. Marques, D. Soares, J.M. Rocha, P.J. Almeida, J.C. Sampaio-Fernandes & M.H. Figueiral

Local anesthetic administration—a rare necrotic ulcer on the palate: A case report 271
J.S. Marques, D. Soares, J.M. Rocha, P. Ferrás, J.C. Reis Campos & M.H. Figueiral

Retention of metal clips in overdentures 275
M.J. Roxo, M. Sampaio-Fernandes, P. Vaz, F. Góis, J.C. Reis Campos & M.H. Figueiral

Implant-tooth fixed supported prosthesis: A review 279
R. Batista, A. Moreira, M. Sampaio-Fernandes, P. Vaz, J.C. Sampaio-Fernandes & M.H. Figueiral

Biomechanical behavior of dental implants—photoelastic analysis 285
V.N. Gomes, D. Tripak, S. Oliveira, J.C. Reis Campos & M.H. Figueiral

Author index 293

Biodental Engineering V – Belinha et al. (Eds)
© 2019 Taylor & Francis Group, London, ISBN 978-0-367-21087-8

Preface

Dentistry is a branch of medicine with peculiarities and diverse areas of action, being commonly considered as an interdisciplinary area. The development, validation and clinical use of better and more advanced techniques and technologies has led to greater demand and more interest.

Biodental Engineering V contains the full papers presented at the 5th International Conference on Biodental Engineering (BIODENTAL 2018, Porto, Portugal, 22–23 June 2018). The conference had two workshops, one of them dealing with computational imaging combined with finite element method, the other dealing with bone tissue remodelling models. Additionally, the conference had three special sessions and sixty contributed presentations.

The topics discussed in **Biodental Engineering V** include:

- Aesthetics
- Bioengineering
- Biomaterials
- Biomechanical disorders
- Biomedical devices
- Computational bio-imaging and visualization
- Computational methods
- Dental medicine
- Experimental mechanics
- Signal processing and analysis
- Implantology
- Minimally invasive devices and techniques
- Orthodontics
- Prosthesis and orthosis
- Simulation
- Software development
- Telemedicine
- Tissue engineering
- Virtual reality

The purpose of the Series of BIODENTAL Conferences on Biodental Engineering, initiated in 2009, is to perpetuate knowledge on bioengineering applied to dentistry, by promoting a comprehensive forum for discussion on recent advances in related fields in order to identify potential collaboration between researchers and end-users from different sciences.

The conference co-chairs would like to take this opportunity to express their gratitude to the conference sponsors, all members of the conference scientific committee, invited lecturers, session-chairs and to all authors for submitting and sharing their knowledge.

J. Belinha
R.M. Natal Jorge
J.C. Reis Campos
Mário A.P. Vaz
João Manuel R.S. Tavares

Biodental Engineering V – Belinha et al. (Eds)
© 2019 Taylor & Francis Group, London, ISBN 978-0-367-21087-8

Acknowledgements

The editors and the Conference co-chairs acknowledge the support towards the organization of the 5th International Conference on Biodental Engineering BIODENTAL 2018 and the publishing of this Book of Proceedings to the following organizations:

- Universidade do Porto (UP)
- Faculdade de Engenharia da Universidade do Porto (FEUP)
- Faculdade de Medicina Dentária da Universidade do Porto (FMDUP)
- Instituto Politécnico do Porto (IPP)
- Instituto Superior de Engenharia do Porto (ISEP)
- Instituto de Ciência e Inovação em Engenharia Mecânica e Engenharia Industrial (INEGI)
- Laboratório de Biomecânica do Porto (LABIOMEP)
- Fundação para a Ciência e a Tecnologia (FCT)
- Project NORTE-01-0145-FEDER-000022—SciTech—Science and Technology for Competitive and Sustainable Industries, cofinanced by Programa Operacional Regional do Norte (NORTE2020), through Fundo Europeu de Desenvolvimento Regional (FEDER)
- Associação Portuguesa de Mecânica Teórica Aplicada e Computacional (APMTAC)
- Câmara Municipal do Porto
- Espaço Atmosfera M—Associação Mutualista Montepio
- Centros auditivos Widex

Biodental Engineering V – Belinha et al. (Eds)
© 2019 Taylor & Francis Group, London, ISBN 978-0-367-21087-8

Scientific committee

All works submitted to BIODENTAL 2018 were evaluated by an International Scientific Committee composed by 58 expert researchers from recognized institutions:

André Correia, *Instituto de Ciências da Saúde, Viseu, UC Portuguesa, Portugal*
António Completo, *Universidade de Aveiro, Portugal*
Carla Roque, *IDMEC, Portugal*
Cláudia Barros Machado, *CESPU, Portugal*
Cornelia Kober, *Hamburg University of Applied Sciences, Germany*
Daniela Iacoviello, *Sapienza University of Rome, Italy*
Elza Maria Morais Fonseca, *Instituto Politécnico do Porto, Portugal*
Estevam Las Casas, *Universidade Federal de Minas Gerais, Brazil*
Fernanda Gentil, *IDMEC—FEUP, Portugal*
Gerhard A. Holzapfel, *Graz University of Technology, Austria*
Helena Figueiral, *FMDUP, Portugal*
Ioannis Misirlis, *University of Patras, Greece*
João Batista Novaes Júnior, *Universidade Federal de Minas Gerais, Brazil*
João Eduardo P.C. Ribeiro, *Instituto Politécnico de Bragança, Portugal*
João Manuel Tavares, *FEUP, Portugal*
João Paulo Flores Fernandes, *University of Minho, Portugal*
Joaquim Gabriel, *Universidade do Porto, Portugal*
Jorge Belinha, *Instituto Politécnico do Porto, Portugal*
John Middleton, *Cardiff University, UK*
Kazem Alemzadeh, *University of Bristol, UK*
Leopoldo Forner Navarro, *Universitat de València, Spain*
Luis Geraldo Vaz, *UNESP, Brazil*
Marco Parente, *FEUP, Portugal*
Maria Cristina Manzanares Céspedes, *Universitat de Barcelona, Spain*
Mário Vaz, *FEUP, Portugal*
Mildred Ballin Hecke, *Universidade Federal do Paraná, Brazil*
Pablo Jesús Rodríguez Cervantes, *Universitat Jaume I, Spain*
Paula Vaz, *FMDUP, Portugal*
Paulo Alexandre Gonçalves Piloto, *Instituto Politécnico de Bragança, Portugal*
Paulo Melo, *FMDUP, Portugal*
Paulo Rui Fernandes, *Instituto Superior Técnico, Portugal*
Pedro Martins, *INEGI, Portugal*
Pedro Miguel Gomes Nicolau, *University of Coimbra, Portugal*
Reis Campos, *FMDUP, Portugal*
Renato Natal Jorge, *FEUP, Portugal*
Sampaio Fernandes, *FMDUP, Portugal*
Stephen Richmond, *Cardiff University, UK*
Yongjie (Jessica) Zhang, *Carnegie Mellon University, USA*
António Ramos, *Universidade de Aveiro, Portugal*
Henrique Almeida, *Instituto Politécnico de Leiria, Portugal*
Teresa Pereira Leite, *USF Alcaides, Portugal*
Vicente Campos, *CHLC Lisboa, Portugal*
Margarida Sampaio Fernandes, *FMDUP, Portugal*
Fernando Guerra, *Universidade de Coimbra, Portugal*

Patrícia Fonseca, *Instituto de Ciências da Saúde, Viseu, UC Portuguesa, Portugal*
Amaya Pérez del Palomar, *University of Zaragoza, Spain*
Urbano Santana-Mora, *University of Santiago de Compostela, Spain*
Urbano Santana-Penin, *University of Santiago de Compostela, Spain*
Mª Jesús Mora, *University of Santiago de Compostela, Spain*
Filipe Silva, *University of Minho, Portugal*
Sílvia Barbeiro, *University of Coimbra, Portugal*
Susana Oliveira, *FMDUP, Portugal*
José Mario Rocha, *FMDUP, Portugal*
Eduardo Campos, *BySteel, UK*
Teresa Oliveira, *FMDUP, Portugal*
César Leal Silva, *FMDUP, Portugal*
Henrique Campos, *HXC-France*

Numerical analysis of titanium hybrid-plates in atrophic maxilla

M. Prados-Privado
Carlos III University, Madrid, Spain
ASISA Dental SA, Madrid, Spain

H. Diederich
Private Practice, Luxembourg, Luxembourg

S.A. Gehrke
BioTecnos, Montevideo, Uruguay

J.C. Prados-Frutos
Rey Juan Carlos University, Madrid, Spain

ABSTRACT: The use of osseointegrated implants in severely atrophied maxilla has important limitations. Two different titanium hybrid-plates are evaluated with finite elements as another viable alternative for atrophic maxilla rehabilitation. The three-dimensional model analyzed is based on a real clinical case. An axial force of 100 N was applied in each plate. The model was subjected to a rigid fixation restriction in the upper and lateral maxilla to prevent displacement in the x, y and z axes. A non-penetration condition between plates and maxilla was added to prevent interferences during the execution process. Von Mises stresses on plates and principal stress on maxilla were obtained with a maximum value of 180 MPa in plates and 80 MPa in maxilla. According to these results, it is possible to conclude that this technique can be considered a viable alternative for atrophic maxilla rehabilitation although it is necessary more studies to corroborate the clinical results.

1 INTRODUCTION

The reconstruction of an atrophic maxilla has been always a challenge because of anatomical and clinical factors (Ali et al. 2014, van der Mark et al. 2011). The most common techniques in atrophic maxilla rehabilitation are bone grafting (Chiapasco et al. 2014), pterygoid (Cucchi et al. 2017) or zygomatic implants (Aparicio et al. 2014), bone regeneration (Gultekin et al. 2017, Kaneko et al. 2016) and, finally, short implants (Alqutaibi et al. 2016).

Hard tissue augmentation provides an adequate bone volume for ideal implant placement and to support soft tissue for optimal esthetics and function. Zygomatic implants present a viable alternative because of their design and length. Pterygoid implants have the advantage of allowing anchorage in the pterygomaxillary region, eliminating the need for sinus lifts or bone grafts. And, finally, short implants are widely used because of their efficiency on implant treatment in atrophic jaw and maxilla (Anitua et al. 2008, Anitua et al. 2014).

The protocol employed in this study is called Cortically Fixed @ Once (CF@O). It is an alternative to conventional implant placement for atrophied maxilla and mandible. This technique has its origins in basal implantology, which was developed by Dr. Scortecci in the early 1980's when he proposed the Diskimplant® (Scortecci & Bourbon 1990).

The aim of this study is to evaluate the biomechanical behavior of CF@O plates on a completely edentulous and atrophic maxilla.

2 MATERIAL AND METHODS

The three-dimensional model analyzed in this study correspond to the real clinical case shown in Figure 1.

Figure 1 represents the final solution to a real case which was employed in a 58-year-old female

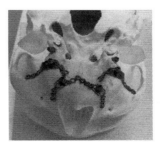

Figure 1. Model employed to reproduce the 3D finite element model.

who wanted fixed teeth in the maxilla in a compromised bone.

2.1 Plates

The plates used in the CF@O protocol are very thin, lightweight and highly flexible and therefore may be adapted to any bone anatomy.

In this study two plates have been employed, which are detailed in Figure 2, where HENGG means Highly Efficient No Graft Gear:

The HENGG-1 plate is appropriated for atrophied maxilla. The HENGG-2 plate is recommended for premaxilla, and the retromolar region.

2.2 Finite element model

Geometry of the maxilla was obtained using CT and transformed to STL format. Maxilla file was imported to SolidWorks 2016 (Dassault Systèmes, SolidWorks Corp., Concord, MA, USA), where the assembly with the four plates was done. All three-dimensional plates were adjusted to the anatomic characteristics of the maxilla. The final reconstruction of the three-dimensional model is detailed in Figure 3.

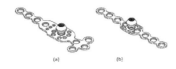

Figure 2. Plates employed in this study: (a) HENGG-1 and (b) HENGG-2.

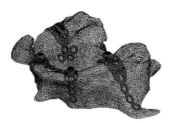

Figure 3. Three-dimensional assembly.

Table 1. Material properties.

	Modulus of elasticity	Poisson's ratio
Plates (Titanium Grade II) (Boyer et al. 1994)	105 GPa	0.37
Cortical bone (Bhering et al. 2016)	13.7 GPa	0.3
Trabecular bone (Bhering et al. 2016)	1.37 GPa	0.3

All materials were considered isotropic, linear, elastic and homogeneous with the properties detailed in Table 1.

2.3 Mesh, boundary conditions and loading configuration

The 3D model was meshed in SolidWorks 2016 (Dassault Systèmes, SolidWorks Corp., Concord, MA, USA) with a fine mesh and all regions of stress concentration that were of interest were manually refined. The convergence criterion was a change of less than 5% in von Mises stress in the model (Peixoto et al. 2017).

A rigid fixation restriction in the upper and lateral maxilla to prevent displacement in the x, y and z axes was applied. A non-penetration condition was also added to prevent interferences between plates and maxilla during the execution. Finally, an axial load of 100 N (Shimura et al. 2016) was directly applied to the area where the prosthesis is fixed to the plate.

3 RESULTS

Figure 4 shows the von Mises stress on plates. The difference between the maximum von Mises stress in HENGG-1 right and left plates is 3%, while the difference between HENGG-2 right and left is 2%.

In view of Figures 5 and 6, which are the plates placed on the molar region, it can be seen that the plate located in the left of the maxilla has bigger stresses on the area situated in the palate than the plate located in the right of the maxilla.

Figures 7 and 8, which represent the plates placed on the premaxilla, detail that both plates have the highest stresses on the area situated in the palate.

All plates showed a similar distribution patterns of maximum principal stress over the atrophic maxilla.

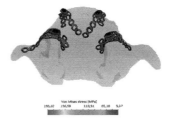

Figure 4. Stress distribution on plates [MPa].

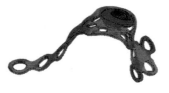

Figure 5. Stress distribution on plate HENGG-1 left.

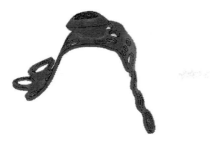

Figure 6. Stress distribution on plate HENGG-1 right.

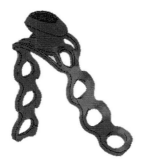

Figure 7. Stress distribution on plate HENGG-2 left.

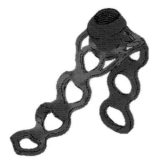

Figure 8. Stress distribution on plate HENGG-2 right.

The difference of principal stress value between the four regions in contact with plates is a 5%, with a mean maximum value of 80 MPa in plates' region.

4 DISCUSSION

The biomechanical behavior of CF@O plates on a completely edentulous and atrophic maxilla has been evaluated employing finite element methods.

The accuracy of results in numerical studies depends on the precision of the model analyzed, the material properties and the constraining conditions (Van Staden et al. 2006). CT was used to obtain the geometry of the atrophic maxilla while plates were provided by the manufacturer.

This study has some limitations and assumptions. All materials were considered homogeneous, isotropic, and linearly elastic. Although these assumptions do not occur in clinical practice, they are common in finite element studies due to the challenges in establishing the properties of living tissues. These assumptions are consistent with other numerical studies (Prados-Privado et al. 2017, Almeida et al. 2015). Another limitation was the use of static loads although cyclic loads occur during chewing movements. This limitation is also validated in the several finite element analyses to study biomechanical behavior (Gümrükçü et al. 2017). However, this study analyzed biomechanical behavior of a new alternative to conventional treatments for atrophic maxilla.

There are several studies available in the literature that employed different techniques to treat edentulous and atrophic maxilla, such as basal disk implants (Odin et al. 2012) or bone augmentation (Baldan et al. 2017).

Küçükkurt et al. compare the biomechanical behavior of different sinus floor elevation for dental implants placement (Küçükkurt et al. 2017). Under the condition of vertical loadings, von Mises stresses in mesial implants were lower than our results in plates in the case of lateral sinus lifting. However, plates analyzed in this study obtain lower von Mises stresses than prosthetic distal cantilever application and short implant placement. Regarding to distal implants, our plates obtained lower stresses than prosthetic distal cantilever.

Ultimate stress limits in cortical bone have been described as 170 MPa in compression and 100 MPa in tension (Pérez et al. 2012). Based on these limits, the values observed in this model were lower than those considered physiologic to bone tissue.

A good biomechanical behavior of plates is understood when a homogeneous stress is transferred to the bone. In this case, the maximum difference between all four plates' region is 5%, meaning that the principal stress transferred from plates to maxilla can be considered homogeneous.

Küçükkurt et al. obtained similar maximum principal stress in maxilla than our results in the case of short implant placement and higher principal stress than our results in prosthetic distal cantilever application (Küçükkurt et al. 2017).

Further studies simulating these titanium hybridplates alternatives for atrophic maxilla and jaw that include dynamic forces that occur during chewing and consider the anisotropic and regenerative properties of bone are needed. Furthermore, some *in vivo* clinical trials are necessary to validate the model and to confirm the efficiency of this protocol. A numerical study of the combination of prosthesis-plates-implant under different functional conditions (bruxism and other parafunctions) just like the antagonist arcade. Finally, a simulation of blood flow and bone regeneration around the plates is also necessary.

5 CONCLUSION

Based on the results provided by this numerical analysis, it is possible to conclude that in terms of clinical application, these titanium hybrid-plates have a better behavior than conventional treatments as prosthetic distal cantilever application and short implant placement. Titanium hybrid-plates distributed load to the maxilla with similar values as the case of short implants but with higher values than prosthetic distal cantilever application. In any case, resistance limits of bone and titanium were not exceeded. Finally, this technique can be considered a viable alternative for atrophic maxilla rehabilitation although it is necessary more studies to corroborate the clinical results.

REFERENCES

Ali, S., Karthigeyan, S., Deivanai, M., Kumar, A. 2014. Implant Rehabilitation For Atrophic Maxilla: A Review. *The Journal of Indian Prosthodontic Society* 13(3): 196–207.

Almeida, E.O., Rocha, E.P., Júnior, A.C.F., Anchieta, R.B. et al. 2015. Tilted and Short Implants Supporting Fixed Prosthesis in an Atrophic Maxilla: A 3D-FEA Biomechanical Evaluation. *Clinical Implant Dentistry and Related Research* 17(Suppl 1): e332–e342.

Alqutaibi, A.Y., Altaib, F. 2016. Short Dental Implant Is Considered as a Reliable Treatment Option for Patients with Atrophic Posterior Maxilla. *Journal of Evidence-Based Dental Practice* 16(3): 173–175.

Anitua, E., Orive, G., Aguirre, J.J., Andía, I. 2008. Five-Year Clinical Evaluation of Short Dental Implants Placed in Posterior Areas: A Retrospective Study. *Journal of Periodontology* 79(1): 42–48.

Anitua, E., Piñas, L., Begoña, L., Orive, G. 2014. Long-Term Retrospective Evaluation of Short Implants in the Posterior Areas: Clinical Results after 10–12 Years. *Journal of Clinical Periodontology* 41(4): 404–411.

Aparicio, C., Manresa, C., Francisco, K., Claros, P., Alández, J., González-Martín, O. et al. 2014. Zygomatic Implants: Indications, Techniques and Outcomes, and the Zygomatic Success Code. *Periodontology 2000* 66(1): 41–58.

Baldan, R.C.F., Coracin, F.L., Lins, L., Mello, W.R., Santos, P.S. 2017. Atrophic Maxilla Reconstruction With Fresh Frozen Allograft Bone, Titanium Mesh, and Platelet-Rich Fibrin: Case Report. *Transplantation Proceedings* 49(4): 893–897.

Bhering, C.L.B., Mesquita, M.F., Kemmoku, D.T., et al. 2016. Comparison between All-on-Four and All-on-Six Treatment Concepts and Framework Material on Stress Distribution in Atrophic Maxilla: A Prototyping Guided 3D-FEA Study. *Materials Science & Engineering. C, Materials for Biological Applications* 69: 715–725.

Boyer, R., Welsch, G., Collings, E.W. 1994. *Materials Properties Handbook: Titanium Alloys.* Ohio: ASM International.

Chiapasco, M., Zaniboni, M. 2014. Methods to Treat the Edentulous Posterior Maxilla: Implants With Sinus Grafting. *Journal of Oral and Maxillofacial Surgery* 67(4): 867–871.

Cucchi, A., Vignudelli, E., Franco, S., Corinaldesi, G. 2017. Minimally Invasive Approach Based on Pterygoid and Short Implants for Rehabilitation of an Extremely Atrophic Maxilla. *Implant Dentistry* 26(4): 1–6.

Gultekin, B.A., Cansiz, E., Borahan, M.O. 2017. Clinical and 3-Dimensional Radiographic Evaluation of Autogenous Iliac Block Bone Grafting and Guided Bone Regeneration in Patients With Atrophic Maxilla. *Journal of Oral and Maxillofacial Surgery* 75(4): 709–722.

Gümrükçü, Z., Korkmaz, Y.T., Korkmaz, F.M. 2017. Biomechanical Evaluation of Implant-Supported Prosthesis with Various Tilting Implant Angles and Bone Types in Atrophic Maxilla: A Finite Element Study. *Computers in Biology and Medicine* 86: 47–54.

Kaneko, T., Nakamura, S., Hino, S., Norio, H., Shimoyama, T. 2016. Continuous Intra-Sinus Bone Regeneration after Nongrafted Sinus Lift with a PLLA Mesh Plate Device and Dental Implant Placement in an Atrophic Posterior Maxilla: A Case Report. *International Journal of Implant Dentistry* 2(1): 16.

Küçükkurt, S., Alpaslan, G., Kurt, A. 2017. Biomechanical Comparison of Sinus Floor Elevation and Alternative Treatment Methods for Dental Implant Placement. *Computer Methods in Biomechanics and Biomedical Engineering* 20(3): 284–293.

Odin, G., Misch, C.E., Binderman, I., Scortecci, G. 2012. Fixed Rehabilitation of Severely Atrophic Jaws Using Immediately Loaded Basal Disk Implants After In Situ Bone Activation. *Journal of Oral Implantology* 38: 611–616.

Peixoto, H.E., Camati, P.R., Faot, F., Sotto-Maior, B. et al. 2017. Rehabilitation of the Atrophic Mandible with Short Implants in Different Positions: A Finite Elements Study. *Materials Science & Engineering. C, Materials for Biological Applications* 80: 122–128.

Pérez, M.A., Prados-Frutos, J.C., Bea, J.A., Doblaré, M. 2012. Stress Transfer Properties of Different Commercial Dental Implants: A Finite Element Study. *Computer Methods in Biomechanics and Biomedical Engineering* 15: 263–273.

Prados-Privado, M., Bea, J.A., Rojo, R., Gehrke, S.A., Calvo-Guirado, J.L., Prados-Frutos, J.C. 2017. A New Model to Study Fatigue in Dental Implants Based on Probabilistic Finite Elements and Cumulative Damage Model. *Applied Bionics and Biomechanics.* 2017: 1–8.

Shimura, Y., Sato, Y., Kitagawa, N., Omor, M. 2016. Biomechanical Effects of Offset Placement of Dental Implants in the Edentulous Posterior Mandible. *International Journal of Implant Dentistry* 2(1):17.

Scortecci, G. & Bourbon, B. 1990. [Dentures on the Diskimplant]. *Revue Francaise Des Prothesistes Dentaires* 13: 31–48.

van der Mark, E.L., Bierenbroodspot, F., Baas, EM., de Lange, J. 2011. Reconstruction of an Atrophic Maxilla: Comparison of Two Methods. British *Journal of Oral and Maxillofacial Surgery* 49(3): 198–202.

Van Staden, R.C., Guan, H., Loo, Y.C. 2006. Application of the Finite Element Method in Dental Implant Research. *Computer Methods in Biomechanics and Biomedical Engineering* 9(4): 257–270.

Effects of introducing gap constraints in the masticatory system: A finite element study

S.E. Martinez Choy, J. Lenz & K. Schweizerhof
Institute for Mechanics, Karlsruhe Institute of Technology (KIT), Karlsruhe, Germany

H.J. Schindler
Department of Prosthodontics, Dental School, University of Würzburg, Würzburg, Germany

ABSTRACT: Disorders in the Temporomandibular Joint (TMJ) are common among the population. In this study, the influence of mechanical gap constraints on the behavior of the TMJ were investigated with the help of a finite element model of the human masticatory system. The finite element model was run as a transient problem that incorporates the dynamic behavior of the jaw, particularly the displacement of the articular disc during jaw motion. Rigid spacers were placed on the molars at each side of the mandible, creating a displacement constraint. Different gaps were introduced by changing the vertical position of one of the rigid spacers. The introduction of a gap raises the biting force at the ipsilateral side and the joint force at the contralateral side. The change of force distribution rotates the jaw slightly and changes the distribution of stresses at the ipsilateral side and increases the stress magnitude at the contralateral side.

1 INTRODUCTION

The temporomandibular joint (TMJ) is a synovial joint which articulates the jaw to the skull. It is composed principally by the mandibular condyle, the mandibular fossa, the articular disc, the capsule, the ligaments and the lateral pterygoid muscle. The articulating surfaces of the condyles and the mandibular fossa are covered with articular cartilage, which together with the synovial fluid allows for a very low coefficient of friction and a uniform transmission of compressive forces to the bone (Radin et al. 1971). The articular cartilage of the TMJ contains both collagen fibers type I and type II, which classifies it as fibrocartilage. Due to the low permeability of the tissue, compression forces rapidly increase fluid pressure, which in turn carries the major part of the load through hydrostatic pressurization (Mow et al. 2005). The collagen fibers of the cartilage, on the other hand, resist the stretching of the tissue from tensile forces (Hukins et al. 1984). The articular disc, also composed of fibrocartilage, lies between the mandibular condyle and the fossa, dividing the synovial joint in two. It distributes loads and dissipates the energy caused from impact loads. The disc allows for relative motion between the condyle and the temporal bone. In the case of the condyle, both translational and rotational motions are possible. The articular disc is connected to the articular surfaces through the joint capsule. The attachments of the joint capsule can be divided as shown in Figures 1–2 into medial, lateral, anterior and posterior attachments. These attachments give the disc a range of movement and at the same time avoid extreme displacements that may result in the dislocation of the disc.

The temporomandibular ligament supports the joint when high posterior forces occur and limits the posterior displacement of the mandible. It also

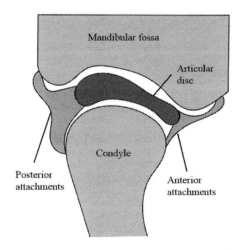

Figure 1. Sagittal view of the Temporomandibular Joint (TMJ) where the anterior and posterior attachments of the joint capsule are shown.

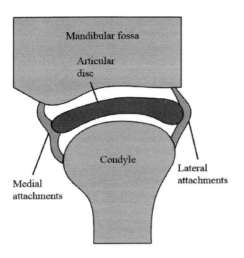

Figure 2. Coronal view of the Temporomandibular Joint (TMJ) where the medial and lateral attachments of the joint capsule are shown.

constraints the condyle during opening (Osborn et al. 1989). It is composed of two bundles of fibers which attach at the zygomatic arch and the neck of the mandible. The lateral pterygoid muscle attaches to the condyle, and in the majority of cases, also directly to the articular disc. The lateral pterygoid muscle is the main responsible for the anterior incursion of the condyle and the disc.

The complexity of the joint makes it very susceptible to problems and disorders. Around 20–30 percent of the population are affected by some type of temporomandibular disorder (TMD), such as pain, clicking, bruxism, limited mobility, articular disc dislocation, etc. (Macfarlane et al. 2002, Llodra-Calvo et al. 2000). One of the most frequent treatments employed for TMD is splint therapy (Ebrahim et al. 2012), with more than 3 million splints made just for the United States. The purpose of the splint is to create a mechanical obstruction in order to restrict dysfunctional forces. Differences in muscle recruitment and activation levels when gap variations are introduced in the masticatory system were studied by Schindler et al. (2009). Based on experimental results (Schindler et al. 2009) and clinical evidence, it has recently been hypothesized that, by means of oral splints, lowering the contact between antagonistic teeth of the dentition opposite to the painful side, might reduce joint loading and, as a result, relieve joint pain.

In the present work, a finite element model that incorporates the different parts of the TMJ, as well as the rest of the components of the human masticatory system, was employed in order to closely study the behavior of the TMJ during the introduction of gap variations. The model was run as a dynamic problem, to accurately capture the relative displacements that the components of the TMJ undergo. These displacements are crucial to determine how the TMJ and its different structures respond to given loads.

2 MATERIALS AND METHODS

The study was carried out with the help of an elaborate finite element (FE) model that comprises all essential components of the stomatognathic system. The components of this model and corresponding material parameters are described in Martinez et al. (2017). Rigid spacers were placed at the second molars in different configurations in order to create the gap variations with the respective muscle activation being employed. In total, four cases are analyzed, with a gap of 0, 100, 200 and 300 μm introduced at the right second molar.

2.1 *Periodontal ligament, bone, teeth and muscles*

The geometry of the PDL was obtained by means of Boolean operations and has a thickness of 0.25 mm. The PDL was modeled using a hyperelastic first-order Ogden material model. Both the cortical and cancellous bone were obtained through a segmentation process. Cortical bone exhibits anisotropic behavior, having different elastic moduli in the longitudinal and radial directions with respect to the axis of the bone (Lettry et al. 2003). Nevertheless, a linear elastic isotropic material model was used for both types of bone in this work.

The jaw muscles present in our model are the lateral pterygoid, digastric, masseter, temporalis and medial pterygoid. Muscles are composed by two entities, one representing the fibrous part and the other the tendon. Hill's muscle model was employed to represent the fibers and an inextensible wire to represent the tendons, because they undergo very small deformation and may, for this reason, be ignored. In total, eight truss elements represent the following muscles (on each side): Anterior and posterior temporalis, superficial and deep masseter, superior and inferior lateral pterygoid, medial pterygoid and digastric. Muscle fibers are composed by myofibrils. In the case of striated muscles, the myofibrils are arranged into contractile units called sarcomeres. Forces produced by this type of muscle are influenced by the length of their sarcomeres (force-length relationship) and their contraction velocities (force-velocity relationship). Additionally, the muscle exhibits a passive elastic force when stretched. In our model, the characteristic curves of the muscle are taken from van Ruijven & Weijs (1990).

2.2 Rigid spacers

Rigid spacers were placed in both sides at the second molar of the mandible. The structures represent the resistance provided by the force measuring devices in the investigation performed by Schindler et al. (2009). The spacer at the right side of the mandible is then lowered to create a gap with respect to the opposite side. The spacers have a thickness of 2 mm.

2.3 Temporomandibular Joint (TMJ)

Several strategies have been employed to model the TMJ. In order to accurately capture its behavior, focus was given to works where the geometry of the articular disc and its relative movement to the condyle were modeled. Koolstra and van Eijden meticulously studied the TMJ. They created a model (Koolstra et al. 2005) that uses a combined FE and rigid body analysis, where the joint consists of an articular disc and cartilage tissue represented with solid finite elements, while the jaw is modeled as a rigid body. In this model, the disc is attached to the condyle by means of inextensible wires, which represent the lateral and medial attachments of the joint capsule. Displacements in this model are a result of forces that originate from the activation of the muscles, which were also closely studied by Koolstra & van Eijden (1988). These authors also studied the viscoelastic behavior of the articular disc, where its decay constants were determined (Koolstra et al. 2007).

Perez et al. carried out numerous investigations of the TMJ (2006a, 2006b, 2007). In their studies, the TMJ consists of the articular disc and the lateral and medial attachments, which are represented with solid elements as part of the geometry of the disc. The attachments connect the condyle to the disc and allow the displacement of the disc. A poroelastic material model is used with different parameters for the anterior, middle and posterior parts of the disc. The cartilage tissue is omitted in their model.

In the present work, the TMJ FE model consists of: an articular disc, the cartilage of the fossa, the cartilage of the condyle, the lateral, medial, posterior and anterior attachments of the disc and the temporomandibular ligament. All components are deformable, with the exception of the medial and lateral attachments. The superior part of the cartilage of the fossa was constrained, as the mandibular fossa was modeled as a rigid body.

2.3.1 Articular disc and cartilage

Since soft tissue is not visible in CT-scans, the geometry of the articular disc was not obtained through a segmentation process. Its creation involved several iterations of manually sculpting the shape following anatomy books while ensuring that it would fit smoothly between the surfaces of the fossa and the condyle. This resulted in an articular disc with a thickness that is more regular than what is observed in reality, as the disc thickness varies considerably between its anterior, middle and posterior part. The articular disc was meshed with over 11.000 hexahedral elements. The geometry for the articular cartilage of both the mandibular fossa and the condyle was created with an offset operation of 0.5 mm (Hansson et al. 1977). The cartilage of the fossa and the condyle are included because of their role in evenly distributing the forces to the bone. A Mooney-Rivlin hyperelastic material model whose parameters were taken from Koolstra & van Eijden (2005) is used for the cartilage and articular disc. The viscoelastic behavior of the disc was also included, with decay constants taken from Koolstra et al. (2007). Node-to-Surface contact elements are used to define the contact between the disc and the cartilage of the fossa, as well as for the contact between the disc and the cartilage of the condyle. In both cases, friction was defined as non-existent since frictional forces are minimal due to the presence of the synovial fluid.

2.4 Attachments and ligaments

The jaw experiences a significant posterior force when the closing muscles are activated. Koolstra activated the lateral pterygoid muscles, in order to bring the system into balance and avoid the disc from dislocating. The measurement of muscle activation levels in Schindler et al. (2009) shows that the lateral muscles are mostly inactive during the biting process.

To ensure joint stability during strong muscle forces, inclusion of the posterior and anterior attachments of the capsule, as well as the temporomandibular ligament was deemed necessary. All attachments and ligaments were modeled using trusses with a material model that only produces resistance during tension. The attachments of the capsule were represented each with a pair of trusses, except the posterior inferior attachments of the capsule, where pulley elements were employed to keep the trusses on the surface of the condyle, in order to produce an appropriate response from the fiber (Figure 3). The temporomandibular ligament was modeled using a pair of trusses in order to represent the deep and superficial part, which are differently oriented. The extent of the trusses was estimated from the area covered by the attachments on the disc. This area was further calibrated a) to ensure that the range of movement of the joint was not unrealistically limited, and b) at the same time to provide the stability required during strong muscle forces. The area of the trusses for the attachments is of approximately

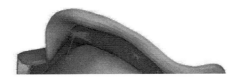

Figure 3. Configuration of the TMJ: cartilage of the fossa, articular disc and cartilage of the condyle modeled using solid elements. Anterior, posterior, medial and lateral attachments, as well as temporomandibular ligament represented with truss elements.

12 mm^2. Similarly for the temporomandibular ligament, the area of its trusses was estimated to be around 15 mm^2.

The attachments of the capsule were given an elastic modulus from the stress-strain curve obtained by Tanaka (2003). However, the inferior posterior and the superior anterior attachments are tense when the mouth is closed (which is the initial configuration of the model). For this reason, a positive offset, determined by measuring the length of the truss during jaw opening (when the fibers are relaxed) was set. Since the task of the medial and lateral attachments of the capsule is to keep the disc on the surface of the condyle, they were modeled as inextensible wires as in Koolstra et al. (2005). The temporomandibular ligament was modeled using the material parameters from Perez (2006).

3 RESULTS

3.1 Variational gap constraint

The configuration for the study can be observed in Figure 4. The rigid body as model for the stiff spacer on the contralateral side remains in the same position for each case, while the rigid body on the ipsilateral side is lowered by 0, 100, 200 or 300 µm. For this task, the jaw is opened slowly from 0 to 225 ms, resulting in a gap between the first molars of circa 5 mm, just enough to bring the lower molars below the rigid bodies. At this point, the contact elements become active and low magnitudes are set for the closing muscles, until a time of 430 ms. These two phases are performed in order to minimize the kinetic energy in the model and avoid sudden movements or impacts. The closing muscles are then activated to their final magnitudes. These magnitudes (Table 1) are the average of the activation levels needed to produce a total biting force of 150 N, which were experimentally measured by Schindler et al. (2009).

In Figure 5, the resulting forces on the joint and on the rigid spacers can be observed. Employing the average activation levels produced in the case

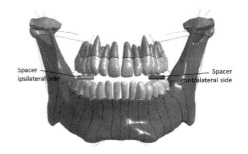

Figure 4. Variational gaps were introduced with spacers (rigid bodies). The ipsilateral side is displaced downwards in each case.

Table 1. Normalized average activation levels of the muscles to produce a bite force of 150 N for each introduced gap.

Muscle	Gap between spacers			
	0	100	200	300 [µm]
Temporalis anterior I	0.38	0.37	0.34	0.36
Temporalis posterior I	0.39	0.20	0.19	0.18
Masseter I 1.15	0.13	0.18	0.17	0.25
Medial pterygoid I	0.07	0.05	0.06	0.06
Lateral pterygoid I	0.00	0.01	0.01	0.01
Temporalis anterior C	0.36	0.37	0.33	0.31
Temporalis posterior C	0.38	0.20	0.17	0.14
Masseter C	0.15	0.20	0.19	0.22
Medial pterygoid C	0.09	0.07	0.10	0.10
Lateral pterygoid C	0.00	0.02	0.01	0.04

I: Ipsilateral; C: Contralateral.

of 0, 100, 200 and 300 µm, a resulting force of 170, 164, 150 and 156 N, respectively. The largest percent error, considering a target force of 150 N, is of 13%, which can be attributed to the use of activation levels of the muscles that were averaged between patients. As expected, as the gap increases the distribution of forces change, with a higher share being shifted to the ipsilateral rigid body and the contralateral joint.

Stresses on the ipsilateral disc are shown in Figure 6. It can be observed that when no gap is introduced, the stresses occur between the middle and the posterior part of the disc. In this case, both condyles are positioned in a very stable position, since no further posterior displacement is possible due to the TMJ ligament and the attachments of the disc, as well as the resulting force on the mandible having a posterior direction. Additionally, a large area of the articular disc is in contact with both the condyle and the mandibular fossa, which allows for a better distribution of the forces in the joint. As the

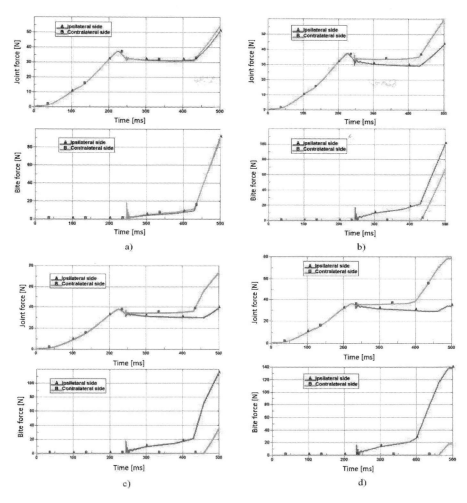

Figure 5. Forces on the joint and the rigid spacers (bite force), when both sides are even (a), and when a gap of 100 (b), 200 (c) and 300 μm (d) is introduced.

gap increases, stresses in the ipsilateral joint continuously shift to the center of the disc. The rising forces in the contralateral side increase the compressive stresses, with the compressive stress reaching a magnitude of −1.67, −1.73, −1.79 and −1.86 MPa.

4 DISCUSSION

Changes in the force distribution, between the joints and the biting points, when gaps are introduced are very similar to those observed in the experimental measurements of Schindler et al. (2009). The contralateral side overcomes the introduced gap through, mostly, the deformation of the articular disc. The model shows that further widening of the gap would be too difficult to overcome, since forces in the contralateral rigid body are minimal while the force in the contralateral joint already surpasses by more than twice the amount found in the ipsilateral joint. When the gap is introduced, a decrease in the activity of the temporalis muscle occurs, while activity in the masseter muscle increases. This phenomenon, along the reduced forces that occur in the ipsilateral joint, lowers the posterior displacement of the ipsilateral condyle and shifts the stresses to the center of the disc. On the other hand, the higher forces withstood by the contralateral joint deform its disc and displace the condyle posteriorly. As a result, in all cases the contralateral condyle is held at its most posterior position by the TMJ ligament and disc attachments.

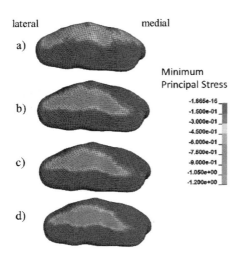

Figure 6. Third principal stresses of the ipsilateral articular disc (front view) during a target bite force of 150 N and a gap of 0 (a), 100 (b), 200 (c) and 300 (d) μm.

Subsequently, stress distribution is very similar but with different magnitudes.

Concerning the modeling with FE, improvements on the details of the geometry of the disc could be performed with the help of MRI-scans to take into account its varying thickness. The material parameters of the articular disc can be further calibrated in order to achieve resulting forces that are closer to those observed in the literature (Schindler et al. 2009), improving the overall behavior of the model.

5 CONCLUSIONS

The simulations performed with the model confirm that the introduction of mechanical constraints change significantly the distribution of forces in the system, allowing, for instance, oral splints to shift compressive stresses in the joints to different parts of the disc as well as limiting the forces on one of the joints. The increase of contact between antagonistic molars at one side of the mandible will result in a reduction of forces at that side of the joint and shift the loads to the opposite joint.

REFERENCES

Ebrahim, S., Montoya, L., Busse, J.W., Carrasco-Labra, A., Guyatt, G.H. 2012. The effectiveness of splint therapy in patients with temporomandibular disorders: A systematic review and meta-analysis. *The Journal of the American Dental Association* 143: 847–857.

Hansson, T., Öberg, T. 1977. Arthrosis and deviation in form in the temporomandibular joint: A macroscopic study on a human autopsy material. *Acta Odontologica Scandinavica* 35:167–874.

Hukins, W., Aspden, R., Yarker, Y. 1984. Fiber reinforcement and mechanical stability in articular cartilage. *Engineering in Medicine* 13: 153–156.

Koolstra, J.H. & van Eijden, T.M.G.J., Weijs, W.A., Naeije, M. 1988. A three-dimensional mathematical model of the human masticatory system predicting maximum possible bite forces. *Journal of Biomechanics* 21:563–576.

Koolstra, J.H. & van Eijden, T.M.G.J. 2005. Combined finite-element and rigid-body analysis of human jaw joint dynamics. *Journal of Biomechanics* 38:2431–2439.

Koolstra, J.H. & van Eijden T.M.G.J 2007. Consequences of Viscoelastic Behavior in the Human Temporomandibular Joint Disc. *J Dent Res* 2007 86:1198–1202.

Lettry, S., Seedhom, B.B., Berry, E., Cupponea, M. 2003. Quality assessment of the cortical bone of the human mandible. *Bone* 32:35–44.

Llodra-Calvo, J.C., Bravo-Pérez, M., Cortés-Martinicorena, F.J. 2000. Encuesta de Salud Oral en España. *Revista Consejo Odontólogos Estomatólogos* 7:19–63.

Macfarlane, T.V., Blinkhorn, A.S., Davies, R.M., Kincey, J. Worthington, H.V. 2002. Oro-facial pain in the community: prevalence and associated impact. *Community Dentistry and Oral Epidemiology* 30: 52–60.

Martinez Choy, S.E., Lenz, J., Schweizerhof, K., Schmitter, M., Schindler, H.J. 2017. Realistic kinetic loading of the jaw system during single chewing cycles: a finite element study. *Journal of Oral Rehabilitation* 44:375–384.

Mow, V.C., Huiskes, R. 2005. *Basic Orthopaedic Biomechanics and Mechanobiology*. Philadelphia: Lippincott Williams & Wilkins.

Osborn, J.W. 1989. The temporomandibular ligament and the articular eminence as constraints during jaw opening. *Journal of Oral Rehabilitation* 16: 323–333.

Perez del Palomar, A., Doblare, M. 2006a. The effect of collagen reinforcement in the behaviour of the temporomandibular joint disc. *Journal of Biomechanics* 39:1075–1085.

Perez del Palomar, A., Doblare, M. 2006b. Finite element analysis of the temporomandibular joint during lateral excursions of the mandible. *Journal of Biomechanics* 39:2153–2163.

Perez del Palomar, A., Doblare, M. 2007. An accurate simulation model of anteriorly displaced TMJ discs with and without reduction. *Medical Engineering & Physics* 29:216–226.

Radin, E.L., Paul I.L. 1971. Response of Joints to Impact Loading. *Arthritis and Rheumatism* 14(3): 356–362.

van Ruijven, L.J., Weijs, W.A. 1990. A new model for calculating muscle forces from electromyograms. *European Journal of Applied Physiology* 61: 479–485.

Schindler, H.J., Lenz, J. Türp, J.C., Schweizerhof, K., Rues, S. 2009. Small unilateral jaw gap variations: equilibrium changes, co-contractions and joint forces. *Journal of Oral Rehabilitation* 36:710–718.

Tanaka, E., Hanaoka, K., Tanaka, M., van Eijden, T., Iwabe, T., Ishino, Y., Sasaki, A., Tanne K. 2003. Viscoelastic properties of bovine retrodiscal tissue under tensile stress-relaxation. *Eur J Oral Sci* 111:518–522.

Biodental Engineering V – Belinha et al. (Eds)
© 2019 Taylor & Francis Group, London, ISBN 978-0-367-21087-8

Influence of temperature on the dimensional stability of an addition silicone

Carlos F. Almeida
Institute of Health Sciences, Portuguese Catholic University, Viseu, Portugal

Filipe Dantas, Ana Portela, Mário Vasconcelos & J.C. Reis Campos
Faculty of Dental Medicine, Porto University, Portugal

ABSTRACT: Dental Impression Materials are used in many stages of dental prosthesis construction and can be classified as: rigid, thermoplastic, or elastic. Elastic Materials are those that remain in an elastic state after removal of the oral cavity. Addition silicones are one of the most utilized in the elastic group. Thus being, the aim of this study is to assess the influence of temperature on the dimensional stability of an addition silicone. Six casts of specimen metal were done and pairs of samples were submitted to warm (60°C), cold (10°C) and environmental temperature (22°C). They were then measured at intervals of 1, 5, 24 and 48 hours after the printing. We experimentally proved that silicone at 60°C showed the highest volumetric contraction, comparing to a slight shrinkage registered at the temperature of 22°C; at the lowest temperature (10°C) there were practically no dimensional changes to the models used. As temperature interferes with the dimensional stability of silicone, you need to manipulate and store it under stable conditions to ensure reliability. The shift from cast to plaster must be made as soon as possible (1 hour). When such is not possible, the best method to ensure the preservation of the dimensional stability of an impression is to place it in a refrigerated environment (for no longer than five hours).

1 INTRODUCTION

Dental impression materials are modulating materials often used in dental practice to reproduce hard structures and adjacent tissues. (Corso et al., 1998, Chen et al., 2004, Hassan, 2006).

Ideal impression materials must have a set of characteristics, such as biocompatibility, fluidity and viscosity, suitable for adaptation to the oral tissues and the supporting structure, ability to harden in the oral environment, be removed from the oral cavity without distortion or breakage, simple use, rapid hardening, dimensional stability in the presence of moisture and temperature, among others. (Giordano, 2000, Kim et al., 2001).

Dimensional stability can be defined as the ability of a material or substance to maintain its original shape for a certain period of time and under specific conditions such as temperature, humidity and pressure, among others. (Fano et al., 1992, Faria et al., 2008).

This property may be affected by several factors, such as the contraction induced by temperature, the reaction by polymerization, or the contraction due to loss of volatile products. (Amin et al., 2009, Berg et al., 2003).

The polymerization reaction may take considerable time to complete, thus being regarded as one of the most crucial factors in terms of dimensional changes of impressions. Moreover, the same study found that the evaporation/loss of constituents is the second cause. (Endo and Finger, 2006, Fano et al., 1992).

In the market, there are a high variety of materials with different individual characteristics. The most commonly used are irreversible hydrocolloid and elastomeric (e.g. addition silicones, polyesters and polysulfides). (Kim et al., 2001; Pamenius and Ohlson, 1992).

Addition silicones are the most used within the group of elastomers. They consist in polymers with large molecular chains that take place when subjected to great stress. Their fundamental characteristic is a good dimensional stability over time. Polyvinylsiloxane are characterized by their excellent dimensional accuracy and stability over the long term. (Chen et al., 2004, Perry, 2013, Rubel, 2007).

Thanks to these intrinsic characteristics of high stability (as well as their elastic behaviour and high functional performance in the oral cavity), addition silicones are, according to literature, a wise choice in dental context. (Chen et al., 2004, Rubel, 2007).

Scientific research has concentrated considerable efforts in the creation and improvement of printing techniques, comparing brands and materials. However, one should not ignore the temperature differences that casts frequently undergo at the clinic, during storage, during transport to the laboratory, or even inside it. These should be taken into account since they can influence the end result of the impression casts. (Corso et al., 1998, Forrester-Baker et al., 2005).

The purpose of this study is to evaluate the dimensional stability alterations with the influence of different storage temperature.

2 MATERIAL AND METHODS

The silicone selected for this experimental procedure was a light body addition silicone (Affinis Precious Silver, Coltene, Switzerland).

Impressions were made using a metallic cylindrical provet (Fig. 1) comprising a base and a lid. The silicone was placed at the base so the reference lines would be imprinted in it. The silicone was applied to the interior of the provet with the aid of a self-mixing cartridge gun with a disposable tip. This was conducted according to the recommendation of the American Dental Association No. 19 and ISO—International Standard 4823.

The provet was previously heated to 37°C to simulate the temperature of the oral cavity. This was filled with silicone. After two minutes the cast was removed.

All procedures complied with the manufacturer's instructions for handling the material.

Thirty casts were done. Ten were placed at 10°C (in a refrigerator), ten others at a temperature of 60°C (incubator). The remaining ten were left at room temperature (22°C). The temperature was recorded over time with the aid of a thermometer. Subsequently, we proceeded to read the lines AB and CD (Fig. 1) after 1, 5, 24 and 48 hours respectively.

For each impression, two readings were performed (AB and CD) with the aid of an electronic magnifying glass (32x magnification Wild-Heerbrugg Makroskop type M420, Germany), attached to a Leica camera with "LAS" Software (Leica Microsystems: Leica Application Suite V.3.8.0). All measurements were carried out by the same operator.

Statistical analysis was performed using the statistical analysis program SPSS ® v.24.0 (Statistical Package for the Social Sciences).

The data were statistically analyzed with non-parametric tests, according to Mann-Whitney, Kruskal-Wallis e Wilcoxon ($\alpha = 0.05$).

3 RESULTS

The results of the various readings are presented in Table 1 and a global representation in Figure 2.

The results prove that an addition silicone at 60°C presents the highest volumetric contraction with significant result ($p < 0.005$), compared to a slight shrinkage registered at 22°C ($p = 0.04$). At the lowest temperature (10°C), there were virtually no dimensional changes worth mentioning ($p = 0.475$). There are no significant changes when comparing between storing in 22°C or 10°C over time. A significant difference result was obtained

Table 1. Measurements of the experiment varying over time and with temperature (distance in μm).

°C/Time	1 h	5 h	24 h	48 h
60°C	6809.46	6511.04	6121.25	5577.27
22°C	6580.78	6563.51	6537.75	6431.29
10°C	6606.57	6609.85	6625.32	6678.28

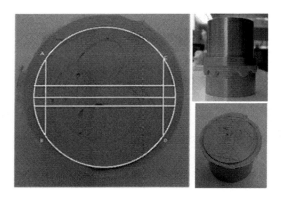

Figure 1. Schematic representation of the reference lines and preparation of an addition silicone sample.

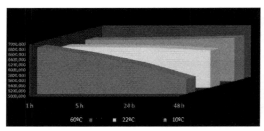

Figure 2. Global representation of the results.

overtime with the storage at 60°C (p = 0.01), compared with the other groups.

4 DISCUSSION

Addition silicones are considered one of the most reliable impression materials for printing on Fixed and Removable Prosthodontics. (Hassan, 2006, Perry, 2013).

By looking carefully at the results, we can easily understand that the silicone kept at the temperature of 60°C recorded the largest contraction in volume compared to the ones kept at other temperatures. This was probably the result of the constant release or continuous loss of volatiles. On the other hand, observing their behavior at room temperature (22°C), we find that there is a slight contraction; after 48 hours it is approximately 150 micrometers, which is negligible.

Regarding the lowest temperature (10°C) we prove that during the first 5 hours there was virtually no change in terms of the two-dimensional models in question. However, after 24–48 hours, a very slight increase (about 68 μm) can be observed.

Kim et al. publish results very similar to those obtained in this study. The authors observed that after 26 hours—low temperature (4°C)—there was an increase of 27 micrometers; at room temperature (23°C), a contraction of 19 μm was observed; at high temperature (40°C), a contraction of around 14 micrometers was registered. In general, taking into account that the models of these authors were subjected to an extra "thermal shock" the results are congruent with ours. (Kim et al., 2001).

Other studies demonstrated dimensional stability over time at room temperature and found that over two readings (5 and 24 hours) after completion of the model, there was a contraction that culminated in a decrease in the length of the models. (Fano et al., 1992).

To link all this information, we conclude that the addition silicone impression is a dimensionally stable material, although there are minor changes over time (especially at higher temperatures). In cold conditions or at room temperature, it preserved its volumetric and dimensional properties well, has proven to be a material of choice for dental arch printing.

However, and despite its splendid features, the more accurate relining method is to make the transition from cast to plaster as soon as possible (preferably within the first hour). When such is not possible, the best method to ensure stability and avoid shrinkage onset is to place it in a refrigerated environment and dispatch it to a dental lab in a period that does not exceed 5 hours.

5 CONCLUSIONS

Based on our results, and considering its limitations (namely the ones inherent to an in vitro study) we conclude the following:

- Temperature plays a key role in the stability of addition silicones.
- After impression, control temperature is vital in storage and transportation of a cast.
- A cast should be done imperatively before 5 hours.

REFERENCES

Amin, W.M., Al-Ali, M.H., Al Tarawneh, S.K., Taha, S.T., Saleh, M.W. & Ereifij, N. 2009. The effects of disinfectants on dimensional accuracy and surface quality of impression materials and gypsum casts. *J Clin Med Res,* 1, 81–9.

Berg, J.C., Johnson, G.H., Lepe, X. & Adan-Plaza, S. 2003. Temperature effects on the rheological properties of current polyether and polysiloxane impression materials during setting. *J Prosthet Dent,* 90, 150–61.

Chen, S.Y., Liang, W.M. & Chen, F.N. 2004. Factors affecting the accuracy of elastometric impression materials. *J Dent,* 32, 603–9.

Corso, M., Abanomy, A., Di Canzio, J., Zurakowski, D. & Morgano, S.M. 1998. The effect of temperature changes on the dimensional stability of polyvinyl siloxane and polyether impression materials. *J Prosthet Dent,* 79, 626–31.

Endo, T. & Finger, W.J. 2006. Dimensional accuracy of a new polyether impression material. *Quintessence Int,* 37, 47–51.

Fano, V., Gennari, P.U. & Ortalli, I. 1992. Dimensional stability of silicone-based impression materials. *Dent Mater,* 8, 105–9.

Faria, A.C., Rodrigues, R.C., Macedo, A.P., Mattos Mda, G. & Ribeiro, R.F. 2008. Accuracy of stone casts obtained by different impression materials. *Braz Oral Res,* 22, 293–8.

Forrester-Baker, L., Seymour, K.G., Samarawickrama, D., Zou, L., Cherukara, G. & Patel, M. 2005. A comparison of dimensional accuracy between three different addition cured silicone impression materials. *Eur J Prosthodont Restor Dent,* 13, 69–74.

Giordano, R., 2nd 2000. Impression materials: basic properties. *Gen Dent,* 48, 510–2, 514, 516.

Hassan, A.K. 2006. Dimensional accuracy of 3 silicone dental impression materials. *East Mediterr Health J,* 12, 632–6.

Kim, K.M., Lee, J.S., Kim, K.N. & Shin, S.W. 2001. Dimensional changes of dental impression materials by thermal changes. *J Biomed Mater Res,* 58, 217–20.

Pamenius, M. & Ohlson, N.G. 1992. Determination of thermal properties of impression materials. *Dent Mater,* 8, 140–4.

Perry, R. 2013. Dental impression materials. *J Vet Dent,* 30, 116–24.

Rubel, B.S. 2007. Impression materials: a comparative review of impression materials most commonly used in restorative dentistry. *Dent Clin North Am,* 51, 629–42, vi.

Biodental Engineering V – Belinha et al. (Eds)
© 2019 Taylor & Francis Group, London, ISBN 978-0-367-21087-8

Computational analysis for stress intensity factor (KI) measuring in metal-ceramic interface

Elza M.M. Fonseca
LAETA, INEGI, Polytechnic Institute of Porto, ISEP, Porto, Portugal

Joana F. Piloto
Faculty of Dental Medicine, University of Porto, Porto, Portugal

Maria G. Fernandes
3B's Research Group, University of Minho, Portugal

R.M. Natal Jorge
LAETA, INEGI, Faculty of Engineering, University of Porto, Porto, Portugal

ABSTRACT: The purpose of this work is to study the effect of cracks on the behavior of SIF (KI) in single edge crack of a bi-material interface, as metal-ceramic dental application. Metals, alloys, ceramics and others materials have been used in dentistry as restorative materials. However, a challenging aspect in ceramic materials is their restricted loading capability due to the low fracture toughness. In this work, the finite element method was used to evaluate the SIFs and to model a single edge crack in a metal (NiCr) and ceramic (KKM95-VITA) model subjected mode I loading.

1 INTRODUCTION

For fracture analysis there are two used approaches: the stress intensity factor analysis or the energy criterion approach. The two types of fracture considered, from a macroscopic point of view, are the plane and the inclined fracture. The plane fracture corresponds to a flat fracture surface perpendicular to the direction of maximum principal stress (Nik 2014). The inclined fracture presents a crack angle in the transverse direction to the propagation (Nik 2014).

The crack geometries, with radius of curvatures approaching zero at the crack tip, produce high stress levels. The stresses in the immediate neighborhood of a crack tip in a linearly elastic plane tend to infinity proportional to the reciprocal of the square root of the distance from the crack (Esben 1970). This occurs even at low load levels, and failure measures such as von Mises, Tresca, or other criteria are not appropriate.

The stress intensity factor (SIF), according K mode, was first proposed by Irwin (1957) and can be thought of the effective local stress at the crack tip measuring (Xian-Kui and James, 2012). SIF is designated by the loading mode, such as KI (crack opening mode), KII (in plane shear mode), KIII (out of plane shear mode) or a mixed mode loading, where the crack is subjected to all loading modes combination, expressed in $MPam^{1/2}$. An increasing SIF indicates the stress near the crack tip is increasing. With this linear elastic fracture mechanics approach of characterizing the crack tip stresses, small amounts of plasticity may be viewed as taking place within the crack tip stress field and neglected for the characterization (Paris and Sih, 1965).

Stress intensity factor, K can be calculated using closed form solutions, finite element method, experimental tests or other methods. The solutions transmit the remote loading, specimen geometry and the crack size with the stress intensity factor, K.

The use of SIF in design involves knowledge of the critical stress intensity factor (K_{IC}) or fracture toughness, as a mechanical property that measures the material resistance to fracture, and can vary with temperature, component thickness and strain rate.

Fracture toughness is used in the assessment of structural integrity, damage tolerance design, fitness for service evaluation, and residual strength analysis (Nik 2014), (Xian-Kui and James, 2012).

Metals, alloys, ceramics and others materials have been used in dentistry as restorative materials. Metal and ceramic restorations are widely used in dentistry. Nevertheless, restorations fracture usually occurs and the incidence of porcelain fracture was the second most common cause of metallic-ceramic fixed partial denture replacement (Rola et al. 2013). The interface between metal and ceramic is often the weakest point of these devices. Different technical factors, as geometric, metal design, porcelain thickness, material defects, material compatibility, technique fixation, are the most important matters in contributing to the formation of internal or external cracks (Ismail 2014), (Rola et al. 2013). However, a challenging aspect in ceramic materials is their restricted loading capability due to the low fracture toughness (Qing Li et al. 2006). This has become a most important problem limiting the use of ceramic materials to completely replace metals in dental restorations (bridges), where the level of tensile stress is higher (Qing Li et al. 2006). It would be desired if the crack initiation can be anticipated and evaluated prior to the bridge construction, thus providing criteria for an improved design (Qing Li et al. 2006).

Structural, experimental and numerical approaches have been adopted to assess prior to the bridge construction. Some investigations reported by Kelly et al. (1990) showed that the failures expected occurred in bridge connectors that link the pontic to the abutment, with approximately 70–78% initiating from the interface between the core and aesthetic ceramics. More recently, significant effort has also been dedicated to the study of fracture mechanism of dental ceramic constructions (Ariel et al. 2001).

The finite element method (FEM), as a numerical approach, is the useful method to vary interfacial strength and material properties and to reveal detailed stresses level in dental restorations, as dental bridges.

The purpose of this work is to study the effect of cracks on the behavior of SIF (KI) in single edge crack of a bi-material interface, as metal-ceramic dental application, using FEM analysis.

2 MATERIAL AND METHODS

2.1 Methodologies

FEM generally applied to elastic problems, was used to evaluate the SIFs and to model a plain stress single edge crack in a metal (Ni-Cr) and ceramic (KKM95-VITA) model subjected mode I loading. For this analysis, a singular element is used around the crack tip.

The fracture predicted from a computational analysis shows a good agreement with the existing experimental observations from other authors.

Four-point bending test was simulated with a sample total size of (B = 6,5; W = 10,50; S = 60) mm. The dimension S is the distance L = 40 mm between the supports and two end distances C = 10 mm until the edge.

In the numerical model, to simulate the bending test, two concentrated loads P = 74,5804 N were introduced in the opposite side to the crack tip, between a distance equal to 20 mm. The applied force P is resulting from a load-displacement ASTM E-399 test (2003).

The numerical simulations were performed as two dimensional under plane stress conditions, as a good approximation for a three-dimensional model. The crack length (a = 5,25 mm) and the position are important factors to consider in the analysis.

The geometric configuration and materials disposition are shown in Figure 1 in conjunction with the generated mesh. The metal (Ni-Cr) has a width equal to 6 mm and ceramic (KKM95-VITA) equal to 3 mm.

2.2 Determination of SIF using FEM

For computational model in 2D analysis a quadratic element is common in use. In fracture mechanics the crack tip is meshed and elements surrounding were applied.

The first row of elements around the crack tip should be singular which the mechanical stress is infinite. The stress state near the crack tip is inhomogeneous, and the plastic deformation will be occurring at very small load. Automatically generated around a keypoint assigns element division sizes, where the first row of elements should have a radius of approximately crack length/8 or smaller, as represented in Figure 2.

2.3 Material properties

For computational model, isotropic properties were taken and presented in Table 1. Table presents the Young Modulus, Poisson ratio, the ultimate stress and the toughness of the material.

2.4 K_{IC} Determination

The analytical method of fracture mechanics is conservative approach to solution of cracks in the material.

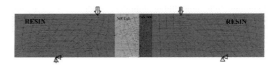

Figure 1. Single edge crack in a metal-ceramic mesh model.

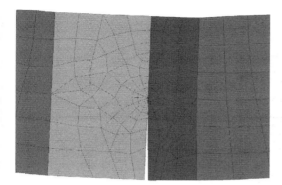

Figure 2. Crack tip model.

Table 1. Material properties.

Material	E, MPa	υ	σ_r, MPa	K_{IC}, MPam$^{0.5}$
Ni-Cr alloy Wironia light from www.bego.com	200000	0,33	470	40
Ceramic VMK 95 from www.vita-zahnfabrik.com	91000	0,25	85	0,67
Resin Epoxy Resin from www.epoxyworktops.com	2952,76	0,3		

The linear elastic fracture mechanics is based on empirical formula for the SIF in terms of the boundary conditions.

The SIF can be calculated analytically for a central crack by the following Equations 1 and 2 (Rooke and Cartwright 1976).

$$K_{IC} = \frac{3PC\sqrt{\pi a}}{BW^2} F\left(\frac{a}{W}\right) \quad (1)$$

$$F\left(\frac{a}{W}\right) = 1,12 - 1,39\left(\frac{a}{W}\right) + 7,32\left(\frac{a}{W}\right)^3 - 13,1\left(\frac{a}{W}\right)^3 + 14\left(\frac{a}{W}\right)^4 \quad (2)$$

The obtained analytical value K_{IC} was equal to 0,598443 MPam$^{0.5}$.

According some investigations in five normalized ASTM tests with metal-ceramic samples, an average value equal to 0,44 MPam$^{0.5}$ was obtained (Livia 2013).

3 RESULTS AND DISCUSSION

3.1 *Comparison*

For post processing part, the numerical results of stress intensity factors and the stress distribution were obtained. A local crack tip coordinate system must be activated for the obtained results of the mixed-mode stress intensity factors KI, KII or KIII, as represented in Figure 3.

The maximum principal stress has a great value in ceramic material, and a different behavior in comparison with metal (Ni-Cr) part. The crack propagation occurs with large intensity in the ceramic material. The interface between the two materials, where the crack zone is activated, doesn't present critical stresses values.

Table 2 permits to identify the calculated numerical values of SIF, for KI mode, to the full crack model.

According KI determination for each material, the obtained average is equal to 0,515 and close to the analytical and experimental investigations presented in Table 3.

Other verification is the comparison between the calculated SIF and the material parameter K_{IC}. For Ni-Cr alloy and ceramic materials the fracture toughness is presented in Table 1.

As a conclusion, if the calculated SIF is smaller as the fracture toughness of used material, then the crack will not be grown and rests stabile (Stefan 2014).

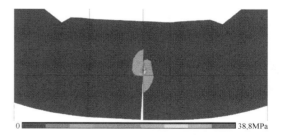

Figure 3. Numerical results in single edge crack model (KI), maximum principal stress.

Table 2. Numerical calculation: Mixed-Mode SIF (Plane Stress, Full crack model).

Material	KI, MPam$^{0.5}$
Ni-Cr alloy	0,70800
Ceramic	0,32214

Table 3. KI comparison.

Comparison of results	KI, MPam$^{0.5}$
Numerical average	0,51507
Analytical	0,59844
Investigations (Livia 2013)	0,4400

In the present study the K_{IC} for ceramic material is equal to 0,67 MPam$^{0.5}$, very close to the calculations in ceramic-metal model.

The results and the methodology presented are significant for understanding the fracture strength in metal-ceramic interface dental models, providing important data for the clinical application.

4 CONCLUSIONS

The fracture predicted from a computational analysis shows a good agreement with the existing experimental observations from other authors.

This paper presents a solution of SIF obtained numerically in metal-ceramic material. The results and the methodology presented are significant for understanding the fracture strength in metal-ceramic dental models, providing important data for the clinical application.

This type of conclusions could be used by dentists to improve bridges design and chosen materials.

Future work using other materials, dimensions and crack position could be used to demonstrate the numerical methods efficiency in these applications.

REFERENCES

Ariel J. Raigrodski DMD, MS, Gerard J. Chiche DDS. 2001. The safety and efficacy of anterior ceramic fixed partial dentures: A review of the literature. *The Journal of Prosthetic Dentistry* 86(5): 520–525.

ASTM E399-90, 2003: Standard Test Method for Plane-Strain Fracture Toughness of Metallic Materials, ASTM Standards, Vol 03.01.

Esben Byskov. 1970. The Calculation of Stress Intensity Factors Using the Finite Element Method with Cracked Elements. *Int. J. Fracture Mechanics* 6(2): 159–167.

Ismail, A.E. 2014. Stress Intensity Factors of Eccentric Cracks in Bi-Material Plates. *Applied Mechanics and Materials* 663: 98–102.

Kelly, J.R., J.A. Tesk and J.A. 1995. Failure of All-ceramic Fixed Partial Dentures in vitro and in vivo: Analysis and Modeling. *Journal of Dental Research* 74(6): 1253–1258.

Livia Goulart Tovar, 2013. Análise Computacional de Propagação de Trinca em Interface de Corpo de Prova Metalocerâmico. Universidade Federal do Rio de Janeiro, DEM/POLI/UFRJ.

Nik Ismail. 2014. Stress Intensity Factors of Edge Cracks in Dissimilar Joint Plates. *Thesis*, Univ. of Malaysia.

Paris P, Sih G. 1965. Stress Analysis of Cracks. *67th Annual Meeting of the ASTM*.

Qing Li, Ionut Ichim, Jeff Loughran, Wei Li, Michael Swain, Jules Ki. 2006. Numerical Simulation of Crack Formation in All Ceramic Dental Bridge. *Key Engineering Materials* 312: 293–298.

Rola M. Shadid, Nasrin R. Sadaqah, Layla Abu-Naba, Wael M. Al-Omari. 2013. Porcelain fracture of metal-ceramic tooth-supported and implant-supported restorations: A review. *Open Journal of Stomatology* 3: 411–418.

Rooke, D.P., D.J. Cartwright. 1976. Compendium of Stress Intensity Factors, London HMSO.

Stefan Hajdu. 2014. The Investigation of the Stress State near the Crack Tip of Central Cracks Through Numerical Analysis. *Procedia Engineering* 69: 477–485.

Xian-Kui Zhu, James A. Joyce. 2012. Review of fracture toughness (G, K, J, CTOD, CTOA) testing and standardization. *Eng. Fracture Mechanics* 85:1–46.

Thermal stimulation of dentinal tubules

Paulo A.G. Piloto
Polytechnic Institute of Bragança, Bragança, Portugal

Joana F. Piloto
Faculty of Dental Medicine, University of Porto, Porto, Portugal

ABSTRACT: Dentine is a permeable mineralised tissue, made with a special geometry. The geometry presents micro tubules with variable dimensions and densities. Dentine can be subdivided into four different classes, depending on the number and shape of the tubules. Dentine can be directly exposed to high or low temperature, when the tooth is under restoration or due to gingival retraction. This temperature variation can induce pain into the patient. This investigation aims to validate the numerical model using experimental data obtained from tests developed in dog teeth. According to this investigation, the rate of temperature, threshold temperature and the neural activity are correlated allowing for a positive correlation between the thermal stimulus and pain.

1 INTRODUCTION

The geometry of dentine presents micro tubules with variable dimensions and densities. According to Coutinho et al (2007), dentine can be subdivided into four different classes, depending on the number and shape of the tubules. Dentine presents a heterogeneous structure but the morphology is almost regular. This work considers the study of the region near the cusps (class II). Dentine can be directly exposed to high or low temperature, when the tooth is under restoration or due to gingival retraction. This temperature variation can induce pain into the patient. Thermal stimuli is normally used in clinical dentistry as a means of evaluating teeth vitality. Thermal stimuli using both heating and cooling are used as diagnostic to distinguish between a normal, inflamed or necrotic pulp. Some receptor neurons of the pulp are situated in the region of the pulpodentinal junction, being these receptors the first sensory structures to respond to external thermal stimulation.

There are several relations between thermal stimuli and pain across the literature. According to Matthews (1977), the threshold value for pain due to high temperature is 45°C and the threshold value due to low temperature is 27°C.

This investigation aims to validate the numerical model using experimental data obtained from tests developed by Matthews (1977) in dog teeth. According to this investigation, the temperature and the electrical activity of two electrodes, located in contact with the pulp region, were measured, allowing for a positive correlation between the thermal stimulus and pain.

2 MATERIAL AND METHODS

The finite element method is used to analyse the effect of the thermal stimulation. The thermal stimulation intends to understand how individual nerves from dentine or pulp region react to the variation of the temperature in the exposed surface of dentine (pain cause). Different thermal stimuli were considered (cooling, cooling after heating, heating, and heating after cooling), see Figure 1.

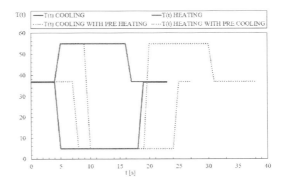

Figure 1. Thermal stimuli to the exposed surface of dentine.

Table 1. Thermal stimuli applied to the exposed dentine.

Thermal stimuli	Temperature level and (duration)
Cooling	+5°C (13 s)
Cooling + pre heating	+55°C (4 s) +5°C (14 s)
Heating	+55°C (11 s)
Heating with pre cooling	+5°C (11 s) +55°C (10 s)

Table 1 summarises the four different thermal stimuli, with the definition of the temperature level and time duration.

Cooling stimulus is defined by a temperature level of +5°C during 13 s, with a cooling rate of 32°C/s. The heating stimulus is defined by a temperature level of +55°C during 11 s, with a heating rate of 18°C/s. The cooling stimulus with pre heating is characterized by a temperature level of +55°C during 4 s followed by a temperature level of +5°C during 14 s, using a heating rate of 18°C/s and a cooling rate of 50°C/s. The heating stimulus after pre cooling is characterized by a temperature level of +5°C during 11 s and a temperature of +55°C during 10 s, using a cooling rate of 32°C/s and a heating rate of 50°C/s. The initial and final temperature of the exposed surface of dentine was always kept to 37°C.

The thermal analysis is governed by second order partial differential equation for energy, Eq. 1, that must be solved in the dentine region. T represents the main state variable (temperature in dentine region), λ represents the thermal conductivity, ρ is the specific mass and C_p is the specific heat. The boundary conditions are defined in the exposed side with a prescribed temperature T(t). A convective boundary condition is also applied in the pulp region (unexposed side), using the convective heat flux coefficient of 4 W/m² K and a bulk temperature of 37°C. The effect of the dentinal fluid in the tubules is simulated by a convective boundary condition, using the same convective heat flux coefficient with an average bulk temperature equal to [T(t)+37]/2, both represented by Eq. 2. The initial temperature was always considered equal to 37°C. The external surface of dentine is consider adiabatic.

$$\vec{\nabla} \bullet \left(-\lambda \vec{\nabla} T\right) = \rho . C_p . \frac{\partial T}{\partial t} \quad (1)$$

$$\left(-\lambda \vec{\nabla} T\right) \bullet \vec{n} = \alpha_c \left(T - T_\infty\right) \quad (2)$$

The geometry of this dentine model was modified to facilitate the construction of the model, based on the density of dentinal tubules (Coutinho et al, 2007). Tubules present a diameter equal to 1 µm, with a distance between them of 6 µm and a volume fraction of 4%, see Figure 2. This Figure compares only a small region of the model, with a real image obtained from electron scanning microscopy from samples of young adults (third molars), representing a square dimension of 20 µm.

Figure 3 represents the geometry and the boundary conditions for the thermal simulation, using a three-dimensional model. The main dimensions are: 100 (width) × 100 (height) × 2000 µm (depth) and this model uses 1 326 837 nodes and 953 500 elements. The mesh is made of solid finite elements (SOLID70), which have eight nodes per element with a single degree of freedom at each node (temperature). The conductivity matrix uses linear interpolating functions and a full integration method (2 × 2 × 2).

The thermal properties were measured by Brow et al. (1970), considering the specific heat equal to 1590 J/kgK, the conductivity equal to 0.48 W/mK and the specific mass equal to 1960 kg/m³. The thermal analysis of dentine region depends mainly on the thermal properties of the materials involved, which present also a large variability, according to data reported in Lin et al. (2011, 2010). The geometry of dentinal tubules also affects the temperature field in this region. A fluid structure interaction is expected in the dentine region. This fluid structure interaction is modelled herein by a convective bidirectional heat transfer between the fluid region

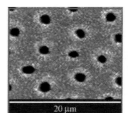

a) Real image (Coutinho et al, 2007).   b) Part of the finite element model (20 µm).

Figure 2. Small region of the model compared with real class II region (Coutinho et al, 2007).

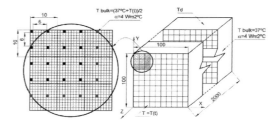

Figure 3. Three dimensional model for dentine (dimensions in µm).

(dentinal fluid) and the solid region (dentine). According to the hydrodynamic theory, thermal stimulation causes dentinal fluid motion. The sense of the motion depends on the type of stimuli. Hot stimulus causes inward fluid motion toward the pulp, while cold stimulus causes outward motion of the fluid. This model only includes the behaviour of the solid region but takes into account the thermal effect of the fluid. The simulation time depends on the duration of the stimuli. The typical time increment used in numerical simulation is 1 s, with the possibility to be reduced to 0.1 s.

3 RESULTS AND DISCUSSION

The heat flux changes according to the thermal stimulus. When the exposed surface is submitted to cold stimulus, the main heat flux direction comes from the pulp region to the exposed side of dentine. There is also an important heat flux (in the orthogonal direction) from the dentinal fluid to the dentin near the exposed region and in reverse sense near the pulp region. Figure 4 represents the temperature field of the dentine, when submitted to the cooling stimulus, for time equal 10 s.

Figures 5–7 represent two slices from the complete model, corresponding to the position $z = -100$ μm (first slice) and $Z = -1900$ μm (second slice). Each slice has a thickness of 20 μm. The amount of heat flux is represented in each direction of space (X,Y and Z). A positive number means that the heat flux flows in positive direction and a negative heat flux means that it flows in negative direction. The heat flux analysis is only represented for the cold stimulus. The heat flux in X and Y directions is leaving the dentinal tubules towards the dentin region, as can be seen for the first slice. In the second slice, near the pulp region, the heat

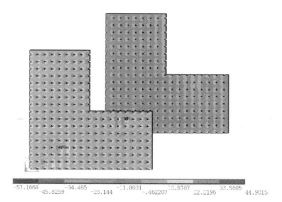

Figure 5. Heat flux in X direction (W/m^2) for cold stimulus (time = 10 s).

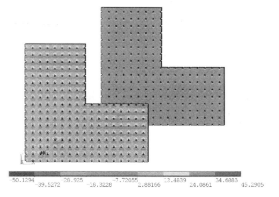

Figure 6. Heat flux in Y direction (W/m^2) for cold stimulus (time = 10 s).

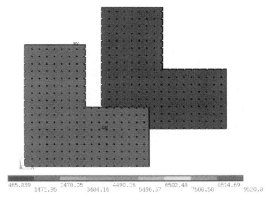

Figure 7. Heat flux in Z direction (W/m^2) for cold stimulus (time = 10 s).

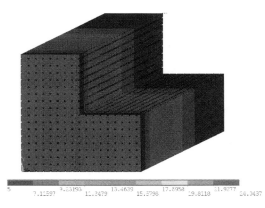

Figure 4. Temperature field (°C) for cold stimulus (time = 10 s).

flux flows in reverse sense. This is because the average temperature of the dentinal fluid is 21°C, while the average temperature of the fist slice is 7°C and the average temperature of the second slice is 24°C, see Figures 5–6.

The heat flux in Z direction is the biggest one and is well aligned in both slices. In both slices, the heat flux is positive, meaning that heat is flowing from the pulp region to the exposed surface of dentine, see Figure 7.

After the removal of the cooling stimulus, the temperature of the dentine increases, trying to stablish the thermodynamic equilibrium. This process requires more than 4 s.

Figure 8 represents the temperature field for time equal to 15 s. This temperature field is the result of the cold stimulus after a short period of pre heating. For this particular time, the average temperature of the dentinal fluid is 21°C. This means that this fluid is heating the exposed region, trying to deliver some heat flux to the exposed side of dentine and still trying to remove heat flux from the region of the dentine closer to the pulp region. The unexposed surface of dentine will decrease the temperature to a minimum of 18°C at time equal to 23 s.

When the exposed surface is submitted to hot stimulus, the main heat flux direction comes from the exposed side of dentine region to the unexposed side of dentine, see Figure 9 for time equal to 10 s. The dentinal fluid is being heated near the region of the exposed dentinal surface and cooled near the unexposed region of dentine.

After the removal of the hot stimulus, the temperature of the dentine decreases, trying to stablish the thermodynamic equilibrium. This process requires more than 6 s.

Figure 10 represents the temperature field for time equal to 25 s. This temperature field is the result of the hot stimulus after a short period of pre cooling. The average temperature of the dentinal fluid is 46°C, which means that this fluid is

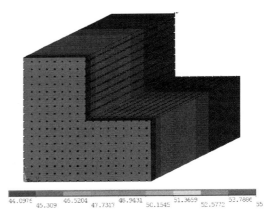

Figure 9. Temperature field (°C) for hot stimulus (time = 10 s).

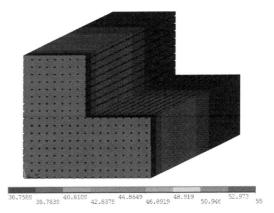

Figure 10. Temperature field (°C) for hot stimulus after pre cooling (time = 25 s).

trying to remove some heat from the exposed dentine and is trying to deliver this heat in the dentine region near to the pulp region. This heat flux is important to keep the temperature of the unexposed side sensitive to the temperature variation of the exposed side; otherwise, the thermal inertia of the unexposed dentine would be higher.

The pulp makes recognition of the outside aggressors by sensory afferent nerve fibres (specific receptors of the pain), known as Aβ-fibres, Aδ-fibres and C-fibres. Aβ-fibres are myelinated, exist in small quantity and have large-diameter. Aδ-fibres are lightly myelinated, they have medium-diameter and they are found to be fast conducting afferents with a low excitability threshold. These fibres might respond without any existing lesion and have a peripheral location comparing to C-fibres. The C-fibres have slow conduction velocities and a high excitability threshold value.

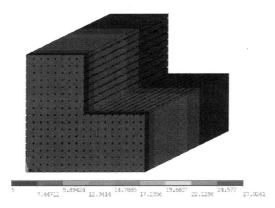

Figure 8. Temperature field (°C) for cold stimulus after pre heating (time = 15 s).

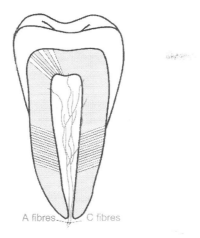

Figure 11. Scheme showing the distribution of intradental A fibre and C fibres.

Aδ-fibres are responsible for recognizing electric and cold stimuli that might induce instant sharp pain. The C-fibres are located on a deeper location of the pulp region, responding only towards intense hot stimulus. The major type of fibres mediating tooth pain sensations are Aδ-fibres and C-fibres (Le Fur et al. 2017), see Figure 11.

The pain produced under thermal stimuli may be attributed to the activation of thermal sensitive receptors (TRPV1 – warm receptor and TRPM8 – cold receptor) (Le Fur et al. 2017, El Karim et al 2011). This activation seems to be caused by the threshold temperature around the warm receptors (Lin et al, 2011) and caused by the high rate of temperature variation in the unexposed surface of dentine for the cold receptor (assuming positive correlation between neural discharge and time derivative of dentinal temperature in the unexposed surface, Td). The pain produced under heating may be attributed to the attainment of a threshold temperature limit. The neural response to cold stimulus differs from the neural response to hot stimulus. Relative long latency is expected in case of hot stimulus, because nerve fibres are less sensitive (Le Fur et al. 2017). The theory used for dentine sensitivity induced by thermal stimulus is still under development. Dentine sensitivity is increased when it is directly exposed to thermal stimulus. The transmission of the stimuli in this region generate nerve impulses that have been registered during several experimental investigations (Le Fur et al. 2017). The neural theory dictates that pulpal nerves are activated by external thermal stimuli and produce electrical signals that are collected by nociceptive receptors (Le Fur et al. 2017). Among them, according to El Karim et al. (2011), the TRPM8 is cold sensitive with a threshold value of $22 \pm 3°C$ and the TRPV1 (warm receptor) is hot sensitive with threshold temperature value of $43 \pm 2°C$.

The sensitive reaction to pure cold stimulus (Figure 12) is significant different from the sensitive reaction to pure cooling with pre heating stimulus (Figure 13). Both figures represent the temperature in the exposed side T(t) and the temperature in the unexposed side Td. The rate of temperature variation (dTd/dt) was calculated, based on the time derivative of Td during the simulation time. The rate of neural discharge is higher for the second case, but in both stimuli the duration of discharge coincides with the maximum rate of temperature variation in the unexposed side of dentine (see dot line in both graphs, with a maximum value between −2 and −3°C/s). According to Lin et al. (2011) this bigger discharge can also be explained by the higher flow rate of the dentinal fluid towards the exposed surface of dentine, by the activation of the mechanical sensitive receptors.

The fibres responsible for the discharge during the hot stimuli are less sensitive. The relatively

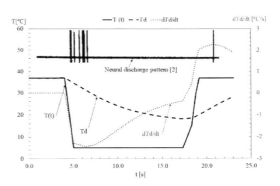

Figure 12. Cold stimulus and thermal reaction at the unexposed surface of dentine, including neural discharge.

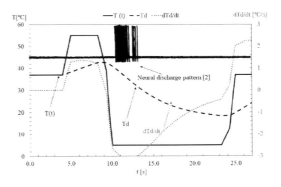

Figure 13. Cold stimulus after pre heating and thermal reaction at the unexposed surface of dentine, including neural discharge.

long latency due to warming conditions seems to be related to the position of that fibres, when the unexposed dentinal surface reaches the threshold temperature value of 43 ± 2°C, during the time being exposed. This observation is in accordance to the temperature evolution of the unexposed dentinal surface, see Figures 14 and 15. The hot stimulus after pre cooling did not keep the unexposed dentinal surface to a temperature level higher than the threshold value. This can justify the difference between both stimuli, because both have almost the same warming duration (10–11 s). The rate of temperature variation in the unexposed side is not activating any thermal sensitive receptors during heating, but the threshold temperature and the duration to the exposed value seems to be correlated with thermal induced pain.

Figure 14 represents the temperature evolution of the unexposed surface of dentine Td during the hot stimulus. The threshold values is also represented (Td=45°C) to underline the discharge activity during this period.

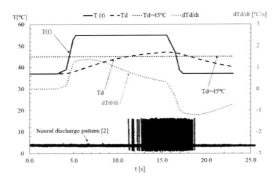

Figure 14. Hot stimulus and thermal reaction at the unexposed surface of dentine, including neural discharge.

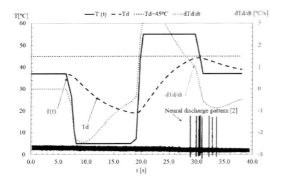

Figure 15. Hot stimulus after pre cooling and thermal reaction at the unexposed surface of dentine, including neural discharge.

Figure 15 represents the temperature variation of the unexposed dentinal surface Td, when submitted to hot stimulus with pre cooling. The unexposed surface of dentine reached the threshold value only for a short period and a lower maximum temperature was predicted.

4 CONCLUSIONS

The thermal simulation of dentinal tubules was investigated by the finite element method, based on the experimental tests developed by Mattews (1977). Four different stimuli were consider without producing irreversible damage. Pure cooling, cooling with pre heating, pure heating and heating with pre cooling were analysed with respect to temperature of the unexposed dentinal surface and with respect to neural discharges recorded at inferior dental nerves. A good correlation was observed for both cold and hot stimulus. According to the results, the cold stimulus can produce pain if the rate of temperature variation next to the pulp region reaches −3°C/s with short latency. The hot stimulus can produce pain if the unexposed dentinal surface is exposed to the threshold temperature of 43 ± 2°C, being the latency and duration in accordance to experimental evidences.

REFERENCES

Brown, W.S., Dewey, W.A., & Jacobs, H.R. 1970. Thermal Properties of Teeth. *Journal of Dental Research*, 49(4), 752–755.

Coutinho, E.T., D'almeida, J.R.M., Paciornik, S. 2007. Evaluation of microstructural parameters of human dentin by digital image analysis. *Materials Research*, v. 10, n. 2: 153–159.

El Karim, I.A., Linden, G.J., Curtis, T.M., About, I., McGahon, M.K., Irwin, C.R., & Lundy, F.T. 2011. Human odontoblasts express functional thermosensitive TRP channels: Implications for dentin sensitivity. *Pain*, 152(10), 2211–2223.

Le Fur-Bonnabesse, A., A. Bodere, C. Helou, V. Chevalier and J.P. Goulet. 2017. Dental pain induced by an ambient thermal differential: pathophysiological hypothesis. *J Pain Res* 10: 2845–2851.

Lin, M., Liu, S., Niu, L., Xu, F., & Lu, T.J. 2011. Analysis of thermal-induced dentinal fluid flow and its implications in dental thermal pain. *Archives of Oral Biology*, 56(9), 846–854.

Lin, M., Xu, F., Lu, T.J., & Bai, B.F. 2010. A review of heat transfer in human tooth—Experimental characterization and mathematical modeling. *Dental Materials*, 26(6), 501–513.

Matthews, B. 1977. Responses of Intradental Nerves to Electrical and Thermal Stimulation of Teeth in Dogs. *The Journal of Physiology* 264.3: 641–664.

Biodental Engineering V – Belinha et al. (Eds)
© 2019 Taylor & Francis Group, London, ISBN 978-0-367-21087-8

Analysis tool of skills' acquisition in fine motor skill

R.D. Lopes, S. Castro & M.J. Ponces
Faculdade de Medicina Dentária, Universidade do Porto, Porto, Portugal

N. Ramos
Institute of Science and Innovation in Mechanical and Industrial Engineering, Porto, Portugal

M. Vaz
Faculty of Engineering, University of Porto, Porto, Portugal

ABSTRACT: Manual skills form only a part of the capabilities required of future dentists, but they are a very important component that should be tested. The purpose of this investigation project is to assess the development of this ability and the acquisition of skills by students of the Faculty of Dental Medicine of University of Porto during the pre-graduate training, considering as primary reference the identification of the initial individual status in what concerns motor maturation. A prototype was developed to allow the monitoring of the acquisition of competences in terms of fine motor skills.

Keywords: Fine motor skill, manual dexterity

1 INTRODUCTION

The acquisition and appropriation of fine motor coordination, which is regulated in the frontal lobes, is called manual intelligence and distinguishes us from other species (Luck 2000). According to Berger et al. (Costa 2013) manual dexterity is defined as the ability to manipulate small objects, to transport them in space and to position them properly in a specific location. In the context of Dental Medicine, the qualitative performance of the daily professional activities is largely determined by the function and by the manual dexterity (Carvalho, 2014). Considering the motor dexterity as the capacity of the individual to be efficient in a certain skill, this characteristic can be acquired and developed through a learning process (Giuliani et al. 2007). When performing a skill, there are different levels or qualitative degrees of performance that are named as dexterity capacity. The development of this competence, through a learning process, is an important formative program content for the future performance with quality of several professions, some of which related to the health sector, particularly the Dental Medicine. The motor dexterity may be in some individuals quite developed and innate, while in others, in contrast, inevitably requires adequate training, implying a more or less exhaustive learning process. The purpose of this investigation project is to assess the development of this ability and the acquisition of skills by students of the Faculty of Dental Medicine of University of Porto during the pre-graduate training, considering as primary reference the identification

of the initial individual status in what concerns motor maturation. A prototype (FIMAT – Fine Motricity Assessment Tool) was developed in order to establish an automated system for the quantitative assessment of skills in the field of fine motor skills. The system will assign a quantitative appreciation of the wire elements performed, and will also provide the necessary gradation to measure the progress in the acquisition of fine motor skills.

Therefore, the application of this system will allow to monitor the acquisition of competences in terms of fine motor skills.

2 MATERIAL AND METHODS

For the execution of wire elements that will later be evaluated in the prototype, it was requested the participation of university students of Dental Medicine, over 18 years old, of both genders, without functional deficiency in the upper limb whose motor dominance it may be right or left. As exclusion criteria was determined any history of fatigue, disease, or musculoskeletal alterations, resulting in a motor and sensory compromise of the upper limbs; repeating students; students over 30 (since there are studies that point out that after the 30 years of age the manual dexterity begins to decrease); students who reject the execution of the exercise; students undergoing recent or frequent use of medications or substances that interfere with the performance of motor skills, such as neuroleptic drugs, alcohol and caffeine; and frequent and intense fine motor activity, namely students of the Computing and Music courses. A previous experimental study was developed through the construction of a pre-prototype that uses a cardboard structure by positioning two cameras Trust® Webcam Spotlight 16429 (Trust International B.V., Dordrecht, Netherlands) to obtain the images of the wire elements. A proper lighting system with LEDs and oriented targets was built in order to promote an even illumination, avoiding reflections and shadows. The structures' images are recorded simultaneously by the cameras using the video recording program ManyCam® (Visacom Media Inc. Brossard, Quebec). This system will use appropriate image processing and software to assign a quantitative value to the wire elements made. The data collected will be stored in a database and will allow not only to identify the main difficulties, but also to know the evolution of each wire element and to readjust the tasks according to the intended objectives.

3 RESULTS

The study intends to evaluate the geometric and dimensional precision of three-dimensional wire structures built from a previous design. The use of a set of conveniently positioned cameras allows to record the orthogonal projections of the structures built. The study allowed to adjust the images so that they could be adapted to the purpose of the study. Camera selection and positioning as well as the adjustment of the lighting system were calibrated. The real dimensions of the system, as well as its functionalities were defined, resulting in the 3D prototype with a mechanical design that allows its manufacturing (Figure 1).

We believe that the results obtained will demonstrate that training, in terms of fine motor skills, contributes effectively to the acquisition of competences in Dental Medicine students. We suspect that the associations that we will find between the types of grip and the quality of motor dexterity will provide us with important data as it relates to the specificity of the individual pedagogical approach to Dental Medicine students.

4 DISCUSSION

The creation of this prototype opens perspectives to the development of pedagogical tools with the intention of training professionals who need, in their areas of activity, additional specific abilities in terms of fine motricity.

In fact, the FIMAT prototype will represent an innovative contribution as it reveals a new tool that comes to technically solve the problem that is the quantitative evaluation of exercises performed in orthodontic wire. Indeed, until now, this evaluation inevitably had a subjective nature, despite the efforts of the evaluators to rely on objective parameters. The prototype was made following an experimental work aimed at creating constant and replicable assessment conditions, and reveals not only pedagogical but also industrial applicability.

5 CONCLUSIONS

Following the creation of the FIMAT prototype, the research team intends to register and patent this tool. In fact, the FIMAT prototype will represent an innovative contribution since it reveals itself as a new tool that technically solves the problem of quantitative evaluation of exercises performed in orthodontic wire. Up to date, this evaluation has inevitably had a subjective nature, despite the efforts of the evaluators to rely on objective parameters. Through the implementation of partnership protocols, not only with the industry, but also with companies in the field of information technology, it is projected the development of a system that, being commercially viable, may represent an important pedagogical tool in the field of assessment and training for professionals from different expert areas.

REFERENCES

Carvalho I. 2014. A Motricidade Fina em Estudantes de Medicina Dentária: comparação entre os estudantes dos 1º e 5º anos [CESPU – MSc Thesis] https://repositorio.cespu.pt/handle/20.500.11816/345.
Costa, A. 2013. O desenvolvimento da motricadade fina: Um estudo de intervenção com crianças em idade pré-escolar. [IPVC – MSc Thesis] http://hdl.handle.net/20.500.11960/1392.
Giulani, M., Lajolo, C., Clemente, L., Querqui, A., Viotti, R., Boari, A and Miani, C. 2007. Is manual dexterity essential in the selection of dental students? *British Dental Journal* Volume 203(3): pg. 149–55. DOI: 10.1038/bdj.2007.688.
Luck, O., Reitemeier, B., Scheuch, K., 2000. Testing of fine motor skills in dental students. *Eur J Dent Educ*, 4: 10–14.

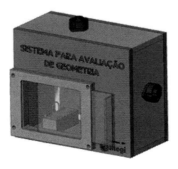

Figure 1. Lateral view of the prototyte.

Biodental Engineering V – Belinha et al. (Eds)
© 2019 Taylor & Francis Group, London, ISBN 978-0-367-21087-8

A new approach in 3D finite element analysis in restorative dentistry

C. Özcan & C. Muraille
Faculty of Odontology, GRESPI, URCA, France

P. Lestriez
GRESPI, URCA, France

Y. Josset
Faculty of Odontology, GRESPI, URCA, France

ABSTRACT: The goal of the study is to design a realistic and accurate three-Dimensional (3D) dental model that does not incorporate approximation for use in Finite Element Analysis (FEA). A segmentation is carried out on the images resulting from a micro-CT acquisition and makes it possible to differentiate the various components of the teeth (enamel, pulp, dentin). Reconstruction does not use Boolean operations, so approximations are avoided. A class II MOD cavity is simulated on the tooth and different types of restorations (ceramic and composite) are set up for finite element calculations. The results showed that the concave parts of the occlusal table, the cavosurface angle of the cavity, the internal angles of the restorations and the cervical area of the tooth are stress concentration areas.

1 INTRODUCTION

The benefits of finite element analysis (FEA) have been demonstrated for many years in dentistry. They allow to obtain an infinite reproducibility of the tests, to override the availability of the raw materials and does not pose an ethical problem like an experimental analysis which requires anatomical parts (Magne & Oganesyan 2009a, Magne 2010, Magne & Schlichting 2011, Yamanel 2009). The analysis makes it possible to calculate the internal stresses of the structures and the interfaces of the components.

In the behavioural analysis of dental restoration materials, the literature shows a lot of diversity. With the development of restorative materials such as composites and adhesive systems that complement them, dentistry seeks to understand and prevent the fracture of these elements as well as those of the dental structures on which they are placed (Ausiello 2001, Magne 2007, Magne 2009). The biggest challenge is to build a coherent and realistic three-dimensional (3D) model to observe the effects of different forces on the system. Depending the anatomical piece chosen this model can be more or less complex. The tooth is a complex structure because it is made of different elements such as pulp, dentin and enamel that have different properties.

The literature proposes models of unitary teeth built with a micro computed tomography (μCT) acquisition of an extracted tooth (Magne & Oganesyan 2009a, b, Magne 2010, Magne & Douglas 1999, Rodrigues et al. 2009). The different

elements that make up the tooth are delimited, and a mask is created for each part. These are superimposed to create the final object (Magne & Douglas, 1999). When the limits of the different parts are in superposition, Boolean operations make it possible to calculate a new approximate limit to each one of them.

The purpose of our study is to build a 3D model of a tooth with more precision without using Boolean operations. This model of a mandibular molar will allow FEA with the simulation of a restoration with different materials in order to observe the constraints occurring in the different dental structures.

2 MATERIALS AND METHOD

2.1 *Micro-CT scanner acquisition*

A healthy mandibular molar was chosen. An acquisition was carried out with a μCT (Model 1076, Skyscan, Kontich, Belgium) microcomputer coupled with a computer (Dell Precision PWS 450 Intel® Xeon, 4 Gb CPU, 3.06 GHz) equipped with SkyScan 1076® software (Skyscan, Kontich, Belgium); with TView® and NRecon® (Skyscan, Kontich, Belgium). The μCT creates a 3D volume of the object by stacking two-dimensional X-ray slices. The instrument was set to scan the entire tooth with an acceleration voltage of 100 kV and a current of 100 μA. The SkyScan 1076® software produced 547 images in 8-bit Tag Image File Format (TIFF) format with horizontal and vertical resolution of 35 μm. The coronal portion of the tooth was selected to generate 276 horizontal sections (cross sections) with a resolution of 464 × 464. The exposure time was 130 ms. The absence of artefacts and/or fault zones on the cross-sectional images was checked for each cut with TView® software. No filter was used to not embed an error in these images. At the end of this control step all the sections (276) were selected for 3D construction of the coronal part of the tooth (Fig. 1).

2.2 Creation of different masks

The stack of scanned sections has been imported into this Amira® image processing software (Visage Imaging®, Germany) to segment the different parts of the dental organ. Enamel, dentin and pulp have different degrees of radio opacities related to their degree of mineralization. The software Amira® allows to delimit each part thanks to the different level of grey expressed on the cuts. The delineation is done pixel by pixel on each section using semi-automatic or manual methods which, by interpolation, extraction and progressive filling of the edges produce masks. A mask for each part was obtained: enamel, dentin and pulp. Subsequently, a mesh is generated to create a 3D-FE model that is imported into another software package (Rapidform®, INUS Technology, Seoul, Korea).

2.3 Simulation of cavity design and different obturation materials

The congruence of the pulp-dentin-enamel junctions has been restored with the RapidForm software (Rapidform®, INUS Technology, Seoul, Korea). 3D surfaces were created taking into account the junction between enamel and dentin and between the pulp and dentine. Thorough cleaning of the tooth has created a closed solid. Unlike the studies found in the literature (Ausiello et al. 2011, Chuang et al. 2011, Magne et al. 2012, Zhang et al. 2016), the final object is not a superposition of the different volumes but a single volume with three materials, composed of different surfaces that represent the joints between the enamel and dentin and between dentin and pulp (Fig. 2a). This technique does not require Boolean operations that generate constraints at the interface joints.

The use of "cutting planes" has made it possible to simulate a class II MOD cavity (Fig. 2b). Finally, the volumetric mesh of the entire model was created and imported into Abaqus® software (Abaqus® Dassault Systèmes® Simulia Corp®, Paris, France). Boundary conditions, material properties were applied, and FE treatment was initiated.

2.4 Finite element analysis of the 3D model

All the nodes of the lower surface of the tooth were constrained in all directions (X, Y and Z), preventing the rigid displacement of the body, in agreement with previous studies (Magne 2007, Magne & Oganesyan, 2009b, Ausiello et al. 2011, Aussiello et al. 2004). In the simulated boundary conditions (Magne 2007, Ausiello et al. 2004), the root zone only marginally affected the overall distribution of coronal stresses. A distributed load on the occlusal surface has been simulated according to previous literature (Magne 2007, Ausiello et al. 2011). It was applied at a pressure (stress) of 562 N, corresponding to 6 N/mm^2 distributed over 70.88 mm^2 of surface of the occlusal surface molar. The constituent materials have all been considered homogeneous, linear, elastic, and isotropic (Ausiello et al. 2001) and their properties are presented in Table 1.

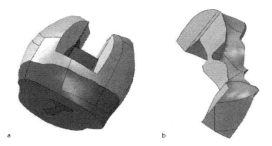

Figure 2. 3D CAD (a) the volumes generated, (b) Class II restoration.

Table 1. Elastic properties of the materials.

	Elastic modulus GPa	Poisson's ratio
Enamel	80	0.30
Dentin	15	0.31
Pulp	0.002	0.45
Resin composite	25	0.30
Ceramic	78	0.28

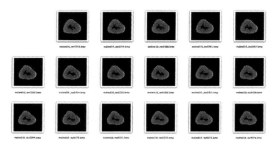

Figure 1. A few of the 276 slices selected.

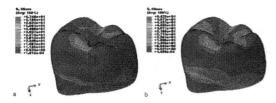

Figure 3. The Von Mises stress (MPa) for the model (a) resin composite restoration, (b) ceramic restoration.

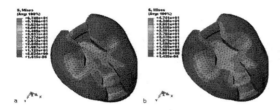

Figure 4. The Von Mises stress (MPa) for the model (a) without resin composite restoration, (b) without ceramic restoration.

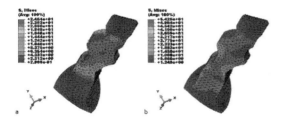

Figure 5. The Von Mises stress (MPa) (a) resin composite restoration, (b) ceramic restoration.

3 RESULTS

No error was generated during the FEA by the 3D model of the molar. Stresses on the concave parts of the occlusal table (grooves, occlusal dimples), especially around the cavosurface angle of the cavity were observed with the application of the load dispersed on the occlusal surface. The internal angles of the cavity under the restoration and the cervical region of the crown are also the seat of stress concentration.

The interfaces between the different constituents of the tooth did not include constraints. The constraints were due to the configuration of the restoration and reconstruction model. The model is therefore more precise and more realistic (Figs. 3–5).

4 DISCUSSION

Actually, very used in multiple fields; FEA have also demonstrated their interest in dentistry. It was after the studies of Farah and Craig in 1973 (Farah & Craig 1973) that the inhomogeneity of the dental structure was considered. It was not until 1978 that the importance of the delimitation and the description of the external surfaces, the coefficients of friction between the different surfaces and the Poisson's ratio found an importance thanks to the studies of Yettram et al. (1976). Finally, in 1983, Rubin et al. (1983) developed the first model in 3D.

In dentistry, the possibility of obtaining a 3D image of the studied structure is an essential step of the FEA (Magne & Oganesyan 2009a, b, Magne 2010, Ausiello et al. 2001, Rodrigues et al. 2009, Ausiello et al. 2011, Ausiello et al. 2005). The X-ray scanning of the structures makes it possible to obtain 2D slices. The latter are stacked automatically thanks to interpolations and a system of coordinates to give a 3D image of the object. The reading of these images is operator dependent. The software programs accompanying acquisition systems make it possible to apply filters to reduce noise and artifacts, but this tends to also lead to the incorporation of errors. To avoid this, it is better to call out an experienced operator who will be able to better interpret these images. The micro CT offers a higher resolution than other dental imaging systems, and the variation between the initial images and the reconstructed solids may be less than 0.6%, although this depends on the parameters of the device during acquisition. Artifacts, hardening of the beam, the model of the instrument are parameters that interfere with the data, which explains the need for qualified operators in the use of this device.

During the FEA step, each software has a more or less easy use, despite the fact that the proposed tools are similar. In the literature (Magne 2007), the description of the 3D model implementation protocol remains vague concerning the problems that may arise. The constraints observed on the limits of the different parts during the superposition of them is one of these problems. Masks are created for each part during the segmentation and then they are superimposed to create the final volume of the object. The congruence of these masks is not perfect, there are mesh overlapping areas or empty areas. These areas are interpreted as errors or constraint concentration points during computations. These are interfacial constraints. Boolean operations have been proposed for the resolution of this problem. These are complex operations that create an approximate, non-overlapping, or empty limit for each mask. However, the result generates distortions and approximations in the model.

The purpose of our study was to provide a more realistic and precise alternative to the protocols described in the literature. The model presented here does not require Boolean operations and therefore does not include any approximations.

This is a more realistic design that is based on the anatomical design of the dental organ. The tooth is then conceived as a single volume composed of different materials. It is only a single object composed of different parts with different properties and not a superposition of three objects.

In agreement with the studies found in the literature, this dental model has been validated with the simulation of a class II cavity MOD restored with different filling materials such as a composite and a dental ceramic. The restored model was subjected to a uniformly distributed load on the occlusal surface of the tooth, and the results obtained correspond to those from the literature.

The cavo-suface angle, the enamel-dentine junction, the concave areas of the occlusal surface and the angles of the cavity were found to be areas of stress concentration.

At present, studies in this field of dentistry face the limitations of µCT acquisition systems accuracy (Magne & Oganesyan 2009a, Magne 2010, Magne 2007, Magne & Douglas 1999, Magne et al. 2012, Magne & Tan 2008) as well as the lack of automation of certain stages of the design. It is clear that much remains to be done to make this model even more realistic and precise. Further studies are underway to determine the ideal cavity design as well as the influence of material thicknesses such as enamel or dentine, the influence of restoration materials and the relationship between these parameters and tooth type tested.

5 CONCLUSION

The purpose of this study was to describe the sequence of software for the construction of a more accurate and realistic dental model for finite element analysis. The realization of a 3D model close to the tooth anatomical concept with a single volume composed of three different materials not using Boolean operations made it possible to avoid the approximations during the calculations.

This model has been validated by obtaining comparable results to the literature data.

REFERENCES

Ausiello P., Apicella A., Davidson C.L., Rengo S., 2001. 3D-finite element analyses of cusp movements in a human upper premolar, restored with adhesive resin-based composites. *Journal Biomechanics* 34: 1269–1277.

Ausiello P., Rengo S., Davidson C.L., Watts D.C., 2004. Stress distributions in adhesively cemented ceramic and resin-composite Class II inlay restorations: a 3D-FEA study. *Dental Materials* 20: 862–872.

Ausiello P., Franciosa P., Martorelli M., Watts D.C., 2011. Numerical fatigue 3D-FE modeling of indirect composite-restored posterior teeth. *Dental Materials* 27: 423–430.

Chuang S.F., Chang C.H., Chen T.Y.F., 2011. Contraction behaviors of dental composite restorations—Finite element investigation with DIC validation. *Journal of the Mechanical Behavior of Biomedical Materials* 4: 2138–2149.

Farah J.W., Craig R.G., 1973. Element stress analysis of an axisymmeric molar. *Journal of Dental Research* 53: 859–864.

Ledley R.H., Huang H.K., 1968. Linear model of tooth displacement by applied forces. *Journal of Dental Research* 47: 427–32.

Magne P., Douglas W.H., 1999. Optimization of resilience and stress distribution in porcelain veneers for the treatment of crown-fractured incisors. *International Journal of Periodontics and Restorative Dentistry* 19: 543–553.

Magne P., 2007. Efficient 3D finite element analysis of dental restorative procedures using micro-CT data. *Dental Materials* 23: 539–548.

Magne P., Tan D.T., 2008. Incisor compliance following operative procedures: a rapid 3-D finite element analysis using micro-CT data. *Journal of Adhesive Dentistry* 10: 49–56.

Magne P., Oganesyan T., 2009a. CT scan-based finite element analysis of premolar cuspal deflection following operative procedures. *International Journal of Periodontics and Restorative Dentistry* 29: 361–369.

Magne P., Oganesyan T., 2009b. Premolar cuspal flexure as a function of restorative material and occlusal contact location. *Quintessence International* 40: 363–370.

Magne P., 2010. Virtual prototyping of adhesively restored, endodontically treated molars. *Journal of Prosthetic Dentistry* 103: 343–351.

Magne P., Schlichting L.H., 2011. Paranhos MPG. Risk of onlay fracture during pre-cementation functional occlusal tapping. *Dental Materials* 27: 942–7.

Magne P., Stanley K., Schlichting L.H., 2012. Modeling of ultrathin occlusal veneers. *Dental Materials* 28: 777–782.

Rees J.S., Hammadeh M., Jagger D.C., 2003. Abfraction lesion formation in maxillary incisors, canines and premolars: a finite element study. *European Journal Oral Sciences* 111: 149–154.

Rodrigues F.P., Li J., Silikas N., Ballester R.Y., Watts D.C., 2009. Sequential software processing of micro-XCT dental-images for 3D-FE analysis. *Dental Materials* 25: 47–55.

Rubin C., Krishanamurity N., Capilouto E., 1983. Stress analysis of the human tooth using three-dimensional finite element model. *Journal of Dental Research* 62: 82–86.

Yamanel K., Çağlar A., Gülşahi K., Özden U.A., 2009. Effects of different ceramic and composite materials on stress distribution in inlay and onlay cavities: 3-D finite element analysis. *Dental Material Journal* 28: 661–670.

Yettram A.L., Wright K.W.J., Pickard H.M., 1976. Finite element stress analysis of the crowns of normal and restored teeth. *Journal of Dental Research* 55: 1004–1010.

Zhang Z., Zheng K., Li E., Li W., Li Q., Swain M.V., 2016. Mechanical benefits of conservative restoration for dental fissure caries. *Journal of the Mechanical Behavior of Biomedical Materials* 53: 11–20.

Biodental Engineering V – Belinha et al. (Eds)
© 2019 Taylor & Francis Group, London, ISBN 978-0-367-21087-8

Biological behavior of titanium, zirconia or PEEK dental implant-abutments

M.B. Sordi, S.N.D. Sarwer-Foner, F.H. Schünemann, K. Apaza-Bedoya,
G.M.P. Juanito, B. Henriques, R.S. Magini & C.A.M. Benfatti
*Center of Research on Dental Implants (CEPID), Federal University of Santa Catarina,
Florianopolis/SC, Brazil*

ABSTRACT: Novel biomaterials such as ceramics and polymers have been introduced in prosthetic implant dentistry offering other properties than those of titanium abutments. There is a concern in the guarantee of a long-term tissue stability to maintain the peri-mucosal seal, such as the cell biocompatibility and adhesion, and the inhibition of biofilm formation around implant-abutments. The aim of this review was to explore the state of art on the biological behaviors of different abutment materials, namely/titanium, zirconia, and Polyetheretherketone (PEEK). Titanium, as the "gold-standard" in oral implantology, is the most widely investigated biomaterial. Nevertheless, in the last decades, zirconia has emerged in the prostheses field as a promising esthetic biomaterial with mechanical properties similar to titanium. In the articles revised in this study, the authors were unable to identify which material presents the most convenient biological behaviors since different methodologies and inconsistent outcomes were found. Further studies should compare biological behavior on titanium, zirconia and PEEK abutments to stablish the specific clinical application and the advantages and disadvantages of each biomaterial.

1 INTRODUCTION

In the recent years, novel materials such as ceramics and polymers have been introduced in prosthetic implant dentistry, offering other properties than those of titanium abutments. There is a concern in assuring long-term tissue stability to maintain the peri-mucosal seal.

Adhesion and proliferation of cells can vary depending on the surface topography (Köunönen et al. 1992). The peri-implant mucosal attachment around abutments plays an important role in the short- and long-term success of dental implants (Gómez-Florit et al. 2014). Previous literature showed that mechanical or biological complications related to implant-abutment joint might increase peri-implant bone loss (Lazzara et al. 2006). Biocompatibility and adhesive properties of supragingival and gingival-passing structure not only make it possible to form functional soft tissues, but also play an important role in maintaining osseointegration (Moon et al. 2013). It was stablished that an ideal implant-abutment should allow rapid fibroblast and epithelial cell proliferation and attachment, but reduce biofilm and bacterial adherence (Nothdurft et al. 2015). Therefore, the inherent properties of the abutment's substrates may affect the nature and course of the relevant biological processes (Köunönen et al. 1992).

The oral cavity represents a challenging environment for all biomaterials since they are exposed to biofilm formation, which negatively affects their long-time performance. The biofilm is a complex microbial community with a large number of species, including bacteria and fungi, that gathers substances from food, saliva and microbial metabolism (Köunönen et al. 1992). The process starts when the implant-abutment is rapidly covered with a salivary protein pellicle. The adsorbed proteins offer a range of binding sites for oral bacteria to attach and initiate the development of a microbial biofilm (Dorkhan et al. 2014a, Rutkunas et al. 2015). Several bacterial species have been related to be involved in the pathogenesis of periodontal and peri-implantar diseases. Microbial adhesions on surfaces are typically tested by *in vitro* models with one or more bacterial strains. However, the oral microbial ecology contains hundreds of species, which is extremely difficult to simulate through *in vitro* studies (Xing et al. 2015).

Indeed, physical and chemical characteristics of implant-abutment surfaces can directly affect bacterial profile accumulated onto them as well as influence the quality of the interface between the prosthetic abutment and the soft tissues (Rigolin et al. 2017). Implant materials cannot completely prevent bacterial adhesion and consequent colonization of the substrate surfaces (Quirynen et al.

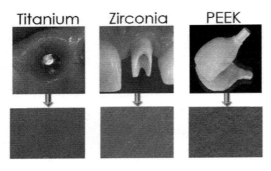

Figure 1. Example of clinical applications and scanning electron microscopy images of titanium, zirconia, and PEEK biomaterials.

2002). Thus, cell biocompatibility and adhesion, as well as inhibition of biofilm formation around prosthetic abutments are properties that elevate the quality of biomaterials when applied clinically.

The literature shows that titanium (Ti) is the most widely used material for implant-abutments, then has become the "gold-standard" in oral implantology due to its excellent mechanical properties and biocompatibility (Gómez-Florit et al. 2014). For a long time and even actually, metallic abutments were considered the best option for customized prosthetic solutions. However, the grey color might impair the esthetics. Hence, different materials that are pure white in color should adequately simulate the color of natural teeth (Linkevicius et al. 2015). In the last decades, zirconia (Zr) has emerged in the prosthetic field as a promising esthetic biomaterial with mechanical properties similar or ever higher when compared to titanium. Polyetheretherketone (PEEK) is a polymer that has been extensively studied in biomedicine for implantation of lost tissues, specifically bone. PEEK is not yet used as prosthetic abutments, despite of being applied for dental implants, provisional prostheses, healing abutments or impressing transfers. Therefore, the purpose of this review was to explore the existing literature of biological behaviors of different abutment materials, specifically titanium, zirconia, and polyetheretherketone (PEEK) (Figure 1).

2 METHODOLOGY

Articles were selected from electronic search on PubMed database. The search strategy was as follows: (peek OR polyetheretherketone OR zirconia OR ZrO_2 OR titanium OR Ti6Al4V) AND (abutment OR prosthetic abutment OR dental components) AND (biological properties OR biological response OR biological behavior OR cell viability OR cell proliferation OR biofilm). Articles in English language from the past 5 years were selected. Clinical, *in vivo* and *in vitro* studies, and literature reviews were included.

3 RESULTS AND DISCUSSION

Overall, 36 relevant articles were selected from a sample of 123 studies resulted from the search strategy, in which 20 were *in vitro* studies, 8 were clinical trials, and 8 were systematic or literature reviews. Summaries on the main outcomes of experimental studies are found on Tables 1 and 2. Only one article contemplated PEEK applications, while all others assessed titanium, zirconia, or even compared both materials. Titanium, as the "gold-standard" in oral implantology, were the most investigated biomaterial.

3.1 *Titanium*

Metal and their alloys have long been used in dentistry. The disadvantage of using metals, besides esthetics, is the adverse reactions of organism. The sources for these reactions are mainly metal ions release during corrosion process that infiltrate the surrounding tissues (Benaszek et al. 2016). Implant surfaces are composed of chemical elements, which may degrade under different temperatures or suffer damage from the forces applied to them. The release of such chemical elements may result in inflammation of the periodontal tissue. Moreover, the surface characteristics may be altered, favoring biofilm development, which will further increase inflammation (Avila et al. 2013). Nevertheless, metals are very likely to be applied in dental prostheses for a long time, since there are few alternative materials of comparable properties, such as resistance and durability (Benaszek et al. 2016).

In order to increase the biological tolerance of metals, as well as improve cell adhesion and reduce biofilm accumulation, different modifications of external metal surfaces, especially on Ti, are being proposed. Nowadays, it is already known that implant-abutment surfaces should be modified not just to reduce microbial adhesion but also to reduce the chemical elements released by the surfaces over time in addition to increase keratinocytes, fibroblasts and osteoblasts adhesion (Avila et al. 2013, Dorkhan et al. 2014a). Regarding Ti, the main concerning's are about the differences between machined or rough surfaces. Previous clinical study, indicate that the safety of hydrophilic acid etched titanium abutments is equivalent to that noted for standard machined abutments (Schwarz et al. 2013). In addition, modern nanostructured titanium surfaces have been also applied, since

Table 1. Summary of the *in vitro* studies evaluating biological aspects of implant-abutment materials.

Author (year)	Materials	Methodology	Biological response
Moon et al. (2013)	Disks of machined titanium, polished titanium, titanium coated with titanium nitride, machined zirconia, and polished zirconia.	Morphologies of cultured human gingival fibroblasts cultured on the samples were observed by scanning electron microscopy. Biocompatibility and focal adhesion were evaluated by ultrasonic wave application and cell viability assay. Focal adhesion linker proteins expression levels were assessed by RT-PCR and western blot.	Little difference in biocompatibility and adhesion strength of fibroblasts was found among the surface conditions and materials. Strength of adhesion of fibroblasts to transmucosal abutment surfaces increases with time and it seemed to be related to expressions of focal adhesion linker proteins.
Dorkhan et al. (2014a)	Titanium discs with three different surfaces: 1) Commercially pure titanium (control), 2) Anodic oxidation on commercially pure titanium, and 3) Anodic oxidation on titanium alloy (TiAl6V4).	The surfaces were characterized by SEM. The number of adhered cells and binding strength, as well as vitality of fibroblasts and keratinocytes were evaluated using confocal scanning laser microscopy after staining with Live/Dead Baclight. To evaluate the effect of bacteria on adherence and vitality, keratinocytes were co-cultured with a four-species streptococcal consortium.	The vitality and level of cellular adherence to the nanostructured surfaces was similar to that on CpTi. Co-culture with streptococci reduced the number of keratinocytes on all the surfaces to approximately the same level and caused cell damage, suggesting that commensal bacteria could affect cellular adherence to abutments.
Dorkhan et al. (2014b)	Disks with surfaces prepared by anodic oxidation on commercially pure titanium or titanium alloy were used as test surfaces. Disks of machined commercially pure titanium were used as control.	Adherence of early colonizing *Streptococcus gordonii*, *Streptococcus oralis*, *Streptococcus mitis* and *Streptococcus sanguinis* to saliva-coated anodically oxidized surfaces was compared with that on commercially pure titanium. The biofilm formation was evaluated by fluorescence microscopy.	The adherence of early colonizers was lower on anodized than on commercially pure titanium surfaces, a factor which contributes significantly to overall biofilm formation on implant surfaces.
Kim et al. (2014)	Six experimental disks surfaces: titanium alloy (smooth machined), cobalt-chrome-molybdenum alloy, titanium nitride-coated titanium, anodic-oxidized titanium, composite resin-coated titanium, and zirconia. Culture plate surface was the control.	Surface roughness, developed interfacial area ratio, and water contact angle were measured. Human gingival fibroblast attachment and proliferation after 3 and 7 days were observed.	On day-3, control group showed significantly greater proliferation than all experimental groups. On day-7, titanium nitride-coated titanium, anodic-oxidized titanium, zirconia, and control groups exhibited twice the number of cells compared to other groups.
Liu et al. (2014)	Abutments of pristine zirconia and polydopamine-coated zirconia.	The responses of human gingival fibroblasts to polydopamine-coated zirconia were analyzed. The adhesion of *Streptococcus gordonii* and *Streptococcus mutans* to zirconia after polydopamine coating was also assessed.	Polydopamine seems to influence to fibroblasts behavior and reduce bacterial adhesion on zirconia abutments.

(Continued)

Table 1. (Continued)

Author (year)	Materials	Methodology	Biological response
Xing et al. (2014)	Titanium disks.	Cathodic polarization was used to modify titanium samples. Three acid was used: oxalic acid, tartaric acid and acetic acid.	Changes in surface topography and hydrophilicity did not significantly influence human gingival fibroblasts growth.
Hahnel et al. (2015)	Titanium, zirconia, and polyetheretherketone (PEEK) disks. Polymethylmethacrylate (PMMA) were the control.	After the simulation of salivary pellicle formation, multispecies biofilm formation was initiated by suspensions of *Streptococcus gordonii*, *Streptococcus mutans*, *Actinomyces naeslundii*, and *Candida albicans* for 20 or 44 hours. Viable microbial biomass adherent to the samples and the percentage of dead microorganisms in the different biofilms were determined.	Biofilm formation on PEEK is equal or lower than on the surface of conventionally applied titanium or zirconia abutments.
Lee et al. (2015)	Titanium disks.	Disks were polished with no dimples (control), had 5-μm dimples at 10-μm intervals, and had 5-μm dimples at 25-μm intervals in the polished surfaces. Human gingival squamous cell carcinoma cells and human lung fibroblasts were used in cell proliferation assays, adhesion assays, immunofluorescent staining of adhesion proteins, and morphological analysis by SEM.	The adhesion strength of epithelial cells was higher on surfaces with 5-μm laser dimples than on polished surfaces. However, epithelial cells and fibroblasts around the laser dimples appeared larger and showed increased expression of adhesion proteins.
Nothdurft et al. (2015)	Machined (no surface modification), smooth (polished), and rough zirconia and titanium alloy cylinders.	Fibroblasts and epithelial cells grown on the samples were investigated 24 and 72 hours after seeding and counted using fluorescence imaging. To investigate adhesion, the abundance and arrangement of the focal adhesion protein vinculin were evaluated by immunocytochemistry.	Fibroblasts exhibited significant higher proliferation rates on zirconia than titanium alloys. Cell spreading was generally higher on polished and machined surfaces than on sandblasted surfaces. Rough surfaces provided favorable properties in terms of cellular adhesion of fibroblasts but not of epithelial cells. Fibroblast and epithelial cell responses were influenced by the material and surface topography.
Rutkunas et al. (2015)	Commercial pure titanium (Grade 2), zirconium oxide ceramic, chrome-cobalt alloy, and dental gold alloy disks.	Gingival fibroblasts were cultured on the tested materials and subjected to lateral shear forces by applying 300 and 500 rpm shaking intensities. Focal adhesion kinase expression and phosphorylation in cells grown on the specimens were registered by cell-based ELISA.	There was a tendency of fibroblast adhesion strength to decrease in the following order: sandblasted titanium, polished titanium, sandblasted zirconium oxide, polished zirconium oxide gold–alloy, chrome–cobalt alloy. Higher levels of proteins were registered in fibroblasts grown on roughened titanium.

Avila et al. (2016a)	Abutments of titanium and zirconia, and bovine enamel (control group).	Biofilm formation was analyzed by growing Porphyromonas gingivalis and Fusobacterium nucleatum as monospecies and mixed species biofilms on the surfaces. The mean roughness (Ra) and surface free energy were evaluated. Mature biofilm (7 days) was analyzed quantitatively and qualitatively by colony-forming unit and confocal laser scanning microscopy.	Zirconia abutment surfaces showed a decrease in anaerobic biofilm compared with titanium and bovine enamel.
Avila et al. (2016b)	Machined pure titanium and yttrium-stabilized zirconia discs, and bovine enamel discs (control group).	*Streptococcus mutans* and *Porphyromonas gingivalis* were cultured. To investigate the influence of material surfaces on bacterial adhesion, surface free energy (SFE), optical profilometry, atomic force microscopy (AFM), and energy dispersive X-ray spectroscope (EDX) were performed.	Bacterial adhesion on titanium was lower than that on zirconia, independent of the bacterial species or Gram-positive or Gram-negative status, but it was consistently higher on bovine enamel. The presence of polar and non-polar components might explain the greater numbers of bacteria on bovine enamel compared to other surfaces.
Banaszek et al. (2016)	Cylindrical samples nickel chromium alloy coated with titanium nitrocarbide (C, N) layers with different content of C and N. Control group has no layers.	The samples were stored in an experimental medium with antibiotics for 30 days. Endothelial cells were incubated for 24 and 96 hours, after all cell viability was determined using MTT method.	During incubation of endothelial cells with coated samples, the number of cells was significantly higher than the number with uncoated samples. The best cell viability was obtained from samples with 51.94% titanium, 28.22% C and 19.84% N.
Brunot-Gohin et al. (2016)	Square samples of lithium disilicate and zirconium oxide ceramics, both raw and polished. A cell culture-treated plastic was used as control.	Physicochemical characteristics were analyzed by contact angle measurements, scanning white-light interferometry, and scanning electron microscopy. Epithelium cells were cultured to simulate peri-implant soft tissue. Samples contact angle, hydrophobicity, roughness, and cell migration/adhesion were analyzed.	The best cell migration was observed on zirconia surfaces. However, cell adhesion was drastically lower on polished zirconia than on both raw and polished lithium disilicate. Evaluating various Surface topographies of lithium disilicate showed that increasing surface roughness improved cell adhesion.
Esfahanizadeh et al. (2016)	Discs of Laser-Lok, titanium, and zirconia.	Human gingival fibroblasts were cultured on different abutment materials. Cell morphology, proliferation rate, and interleukin 10 (IL-10), tumor necrosis factor alpha (TNFα), fibronectin, and integrin gene expressions were assessed by electron microscopy, methyl thiazol tetrazolium (MTT) assay, and real-time polymerase chain reaction (PCR), respectively.	Human gingival fibroblasts on Laser-Lok surfaces had a more mature morphology and greater proliferation and differentiation as compared to those on zirconia and titanium surfaces.

(*Continued*)

Table 1. (Continued)

Author (year)	Materials	Methodology	Biological response
Okabe et al. (2016)	Commertially pure titanium, ceria-stabilized zirconia/ alumina nano-composite, yttria-stabilized zirconia, and alumina oxide disks.	Human oral epithelial cells were cultured on the disks and the adhesion properties of zirconia materials regarding cell attachment, morphology, and mRNA expression of adhesion molecules were assessed and compared with titanium and alumina.	Morphology of cells attached to specimens was similar among all groups. The viable cell numbers on zirconia and alumina after 24 hours were significantly higher than for titanium. Zirconia may support binding of epithelial cells through hemidesmosomes comparable with titanium.
Pabst et al. (2016)	Zirconia disks (CAD-CAM). Control was the tissue culture polystyrene.	Human gingival fibroblasts and oral keratinocytes were cultured. Cell viability was analyzed by MTT, migration ability was detected by scratch assay, and ToxiLight assay was used to analyze the apoptosis rate.	The cell viability and migration ability of keratinocytes were negatively influenced by CAD/CAM zirconia, whereas fibroblasts was overall not negatively influenced.
Alrabeah et al. (2017)	Titanium abutments.	The effect of different concentrations of metal ions (titanium, aluminum, vanadium, cobalt, chromium and molybdenum) released from different implant abutment couples on osteoblastic cell viability, apoptosis and expression of genes related to bone resorption.	Metal ions in concentrations representing the platform-matched groups led to a reduction in cell viability.
Avila et al. (2017)	Disks of machined pure titanium and yttrium-stabilize zirconia.	Initial adherent bacteria and biofilm formation were evaluated after 16 and 48 hours by incubating the disks in a rich medium containing saliva-derived oral microbial community.	The initial attachment phase and biofilm formation are affected by substrate type, with zirconia accumulating significantly more bacteria and biofilm on the material surfaces than titanium.
Rigolin et al. (2017)	Titanium and zirconia disks. Bovine enamel and glass cover slips disks were positive and negative controls.	Cell morphology and viability after 1 and 24 hours were analyzed using gingival epithelial cells.	Roughness and surface free energy had no effect on the cell viability data or on their interaction. Cells attachment and spreading increased after 24 hours on titanium and zirconia than on bovine enamel.

Table 2. Summary of the clinical studies evaluating biological aspects of implant-abutment materials.

Author (year)	Materials	Methodology	Biological response
Harder et al. (2013)	Two-piece titanium implants carrying ball attachments.	Biofilm and non-adherent microbial samples are cultured and analyzed by conventional biochemical testing, MALDI-TOF MS, and 16 s rDNA gene sequencing.	103 species detected: 27 on biofilm, 33 on non-adherent microbial, and 43 on both. Two-piece dental implants harbored a broad spectrum of gram-positive and gram-negative aerobes and anaerobes, especially rods and cocci, confirming bacterial translocation from the oral cavity to intraimplant cavities.
Nascimento et al. (2013)	Machined or cast titanium, and zirconia disks.	Participants used intraoral splints containing four disks of the same substrate for 24 hours. Two discs were located in the anterior region and two in the posterior region. DNA checkerboard hybridization method was used to detect and quantify five different Candida species. Data on the surface roughness and the total area of discs covered by formed biofilm were also provided to correlate the species and biofilm found between different substrates.	Cast and polished titanium presented the higher bacterial mean counts, followed by machined pure titanium and zirconia. *Candida albicans* and *Candida krusei* were not detected in the zirconia group. The region of disk placement did not show differences in relation to Candida adhesion.
Schwarz et al. (2013)	Healing abutments of 1) hydrophobic machined titanium, 2) hydrophilic acid etched titanium, or 3) hydrophilic acid etched titanium-zirconium alloy.	Healing abutments and a limited soft tissue biopsy were harvested and processed for histological analysis on epithelial and connective tissue contact to the abutments.	Hydrophilic acid etched surfaces have the potential to enhance soft tissue adhesion at the transmucosal aspect.
Bressan et al. (2014)	Titanium healing abutments.	Fifty healing abutments were placed in 34 patients 1 week after implant surgery (test group). After 7 days, 50 healing abutments were placed in the same implant sites and removed 1 week after (control group). During the 2 testing periods, patients were instructed to apply chlorhexidine mouth rinsing and no brushing (test); or no chlorhexidine mouth rinsing and no brushing (control). SEM were used to quantify bacterial plaque.	Chlorhexidine mouth rinsing significantly limited plaque formation on healing abutments, being a valid contribution to mechanical brushing in early phases of plaque control.

(*Continued*)

Table 2. (Continued)

Author (year)	Materials	Methodology	Biological response
Nascimento et al. (2014)	Abutments of machined titanium, cast titanium, and zirconia.	Each individual used an intraoral splint containing four disks of the same tested substrate, two located in the anterior and two in the posterior palate during 24 hours. DNA checkerboard hybridization method was used to identify and quantify 38 bacterial species colonizing formed biofilm on substrates.	Cast titanium presented the higher mean bacterial counts, followed by machined titanium and zirconia samples. No significant differences were found in relation to bacterial adhesion between anterior and posterior region.
Kheur et al. (2016)	Zirconia and titanium abutments.	Human cytomegalovirus 1 and Epstein–Barr virus 1 were evaluated in clinically-healthy peri-implant sites: submarginal plaque biofilm at one titanium and one zirconia abutment, one healthy tooth site, and serum using polymerase chain reaction assays.	Epstein-Barr was detected at the titanium abutment in 60% of participants, but in none at their zirconia abutments. Cytomegalovirus was detected at the titanium abutments in 90% of participants, and at the zirconia abutments in 70% of participants.
Nascimento et al. (2016)	Pre-machined zirconia and pre-machined titanium abut-ments.	Probing depth, clinical attachment level, bleeding on probing, and marginal bone level were evaluated over time and correlated with biofilm formation. DNA-Checkerboard and 16S-rDNA-Pyrosequencing were used to quantify and determine species identity.	Species common to all sites belonged to genera *Fusobacterium*, *Prevotella*, *Actinomyces*, *Porphyromonas*, *Veillonella* and *Streptococcus*. Pathogenic and non-pathogenic species were detected colonizing oral sites in both materials. Titanium presented the highest total microbial count and higher counts of pathogenic species.
Freitas et al. (2018)	Titanium and zirconia abutments.	Biofilm was collected from implant-retained restorations after 1, 3, and 6 months.	Titanium and zirconia abutments and teeth showed similar total numbers of operational taxonomic units colonizing surfaces over time. *Firmicutes*, *Proteobacteria*, *Fusobacteria*, *Bacteroidetes*, and *Actinobacteria* were the most prevalent phyla.

improved adherence of keratinocytes and fibroblasts were noted on anodized Ti surfaces compared to commercially pure Ti. Hence, nanostructured surfaces offer promising properties for enhancement of implant-abutment integration with the soft-tissues; however, this process may be negatively affected by the presence of commensal oral bacteria (Dorkhan et al. 2014a).

It was studied that *Streptococcus mutans* performes initial adhesion on titanium surfaces supported by glycoprotein such as mucin or polysaccharides (Souza et al. 2013). In addition, *Candida albicans* has been shown to be present in several sites in studies assessing microbiota from healthy and failed implants (do Nascimento et al. 2013). The use of chlorhexidine demonstrated statistically significant differences on biofilm formation on Ti abutment surfaces in comparison with no treatment. However, mechanical brushing is still considered the best way for biofilm disruption (Bressan et al. 2014).

3.2 *Zirconia*

Esthetic implant-abutments possess light dynamic qualities comparable to natural teeth. However, these esthetic abutments must contain biological properties to allow the healing around crown and gingiva, thus requiring significant roughness of the material, leading to improved cell adhesion. Additionally, they should preferably avoid biofilm formation (Brunot-Gohin et al. 2016).

Zr has been introduced in implant dentistry as an alternative to titanium, since it provides a better esthetic outcome. However, the surface of Zr is bioinert and difficult to modify. The researches on the use of Zr as biomaterial started about 40 years ago (Piconi et al. 1999). Along the time, several physical and chemical surface modification techniques have been developed to enhance the bioactivity of Zr in terms of tissue reactions, such as optimizing the surface texture, like sandblasting (Bacchelli et al. 2009), acid-etching (Flamant et al. 2016), laser application (Moura et al. 2017), and different coatings (Pardun et al. 2015). Modified surface of Zr abutments have shown higher epithelial and connective tissue abutment contact as compared to similarly treated Ti abutments, supporting Zr greater biocompatibility (Piconi et al. 1999). Interestingly, Zr for CAD/CAM-based implant-abutment have different chemical compositions.

Since Zr are in close contact to oral soft-tissues such as marginal keratinized gingiva, it is primordial to analyze if this biomaterial has influence on oral soft-tissue cells, such as fibroblasts or keratinocytes. In this context, oral keratinocytes represent the dominating cell line of the marginal, keratinized gingiva, whereas gingival fibroblasts create the extracellular matrix, collagen, and the stroma downstream of the covering keratinocyte layer (Pabst et al. 2016).

3.3 *PEEK*

For esthetic considerations, zirconia abutments are already frequently used as implant-abutments. Nonetheless, some studies have showed that PEEK has being increasingly employed as abutment material in contemporary implant dentistry. PEEK is a polymeric thermoplastic material with numerous favorable properties, including mechanical properties similar to the bone, chemical inertness and biological compatibility (Kern et al. 2012, Fuhrmann et al. 2014). From a microbiological point of view, considering that connective tissue seal to dental abutment is crucial for peri-implant health, there is almost no scientific evidence available in the literature regarding the formation of biofilms on PEEK's surfaces, but the existing few studies reported favorable properties as definite abutment material.

3.4 *Comparison among materials for implant-abutments*

A summary on the main points of the studies resulted from the present search strategy is presented on Tables 1 and 2.

Physico-chemical characteristics from different materials affect the pathogenic bacterial adhesion. Regarding mixed bacterial species biofilm, the number of microorganisms and the density of the biofilm on Zr were lower than on Ti and bovine enamel (Avila et al. 2016). Additionally, confocal microscopic images revealed that bacterial colonization on bovine enamel was clearly characterized by larger, taller and more widespread microcolonies in comparison to the Ti and Zr surfaces for both *S. mutans* and *P. gingivalis* (Avila et al. 2016b). However, it was suggested that bacterial adhesion on Ti was lower than that on Zr, independent of the bacterial species or Gram-positive or Gram-negative status, though it was consistently higher on bovine enamel than on abutment materials (Avila et al. 2016b). Also, when analyzing the total number of bacteria adhered biofilm to different materials, more bacterial accumulation was observed on Zr surfaces (Avila et al. 2017).

Usually, when comparing different materials, the variable roughness is eliminated to maintain the homogeneity of the groups at a Ra of about 0.2 mm (Avila et al. 2016, Esfahanizadeh et al. 2016). Ti and Zr are hydrophobic materials. Hydrophobic attractive forces and electrostatic charge interactions between surfaces and bacteria play a key role in biofilm formation. Most bacteria have many ionizable groups on their surfaces, which confer a negative charge, particularly during the early stationary phase of bacterial growth. However, the charge that is present on the surface of some types of bacteria can create a hydrophobic effect via nonpolar molecules and result in an affinity for other hydrophobic surfaces, such as Ti and Zr. This characteristic explains why some bacterial species preferentially interact with certain materials and why the findings reported in the literature are inconsistent depending on the type of bacterial species assessed (Avila et al. 2016b). Interestingly, an *in vitro* study suggested that roughness and surface free energy did not influence the bacterial adhesion on Ti and Zr disks. Moreover, the rough surfaces provided favorable properties in terms of cell adhesion of fibroblasts—but not of epithelial cells, especially on Zr than on Ti disks (Rigolin et al. 2017). A clinical study evaluated individuals with Ti or Zr implant-abutments. In both materials, the most prevalent species were Gram-negative bacteria belonging mainly to the phylum *Proteobacteira*, which includes the *Neisseriaceae* and *Campylobacteraceae* families, followed by the phyla *Firmicutes* and *Actinobacteria* and *Bacteroidetes*. Pathogenic and non-pathogenic species were detected colonizing oral sites in both materials. Titanium-related sites presented the highest total microbial count and higher counts of pathogenic species (Nascimento et al. 2016). Clinically, mean probing depths around Ti abutments were slightly deeper than around Zr abutments after 3 months (van Brakel et al. 2011).

Laser irradiation has been recently employed to alter the microtopography of the implant and abutment surfaces. Laser surfaces are more biocompatible with fibroblasts compared to Ti and Zr surfaces. Better adhesion of fibroblasts to laser-modified surfaces can result in more favorable soft tissue seal around dental implants (Esfahanizadeh et al. 2016).

An *in vitro* study reported that the adhesion and proliferation of oral streptococci is similar for surfaces of PEEK and conventional composite resin (Kolbeck et al. 2013). Although, another study that investigated microbial issues on PEEK and titanium implant-abutments identified similar microbial counts and levels of periodontal pathogens in the peri-abutment region of the biomaterials (Volpe et al. 2008). If comparing PEEK, Zr and Ti, the biofilm formation on PEEK's surface is equal or lower than the other materials (Hahnel et al. 2015).

3.5 *Final remarks*

Previously, most researches have concentrated on the optimization of osseointegration. More recently the focus has shifted in the development of biomaterials that enhance the formation of a peri-implant soft tissue barrier. In the oral cavity, implant-abutments protruding through the oral mucosa are exposed to a complex environment containing saliva and gingival exudate, as well as microorganisms. After placement, the abutment surface rapidly becomes colonized by oral bacteria which can compete with epithelial and connective tissue cells for binding to the surface (Dorkhan et al. 2014a). Understanding the influence of materials surfaces on cell and bacterial adhesion will help future development of new materials or surface treatments, in order to improve peri-implant soft-tissue seal and to reduce adhesion of pathogenic microorganisms on dental implant-abutments (Avila et al. 2014).

4 CONCLUSION

The authors were unable to identify which material presents the best biological behavior since different methodologies and inconsistent outcomes were found. Further studies should compare biological behavior on titanium, zirconia and PEEK abutments to establish the specific clinical application and the advantages and disadvantages of each biomaterial.

REFERENCES

[1] Alrabeah GO, Brett P, Knowles JC, Petridis H. The effect of metal ions released from different dental implant-abutment couples on osteoblast function and secretion of bone resorbing mediators. *Journal of Dentistry*. 2017;66(June):91–101.

[2] Bacchelli B, Giavaresi G, Franchi M, et al. Influence of a zirconia sandblasting treated surface on peri-implant bone healing: An experimental study in sheep. *Acta Biomaterialia*. 2009;5(6):2246–2257.

[3] Bächle M, Butz F, Hübner U, Bakalinis E, Kohal RJ. Behavior of CAL72 osteoblast-like cells cultured on zirconia ceramics with different surface topographies. *Clinical Oral Implants Research*. 2007;18(1):53–59.

[4] Banaszek K, Wiktorowska-Owczarek ANNA, Kowalczyk E, Klimek L. Possibilities of applying Ti (C, N) coatings on prosthetic elements: research with the use of human endothelial cells. *Acta of bioengineering and biomechanics*. 2016;18(1).

[5] Bressan E, Tessarolo F, Sbricoli L, Caola I, Nollo G, Di Fiore A. Effect of chlorhexidine in preventing plaque biofilm on healing abutment: a crossover controlled study. *Implant dentistry*. 2014; *23*(1), 64–68.

[6] Brunot-Gohin C, Duval JL, Verbeke S, Belanger K, Pezron I, Kugel G, Egles C. Biocompatibility study of lithium disilicate and zirconium oxide ceramics for esthetic dental abutments. *Journal of periodontal & implant science*. 2016; *46*(6), 362–371.

[7] De Avila ED, De Molon RS, Lima BP, Lux R, Shi W, Junior MJ, de Assis Mollo Junior F. Impact of physical chemical characteristics of abutment implant surfaces on bacteria adhesion. *Journal of Oral Implantology*. 2016a; *42*(2), 153–158.

[8] de Avila ED, Avila-Campos MJ, Vergani, CE, Spolidório DMP, de Assis Mollo Jr F. Structural and quantitative analysis of a mature anaerobic biofilm on different implant abutment surfaces. *Journal of Prosthetic Dentistry*. 2016b; *115*(4), 428–436.

[9] de Avila ED, de Molon RS, Palomari Spolidorio DM Implications of surface and bulk properties of abutment implants and their degradation in the health of periodontal tissue. *Materials*. 2013; *6*(12), 5951–5966.

[10] de Avila ED, Vergani CE, Junior FAM, Junior MJ, Shi W, Lux R. Effect of titanium and zirconia dental implant abutments on a cultivable polymicrobial saliva community. *Journal of Prosthetic Dentistry*. 2017; *118*(4), 481–487.

[11] de Freitas AR, Silva TSDO, Ribeiro RF, de Albuquerque Junior RF, Pedrazzi V, Do Nascimento C. Oral bacterial colonization on dental implants restored with titanium or zirconia abutments: 6-month follow-up. *Clinical Oral Investigations*. 2018:1–9.

[12] do Nascimento C, Pita MS, Pedrazzi V, de Albuquerque Junior RF, Ribeiro RF. In vivo evaluation of Candida spp. adhesion on titanium or zirconia abutment surfaces. *Archives of oral biology*. 2013;58(7):853–861.

[13] Dorkhan M, Hall J, Uvdal P, Sandell A, Svensäter G, Davies JR. Crystalline anatase-rich titanium can reduce adherence of oral streptococci. *Biofouling*. 2014a;30(6):751–759.

[14] Dorkhan M, Yücel-Lindberg T, Hall J, Svensäter G, Davies JR. Adherence of human oral keratinocytes and gingival fibroblasts to nano-structured titanium surfaces. *BMC oral health*. 2014b; (1), 75.

[15] Esfahanizadeh N, Motalebi S, Daneshparvar N, Akhoundi N, Bonakdar S. Morphology, proliferation, and gene expression of gingival fibroblasts on Laser-Lok, titanium, and zirconia surfaces. *Lasers in medical science*. 2016; *31*(5), 863–873.

[16] Fuhrmann G, Steiner M, Freitag-Wolf S, Kern M. Resin bonding to three types of polyaryletherketones (PAEKs)—Durability and influence of surface conditioning. *Dental Materials*. 2014;30(3):357–363.

[17] Flamant Q, Anglada M. Hydrofluoric acid treatment of dental zirconia. Part 2: effect on flexural strength and ageing behavior. *Journal of the European Ceramic Society*. 2016;36(1):135–145.

[18] Gómez-Florit M, Ramis JM, Xing R, et al. Differential response of human gingival fibroblasts to titanium- and titanium-zirconium-modified surfaces. *Journal of Periodontal Research*. 2014;49(4):425–436.

[19] Hahnel S, Wieser A, Lang R, Rosentritt M. Biofilm formation on the surface of modern implant abutment materials. *Clinical Oral Implants Research*. 2015;26(11):1297–1301.

[20] Harder S, Podschun R, Grancicova L, Mehl C, Kern M. Analysis of the intraimplant microflora of two-piece dental implants. *Clinical Oral Investigations*. 2013;17(4):1135–1142.

[21] Kern M, Lehmann F. Influence of surface conditioning on bonding to polyetheretherketon (PEEK). *Dental Materials*. 2012;28(12):1280–1283.

[22] Kheur M, Harianawala HH, Sethi T, Kheur S, Acharya A, Mattheos N. Human cytomegalovirus-1 and Epstein-Barr virus-1 viral colonization of titanium and zirconia abutments: a split-mouth study. *Journal of investigative and clinical dentistry*. 2016;7(4):396–400.

[23] Kim Y-S, Ko Y, Kye S-B, Yang S-M. Human Gingival Fibroblast (HGF-1) Attachment and Proliferation on Several Abutment Materials with Various Colors. *The International Journal of Oral & Maxillofacial Implants*. 2014;29(4):969–975.

[24] Kolbeck C, Sereno M, Rosentritt M, Handel G. Biofilm formation on polyetheretherke—tone surfaces and cleaning options. *IADR Seattle, No 2353*. March 2013.

[25] Köunönen M, Hormia M, Kivilahti J, Hautaniemi J, Thesleff I. Effect of surface processing on the attachment, orientation, and proliferation of human gingival fibroblasts on titanium: Attachment of Fibroblasts on Titanium. *Journal of Biomedical Materials Research*. 1992;26(10):1325–1341.

[26] Lazzara RJ, Porter SS. Platform switching: a new concept in implant dentistry for controlling postrestorative crestal bone levels. *The International journal of periodontics & restorative dentistry*. 2006;26(1):9–17.

[27] Lee D-W, Kim J-G, Kim M-K, et al. Effect of laser-dimpled titanium surfaces on attachment of epithelial-like cells and fibroblasts. *The Journal of Advanced Prosthodontics*. 2015;7(2):138.

[28] Linkevicius T, Vaitelis J. The effect of zirconia or titanium as abutment material on soft peri-implant tissues: A systematic review and meta-analysis. *Clinical Oral Implants Research*. 2015;26:139–147.

[29] Moon Y-H, Yoon M-K, Moon J-S, et al. Focal adhesion linker proteins expression of fibroblast related to adhesion in response to different transmucosal abutment surfaces. *The journal of advanced prosthodontics*. 2013;5(3):341–350.

[30] Moura CG, Pereira R, Buciumeanu M, et al. Effect of laser surface texturing on primary stability and surface properties of zirconia implants. *Ceramics International*. 2017;(July).

[31] Nascimento C do, Pita MS, Santos E de S, et al. Microbiome of titanium and zirconia dental implants abutments. *Dental materials/official publication of the Academy of Dental Materials*. 2016;32(1):93–101.

[32] Nothdurft FP, Fontana D, Ruppenthal S, et al. Differential Behavior of Fibroblasts and Epithelial Cells on Structured Implant Abutment Materials: A Comparison of Materials and Surface Topographies. *Clinical implant dentistry and related research*. 2015;17(6):1237–1249.

[33] Okabe E, Ishihara Y, Kikuchi T, et al. Adhesion Properties of Human Oral Epithelial-Derived Cells to Zirconia. *Clinical implant dentistry and related research*. 2016;18(5):906–916.

[34] Pardun K, Treccani L, Volkmann E, et al. Magnesium-containing mixed coatings on zirconia for dental implants: mechanical characterization

and in vitro behavior. *Journal of Biomaterials Applications*. 2015;30(1):104–118.

[35] Piconi C, Maccauro G. Zirconia as a Biomaterial. *Biomaterials*. 1999:95–1081–25.

[36] Quirynen M, De Soete M, van Steenberghe D. Infectious risks for oral implants: a review of the literature. *Clinical Oral Implants Research*. 2002;13(1):1–19.

[37] Rigolin MSM, de Avila ED, Basso FG, Hebling J, Carlos CA, Mollo Junior F de A. Effect of different implant abutment surfaces on OBA-09 epithelial cell adhesion. *Microscopy Research and Technique*. 2017;80(12):1304–1309.

[38] Rutkunas V, Bukelskiene V, Sabaliauskas V, Balciunas E, Malinauskas M, Baltriukiene D. Assessment of human gingival fibroblast interaction with dental implant abutment materials. *Journal of materials science Materials in medicine*. 2015;26(4):169–169.

[39] Souza JCM, Ponthiaux P, Henriques M, et al. Corrosion behaviour of titanium in the presence of Streptococcus mutans. *Journal of Dentistry*. 2013;41(6):528–534.

[40] Schwarz F, Mihatovic I, Becker J, Bormann KH, Keeve PL, Friedmann A. Histological evaluation of different abutments in the posterior maxilla and mandible: an experimental study in humans. *Journal of clinical periodontology*. 2013; 40(8), 807–815.

[41] Tetè S, Zizzari V. Collagen Fiber Orientation Around Machined Titanium and Zirconia Dental Implant Necks: An Animal Study. 2008:7.

[42] van Brakel R, Cune MS, van Winkelhoff AJ, de Putter C, Verhoeven JW, van der Reijden W. Early bacterial colonization and soft tissue health around zirconia and titanium abutments: an in vivo study in man: Bacterial colonization and soft tissue health around zirconia and titanium. *Clinical Oral Implants Research*. 2011;22(6):571–577.

[43] Volpe S, Verrocchi D, Andersson P. Comparison of early bacterial colonization of PEEK and titanium healing abutments using real-time PCR. *Applied Osseointegration Research*. 2008;6:54–56.

[44] Xing R, Lyngstadaas SP, Ellingsen JE, Taxt-Lamolle S, Haugen HJ. The influence of surface nanoroughness, texture and chemistry of TiZr implant abutment on oral biofilm accumulation. *Clinical oral implants research*. 2015;26(6):649–656.

[45] Xing R, Salou L, Taxt-Lamolle S, Reseland JE, Lyngstadaas SP, Haugen HJ. Surface hydride on titanium by cathodic polarization promotes human gingival fibroblast growth. *Journal of Biomedical Materials Research—Part A*. 2014;102(5):1389–1398.

Biodental Engineering V – Belinha et al. (Eds)
© 2019 Taylor & Francis Group, London, ISBN 978-0-367-21087-8

Dental implants fatigue life: A probabilistic fatigue study

M. Prados-Privado
Carlos III University, Madrid, Spain
ASISA Dental, Madrid, Spain

S.A. Gehrke
BioTecnos, Montevideo, Uruguay

R. Rojo & J.C. Prados-Frutos
Rey Juan Carlos University, Madrid, Spain

ABSTRACT: The aim of this study was to analyze the mechanical behavior of five titanium dental implants with a hexagonal external connection. Two *in vitro* studies were performed: a compression test and a dynamic loading test. Then a probabilistic approach based on Markov chains and cumulative damage model was computed. Load and Young's modulus was chosen as random variables. Results obtained by this mathematical model provided the principal statistics of the fatigue life of dental implants and the cumulative probability function. Results obtained by the mechanical test and the theoretical model are in accordance. Therefore, this study provides a novel approach to study and design fatigue life in dental implants.

1 INTRODUCTION

Dental implants have become a common practice in different clinical situations in the last few years (Tian et al. 2012). This technique to replace loss teeth has more than a 90% success rate (Gherke et al. 2014) but, occasionally, prosthetic implants fail because of mechanical or biological causes (Manda et al. 2009). Therefore, a good long-term evaluation of dental implants is essential for acquiring as much information as possible about causes of implant success and failure.

Even though dental implants must support a lot of cyclic loads during their life, most of *in vitro* studies available in the literature are made with quasi-static loads (Ayllón et al. 2014, Coray et al. 2016). Implants designs which are available in the market must comply with the quality requirements defined by ISO 14801. This standard detail how the fatigue test of dental implants must be conducted to get the certification (ISO 2007).

Compression tests are the most common mechanical analysis in dentistry literature. The goal of these kind of studies is to determine the maximum load that the implant can withstand. However, these mechanical tests do not simulate the masticatory function so that other tests should be applied to simulate more real situations (Coray et al. 2016). Fatigue testing exposes implant components to cyclic loading. Dental literature does not present controlled and standardized environment

for cyclic loading conditions. Also, due to the randomness of the fatigue phenomenon, a probabilistic study should be included to fully characterize the mechanical behavior of implants.

This study presents an alternative to the traditional fatigue life approach. This paper employs a probabilistic fatigue *in silico* model on dental implants and their components, considering as random variables the material data and the loading configurations from an *in vitro* study. The main novelty of this paper is that, unlike most of the previous finite element analysis, this study was done with a probabilistic point of view, based on Probabilistic Finite Element Method and a cumulative damage model, which is based on Markov chains (Prados-Privado et al. 2016).

2 MATERIAL AND METHODS

2.1 Dental implants analyzed

Ten OXTEIN N6 implants (Rimini, Italy) are analyzed in this study (Fig. 1). These implants are made of Ti6Al4V with a 3.5 mm diameter, 10 mm length and external connection. These ten implants were randomly divided into two groups (n = 5): one group was exposed to a compressive mechanical test and the other group was exposed to a cycling loading test.

According to the manufacturer's recommendation, the abutment was connected to the implant with

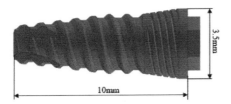

Figure 1. OXTEIN N6 dental implant.

a torque of 30 Ncm. The components were retightened 10 minutes later the initial torque (Hoyer et al. 2001). All implants were immersed in a rigid epoxy resin model GIV (Polipox, São Paulo, Brazil) with a Young's modulus similar to cortical bone, using cylindrical acrylic tubes with a 20mm in diameter. The sets (implant/abutment) were immersed, leaving 3 mm of the exposed implant to reproduce bone loss, according to the international guidelines (ISO 2007).

2.2 Compressive test

With this mechanical test it is possible to determine the maximum load that implants can support. This fracture test was done according to ISO guidelines: an angle of $30 \pm 2°$ with respect to the applied load, with 3 mm of the exposed implant, reproducing bone loss. All tests were carried out at the Testing Laboratory of Biomechanics (Biotecnos, Montevideo, Uruguay) at a test speed of 1mm/min.

2.3 Dynamic loading test

Samples were placed on a chewing simulator (BioPDI, São Carlos, Brazil). All of them were subjected to 360.000 cycles of 150 ± 10 N of controlled axial force were applied at 4 Hz (Gehrke et al. 2015, Gehrke et al. 2016).

2.4 Probabilistic fatigue model

Due to the probabilistic nature of the fatigue in dental implants, the use of probabilistic methods is justified. However, most of the studies that analyzed fracture and fatigue in dental implants are made from a deterministic point of view (Prados-Privado et al. 2016).

In this study, the randomness of the titanium Young's modulus and loads were considered, due to its influence on the life of the structural components (Madsen et al. 1986).

In this study, we will focus on the first stage (nucleation stage). To study crack nucleation process are based on the local strain approach. Authors have chosen the B-K unit step model due to its adaptation to the nucleation stage. Authors refer to Prados-Privado et al. (2016) for further details.

3 RESULTS

3.1 Compressive test results

All implants fractured in the first implant thread, at the level of the embedding resin, as shown in Figure 2.

The failure load was $F = 999,56 \pm 29,75$ N.

3.2 Dynamic loading test results

After applying 360,000 cycles with a 150 N, no deformations nor cracks were observed in any samples (Fig. 3).

3.3 Probabilistic fatigue results

The load and the elasticity modulus of titanium were chosen as random variables. A load of 150 ± 10 N and a Young's modulus of 100 ± 10 GPa were employed.

After solving the mathematical model, a mean life of 552,626 cycles and a variance of the fatigue life of 25,26 cycles^2 was obtained.

In view of these results obtained by this probabilistic approach, it is possible to conclude that OXTEIN N6 implant can support 360,000 cycles without any failure as detailed previously and, also, can support a higher life than that obtained by the numerical fatigue analysis.

A Probability Transition Matrix (PTM) was constructed with the following data: a matrix dimension of 13, a probability of remaining in the same damage cycle, p, of 0.97 and a probability of jumping to the next damage cycle, q, of 0.03.

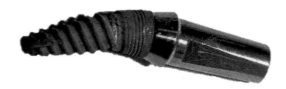

Figure 2. Dental implant after compressive test.

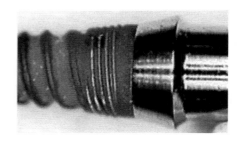

Figure 3. Dental implant after dynamic loading test.

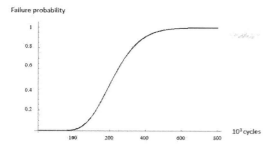

Figure 4. Cumulative probability function.

Finally, this probabilistic methodology allowed us to determine the probability of local failure of the implant for a specific number of load cycles. The cumulative probability function has been represented in Figure 4.

4 DISCUSSION

This study has analyzed the mechanical behavior of 10 titanium dental implants (ø3.5 mm) with a hexagonal external connection.

Implants were first exposed to a compressive load test until failure with the aim of obtaining the maximum load. Then, dental implants were exposed to 360,000 cycles and cracks were evaluated. Finally, the mathematical model was computed. Results obtained by this model are in accordance with those obtained by the dynamic loading test.

However, this study has some limitations, like that we cannot verify our results with an *in vivo* study. Therefore, we cannot keep in mind other biological factors such as bacterium, corrosion or osseointegration (Sridhar et al. 2015).

To the authors' best knowledge, there are no studies published in the literature with a complete mechanical characterization and a probabilistic approach. It is possible to include the effect of the variability of different parameters in this new mathematical model.

Despite the high success rate of these treatments, an expert knowledge of the biomechanical behavior of the implants is crucial to avoid mechanical failures during the design process (Gupta et al. 2015). Mechanical compression tests are common in dental studies. Marchetti *et al.* analyzed five internal connection implants of 3,8 mm in diameter and 12 mm in length with a maximum load after break of 430 ± 35.66 N (Marchetti et al. 2016). There were significant differences in the maximum fracture load between the different commercial implants. Those values varied from 600 N in an internal hexagon connection to 1200 N in an external connection. These mechanical studies have the aim of knowing the maximum fracture load of different dental implants (Alsahhaf et al. 2017, Patankar et al. 2016). The implant analyzed in this study, OXTEIN N6, obtained a maximum load fracture of 999 ± 29,75 N. The mean fracture loads in this study exceeded the physiologic maximum posterior masticatory force of approximately 900 N (Takata et al. 2018).

This research provides a new method that engineers can employed during the design stage, and clinicians could also employ it if they would like to know long-term behavior of different implants, especially in those cases with a compromise bone or parafunctions habits.

Future works should evaluate the effect of different bone densities and the geometry of the implants.

5 CONCLUSIONS

This study presents a mechanical characterization of an external dental implant and, as a novelty, obtained the probability of failure under certain conditions employing a probabilistic approach.

REFERENCES

Alsahhaf, A., Spies, B.C., Vach, K., Kohal, R.-J. 2017. Fracture resistance of zirconia-based implant abutments after artificial long-term aging. *Journal of the Mechanical Behavior Biomedical Materials* 66: 224–232.

Ayllón, J.M., Navarro, C., Vázquez, J., Domínguez, J. 2014. Fatigue life estimation in dental implants. *Engineering Fracture Mechanics* 123: 34–43.

Coray, R., Zeltner, M., Özcan, M. 2016. Fracture strength of implant abutments after fatigue testing: A systematic re-view and a meta-analysis. *Journal of the Mechanical Behavior of Biomedical Materials* 62: 333–346.

Gehrke, S.A., Souza dos Santos Vianna, M., Dedavid, B.A. 2014. Influence of bone insertion level of the implant on the fracture strength of different connection designs: an in vitro study. *Clinical Oral Investigations* 18(3): 715–720.

Gehrke, S.A., De Carvalho Serra, R. 2015. Load fatigue performance of conical implant-abutment connection: effect of torque level and interface junction. *Minerva Stomatologica* 64(1): 1–7.

Gehrke, S.A., Poncio da Silva, P.M., Calvo Guirado, J.L. et al. 2016. Mechanical behavior of zirconia and titanium abutments before and after cyclic load application. *Journal of Prosthetic Dentistry* 116(4): 529–535.

Gupta, S., Gupta, H., Tandan, A. 2015. Technical complications of implant-causes and management: A comprehensive review. *National Journal of Maxillofacial Surgery* 6(1): 3–8.

Hoyer, S.A., Stanford, C.M., Buranadham, S. et al 2001. Dynamic fatigue properties of the dental implant–

abutment interface: Joint opening in wide-diameter versus standard-diameter hex-type implants. *Journal of Prosthetic Dentistry* 85(6): 599–607.

ISO 14801 2007. *Dentistry. Implants. Dynamic fatigue test for endosseous dental implants.* Geneva: International Organization for Standardization.

Manda M.G., Psyllaki, P.P., Tsipas, D.N., Koidis, P.T 2009. Observations on an in-vivo failure of a titanium dental implant/abutment screw system: A case report. *Journal of Biomedical Materials Research Part B: Applied Bio-materials* 89B(1): 264–273.

Madsen, H.O., Krenk, S., Lind, N.C. 1986. *Methods of Structural Safety.* Englewood Cliffs: Prentice-Hall.

Marchetti, E., Ratta, S., Mummolo, S. et al 2016. Mechanical Reliability Evaluation of an Oral Implant-Abutment System According to UNI EN ISO 14801 Fatigue Test Protocol. *Implant Dentistry* 25(5): 613–618.

Patankar, A., Kheur, M., Kheur, S., et al 2016. Fracture Resistance of Implant Abutments Following Abutment Alterations by Milling the Margins: An In Vitro Study. *Journal of Oral Implantology* 42(6): 464–468.

Prados-Privado, M., Prados-Frutos, J.C., Calvo-Guirado, J.L., Bea, J.A 2016. A random fatigue of mechanize titanium abutment studied with Markoff chain and stochastic finite element formulation. *Computer Methods in Biomechanics and Biomedical Engineering* 19(15): 1583–1591.

Sridhar, S., Wilson, T.G. Jr, Palmer, K.L. et al 2015. In Vitro Investigation of the Effect of Oral Bacteria in the Surface Oxidation of Dental Implants. *Clinical Implant Dentistry and Related Research* 17(Suppl 2): e562–e575.

Takata, H., Komine, F., Honda, J., Blatz, M., Matsumura, H. 2018. An in vitro evaluation of fracture load of implant-supported zirconia-based prostheses fabricated with different veneer materials. *Clinical Oral Implants Research*. 2018 Feb 27.

Tian, K., Chen. J., Yang. J., Huang, W., Wu, D 2012. Angled abutments result in increased or decreased stress on surrounding bone of single-unit dental implants: A finite element analysis. *Medical Engineering & Physics* 34(10): 1526–1531.

Biodental Engineering V – Belinha et al. (Eds)
© 2019 Taylor & Francis Group, London, ISBN 978-0-367-21087-8

Micromorphology, microstructure and micro-Raman spectroscopy of a case of amelogenesis imperfecta

Sebastiana Arroyo Bote
Department Odontostomatology, HUBc, U. Barcelona, Barcelona, Spain

Alfonso Villa-Vigil
Universidad de Oviedo, Oviedo, Spain

M.C. Manzanares Céspedes
Human Anatomy and Embryology Unit, HUBc, U. Barcelona, Barcelona, Spain

Esteban Brau-Aguadé
HUBc-Bellvitge, Universidad de Barcelona, Barcelona, Spain

ABSTRACT: Amelogenesis Imperfecta (AI) affects the quantity and quality of enamel, and it has diverse phenotypes (hypoplastic, hypomadure and hypocalcificated enamel). Our objective was to study the micromorphology, microstructure and micro-Raman spectroscopy of enamel samples with AI of hypoplastic phenotype. Two members of a family were studied. One patient had hypoplastic phenotype of AI and the other did not. Six teeth from the patient with AI and two teeth from the unaffected member were processed. In the samples with AI, the ESEM showed deep fissures and superficial alterations in enamel surface, a decrease on the width of the enamel and a irregular disposition of the heterogeneously calcified enamel prisms. RAMAN spectrometrometry indicated that the spectrometry of the hidroxyapatite crystals in the AI enamel was different from the control sample. This leads us to consider that the classifications based only on clinical aspects are insufficient for a correct understanding of the pathology.

1 INTRODUCTION

Amelogenesis Imperfecta (AI) is characterized by presenting enamel defects, without defects in others tissues (Witkop, 1988). Hereditary defects in the enamel development or environmental exposure to chemicals and drugs can damage the ameloblasts (Ferreira et al., 2005). AI is characterized by its heterogeneous phenotypical clinical patterns of variable severity, as well as for its complex genetype (Wright, 2006; Gibson, 2008; Wang et al., 2013) and/or environmental aetiology (Hedge, 2012; Malik et al., 2012). Based on its heredity and clinical evidences, four types and numerous subtypes of AI were described in 1988 by Witkop (hypoplastic, hypomaturation, hypocalcified AI and a combination of them), and today this is the most widely used classification in the clinical practice. The development of enamel starts with the secretion of the enamel protein matrix by the ameloblasts, followed by its calcification and maturation (Sapp et al., 2005; Malik et al., 2012). Less than 1% of the mature enamel is constituted by organic components, while the mineral components constitute more than a 95%. The enamel

mineral crystals are deposited in compact hexagonal rod-shaped structure, making this tissue the hardest in the human body (Nanci, 2012). Numerous genes have been reported as responsible of the regulation of this complex process (Sapp et al., 2005; Bailleul-Forestier et al., 2008; Lee et al., 2008; Misiadis & Luder, 2011; Luder et al., 2013; Simmer et al., 2013; Wang et al., 2014; Zhang et al., 2015; Prasad et al., 2016). Mutations of AMELX (amelogenin), ENAM (enamelin) (Misiadis & Luder, 2011), COL17A1 (Prasad et al., 2016) and FAM20A (Wang et al., 2014) have been proven as causes of hypoplastic AI, either with smooth or rough enamel; while the AI with hypomature phenotype has been attributed to genetic defects in AMELX, MMP20, KLK4 and WDR72. Hypocalcified AI have been reported to be caused by FAM83H or C4orf26 (Kim et al., 2008; Parry et al., 2012; Luder et al., 2013) in humans. Additionally, some studies indicate that a mutation in one gene could be related to more than one type of AI; thus CNNM4 mutation is related to hypoplastic/hypomineralized types (Lee et al., 2008), DLX3 mutation is related with and hypomature/hypoplastic types (Wang et al., 2014) and C4orf26 hypomineralized-hypoplastic types (Prasad et al., 2016).

Thus, an alteration in the amelogenesis process could induce to one or a combination of the three types of AI: (1) an abnormal appositional of the enamel matrix, insufficient growth and less elongation of the crystals (Coxon et al., 2012), thus causing an hypoplastic enamel, (2) a failure in the hardening of the enamel, because of the non-removal of its organic matrix, causing an hypomature enamel; (3) or an extreme deficiency in mineralization, that causes the hypocalcified AI (Mitsiadis & Luder, 2011). The enamel in the hypoplasic AI is clinically described as thin, with normal hardness, while the hypomature enamel is described as soft and with colour alterations, but with an unaltered thickness, and hypocalcified enamel is described as soft with post-eruptive abrasions (Hu et al., 2007; Mitsiadis & Luder, 2011; Gadhia et al., 2012; Gasse et al., 2013).

The present case is compatible with hypoplastic AI phenotype. However, due to the enamel formation complexity and its different stages until its final mineralization, a failure in one of this steps, could affect the following stages of tissue formation, even though it might not be clinically evident. The goal of this study was to analyse the enamel of a patient with hypoplastic AI phenotype using techniques that allow us to measure the thickness, the degree of mineralization and mineral ultrastructure of the enamel, to find or rule out abnormal tissue mineralization.

2 CASE REPORT

2.1 Materials and methods

The investigation was carried out in complete accordance with all the appropriate legal regulations and with Helsinki Declaration. The characteristics and objective of the study were explained to the patients, before they signed the informed consent.

2.2 Patients and diagnosis

Two different members of a Spanish family (Fig. 1-A) were studied. One of them, a 45 years-old man was clinically diagnosed with hypoplastic AI. The clinical and radiographic situation are exposed in Figure 1-B and 1-C, respectively. His nephew (20 years old), unaffected with AI, was studied as control. Both patients were specifically asked about factors affecting their dental structure during development, such as systemic illnesses and tetracycline or fluoride consumption. The patients were also asked about dental pain related to chemical or thermal stimuli. The recorded clinical data included alterations of the colour and form of the teeth;

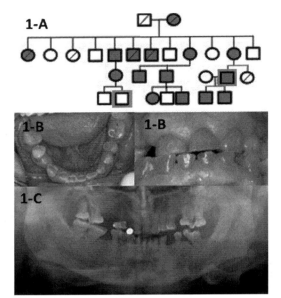

Figure 1. 1-A: Pedigree of the AI kindred, including affected (red) and unaffected (white) family members. The AI patient is marked in blue; the unaffected sibling is signaled in green. 1-B: Clinical phenotype of the patient. The enamel shows an homogeneous aspect, with a smooth, brilliant surface with evident discoloration, and with enamel fractures. All teeth evidence a premature degree of abrasion, visible both in the occlusal and the vestibular view. 1-C: The enamel radiopacity appears normal in the panoramic radiograph, while its thickness is diminished. No morphological alterations (taurodontism, globular crowns, and cervical constriction) are visible.

hardness, excessive wear or absence of enamel, and especially distortions of the enamel surface. Both members of the family, were evaluated clinically. Skin, hair, fingernails and osseous defects related with syndromes or systemic conditions associated with dental diseases were also analysed.

For dental reasons, and for the rehabilitation of the oral function of the patient with AI (Fig. 1-A blue), 6 teeth (two incisors, one premolar and three molars) were extracted and the morphology and ultrastructure of the enamel were studied. Additionally, two permanent teeth (18 and 28) were extracted from the healthy family member (Fig. 1-A, green), for orthodontical reasons, and were used as control.

All the samples were first observed with an Environmental Scanning Electron Microscope (ESEM, Quanta 200, FEI Co, The Netherlands), in order to analyse the enamel surface alterations of the samples without further laboratory process. Teeth were analysed individually under ×150 and ×500 magnification at high vacuum conditions.

Afterwards, all the samples were included in methyl metacrilate polymers as described by Manzanares et al. (2001) and were observed by means of Secondary and Backscattered Electron Microscopy (×25) and energy dispersive X-ray analysis (EDX) (LEO-Leica 20, Cambridge, UK). This permitted to assess the aspect, the thickness and the calcification level of the tissues. Additionally, the samples were analysed through RAMAN spectroscopy (LABRAM HR800) to analyse the structure of the hydroxyapatite crystals.

3 RESULTS

3.1 *For samples with AI*

The ESEM showed that the enamel surface presented various lesions, such as deep linear fissures (Fig. 2: A-1) and irregularly shaped superficial lesions (Fig. 2: A-2). Also, crater shaped defects were found in the enamel surface (Fig. 2: A-3).

Despite the fact that in the clinical exploration the enamel of the incisors appeared homogeneous, two types of enamel anomalies were evidenced by ESEM: lineal fissures and isolated areas with defects (Fig. 2: A-1). Fissures were visible in the vestibular surfaces as deep linear creases, some of

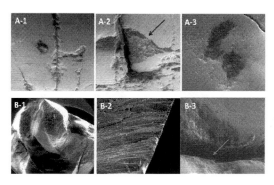

Figure 2. ESEM analysis. **A**. Vestibular surface of incisor teeth with enamel defects: vertical creases and irregularly shaped superficial lesions. **A-1**: ×150 Ramified vertical creases with chirped borders, continuous with surface enamel lesions. **A-2**: Higher magnification of the deep vestibular fissure in A with disruption of the enamel outer layer, evidencing the honeycomb-shaped structure of the enamel prisms. **A-3**: isolated vertical crease, apparently unrelated to the enamel surface geographical defects. **B**. Occlusal view of a molar tooth **B-1**: ×150 magnification with cuspal enamel defects: both deep, vertical creases and surface defects. **B-2**: ×500 the enamel parallel prismatic structure is visible. **B-3**: ×500: deep linear enamel fissure with absence of the enamel outer layer in one of the geographic superficial lesions.

them were unique, and some of them were ramified. Moreover, the more wide fissures presented on the edge an irregular appearance (Fig. 2: A-2), where the loss of the superficial layer of the enamel showed a regularly honeycomb-like shape (Fig. 2: A-2, black arrow). The regular aspect of these defects, were different from the defects of the isolated areas (Fig. 2: A-3, red asterisk), that present an irregular, rough, discoloured surface, where the enamel prismatic structure was not visible.

In the surface of the molars (Fig. 2: B), the ESEM showed altered cusps with deep fissures and fractures, with a severe loss of substance that can be attributed to abrasion. However, in non-occlusive surfaces, defects were also visible (Fig. 2: B-1). When observed perpendicularly to the enamel fractured cusps, parallel and regular disposition of enamel prisms were observed (Fig. 2: B-2). Some fissures appear as deep narrow spaces, breaking the continuity of the enamel surface (Fig. 2: B-3, blue arrow) with only a limited loss of the enamel outer layer. In this type of fissures it was not possible to observe the honeycomb appearance of the enamel prisms described in the incisor fissures (Fig. 2: A-2), however, in the deep aspect of the defects, structures similar to enamel rods were visible. In molars there were isolated areas with defects similar to the ones on the incisors (Fig. 2: B-3, red asterisk). In these lesions, the external layer of the enamel appears to be absent, showing a rough irregular surface defect similar to the ones visible in the incisors.

The BS-SEM analysis showed a reduced thickness of the enamel layer in the molar with pathology, to the point that totally disappear and expose the dentin, in some areas (Fig. 3: A, white arrow). Images obtained from the molar enamel of one unaffected tooth (Fig. 3: B), showed clearly the difference in the thickness of enamel layer between the two molars.

Regarding the ultrastructure of the enamel prisms in occlusal surface of the molar samples, the control sample showed both a regular disposition of the enamel prisms and a regular level of calcification of the enamel layer (Fig. 3: C, black arrow). On the contrary, the enamel layer from the AI teeth showed both an irregular disposition, size and shape of the prisms and a heterogeneous level of calcification (Fig. 3: D, black arrow), evidenced in the different whiteness of the material at the BS-SEM, despite of the presence of the same elements in the EDX analysis in both sample series. However, such alterations were not observed in the dentin-enamel junction of the dental organs studied.

The RAMAN spectrometry was carried out in selected areas of both affected and unaffected teeth. In the affected teeth, measurements were obtained in the apparently healthy enamel surface,

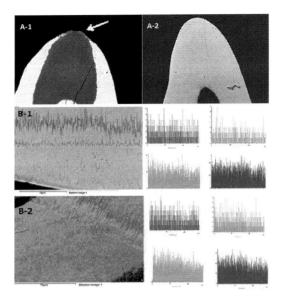

Figure 3. **A-B.** Backscattered images of sections perpendicular to the main axis of the cusp. **3-A.** ×25 corresponding to affected teeth. **3-B** ×25 control teeth. The enamel in the affected tooth is thinner than the one on the control. The arrow in figure 3-A signals the deepest point of the surface enamel defect. **C-D:** Backscattered electron image and EDX analysis of a control sample (3C) and AI tooth sample (3D). The elements analyzed (carbon in red, oxygen Green, calcium blue and phosphorus, purple) are present in both samples. 3C: regular prisms, showing a homogeneous level of calcification. 3D. Irregulars prisms, less orderly disposed and showing different shades of gray, indication an irregular level of calcification.

as well as in the areas of defective enamel (fissures and isolated areas with defects).

In Figure 4: A, it can be observe the spectra obtained in the control sample, the spectrum corresponding to the dentin (Fig. 4: A1, green) and to the enamel (Fig. 4: A2, blue).

In the AI samples, the values obtained for the spectrum in mode "stretching" (vs (PO) of the PO4- at 961 cm) revealed that values obtained in the affected teeth, were identical in position, shape and thickness to those from the control enamel and dentin. This seems to suggest that part of the crystalline structure of the samples is very similar to the one in the controls (Fig. 4:B). However, the spectra of the analysed AI samples revealed a difference in the deformity (δ (OPO) of the PO4−) (Fig. 4: B circle) between 400 and 470 cm^{-1} (which is characteristic of the enamel hydroxyapatite). An evident alteration was visible in the relative intensities of the bands at 430 and 447 cm^{-1} (Fig. 4: B red arrow) respect to the control values (Fig. 4: B blue arrow). These measurements seem to indicate that the hydroxyapatite crystals that are characteristic of the enamel areas of the AI teeth are oriented in a different manner that the ones in the control samples. This was confirmed with the observations

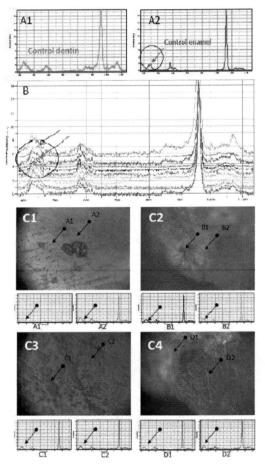

Figure 4. **A:** Spectra from control dentin (A-1) and enamel (A-2). Blue arrow: δ (OPO) of the PO4− between 400 and 470 cm^{-1}, characteristic of the enamel normal hydroxyapatite. **B:** RAMAN spectra of all the observed samples. Values from 900 to 1000 cm^{-1} correspond with the mode "stretching" ν s (PO); between 630 and 570 cm^{-1} and 470 and 400 cm^{-1} correspond to the deformity δ (OPO) of the chemical group PO−. The blue arrow points to the values in the control enamel, and red arrow points to the values of AI enamel **C:** 1-4 selected areas in the samples of AI tooth. Spectra A1, B1, C1 and D1 were obtained in areas with evident morphological lesions (arrows) Spectra A2, B2, C2 and D2 were obtained in apparently unaffected areas (arrows) in the same samples. All spectra are similar, despite the fact of having been obtained in an apparently unaffected or a lesion area.

carried out with Backscattered Electron image and EDX analysis (Figure 3).

Raman spectra was recorded for samples with AI enamel from different anatomical areas. Some of these areas had apparently healthy enamel and other areas had visible structural abnormalities. When comparing the spectra obtained in the surface of the AI enamel (Fig. 4: C) with the ones obtained in the pits or the grooves of the enamel, it was evident that they had similar values and shapes. No differences were observed between the values measured in the clinically described as "enamel lesions" (Fig. 4: C1-4, A1, B1, C1 and D1) respect to the apparently intact enamel in the affected teeth (Fig. 4: C1-4, A2, B2, C2 and D2).

4 DISCUSSION

The alterations taking place during the enamel development that lead to Amelogenesis Imperfecta (AI) are not yet fully known (Zhang et al., 2013). The difficulty on establishing a classification of the AI forms is related to the fact that numerous different phenotypes can be found in clinical practice, and many of them can be due to the same genetic disorder (Gadhia et al., 2012). Also, a great number of genes have been related to the AI (Sapp et al., 2005; Bailleul-Forestier et al., 2008; Lee et al., 2008; Misiadis & Luder, 2011; Wright et al., 2011; Parry et al., 2012; Luder et al., 2013; Simmer et al., 2013; Wang et al., 2014; Zhang et al., 2015; Prasad et al., 2016). Those genetic alterations, however, do not explain neither all the molecular disorders found in the different types of AI nor its varied phenotypes. Thus, it could be more genes responsible for the AI phenotypes that have not yet been identified (Hu et al., 2007). Our report presents a subject with an autosomal dominant inheritance pattern, and a phenotype compatible with the hypoplastic pattern as described by Gadhia et al. (2012), but with an obvious alteration on the orientation and mineralization of the enamel hydroxyapatite crystals, observed by ESEM, BS-SEM, EDX and Raman spectroscopy.

In healthy enamel, hydroxyapatite crystals are distributed in an orderly manner, except at the end zone, both at the palatine and the buccal aspect, and in the fissures, where the crystals appear disordered (Simmons et al., 2011). It has been described in hypomaturated AI the dysplasic enamel has an altered dentino-enamel junction (DEJ) due to the altered orientation of the hydroxyapatite crystals (Hu et al., 2011). No DEJ alterations were found in our AI patient, but the observed altered orientation of the enamel prisms could suggest an alteration characteristic of the hypomaturated AI.

In a first step of enamel formation, the ameloblasts secrete the organic matrix in which hydroxyapatite crystals are loosely deposited (Mitsiadis & Luder, 2011). Alteration in this stage cause a hypoplastic enamel. Subsequently, most of the organic matrix is degraded, while the crystals grow in thickness until they have and ordered organization, thus alteration in this phases causes hypomature and hypomineralized enamel. Our RAMAN results showed that indeed in both the altered and the unaffected areas of the AI enamel, the hydroxyapatite crystals present a different orientation when compared with both the dentin and the enamel of a non-AI patient. These alterations are evident both in the fractured and in the depressed enamel lesions, as well as in the apparently healthy enamel surface. Also, Our BS-SEM results show that the enamel prisms of the affected teeth had an irregular size and shape, as well as a different degree of mineralization when compared with control samples. These characteristics are similar to the hypomature type of AI described by Mitsiadis & Lunder (2011). An altered distribution of the enamel prisms has also been described in hypomineralized AI (Sanchez-Quevedo et al., 2006). Moreover, it has been suggest that mutations of AMELX, a gene related to hypomature type of AI, could be present in patients whose phenotype includes fractured dental crowns (Lee et al., 2011), such as the ones visible in our patient.

The quantitative deficiency of enamel, the vertical furrows and the pits present in our AI samples are compatible with the hypoplastic phenotype. The absence of taurodontism and other size or shape tooth alterations, the finding of ultrastructural evidences of hypocalcification, and hypomaturation in all AI samples from a unique patient, with clinical characteristics of a hypoplastic AI phenotype leads us to consider that the classifications based only and the presence of a clinical aspect of hypoplastic enamel lead us to suggest that our patient's phenotype could represent a different pattern to those nowadays described.

ACKNOWLEDGEMENTS

Authors deny any conflict of interest.

REFERENCES

Bailleul-Forestier I., Molla M., Verloes A. and Berdal A. 2008. The genetic basis of inherited anomalies of the teeth. Part 1: clinical and molecular aspects of non-syndromic dental disorders. *Eur J Med Genet* 51, 273–291.
Coxon T., Brook A., Barron M. and Smith R. 2012. Phenotype-Genotype Correlations in Mouse Models

of Amelogenesis Imperfecta Caused by Amelx and Enam Mutations. *Cells Tissues Organs* 196, 420–430.

Ferreira L., Paiva E., Ríos H., Boj J., Espasa E. and Planells P. 2005. Hipomineralización incisivo molar: su importancia en Odontopediatría. *Odon Pediatr* 13, 54–59.

Gadhia K., McDonald S., Arkutu N. and Malik K. 2012. Amelogenesis imperfecta: an introduction. *Br Dent J* 212, 377–379.

Gasse B., Karayigit E., Mathieu E., Jung S., Garret A., Huckert M., Morkmued S., Schneider C., Vidal L., Hemmerlé J., Sire J. and Bloch-Zupan A. 2013. Homozygous and Compound Heterozygous MMP20 Mutations in Amelogenesis Imperfecta. *J Dent Res* 92, 598–603.

Gibson C. 2008. The amelogenin "enamel proteins" and cells in the periodontium. *Crit Rev Eukaryot Gene Expr* 18, 345–360.

Hegde S. 2012. Multiple Unerupted Teeth with Amelogenesis Imperfecta in Siblings. *North Am J Med Sci* 4, 235–237.

Hu J., Chun Y.H., Al Hazzazzi T. and Simmer J.P. 2007. Enamel Formation and Amelogenesis Imperfecta. *Cells Tissues Organs* 186, 78–85.

Hu Y., Hu J., Smith C., Bartlett J. and Simmer J. 2011. Kallikrein-related peptidase 4, matrix metalloproteinase 20, and the maturation of murine and porcine enamel. *Eur J Oral Sci* 119, 217–225.

Kim J., Lee S., Lee Z., Park J., Lee K., Lee M., Park J., Seo B., Hu J. and Simmer J. 2008. FAM83H Mutations in Families with Autosomal-Dominant Hypocalcified Amelogenesis Imperfecta. *Am J Hum Genet* 82, 89–94.

Lee K.E., Lee S.K., Jung S.E., Song S., Cho S., Lee Z. and Kim J.W. 2011. A novel mutation in the AMELX gene and multiple crown resorptions. *Eur J Oral Sci* 119, 324–328.

Lee S.K., Lee Z.H., Lee S.J., Ahn B.D., Kim Y.J., Lee S.H. and Kim J.W. 2008. DLX3 mutation in a new family and its phenotypic variations. *J Dent Res* 87, 354–357.

Luder H.U., Gerth-Kahlert C., Ostertag-Benzinger S. and Schorderet D.F. 2013. Dental phenotype in Jalili syndrome due to a c.1312 dupC homozygous mutation in the CNNM4 gene. *PLoS One* 8, e78529.

Malik K., Gadhia K., Arkutu N. and McDonald S. 2012. The interdisciplinary management of patients with amelogenesis imperfecta–restorative dentistry. *Bri Dent J* 212, 537–542.

Manzanares M., Franch J., Carvalho P., Belmonte A., Franch T.J.B., Fernandez J., Clèries L. and Morenza J. 2001. BS-SEM evaluation of the tissular interactions between corticalbone and calcium-phosphate covered titanoum implants. *Bulletin du GIRSO* 43, 100–108.

Mitsiadis T. and Luder H. 2011. Genetic basis for tooth malformations: from mice to men and back again. *Clin Genet* 80, 319–329.

Nanci A. 2012. *Ten Cate's Oral Histology. Development, structure and function.* Londres: Mosby.

Parry D.A., Brookes S.J., Logan C.V., Poulter J.A., El-Sayed W., Al-Bahlani S., Al Harasi S., Sayed J., Raïf el M., Shore R.C., Dashash M., Barron M., Morgan J.E., Carr I.M., Taylor G.R., Johnson C.A., Aldred M.J., Dixon M.J., Wright J.T., Kirkham J., Inglehearn C.F. and Mighell A.J. 2012. Mutations in C4orf26, Encoding a Peptide with In Vitro Hydroxyapatite Crystal Nucleation and Growth Activity, Cause Amelogenesis Imperfecta. *Am J Hum Genet* 91, 565–571.

Prasad M.K., Laouina S., El Alloussi M., Dollfus H. and Bloch-Zupan A. 2016. Amelogenesis Imperfecta: 1 Family, 2 Phenotypes, and 2 Mutated Genes. *J Dent Res* 95, 1457–1463.

Sánchez-Quevedo C., Ceballos G., Rodríguez I.A., García J. and Alaminos M. 2006. Acid-etching effects in hypomineralized amelogenesis imperfecta. A microscopic and microanalytical study. *Med Oral Patol Oral Cir Bucal* E11:40–43.

Sapp J., Eversole L. and Wysolki G. 2005. Alteración del desarrollo de la región oral. *Patología Oral y Maxilofacial* 2ª ed. Madrid: Elsevier.

Simmer S., Estrella N., Milkovich R. and Hu J. 2013. Autosomal dominant amelogenesis imperfect associated with ENAM frameshift mutation p.Asn36Ilefs56. *Clin Genet* 83, 195–197.

Simmons L., Al-Jawad M., Kilcoyne S. and Wood D. 2011. Distribution of enamel crystallite orientation through an entire tooth crown studied using synchrotron X-ray diffraction. Eur. *J Oral Sci* 119, 19–24.

Wang S.K., Hu Y., Simmer J., Seymen F., Estrella N., Pal S., Reid B., Yildirim M., Bayram M., Bartlett J. and Hu J. 2013. Novel KLK4 and MMP20 Mutations Discovered by Whole-exome Sequencing. *J Dent Res* 92, 266–271.

Wang S.K., Reid B.M., Dugan S.L., Roggenbuck J.A., Read L., Aref P., Taheri A.P., Yeganeh M.Z., Simmer J.P. and Hu J.C. 2014. FAM20A mutations associated with enamel renal syndrome. *J Dent Res* 93, 42–48.

Witkop C. 1988. Amelogenesis imperfecta, dentinogenesis imperfecta and dentin dysplasia revisited: problems in classification. *J Oral Pathol* 17, 547–543.

Wright J., Torain M., Long K., Seow K., Crawford P., Aldred M.J., Hart P.S. and Hart T.C. 2011. Amelogenesis Imperfecta: Genotype-Phenotype Studies in 71 Families. *Cells Tissues Organs* 194, 279–283.

Wright J. 2006. The molecular etiologies and associated phenotypes of amelogenesis imperfecta. *Am J Med Genet* A 140, 2547–2555.

Zhang C., Song Y. and Bian Z. 2015. Ultrastructural analysis of the teeth affected by amelogenesis imperfecta resulting from FAM83H mutations and review of the literature. *Oral Surg Oral Med Oral Pathol Oral Radiol* 119, e69–76.

Zhang Z., Gutierrez D., Li X., Bidlack F., Cao H., Wang J., Andrade K., Margolis H.C. and Amendt B.A. 2013. The LIM Homeodomain Transcription Factor LHX6. A Transcriptional repressor that interacts with pituitary homeobox2 (PITX2) to regulate odontogenesis. *J Biol Chem* 288, 2485–2500.

Biodental Engineering V – Belinha et al. (Eds)
© 2019 Taylor & Francis Group, London, ISBN 978-0-367-21087-8

Influence of resin composite cement on the final color of fixed rehabilitation

Joana F. Piloto
Faculty of Dental Medicine, University of Porto (FMDUP), Portugal

Claudia A.M. Volpato
Federal University of Santa Catarina, Florianópolis, Brazil

Paulo Rocha, Paulo Júlio Almeida, César Silva & Paula Vaz
FMDUP, Portugal

ABSTRACT: Aesthetic ceramic restorations, such as veneers, inlays, onlays and total crowns, are the basis of nowadays conservative dental medicine. Their success depends mostly on their optical attributes, emphasizing the color and translucency, as well their biocompatibility and good mechanical properties. Literature highlights the necessity of a great combination between translucency and thickness of the resin composite cements, in order to obtain the idealized final color on dental restorations. This *in vitro* study aimed to analyze the influence of the resin composite cement on the final color of an aesthetic fixed prosthodontics rehabilitation, using zirconia as restorative material.

1 INTRODUCTION

Nowadays dental aesthetic concept, the "perfect smile" and "divine facial proportions" are deep-rooted within the present generation, with overvalued tendency in the future (Simões, 2015). Dental medicine go together with this social-stereotyped trend and gives industry the motivation to create and innovate products, drawing a line that reaches great satisfaction from patients and professionals (Ozturk et al., 2013). Prosthodontics and preventive dentistry had determining role, trying to answer these social requirements through studies and clinical trials implementation (Simões, 2015).

Aesthetic ceramic restorations, such as veneers, inlays, onlays and total crowns, are the basis of nowadays conservative dental medicine. Their success depends mostly on their optical attributes, emphasizing the color and translucency as well their biocompatibility and good mechanical properties (Xing et al., 2017, Shillingburg et al., 1986).

Currently, studies found some influencing aspects on the final color restoration, searching for new clinical implications that could arise from the experiments (Turgut and Bagis, 2013). Wenzhong Xing et al. (2017) completed an *in vitro* study regarding the effect of ceramic's thickness and the cement shade on the color matching of ceramic veneers, over a grey dental surface. In the latter, seventy-two dental preparations for veneers were made and

ceramic material (LT, shade A2, IPS e.max Press) was selected to create 0.5 mm and 0.7 mm thickness veneers. Six different colored resin cements were used to apply those ceramic materials on the artificial teeth. The L*a*b* color coordinates were acquired with a spectrophotometer, and the color difference (ΔE_{ab}) was calculated. These authors concluded that the final color restoration was significantly influenced not only by the thickness of ceramic and shades from the resin cement, but also by the tooth areas (Xing et al., 2017).

On the last decade, the ceramic biomaterial zirconia has offered high biocompatibility, aesthetics and mechanical resistance in fixed prosthodontic rehabilitations. Its optical applicability is justified by the high refractive index, low absorption coefficient, its white pigmentation and high opacity in the visible and infrared spectra. Despite the widespread use of zirconia, some issues related to its properties have not yet been fully resolved, such as the stability and longevity of the material (Vagkopoulou et al., 2009).

The space between an indirect fixed restoration and the tooth is commonly filled with a cementing agent. Alluding to the type of adhesion, this material can be classified as adhesive, non-adhesive (mechanical) or micro-mechanics cement. The fixed prosthodontics longevity depends on the right selection of the cement, according to the function and desired properties. The main functions include retention, resistance to restoration and tooth, and marginal adaptation (Garcia, 2014).

The success of fixed restorations, whether partial, total or unitary crowns, depends not only on an adequate diagnosis, treatment plan, adequate design of the preparations, good professional performance and clinical experience, but in many situations, on the choice of the cementing agent and of the technique appropriated to the clinical situation (Garcia, 2014). In addition, it is also known that the optic effect "opalescence" is important for the reproduction of the final color on dental fixed rehabilitations. This property differs according to the type of ceramic, being always smaller in the ceramics than on natural tooth's enamel. It is also being shown that the measurements of color parameters, lightness (L*), chroma (C'), and hue angle (H'), display a strong correlation when diverse instruments measure the color difference (Azer et al., 2011).

In 1973, Sproull described the concept of color with a three-dimensional nature, defining a practical method of measuring and controlling it. The CIELab color system consists of three color attributes: L* (lightness), a* (red-green chroma), b* (yellow-blue chroma). The CIELCh system derives from the previous system and is based on the coordinates of the color: L* (lightness), C* (chroma), h* (hue). Colorimeters and spectrophotometers are used for such measures (Azer et al., 2011). A difference or a color change is determined in the CIELab system with the following equations

$$\Delta E_{ab} = [(\Delta L)^2 + (\Delta a)^2 + (\Delta b)^2]^{1/2} \qquad (1)$$

$$\Delta E_{00} = \left[\left(\frac{\Delta L'}{k_L S_L} \right)^2 + \left(\frac{\Delta C'}{k_c S_c} \right)^2 + \left(\frac{\Delta H'}{k_H S_H} \right)^2 \right. $$
$$\left. + R_T \left(\frac{\Delta C'}{k_c S_C} \right) \times \left(\frac{\Delta H'}{k_c S_C} \right) \right]^{1/2} \qquad (2)$$

In the field of Dental Medicine, equation (1) is more frequently found due to its simplicity. However, equation (2) provides a better comparison of color differences with a visual perception to the human eye. To calculate color compatibility, some researchers measured the color difference (ΔE) between a restoration and the tooth surface or a predefined color. The ΔE is compared with the thresholds of the human eye for perception (ΔE = 2.6) and acceptability (ΔE = 5.5) in order to determine the visibility of the color difference (Azer et al., 2011).

Literature emphasizes the necessity of a great combination between translucency and thickness with the resin composite cements, in order to obtain the idealized final color (Xing et al., 2017).

Some color measurement instruments provide its own analysis and decreases its subjective variables. It also provides a final color determination and a better communication with the dental laboratory. The spectrophotometer is a color measurement tool that measures the spectral light distribution and converts it into color values (tristimulus value) or an internationally accepted numerical value.

The influence of infra structures (color, material and thickness), resin cement and restoration types have been a target for in vitro studies (Perroni et al., 2017). However, the evidence provided through the analysis of clinical cases is frankly sparse.

This *in vitro* study aimed to analyze the influence of resin composite cement on the final color of an aesthetic fixed prosthodontic rehabilitation, using zirconia as restorative material. The null hypothesis states that the color of the composite resin cement does not affect the final color of the zirconia ceramic restoration.

2 MATERIAL AND METHODS

Within this study, twenty samples will be evaluated and divided into two groups (n = 10), according to the color of the composite resin cement used (Bifix SE, universal shade and Bifix SE, shade white) for the cementation of zirconia disk (Zirlux Anterior Multi, universal shade) with a dental composite resin disk (VOCO, GrandioSO—nano-hybrid composite, A5 opaque). Table 1 presents a summary of the relevant information of mentioned materials (Table 1). The Figure 1 exemplifies a methodology schematic representation of this *in vitro* study.

2.1 *Preparation of ceramic samples*

Twenty-five ceramic zirconia disks will be milling with 1,4 mm thickness. After sintering, the disks will be regularized in polishing equipment.

The notorious color transition that's going to mimic the various dental layers (incisal, dentine and cervical) will be obtained. Both surfaces, of each disk, will be polished with a 1000-grain wet silicon carbide abrasive paper, yielding a final thickness of 1 mm, controlled by measurement on the digital micrometer. Those will then be cleaned with ultrasonic on distilled water for 10 minutes, with excess water being withdrawn with absorbent paper. Five of these ceramic disks will be part of the control group for this study.

2.2 *Preparation of dental composite resin samples*

Twenty composite resin disks (shade A5 opaque, VOCO GrandioSO) are going to be prepared with

Table 1. Properties of materials.

Material	Manufacturer	Additional information
Universal nano-hybrid restorative	VOCO GrandioSO	Content of load exceeding 83%. High color stability.
Universal (A2), dual-curing, self-adhesive, luting composite	Bifix SE	Indications: – Definitive cementation of porcelain, resin or metal inlays, onlays, crowns and bridges. – Definitive cementation of metallic dental posts, ceramic or fiber reinforced posts.
Ceramic zirconia material	Zirlux Anterior Multi	Indications: – Total crowns – Bridges of 2–3 elements – Veneers

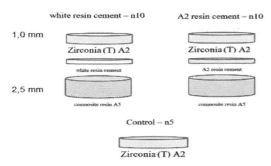

Figure 1. Methodology schematic representation.

the ultimate aim of representing the dentin surface of the natural tooth. For this purpose, it will be used a Porcelain Sampler as a template to obtain each of the twenty composite resin disks, ending with a final thickness of 2,5–2,7 mm and a diameter of 10,0–10,5 mm per disk These will then be light cured under a light intensity of 1,700 mW/cm^2, 7 watts (Technoflux), 40 seconds on the disks' exposed side when placed on the Porcelain Sampler, followed by light curing on the other side for 40 seconds, when individualized from the mold. The surfaces' polishing will be achieved with a 1000-grain wet silicon carbide abrasive paper adjusting the thickness of each disk to 2,5 mm, with proper millimetric control of the digital micrometer.

2.3 Adhesive cementation of ceramic disks on composite resin disks

The etching with 37% phosphoric acid gel will be applied on the bonding surface from the composite resin disks. The bonding side of the zirconia disks will be treated with a 9% hydrofluoric acid and covered with a layer of silane (ceramic primer). Each composite disk will randomly match with a zirconia disk, thereby obtaining twenty pairs of samples. These combinations will be accomplished through the adhesive cementation of each pair. Ten pair samples will be individually cemented with Bifix SE, universal shade (A2), and the other ten with Bifix SE shade white opaque, always according to the manufacturer's instructions. Proceeding this process, light curing will take 20 seconds, followed by the removal of excess polymerized cement with a finishing diamond drill bit. The final polishing of the twenty samples will certainly be achieved with a large polisher cup.

2.4 Color analysis

Color values will be analyzed in both twenty pairs of cemented disks and in the five zirconia disks constituting the control group. To measure these color parameters, a calibrated clinical spectrophotometer shall be used and prepared according to the manufacturer's instructions.

2.5 Calculation of color difference

The color parameters of CIE values L*a*b* shall be analyzed in all measurements made. The CIE color difference will be calculated with the following equation: $\Delta E_{ab} = [(\Delta L)^2 + (\Delta a)^2 + (\Delta b)^2]^{1/2}$.

2.6 Statistical analysis

The 1-way ANOVA ($P < 0.05$) will be used for subsequent statistical analysis. Multiple comparisons are going to be performed by Tukey's Test.

REFERENCES

Azer, S.S., Rosenstiel, S.F., Seghi, R.R. & Johnston, W.M. 2011. Effect of substrate shades on the color of ceramic laminate veneers. *J Prosthet Dent*, 106, 179–83.

Garcia, D.R.S. 2014. *Cimentação Adesiva em Prótese Fixa*. Universidade Fernando Pessoa.

Ozturk, E., Chiang, Y.C., Cosgun, E., Bolay, S., Hickel, R. & Ilie, N. 2013. Effect of resin shades on opacity of ceramic veneers and polymerization efficiency through ceramics. *J Dent*, 41 Suppl 5, e8–14.

Perroni, A.P., Bergoli, C.D., Dos Santos, M.B.F., Moraes, R.R. & Boscato, N. 2017. Spectrophotometric analysis of clinical factors related to the color of ceramic restorations: A pilot study. *J Prosthet Dent*, 118, 611–616.

Shillingburg, H.T., Hobo, S. & Whitsett, L.D. 1986. *Fundamentos de prótese fixa*, Quintessence.

Simões, M.B.S.E. 2015. *Estética dentária: perceção e preconceitos sociais*. mestrado integrado, instituto superior de ciências da saúde egas moniz.

Turgut, S. & Bagis, B. 2013. Effect of resin cement and ceramic thickness on final color of laminate veneers: an in vitro study. *J Prosthet Dent*, 109, 179–86.

Vagkopoulou, T., Koutayas, S.O., Koidis, P. & Strub, J.R. 2009. Zirconia in dentistry: Part 1. Discovering the nature of an upcoming bioceramic. *Eur J Esthet Dent*, 4, 130–51.

Xing, W., Chen, X., Ren, D., Zhan, K. & Wang, Y. 2017. The effect of ceramic thickness and resin cement shades on the color matching of ceramic veneers in discolored teeth. *Odontology*, 105, 460–466.

Biodental Engineering V – Belinha et al. (Eds)
© 2019 Taylor & Francis Group, London, ISBN 978-0-367-21087-8

Clinical determination of chewing side

I. Fediv & A. Carvalho
Institute of Health Sciences, Universidade Católica Portuguesa, Viseu, Portugal

A. Correia & P. Fonseca
Centre of Interdisciplinary Research in Health, Institute of Health Sciences, Universidade Católica Portuguesa, Viseu, Portugal

ABSTRACT: The main aim of this work is to identify the chewing side by clinic determination of the functional masticatory angle. 70 individuals (58,6% female; 41,4% male) were evaluated. The data were achieved by questionnaire and by clinical examination. The collected data were introduced and analyzed in IBM-SPSS® software, considering a significance level of 5%. We found a statistically significant relation ($p \leq 0,05$) between the preferential chewing side and the functional masticatory angle. Bilateral masticators have similar functional masticatory angle and unilateral ones do it for the side with a lower functional masticatory angle. Since most patients do not recognize their preferential chewing side and that it has important functional repercussions that can affect all the components of the stomatognathic system, the simple and rapid clinical determination of the functional masticatory angle indicates the patient's preferential chewing side.

1 INTRODUCTION

Chewing as a primary function of the stomatognathic system, is a complex activity that can influence the general quality of the individual: good masticatory efficacy is directly related to a correct and healthy diet and, consequently, a better quality of life [Yamashita et al. (1999); Moynihan et al. (2000)].

Planas (1988) states that chewing must be bilateral for harmonious facial development. An atypical stimulus may lead to unequal or asymmetrical growth of the face.

The literature demonstrates that alterations in masticatory movements may lead to transformations in important structures, namely the osseous bases, masticatory muscles, TMJ, teeth, periodontium and afferent and efferent nerve pathways, resulting, in the last instance, in an imbalance of the whole face [Ferrario (2006) et al.; Barcellos et al. (2011)].

Although ideally mastication should be alternate bilaterally, it is known that large part of the population has preference for one side, called Preferential Chewing Side (PCS) [Planas (1988); Martinez-Gomis et al. (2009); Ved et al. (2017)].

The determination of PCS can be done by direct observation of chewing [Pond et al. (1986)], by electromyography [Neto et al. (2004)] or by the chewing gum test and visual inspection of the first masticatory cycle [Nissan et al. (2009)].

The main aim of this work is to identify the preferential chewing side by clinic determination of the functional masticatory angle (FMA) as defined by Planas (1988).

2 MATERIAL AND METHODS

The authors performed a cross-sectional observational epidemiological study with 70 patients (58,6% women and 41,4% men) in the dental clinic of the Institute of Health Sciences from Portuguese Catholic University.

General data were collected by questionnaire such as gender, age and chewing side patient's perception. PCS and FMA were achieved by clinical examination.

Through the chewing gum test we determined the preferential side of initial chewing and of continuous mastication (10 cycles). They were classified as predominantly unilateral right, unilateral left or bilateral.

The measurement of the functional masticatory angle was performed with an orthometer, a protractor and a millimeter ruler, recording the angle formed in the midline by intercepting the trajectory followed by the lower central incisor in the lateral movement with a horizontal plane parallel to the occlusal plane (Figures 1–3).

All ethical and legal procedures were respected and the collected data were introduced and analyzed

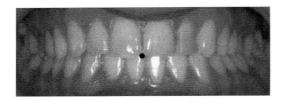

Figure 1. Maximum intercuspation and incisor point registration.

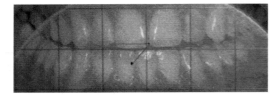

Figure 2. Right functional masticatory angle.

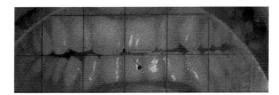

Figure 3. Left functional masticatory angle.

in IBM SPSS Statistics® (version 24) software considering the significance level of 5% and the independence of the variables the null hypothesis.

3 RESULTS

The mean age of the 70 patients observed was 27 ± 12 years, ranging from 16 to 69 years old.

Twenty patients (28,6%) not have perception of the chewing side, 15,7% (n = 11) reported chewing preferentially to the left, 30% (n = 21) preferentially chewing on the right and 25,7% (n = 18) stated chewing bilaterally.

Most patients (67,1%; n = 47) directed the first masticatory reflex to the right side. Regarding the predominant chewing side (10 cycles), 22,9% (n = 16) of the patients presented bilateral mastication, in 28,6% (n = 20) left side is predominant and the right side in 48,6% (n = 34).

The authors found no relation with statistical significance between the gender of the patient and the preferential side of mastication ($p = 0,324$), the first masticatory reflex ($p = 0,785$) nor with predominant chewing side ($p = 0,436$).

For the 70 patients under study, the left FMA (mean = 29,4 ± 12,4 degrees) was higher than the

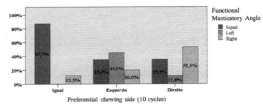

Figure 4. Sample distribution according to the PCS and the FMA.

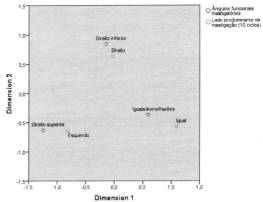

Figure 5. Correspondence analysis between the categories of variables studied PCS and FMA.

right one (mean = 27,5 ± 11, 1 degrees). 47,1% (n = 33) of patients presented equal or similar angles (right and left); 34,3% (n = 24) had a superior FMA at left and 18,6% (n = 13) at right.

We found a statistically significant relation ($p = 0,000$) between the PCS and the FMA. Bilateral masticators have similar functional masticatory angles (right and left) and unilateral ones do it for the side with a lower FMA (Figure 4).

The existence of the following correlations can be affirmed (Figure 5):

1–Equal or similar FMA/bilateral chewing;
2–Right FMA higher/left unilateral mastication;
3–Right FMA lower/right unilateral chewing.

4 DISCUSSION

Similarly to other authors [Jiang et al. (2015); Flores-Orozco et al. (2016); Yamasaki (2016)] and in order to evaluate PCS, we used the chewing gum test and opted for the direct observation of chewing described by McDonnell et al. (2004) and employed in several masticatory studies [Flores-Orozco et al. (2016); Diemberg et al. (2008)]. Already Neto et al. (2004) show a concordance in 83% of the observations in a comparison study between the electromyographic examination and the visual examination, which suggests that visual inspection, being the simplest method, is perfectly feasible to apply in the evaluation of PCS. The ideal method for day-to-day clinical use should be a simple, replicable, valid method and able to determine PCS quantitatively [Flores-Orozco et al. (2016)].

The most frequent side of directing the first masticatory reflex found by authors is the right one (67,18%). In this sense, our results prove the results achieved by previous studies [Pond et al. (1986); McDonnell et al. (2004); Martinez-Gomis et al. (2009); Ved et al. (2017)].

The relationship found between FMA and PCS confirms the results described by Planas (1988) and by Neto et al. (2000), that is, individuals present masticatory preference on the side where the FMA is smaller.

In our sample, unilateral chewers do it more frequently to the right side (48.6%) which, once again, corroborates previous studies, even under different evaluation protocols [Barcellos et al. (2011); McDonnell et al. (2004); Martinez-Gomis et al. (2009); Ved et al. (2017)].

We were able to confirm the findings of Pedro Planas (1988) regarding PCS's evaluation method through FMA. We also confirmed that the majority of population presents a unilateral chewing pattern.

Since most patients do not recognize their preferential chewing side and that has important functional repercussions that can affect all the components of the stomatognathic system (muscles, bones, joints, teeth and periodontium), the relationship between the chewing side and functional masticatory angle proved with this study can help in oral rehabilitation.

5 CONCLUSIONS

Oral rehabilitation should balance and functionally restore the stomatognathic system, emphasizing its main function: chewing. It was proved that the simple and rapid clinical determination of the FMA indicates the patient PCS and consequently helps the clinician to prevent some musculoskeletal conditions, as well as to diagnosis and plan treatment in oral rehabilitation.

REFERENCES

Barcellos, D.C., Paiva Gonçalves, S.E., Silva, M.A., Batista, G.R., Pleffken, P.R., Pucci, C.R., et al. 2011.

Prevalence of Chewing Side Preference in the Deciduous, Mixed and Permanent Dentitions. *The Journal of Contemporary Dental Practice* 12(5): 339–342.

Diernberger, S., Bernhardt, O., Schwann, C. & Kordass, B. 2008. Self-reported chewing side preference and its associations with occlusal, temporomandibular and prosthodontic factors: results from the population-based Study of Health in Pomerania (SHIP-0). *Journal of Oral Rehabilitation* 35(8): 613–620.

Ferrario, V.F., Piancino, M.G., Dellavia, C., Castroflorio, T., Sforza, C. & Bracco, P. 2006. Quantitative Analysis of the Variability of Unilateral Chewing Movements in Young Adults. *The Journal of Craniomandibular Practice* 24(4): 274–282.

Flores-Orozco, E.I., Rovira-Lastra, B., Peraire, M., Salsench, J. & Martinez-Gomis, J. 2016. Reliability of a visual analog scale for determining the preferred mastication side. *The Journal of Prosthetic Dentistry* 115(2): 203–208.

Jiang, H., Li, C., Wang, Z., Cao, J., Shi, X., Ma, J., et al. 2015. Assessment of osseous morphology of temporomandibular joint in asymptomatic participants with chewing-side preference. *Journal of Oral Rehabilitation* 42(2): 105–112.

Martinez-Gomis, J., Lujan-Climent, M., Palau, S., Bizar, J., Salsench, J. & Peraire, M. 2009. Relationship between chewing side preference and handedness and lateral asymmetry of peripheral fators. *Archives of Oral Biology* 54(2): 101–107.

McDonnell, S.T., Hector, M.P. & Hannigan, A. 2004. Chewing side preferences in children. *Journal of Oral Rehabilitation* 31(9): 855–860.

Moynihan, P.J., Butler, T.J., Thomason, J.M. & Jepson, N.J.A. 2000. Nutrient intake in partially dentate patients: the effect of prosthetic rehabilitation. *Journal of Dentistry* 28(8): 557–563.

Neto, G.P., Bérzin, F. & Rontani, R.M.P. 2004. Identificação do lado de preferência mastigatória através de exame eletromiográfico comparado ao visual. *R Dental Press Ortodon Ortop Facial* 9(4): 77–85.

Nissan, J., Gross, M.D., Shifman, A., Tzadok, L. & Assif, D. 2004. Chewing side preference as a type of hemispheric laterality. *Journal of Oral Rehabilitation* 31(5): 412–416.

Planas, P. (2nd ed) 1988. *Reabilitação Neuro-Oclusal*. Rio de Janeiro: Medsi.

Pond, L.H., Barghi, N. & Barnwell, G.M. 1986. Occlusion and chewing side preference. *The Journal of Prosthetic Dentistry* 55(4): 498–500.

Ved, V.P., Arora, A., Das, D. & Kalra, D. 2017. The Correlation of Unilateral Chewing Habit with Temporomandibular Joint Disorders. *International Journal of Scientific Study* 5(1): 1–4.

Yamashita, S., Hatch, J.P. & Rugh JD 1999. Does chewing performance depend upon a specific masticatory pattern? *Journal of Oral Rehabilitation* 26(7): 547–553.

Yamasaki, Y., Kuwatsuru, R., Tsukiyama, Y., Oki, K. & Koyano, K. 2016. Objective assessment of mastication predominance in healthy dentate subjects and patients with unilateral posterior missing teeth. *Journal of Oral Rehabilitation* 43(8): 575–582.

Biodental Engineering V – Belinha et al. (Eds)
© 2019 Taylor & Francis Group, London, ISBN 978-0-367-21087-8

Finishing and polishing of acrylic resins used in provisional restorations

S. Matos
Institute of Health Sciences, Universidade Católica Portuguesa, Viseu, Portugal

F. Araujo & A. Correia
Centre of Interdisciplinary Research in Health, Institute of Health Sciences, Universidade Católica Portuguesa, Viseu, Portugal

S. Oliveira
Department of Mechanical Engineering and Industrial Management, School of Technology and Management, Polytechnic Institute of Viseu, Viseu, Portugal

ABSTRACT: Provisional restoration is used in fixed prosthodontics to enhance aesthetics and/or function for a limited period of time. It should be replaced by a definitive dental prosthesis. A Polyethyl Methacrylate (PEMA) and a Bis-acrylic resin were selected as test materials in this study. Specimens were divided into eight groups. The roughness of surface was verified in a Hommel Tester T1000 rugosimeter, before and after different techniques of finishing and polishing. Not all measurements were performed, so this study is not yet complete.

1 INTRODUCTION

Interim or provisional restoration are used in fixed or removable prosthodontics to enhance aesthetics and/or function for a limited period of time, after which it should be replaced by a definitive dental prosthesis. (Dale BG 1993).

The success of Rehabilitation with Fixed Prosthesis is only achieved with rigorous attention and effectiveness in each stage of the treatment. (Chalifoux 2014) Interim restorations in dental medicine thus play an important role as they should be as similar as possible to permanent restoration. (Burns, Beck, and Nelson 2003; Chalifoux 2014) The main goal of finishing and polishing techniques in dental restorations is to create aesthetically natural restorations and to harmonize both function and aesthetics with respect to adjacent dental structures. Resurfacing with surface softness and light reflectivity similar to the natural tooth structure thus arise. The properties of the ideal surface are also important for oral hygiene. (Jefferies 2007) Several critical points have been identified in relation to temporary restorations, such as aesthetics, function, speech, periodontal health and occlusion.

Provisional restorations protect prepared teeth, stabilize occlusion, address the patient's aesthetic concerns, and keep the patient comfortable from the initial dental preparation to cementing the final restoration. In addition, they maintain gingival and periodontal health. (Mei et al. 2015).

The main requirements for temporary materials are adequate marginal adaptation, fracture toughness, low thermal conductivity, non-irritating reaction to the dental pulp and gingival tissues, and ease of sanitization. (Ayuso-Montero et al. 2009) The surface roughness of acrylic resins is substantially important because directly affects the tissues in direct contact with the dental structure. Authors further claimed that uneven surfaces protect bacteria from natural removal forces and even from oral hygiene methods. Ideally, a surface with the least roughness is recommended to prevent retention of microorganisms and prevent local infections. (Rahal et al. 2004).

Although it is possible to make temporary restorations by means of preformed polycarbonate or metal crowns (Guler, Kurt, and Kulunk 2005), the materials most used for temporary restorations are self-curing Methacrylate resins and Bis-acrylic resins. (Christensen 1996) Polymethyl Methacrylate (PMMA) and Polyethyl Methacrylate (PEMA) are the first materials being available in Dental Medicine (they appeared in 1940 and 1960, respectively). PMMA has a high coefficient of thermal expansion, has a relatively low cost, but has a strong smell and low durability. PEMA is not so strong, nor as durable and resistant to abrasion as PMMA, but has a less strong smell, generates less heat and shrinks less during polymerization than PMMA, and is more biocompatible. Bis-acrylic is different from methacrylate resins. It has a high resistance because its monomers have a high molecular weight. Regarding methacrylates, they have higher surface hardness, higher wear resistance, better marginal adaptation and less shrinkage. However, the rigid nucleus of the aromatic group (R group) makes the backbone rigid, which will hamper the complete polymerization. (Mei et al. 2015).

The surface of a temporary restoration may be terminated using various techniques, from abrasive disks to polishing pastes. Not all interim restoration finishing methods may work perfectly, depending on the types of materials available. (Guler et al. 2005) Finishing is the process that involves removing marginal irregularities, defining anatomic contours, and smoothing away surface roughness of a restoration. Polishing is the process carried out after the finishing and margination steps of the finishing procedure to remove minute scratches from the surface of a restoration and obtain a smooth, light-reflective luster. The polishing process is also intended to produce a homogeneous surface. (Jefferies 2007) The use of rubber discs is also recommended when compared to the use of varnishes in the tooth preparation. (Borchers, Tavassol, and Tschernitschek 1999) The techniques used during the finishing and polishing of tooth restorative materials not only improves the longevity and aesthetic appearance of the material, but also minimizes plaque accumulation, gingival irritation and secondary caries. (Rahal et al. 2004) It is practically impossible to achieve a highly polished surface due to the characteristics of the materials. By analyzing different studies, it is possible to notice that there is no consensus on the best finishing and polishing technique. (Madhyastha et al. 2015) Aluminum oxide is a chemical compound of aluminum and oxygen. Its hardness makes it suitable for use as an abrasive and as a component in cutting tools. Aluminum oxide is typically produced as particles bonded to paper or polymer disks and strips or impregnated into rubber wheels and points. Fine particles of aluminum oxide can be mixed into a polishing paste to produce smooth, polished surfaces on many types of restorations, including acrylics and composites. (Jefferies 2007) The main requirements for choice of interim materials are an appropriate marginal adaptation, resistance to fracture, low thermal conductivity, non-irritating reaction to the dental pulp and gingival tissues, and ease of cleaning. The surface roughness of acrylic resins is highly relevant because affects the tissues in direct contact with the dental structure. (Burns et al. 2003).

Proper provisional restoration fit, shape, and polish further reduces chances of gingival inflammation. (Jefferies 2007) This study aimed at evaluating the surface roughness of two acrylic resins used for provisional crowns and bridges, before and after finishing and polishing.

2 MATERIAL AND METHODS

2.1 Provisional prosthetic materials

A Polyethyl Methacrylate (PEMA) and a Bis-acrylic resin were selected as test materials in this study, as shown in Table 1. The choice of materials took into account their use in the University Dental Clinic, in Viseu (Portugal).

2.2 Specimen preparation

Using polylactic acid (PLA) molds (20 mm diameter × 3 mm height). (Fig. 1)

All specimens were fabricated by a single operator, according to the manufacturer's instructions.

Forty specimens were fabricated (n = 10).

Specimens of Trim® were divided into four groups:

A – no finishing and polishing;
B – specimens of group A subject to a system of three abrasive discs, of different grades, and prophylactic brush with a paste of pumice and water;
C – no finishing and polishing;
D – specimens of group C subject a goat hair brush with polishing fluid to acrylics.

Specimens of Structure 3® were also divided into four groups:

E – no finishing and polishing;

Table 1. Material of this study.

Product	Manufacturer	Resin type
Trim	Bosworth	PEMA
Structur 3	VOCO	Bis-acrylic

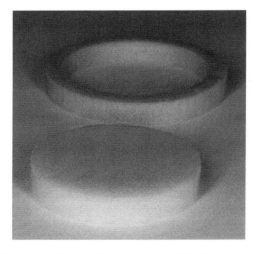

Figure 1. PLA mold and specimen of Trim®.

Table 2. Preliminary results.

Material	Group	Mean of Ra (μm)
Trim	A	2,80
Structur 3	E	0,29

F – specimens of group E subject to a ethanol in their surface, according brand recommendations.

G – no finishing and polishing;

H – specimens of group G subject a goat hair brush with polishing fluid to acrylics.

2.3 Finishing and polishing

The methods of finishing and polishing were carried out for 30 seconds, trying to avoid angulations that could compromise the analysis.

The surface roughness (Ra) was verified in a Hommel Tester T1000 rugosimeter. Five readings per specimen were taken, from the centre of the disc to five points randomly marked on the mold.

3 RESULTS AND DISCUSSION

Preliminary results of this research (Table 2) show that Structur 3® has a smoothest surface compared with Trim®, concerning the Groups A and E (no finishing and polishing).

This initial results predict that finishing and polishing methods will decrease the mean of Ra values about Trim® and probably will promote no significative differences about Structur 3®.

4 CONCLUSION

The surface roughness of the bis-acrylic resin Structur 3® has lower values when compared to the PEMA acrylic resin Trim®.

REFERENCES

Ayuso-Montero, Raul, Jordi Martinez-Gomis, Mar Lujan-Climent, Juan Salsench, and Maria Peraire. 2009. "Influence of Matrix Type on Surface Roughness of Three Resins for Provisional Crowns and Fixed Partial Dentures." *Journal of Prosthodontics* 18(2):141–44.

Borchers, L., F. Tavassol, and H. Tschernitschek. 1999. "Surface Quality Achieved by Polishing and by Varnishing of Temporary Crown and Fixed Partial Denture Resins." *The Journal of Prosthetic Dentistry* 82(5):550–56.

Burns, David R., David A. Beck, and Steven K. Nelson. 2003. "A Review of Selected Dental Literature on Contemporary Provisional Fixed Prosthodontic Treatment: Report of the Committee on Research in Fixed Prosthodontics of the Academy of Fixed Prosthodontics." *Journal of Prosthetic Dentistry* 90(5):474–97.

Chalifoux, Paul R. 2014. "Acrylic and Other Resins: Provisional Restorations." Pp. 197–230 in *Esthetic Dentistry: A Clinical Approach to Techniques and Materials, Third Edition.*

Christensen, G.J. 1996. "Provisional Restorations for Fixed Prosthodontics." *Journal of the American Dental Association (1939)* 127(2):249–52.

Dale BG, Aschheim KW. 1993. *Esthetic Dentistry: Clinical Approach to Techniques and Materials.*

Guler, Ahmet Umut, Safak Kurt, and Tolga Kulunk. 2005. "Effects of Various Finishing Procedures on the Staining of Provisional Restorative Materials." *Journal of Prosthetic Dentistry* 93(5):453–58.

Jefferies, Steven R. 2007. "Abrasive Finishing and Polishing in Restorative Dentistry: A State-of-the-Art Review." *Dental Clinics of North America* 51(2):379–97.

Madhyastha, Prashanthi S., Dilip G. Naik, N. Srikant, Ravindra Kotian, and Kumar Bhat. 2015. "Effect of Finishing/Polishing Techniques and Time on Surface Roughness of Silorane and Methacrylate Based Restorative Materials." *Oral Health Dent Manag* 14(4):212–8. Retrieved (http://www.omicsonline.com/open-access/effect-of-finishing-polishing-techniques-and-time-on-surface-roughness-of-silorane-and-methacrylate-based-restorative-materials-2247-2452-1000810.pdf).

Mei, May, Sam So, Hao Li, and Chun-Hung Chu. 2015. "Effect of Heat Treatment on the Physical Properties of Provisional Crowns during Polymerization: An in Vitro Study." *Materials* 8(4):1766–77. Retrieved (http://www.mdpi.com/1996-1944/8/4/1766/).

Rahal, J.S., M.F. Mesquita, G.E.P. Henriques, and M.A.A. Nóbilo. 2004. "Surface Roughness of Acrylic Resins Submitted to Mechanical and Chemical Polishing." *Journal of Oral Rehabilitation* 31(11):1075–79.

Biodental Engineering V – Belinha et al. (Eds)
© 2019 Taylor & Francis Group, London, ISBN 978-0-367-21087-8

3D analysis of the clinical results of VISTA technique combined with connective tissue graft

D.S. Martins, L. Azevedo & N. Santos
Institute of Health Sciences, Universidade Católica Portuguesa, Viseu, Portugal

T. Marques, C. Alves & A. Correia
Institute of Health Sciences, Universidade Católica Portuguesa, Viseu, Portugal
Centre for Interdisciplinary Health Research, Institute of Health Sciences, Universidade Católica Portuguesa, Viseu, Portugal

ABSTRACT: AIM: To evaluate with precision the percentage of root coverage and the increase of soft tissue volume, in single gingival recessions, treated by VISTA+CTG technique. MATERIAL METHODS: Three patients with Miller Class III single gingival recessions in incisors (maxillary or mandibular) were treated by VISTA+CTG technique. Patient's casts were recorded at baseline (T0), 3 and 6 months after surgery (T1 and T2, respectively). The cast were digitalized by an intra-oral scanner and they were superimposed in Geomagic Control X® to evaluate and quantify the changes occurred in 3D. RESULTS: At 6 months, VISTA+CTG technique ensure a gingival recession reduction as well as mean root coverage (2,49 mm and 81,28% respectively) and a gingival thickness increase (average 1,17± 0,36 mm). CONCLUSIONS: The results shows that the technique utilized was predictable for the treatment of this gingival recessions and may promote with success the root coverage and the gingival thickening, within the follow-up time frame.

1 INTRODUCTION

Gingival recession, which is clinically manifested by an apical displacement of the gingival margin from the cementoenamel junction (CEJ), are common in populations with high oral hygiene standards (Sangnes and Gjermo 1976, Serino, Wennstrom *et al.* 1994, Matas, Sentis *et al.* 2011) or with low oral hygiene standards (Baelum, Fejerskov *et al.* 1986, Loe, Anerud *et al.* 1992) and can leading to root surface exposure. (Wennstrom 1994).

Gingival recession located on buccal surface of the tooth, may be associated with a dehiscence of the buccal bone (Bernimoulin and Curilović 1977, Watson 1984), which may be result of development defects (anatomical) or acquired defects (physiological or pathological). (Geiger 1980) Anatomical defects are composed of a buccal bone fenestration/dehiscence or an abnormal tooth position. (Alldritt 1968) Physiological or pathological defects may be associated with orthodontic movements that makes buccal bone and gingiva thinner. Also, orthodontic movements can be a major risk factor for gingival recession progression, when plaque-induced gingival inflammation or traumatic brushing are present. (Wennstrom, Lindhe *et al.* 1987).

The treatment of gingival recessions is indicated for aesthetic reasons, to reduce root hypersensitivity or to create or augment the keratinized tissue band. (Wennstrom 1994, Wennstrom 1996, Gray 2000, Needleman 2002, Roccuzzo, Bunino *et al.* 2002, Cairo, Pagliaro *et al.* 2008, Chambrone, Sukekava *et al.* 2010) Indications for performing root-covering techniques are tooth abrasion/root caries and inconsistency/disharmony of the gingival margin. (Zucchelli and Mounssif 2015).

Several techniques have been proposed in the field of periodontal plastic surgery to achieve root coverage of denuded root surfaces. Among these techniques, coronally advanced flap is considered to be the gold standard in the treatment of single gingival recessions. (Roccuzzo, Bunino *et al.* 2002).

To treat multiple gingival recessions, mainly in aesthetic zone, Zadeh *et al.* (2011) described a new surgical technique (VISTA – vestibular incision subperiosteal tunnel access). (Zadeh 2011, Chatterjee, Sharma et al. 2015).

Also, it has been suggested that the use of connective tissue graft (CTG) in combination with different techniques for the treatment of the gingival recessions has many advantages, like root coverage and increase of soft tissues volume (Rebele, Zuhr *et al.* 2014). The last has been associated with stability of the position of the gingival margin in the long term. (Ribeiro, Zandim *et al.* 2008, Aroca, Keglevich *et al.* 2010, Agudio, Cortellini *et al.* 2016).

Three-dimensional digital analyses allow a reliable and accurate evaluation of the clinical results in the treatment of gingival recessions. To our knowledge there is only one clinical study (Rebele, Zuhr *et al.* 2014) published in the literature which evaluated the increase of soft tissue volume in the treatment of gingival recessions with a modified microsurgical tunnel technique, described by Zuhr *et al.* (2007).

Also, to our knowledge, there are no studies which used three-dimensional digital analysis to evaluate clinical results obtained by VISTA technique combined with a CTG, in the treatment of Miller Class III, single gingival recessions in incisors (maxillary and mandibular).

Therefore, the aims of this prospective study were to make a 3D digital analysis of the gingival thickening and to evaluate the percentage of root coverage obtained, in order to verify the predictability of the surgical technique described above, in the treatment of this type of gingival recessions.

2 MATERIAL METHODS

2.1 *Study design*

This study is a prospective cohort study, over a period of 6 months. Three evaluation times were made – surgery day (T0), 3 months (T1) and 6 months after surgery (T2) – in which Miller Class III single gingival recessions in incisors (maxillary and mandibular) are treated with VISTA technique combined with connective tissue graft.

The main variable analyzed was gingival thickening obtained on the covered root surface. The secondary variable analyzed was percentage of root coverage.

All patients signed an informed consent prior to the surgery and they were included in the study according to the principles set out in the Declaration of Helsinki, revised in 2000.

2.2 *Researchers and institutions*

All surgical procedures were performed by two periodontologists (T.M. and N.M.S.), guest assistants of Department of Periodontology, Institute of Health Sciences – Viseu, Universidade Católica Portuguesa (UCP), with long experience in periodontal plastic surgery. Surgical interventions were performed at the University Clinic of UCP, Viseu, Portugal.

The main author collected all relevant clinical data from treated patients, performed the digital study of clinical outcomes, and analysed the clinical and volumetric outcomes.

2.3 *Patients sample*

Patients were treated by Department of Periodontics of the Health Sciences Institute – Viseu, at the University Clinic of the Portuguese Catholic University between November 2016 and November 2017.

Six patients with Miller Class III, single gingival recessions in maxillary and mandibular incisors were treated, and three were excluded of this study due to fail follow-up appointments. Thus, only three patients were included in this study.

Patients were recruited according to the following inclusion criteria: age ≥ 18 years, non-smokers, no systemic diseases or pregnancy; periodontal health (no active periodontal disease), including ability to maintain good oral hygiene and control of gingivitis with plaque indexes and bleeding in the oral cavity of less than or equal to 25%; not taking medication that interferes with the health of the periodontal tissues or their healing; no contraindication for periodontal surgery; presence of Miller Class III, single gingival recessions in aesthetic zone, which is equal to or greater than 1 mm and does not exceed 5 mm. Natural and clearly identifiable cemento-enamel junction and not clinical mobility were also inclusion criteria.

Patients were not recruited according to the following exclusion criteria: teeth with root steps, at the level of the cemento-enamel junction (CEJ); presence of crown/root abrasion; teeth with crowns or restorations, at the level of the CEJ; teeth with history of mucogingival or periodontal surgery; use of systemic antibiotics in the last 3 months; use of systemic antibiotics for the prophylaxis of bacterial endocarditis and no signature of informed consent, prior to periodontal plastic surgery.

Due to the sample size, this research is considered as a preliminary study.

2.4 *Preoperative protocol*

According Thalmair, T. *et al.* (2016), before periodontal plastic surgeries, all patients will be informed about the probable cause of their gingival recessions and they have been instructed about correct oral hygiene practices. Thus, they had at least two prophylaxis consultations to remove plaque from teeth and to confirm their ability to maintain adequate and complete oral hygiene.

According to McLeod *et al.* (2009), in the preparation of the surgery, an acrylic stent was made for each patient, from the upper cast model, to fully cover the palate during the initial healing phase of the palatine tissues. The acrylic stent was cleaned and placed in a 0.2% solution of chlorhexidine digluconate until it was placed in the mouth after surgery.

Prior to surgery, patients made a mouthwash with a 0.2% solution of chlorhexidine digluconate, according (Thalmair, Fickl et al. 2016).

2.5 *Surgical protocol*

All patients were treated according to the VISTA technique, described by Zadeh et al. (2011), combined with a connective tissue graft.

A minimally invasive technique was performed, by the use of magnification magnifiers ×4.5 (Carl Zeiss®, Germany) with it own illumination, microsurgical instruments (microsurgical needle holder, mini scalpel handle, anatomical microsurgical clamp and microsurgical scissors) (devemed GmbH®, Germany) and adapted suture materials. (Burkhardt and Hurzeler 2000).

After local anaesthesia, the initial preparation of the tooth to be treated involves scaling and root planning of the exposed root surfaces with hand instruments (Gracey Curets, LM-Instruments Oy, LMDental®, Finland) and odontoplasty to reduce some cervical root prominence, which extended beyond the limits of the alveolar process. The odontoplasty was done with rotary finishing drills (Intensiv Perio Set®, Switzerland). (Zadeh 2011) Roots are conditioned for two minutes with an antibiotic solution based on vibramycin to condition the root surface and to eliminate the smear layer.

VISTA technique begins with a vestibular access incision. In the anterior zone of the maxilla, the preferred location for the incision is the lip frenulum, located in the midline. The incision is made until the periosteum, until a subperiosteal tunnel is made, to expose the vestibular bone cortex and the root dehiscence. This tunnel extends at least one or two teeth beyond the teeth that require root coverage, so as to be able to mobilize the gingival margins and facilitate their coronal repositioning. (Zadeh 2011).

A second surgical site is created after tunnel preparation. A free gingival graft was collected from the lateral palate, with extra-oral desepithelialization, becoming a subepithelial connective tissue graft. (Zucchelli, Mele et al. 2010).

In all cases a suitable size ETCS and a thickness of 1.0–1.5 mm with a MB69 microsurgical blade (Hu-Friedy®, Chicago, IL, USA) was obtained. Immediately after CTG harvesting, pressure is applied to the donor area. (Thalmair, Fickl et al. 2016).

CTG is introduced into the previously prepared tunnel, having been fixed with 6–0 polyamide (Atramat®) suture, at the ends of the tunnel.

The graft used and the mucogingival complex are then advanced coronally and stabilized in the new position with a horizontal mattress suture technique, anchored with flow composite on the buccal surfaces of the treated tooth, to place the gingival margin approximately 2/3 mm to coronal of the cemento-enamel junction of each tooth. (Zadeh 2011).

2.6 *Post-surgical protocol*

According (Rebele, Zuhr et al. 2014, Zuhr, Rebele et al. 2014, Thalmair, Fickl et al. 2016), all patients received 600 mg Ibuprofen® after the end of the surgical procedure to reduce edema caused by the flap preparation.

Patients are instructed to avoid any mechanical trauma and not to brush their teeth, corresponding to the intervened sites, during two weeks.

The prescribed analgesic and anti-inflammatory medication was Ibuprofen® and patients were instructed to rinse with a solution of 0.2% chlorhexidine diglocunate 3 times a day for 2 weeks. Sutures were removed after 10 days.

Two weeks after surgery, patients could begin to brush their teeth mechanically with a soft toothbrush.

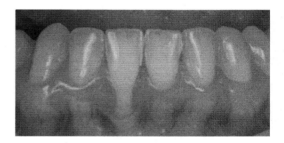

Figure 1. Intraoral frontal photography, at T0, of a Miller class III, single gingival recession, in a mandibular right incisor.

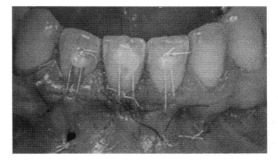

Figure 2. Intraoral frontal photography, immediately after periodontal plastic surgery.

Patients were called after 3 and 6 months to perform follow-up appointments and to receive oral hygiene instructions, to perform hygienic phases (re-evaluation) and to collect the clinical data of interest.

2.7 *Impression protocol*

The impression protocol was adapted from (Rebele, Zuhr et al. 2014).

Alginate impressions were made to the patients at three different times – T0 (before surgery), T1 (3 months after surgery) and T2 (6 months after surgery). Then, were made cast models (Orthodontic Model Mix®, Kerr Dental, USA).

2.8 *Protocol for digital scanning of the cast models and STLs files*

The protocol for digital scanning of the cast models and STLs files was adapted from (Rebele, Zuhr et al. 2014).

The models are meticulously evaluated after alginate impression removal to examine for artefacts in the region of interest. A DentalWings® intraoral scanner (Straumann, Basel, Switzerland) was used to scan the models and consequently generate STL's files, corresponding to each case.

The region of interest was selected by vestibular, in the tooth that present gingival recession. The models were digitalized from the coronal edge of the tooth with recession to 5–6 mm beyond the mucogingival junction and the mesiodistal extension of the scan is of canine to canine.

2.9 *Data transfer from DentalWings® intraoral scanner to Geomagic Control X® software*

The STL files were exported from the DentalWings® intraoral scanner and were imported into Geomagic Control X® software (Geomagic, Inc., North Carolina, USA).

2.10 *Digital models superimposition protocol in Geomagic Control X® software*

STL files of the digital models (T0 and T1 and then T0 and T2) were superimposed.

A strict alignment of the surfaces of the STL files was made for an optimal superimposition with "Align Between Measured Data" and "Best Fit Alignment" functions.

Volumetric evaluation of the gingival thickening in T1 and T2, in relation to T0, was made.

"3D Compare" function create a colour map, in superimposed digital models, in order to quantitatively analyse the three-dimensional changes occurring in the intervened areas and adjacent tissues.

Colour map obtained after digital models superimposition may be interpreted as follows, the green areas correspond to the perfect alignment of the model, after the superimposition. The variation between yellow and red represent different variations of volumetric increase, while the variation between light blue and dark blue represents variations of volumetric decrease. Colour map varies from +2 mm to −2 mm, with a tolerance of ± 0.15 mm.

2.11 *Clinical variables measurement protocol in Geomagic Control X® software*

The STL's files were exported from the DentalWings® intraoral scanner and were imported into Geomagic Control X® software (Geomagic, Inc., North Carolina, USA).

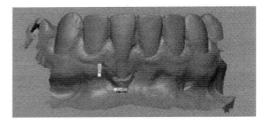

Figure 3. Gingival recession depth measurement, at T0, in Geomagic Control X®.

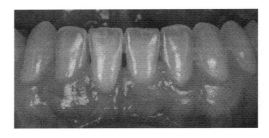

Figure 4. Intraoral frontal photography, at T2, of a treated Miller class III, single gingival recession, in a mandibular right incisor.

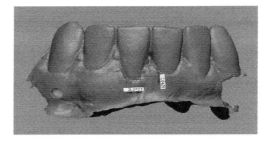

Figure 5. Gingival recession depth measurement, at T2, in Geomagic Control X®.

2.11.1 Gingival recession depth measurement

Gingival recession depth at baseline and residual gingival recessions at T1 and T2 were measured from cemento-enamel junction to free gingival margin at the midpoint of the teeth.

2.11.2 Root coverage percentage calculation

Root coverage percentage is calculated from the formula: (vertical dimension of the preoperative recession – vertical dimension of the postoperative recession)/vertical dimension of the preoperative recession)) × 100 (%).

If the free gingival margin is under the LAC, after the surgery, it is because 100% of root coverage was achieved (complete root coverage).

2.11.3 Gingival thickening evaluation

To study the gingival thickening in T1 and T2, a plane is defined in digital models, so that it passes through the midpoints of the cemento-enamel junction and the buccal free gingival margin. At this stage, we study the points of interest, in which we want to study the local gingival thickening.

In the same section plane mentioned above, a number of cross-sectional planes perpendicular to the plane of vertical section were created, from the cemento-enamel junction to the free gingival margin of the intervened teeth, with a distance of 0,1 mm between each section plane.

The interception of these two 2D planes creates standardized points in each case to assess the gingival thickening of the soft tissues that cover the previously exposed root surface, from cemento-enamel junction to the free gingival margin, and finally, the average of these values obtained, to know the average gingival thickening, in each case.

2.11.4 Intra-examiner reproducibility

The blinded examiner who evaluated the clinical variables, before starting to analyse the cases of this study, was calibrated by a periodontologist, specialist in Geomagic Control X®, with two evaluations, 48 hours apart, in 10 cases of single gingival recessions not included in this study, treated at the University Dental Clinic of UCP.

This evaluation consisted in identification of the gingival zenith, the midpoint of the cemento-enamel junction and consequently in measurement of the depth of the gingival recessions, in the same software.

In all cases, three test measurements were performed. The calibration was only accepted when 90% of the registers were within a difference of 0.1 mm. After this calibration, the examiner started to make the clinical measurements in the cases included in this study.

2.11.5 Statistical analysis

Statistical analysis was done using SPSS 22.0 (Chicago, IL, USA). Descriptive statistics included mean values, standard deviation, frequencies (relative and absolute) and percentages of the clinical variables, in the three moments of evaluation, in each clinical case. The Spearman's correlation coefficient was calculated to verify statistical significance between the recession depth reduction and the mean gingival thickening as well as mean gingival thickening and % RC, at T2. Differences were considered statistically significant for p-values < 0.05.

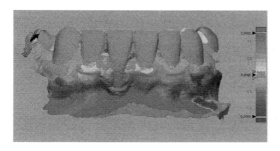

Figure 6. Volumetric evaluation (3D) from the superimposition of the T0 and T2 digital models, in Geomagic Control X®.

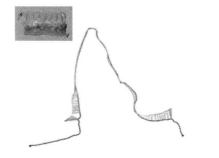

Figure 7. Gingival thickening evaluation (2D) from the section showed. in Geomagic Control X®.

3 RESULTS

3.1 Sample

3 patients (2 females, 1 male) with three Miller Class III, single gingival recessions, were recruited and treated between November 2016 and November 2017. The mean age was 20,67 ± 2,52 years (18–23 years). All patients were treated with VISTA technique and a connective tissue graft (VISTA+CTG technique).

All 3 patients did not miss any of their examinations, participating in the two moments of follow-up to monitor healing dynamics.

3.2 *Defect characteristics at T0 – recession reduction, root coverage and gingival thickness at 3 and 6 months*

Table 2 depicts descriptive statistics for the measured parameters of gingival recession depth (REC) and mean gingival thickness (THK) at baseline, 3 and 6 months.

The clinical outcomes of VISTA+CTG technique, such as recession depth (REC) reduction (mm),% root coverage (RC) and% defects with complete root coverage (CRC) 3 and 6 months after surgery are reported in Table 2.

The sample treated with VISTA+CTG technique comprises 3 gingival recessions with a baseline recession depth of $3,27 \pm 1,33$ mm (1.83–4,44 mm).

At the 6-months follow-up, VISTA+CTG technique obtained a mean root coverage of $81,28 \pm 19,00\%$, a REC reduction of $2,49 \pm 0.58$ mm (corresponding to a mean residual recession depth of 0.78

± 0.85 mm). CRC was detected in 1 out of 3 intervened sites (33,3%) analyzed at 3 and 6 months. The measured THK after 6 months was 1.17 ± 0.36 mm.

3.3 *The relationship of gingival thickness to recession reduction and root coverage*

Spearman's correlation coefficient was used to verify statistical significance between the recession reduction and the mean gingival thickening at T2.

Although there was no significant statistical correlation with those variables, it can be affirmed that there may be a relationship between the greater the gingival thickening and the greater recession reduction at T2.

Regarding the correlation of the mean gingival thickening and% RC at T2, a calculated Spearman's correlation coefficient of $r = -1,000$ revealed a negative correlation of those two variables, that

Table 1. Characterization of the group of patients, with single gingival recessions, treated with VISTA+CTG technique, in T0.

Patient	Age	Tooth	GR Classification	Gingival recession depth (mm) T0
1	21	41	III	3,54
2	18	41	III	1,83
3	23	21	III	4,44
Mean ± SD	20,67 ± 2,52	–	–	3,27 ± 1,33

Legend: GR – gingival recession. SD – standard deviation.

Table 2. Characterization of the evolution of single gingival recessions treated, in T0, T1 and T2.

Patient	GRD (mm) T0	GRD (mm) T1	DRGR (mm) T1	% RC T1	GRD (mm) T2	DRGR (mm) T2	% RC T2
1	3,54	0,55	2,99	84,42	0,64	2,89	81,83
2	1,83	0	1,83	100	0	1,83	100
3	4,44	1,12	3,32	74,85	1,69	2,75	62,01
Mean ± SD	3,27 ± 1,33	0,56 ± 0,56	2,71 ± 0,78	86,42 ± 12,69	0,78 ± 0,85	2,49 ± 0,58	81,28 ± 19,00

Legend: GRD – gingival recession depth, DRGR – depth reduction of gingival recession, % RC – percentage of root coverage, SD – standard deviation.

Table 3. Characterization of the evolution of gingival thickening, from T0 to T1, from T1 to T2 and from T0 to T2.

Patient	Δ GT T0-T1		Δ GT T1-T2		Δ GT T0-T2	
	A (mm)	R (%)	A (mm)	R (%)	A (mm)	R (%)
1	0,951	100	0,03	3,62	0,99	103,62
8	0,9247	100	0,02	2,28	0,95	102,28
9	1,4872	100	0,10	6,84	1,59	106,84
Mean ± SD	1,12 ± 0,32	100 ± 0,00	0,05 ± 0,04	4,25 ± 2,34	1,17 ± 0,36	104,25 ± 2,34

GT – gingival thickening, A – absolute, R – relative. SD – standard deviation.

is, the higher the root coverage values, the smaller the gingival thickening on previously exposed root surfaces.

3.4 *Healing dynamics at surgical treated sites*

The results of volumetric evaluations performed in all 3 patients treated with VISTA+CTG technique in order to monitor healing dynamics from T0 to T1 and T1 to T2 are presented in Table 3. With the post-operative volume gained at T1 being regarded as baseline value of mean gingival thickness (1,12 ± 0,32 corresponds to 100%). The treated sites showed a mean volumetric gain of 104,25 ± 2,34% (corresponding to a mean gingival thickness of 1,17 ± 0,36 mm), from T1 to T2. With regard to post-operative gingival volume changes, the healing process seemed to be accomplished from 3 to 6 months.

4 DISCUSSION

This prospective cohort study is challenging for three clinical reasons. To our knowledge, no clinical study has been published previously that reports 3D analysis of the clinical results of VISTA technique combined with a connective tissue graft. In addition, only one clinical study has been published previously that involves Miller's class III gingival recessions exclusively and also the fact that we are dealing with single gingival recessions in aesthetic zone increases the surgical difficulty (Aroca, Molnar et al. 2013) and the risk of aesthetic failure. (Clauser, Nieri et al. 2003).

Nart, J. *et al.* (2012), in a case series study, evaluated the use of subepitelital connective tissue graft in combination with coronally advanced flap for the treatment of Miller Class II and III gingival recessions in mandibular incisors. At baseline, in Miller Class III gingival recession, mean gingival recession was 5,14 ± 2,41 mm and, after 1 year follow up, the mean gingival recession residual was 0,85 ± 1,06 mm, which corresponds to a gingival recession reduction of 4,29 ± 1,35 mm. They observed that the teeth with Miller Class III gingival recessions obtained a mean root coverage of 86,41 ± 13,70% and a complete root coverage of 42,85%, after 12 months of follow-up. (Nart, Valles et al. 2012).

Aroca, S. *et al.* (2010), in a randomized-clinical trial, evaluated whether a modified tunnel technique with a connective tissue graft, combined with enamel matrix derivative (test group), improve the treatment of multiple class III gingival recessions when compared with the same technique alone (control group). At baseline, in control group, mean gingival recession was 3,2 ± 1,4 mm and, after 1 year follow up, the mean gingival recession residual was 0,6 ± 0,9 mm, which corresponds to a

mean gingival recession reduction of 2,6 ± 0,5 mm. They observed that, in control group, the mean root coverage was 83 ± 26% and the complete root coverage was 40%, from baseline to 1 year post-surgery. (Aroca, Molnar *et al.* 2013).

In our study, we treated Miller class III, single gingival recessions in incisors (maxillary and mandibular) with VISTA technique combined with a connective tissue graft, despite VISTA technique have been described to treat multiple gingival recessions, in aesthetic zone, by Zadeh *et al.* (2011).

At baseline, mean gingival recession was 3,27 ± 1,33 mm and, after 6 months follow up, the mean gingival recession residual was 0,78 ± 0,85 mm, which corresponds to a mean gingival recession reduction of 2,49 ± 0,58 mm. We observed that mean root coverage was 81,28 ± 19,00% and complete root coverage was 33,33%, from baseline to 6 months post-surgery.

Although Nart *et al.* (2012), the group of Miller Class III gingival recessions have on average about 2 mm deeper than the sample of Aroca *et al.* (2013) and our sample, the mean depth of the residual gingival recessions obtained in T2 by all the authors was relatively similar (standard deviation of approximately 0.13 mm).

Regarding to the reduction of gingival recession observed in those three clinical studies, the relationship between the depth of gingival recession at baseline and the final root coverage is a controversial topic in the literature. (de Sanctis and Clementini 2014) There are literature reviews that conclude that a deeper gingival recession is associated with a low percentage of complete root coverage or partial root coverage. (Roccuzzo, Bunino et al. 2002, Clauser, Nieri et al. 2003, Nieri, Rotundo et al. 2009) On the other hand, some clinical studies have observed that deeper recessions present greater reductions when treated. (Zucchelli, Clauser *et al.* 1998, Zucchelli and De Sanctis 2000, Cortellini, Tonetti *et al.* 2009) These latest findings be in accordance with our results and with the results reported by Nart *et al.* (2012) and Aroca *et al.* (2013).

Since Miller (1985), it has been kept in mind that the predictability of root coverage in Miller Class III gingival recessions is uncertain and, thus, Miller stated that this type of gingival recessions only achieved partial coverage and concluded that interdental bone loss is a limiting factor in the predictability of gingival recession treatment. (Miller 1985).

Our study presents promising outcomes according to root coverage, in this type of recessions, and although has been inferior to the percentage of root coverage and to the percentage of complete root coverage outcomes, be in agreement with the observed clinical outcomes of Nart *et al.* (2012) and Aroca *et al.* (2013).

The applied methodology not only allows measurement of soft-tissue volume alterations but also to quantify the gingival thickening that were surgically established above the surfaces of the roots previously exposed. This method offers several great advantages, including its non-invasive character as well as an excellent accuracy and high reproducibility of measurements. (Lehmann, Kasaj *et al.* 2012, Schneider, Ender et al. 2014).

Rebele *et al.* (2014), in a randomized clinical trial, evaluated with a 3D digital measuring methods the healing dynamics and gingival dimensions at sites treated with a tunnel technique and a connective tissue graft or a coronally advacend flap with enamel matrix derivative. They reported that the measured mean gingival thickening after 12 months, in tunnel group, was 1,63 mm.

In our study, mean gingival thickening obtained, after 6 months of healing, was 1.17 ± 0.36 mm. These results show a high difference in relation with results of Rebele *et al.* (2014), which can be explained by the use of different volumetric measurement protocols or more probably related to differences in graft size, as well as the histological composition or the quality (as a consequence of the donor area) of the grafts used. (Zucchelli, Mele *et al.* 2010).

From our results of the gingival thickening, it can be stated with caution that the greater increase of the gingival thickness and the greater recession reduction at T2, being in agreement with results of Rebele *et al.* (2014).

Regarding the correlation of gingival thickening and% RC at T2, our observations are against the findings reported by Rebele *et al.* (2014). In our study, we observed that the higher the root coverage, the smaller the mean gingival thickness on previously exposed root surfaces, which can be explained by the use of different volumetric measurement protocols.

Our volumetric study performed in all 3 patients treated with VISTA+CTG technique in order to monitor healing dynamics of the intervened tissues, from T0 to T1 and T1 to T2, observed a mean gingival thickening of $1,12 \pm 0,32$ at T1 (that corresponds to 100%). The treated sites showed a mean volumetric gain of $104,25 \pm 2,34\%$ (corresponding to a mean gingival thickness of $1,17 \pm 0,36$ mm), from T1 to T2. There was a considerable increase in gingival thickness between T0 and T1, and there was a residual increase until the end of the follow-up period (T2). With regard to post-operative gingival volume changes, the healing process seemed to be accomplished from 3 to 6 months.

5 CONCLUSIONS

In spite of all limitations of this research, such as the reduced sample and follow-up, the following conclusions can be referred:

- The innovative methodology used in this study ensures high metric precision in a volumetric evaluation of clinical results in comparison with traditional measurements methods;
- The results shows that this technique was predictable for the treatment of Miller Class III, single gingival recessions in incisors (maxillary and mandibular), and it may promote with success root coverage (average of $81,28 \pm 19,00\%$) and the increase of gingival thickness (average $1,17 \pm 0,36$ mm), within the follow-up time frame;
- With regard to post-operative gingival volume changes, there were a considerable increase in gingival thickness at 3 months and a residual increase between 3 and 6 months postoperatively. In this way, the healing process seemed to be accomplished from 3 to 6 months.
- It can be verified that the VISTA+CTG technique could increase the gingival thickness considerably and obtained promising results of root coverage in cases of Miller Class III, single gingival recessions. Based on these results, a similar or better behaviour can also be expected in Miller Class I and II gingival recessions, in aesthetic zone.

To reinforce our findings, more clinical studies are needed, with a longer follow-up period and a larger sample of patients. However, this research allowed us to take the first step toward validating the use of the VISTA+CTG technique in Miller Class III, single gingival recessions, in incisors.

REFERENCES

Agudio, G., P. Cortellini, J. Buti and G. Pini Prato (2016). "Periodontal Conditions of Sites Treated With Gingival Augmentation Surgery Compared With Untreated Contralateral Homologous Sites: An 18- to 35-Year Long-Term Study." *J Periodontol* **87**(12): 1371–1378.

Alldritt, W. (1968). Abnormal gingival form, SAGE Publications.

Aroca, S., T. Keglevich, D. Nikolidakis, I. Gera, K. Nagy, R. Azzi and D. Etienne (2010). "Treatment of class III multiple gingival recessions: a randomized-clinical trial." *J Clin Periodontol* **37**(1): 88–97.

Aroca, S., B. Molnar, P. Windisch, I. Gera, G.E. Salvi, D. Nikolidakis and A. Sculean (2013). "Treatment of multiple adjacent Miller class I and II gingival recessions with a Modified Coronally Advanced Tunnel (MCAT) technique and a collagen matrix or palatal connective tissue graft: a randomized, controlled clinical trial." *J Clin Periodontol* **40**(7): 713–720.

Baelum, V., O. Fejerskov and T. Karring (1986). "Oral hygiene, gingivitis and periodontal breakdown in adult Tanzanians." *Journal of periodontal research* **21**(3): 221–232.

Bernimoulin, J.P. and Z. Curilović (1977). "Gingival recession and tooth mobility." *Journal of clinical periodontology* **4**(2): 107–114.

Burkhardt, R. and M.B. Hurzeler (2000). "Utilization of the surgical microscope for advanced plastic periodontal surgery." *Pract Periodontics Aesthet Dent* **12**(2): 171–180; quiz 182.

Cairo, F., U. Pagliaro and M. Nieri (2008). "Treatment of gingival recession with coronally advanced flap procedures: a systematic review." *J Clin Periodontol* **35**(8 Suppl): 136–162.

Chambrone, L., F. Sukekava, M.G. Araújo, F.E. Pustiglioni, L.A. Chambrone and L.A. Lima (2010). "Root-coverage procedures for the treatment of localized recession-type defects: a Cochrane systematic review." *Journal of periodontology* **81**(4): 452–478.

Chatterjee, A., E. Sharma, G. Gundanavar and S.K. Subbaiah (2015). "Treatment of multiple gingival recessions with vista technique: A case series." *J Indian Soc Periodontol* **19**(2): 232–235.

Clauser, C., M. Nieri, D. Franceschi, U. Pagliaro and G. Pini-Prato (2003). "Evidence-based mucogingival therapy. Part 2: Ordinary and individual patient data meta-analyses of surgical treatment of recession using complete root coverage as the outcome variable." *J Periodontol* **74**(5): 741–756.

Cortellini, P., M. Tonetti, C. Baldi, L. Francetti, G. Rasperini, R. Rotundo, M. Nieri, D. Franceschi, A. Labriola and G. Pini Prato (2009). "Does placement of a connective tissue graft improve the outcomes of coronally advanced flap for coverage of single gingival recessions in upper anterior teeth? A multi centre, randomized, double blind, clinical trial." *Journal of clinical periodontology* **36**(1): 68–79.

de Sanctis, M. and M. Clementini (2014). "Flap approaches in plastic periodontal and implant surgery: critical elements in design and execution." *J Clin Periodontol* **41 Suppl 15**: S108–122.

Geiger, A.M. (1980). "Mucogingival problems and the movement of mandibular incisors: a clinical review." *American journal of Orthodontics* **78**(5): 511–527.

Gray, J.L. (2000). "When not to perform root coverage procedures." *J Periodontol* **71**(6): 1048–1050.

Lehmann, K.M., A. Kasaj, A. Ross, P.W. Kammerer, W. Wagner and H. Scheller (2012). "A new method for volumetric evaluation of gingival recessions: a feasibility study." *J Periodontol* **83**(1): 50–54.

Loe, H., A. Anerud and H. Boysen (1992). "The natural history of periodontal disease in man: prevalence, severity, and extent of gingival recession." *J Periodontol* **63**(6): 489–495.

Matas, F., J. Sentis and C. Mendieta (2011). "Ten-year longitudinal study of gingival recession in dentists." *J Clin Periodontol* **38**(12): 1091–1098.

Miller, P.D., Jr. (1985). "Root coverage using the free soft tissue autograft following citric acid application. III. A successful and predictable procedure in areas of deepwide recession." *Int J Periodontics Restorative Dent* **5**(2): 14–37.

Nart, J., C. Valles, S. Mareque, A. Santos, J. Sanz-Moliner and A. Pascual (2012). "Subepithelial connective tissue graft in combination with a coronally advanced flap for the treatment of Miller Class II and III gingival recessions in mandibular incisors: a case series." *Int J Periodontics Restorative Dent* **32**(6): 647–654.

Needleman, I.G. (2002). "A guide to systematic reviews." *J Clin Periodontol* **29 Suppl 3**: 6–9; discussion 37–38.

Nieri, M., R. Rotundo, D. Franceschi, F. Cairo, P. Cortellini and G. Pini Prato (2009). "Factors affecting the outcome of the coronally advanced flap procedure: a Bayesian network analysis." *Journal of periodontology* **80**(3): 405–410.

Rebele, S.F., O. Zuhr, D. Schneider, R.E. Jung and M.B. Hurzeler (2014). "Tunnel technique with connective tissue graft versus coronally advanced flap with enamel matrix derivative for root coverage: a RCT using 3D digital measuring methods. Part II. Volumetric studies on healing dynamics and gingival dimensions." *J Clin Periodontol* **41**(6): 593–603.

Ribeiro, F.S., D.L. Zandim, A.E. Pontes, R.V. Mantovani, J.E. Sampaio and E. Marcantonio (2008). "Tunnel technique with a surgical maneuver to increase the graft extension: case report with a 3-year follow-up." *J Periodontol* **79**(4): 753–758.

Roccuzzo, M., M. Bunino, I. Needleman and M. Sanz (2002). "Periodontal plastic surgery for treatment of localized gingival recessions: a systematic review." *J Clin Periodontol* **29 Suppl 3**: 178–194; discussion 195–176.

Sangnes, G. and P. Gjermo (1976). "Prevalence of oral soft and hard tissue lesions related to mechanical toothcleansing procedures." *Community Dentistry and Oral Epidemiology* **4**(2): 77–83.

Schneider, D., A. Ender, T. Truninger, C. Leutert, P. Sahrmann, M. Roos and P. Schmidlin (2014). "Comparison between clinical and digital soft tissue measurements." *J Esthet Restor Dent* **26**(3): 191–199.

Serino, G., J.L. Wennstrom, J. Lindhe and L. Eneroth (1994). "The prevalence and distribution of gingival recession in subjects with a high standard of oral hygiene." *J Clin Periodontol* **21**(1): 57–63.

Thalmair, T., S. Fickl and H. Wachtel (2016). "Coverage of Multiple Mandibular Gingival Recessions Using Tunnel Technique with Connective Tissue Graft: A Prospective Case Series." *Int J Periodontics Restorative Dent* **36**(6): 859–867.

Watson, P.J. (1984). "Gingival recession." *J Dent* **12**(1): 29–35.

Wennstrom, J.L. (1994). Mucogingival surgery. *Proceedings of the 1st European Workshop on Periodontology*. N.P. Lang and T. Karring. London, Quintessence: 193–209.

Wennstrom, J.L. (1996). "Mucogingival therapy." *Ann Periodontol* **1**(1): 671–701.

Wennstrom, J.L., J. Lindhe, F. Sinclair and B. Thilander (1987). "Some periodontal tissue reactions to orthodontic tooth movement in monkeys." *J Clin Periodontol* **14**(3): 121–129.

Zadeh, H.H. (2011). "Minimally invasive treatment of maxillary anterior gingival recession defects by vestibular incision subperiosteal tunnel access and platelet-derived growth factor BB." *Int J Periodontics Restorative Dent* **31**(6): 653–660.

Zucchelli, G., C. Clauser, M. De Sanctis and M. Calandriello (1998). "Mucogingival versus guided tissue regeneration procedures in the treatment of deep recession type defects." *Journal of periodontology* **69**(2): 138–145.

Zucchelli, G. and M. De Sanctis (2000). "Treatment of multiple recession-type defects in patients with esthetic demands." *J Periodontol* **71**(9): 1506–1514.

Zucchelli, G., M. Mele, M. Stefanini, C. Mazzotti, M. Marzadori, L. Montebugnoli and M. de Sanctis (2010). "Patient morbidity and root coverage outcome after subepithelial connective tissue and de-epithelialized grafts: a comparative randomized-controlled clinical trial." *J Clin Periodontol* **37**(8): 728–738.

Zucchelli, G. and I. Mounssif (2015). "Periodontal plastic surgery." *Periodontol 2000* **68**(1): 333–368.

Zuhr, O., S.F. Rebele, D. Schneider, R.E. Jung and M.B. Hurzeler (2014). "Tunnel technique with connective tissue graft versus coronally advanced flap with enamel matrix derivative for root coverage: a RCT using 3D digital measuring methods. Part I. Clinical and patient-centred outcomes." *J Clin Periodontol* **41**(6): 582–592.

Biodental Engineering V – Belinha et al. (Eds)
© 2019 Taylor & Francis Group, London, ISBN 978-0-367-21087-8

3D analysis of rest seats in clinical environment

M. Pimenta
Institute of Health Sciences, Universidade Católica Portuguesa, Viseu, Portugal

F. Araujo, T. Marques, P. Fonseca & A. Correia
Centre of Interdisciplinary Research in Health, Institute of Health Sciences, Universidade Católica Portuguesa, Viseu, Portugal

ABSTRACT: Introduction: rest seats are used in Removable Prosthodontics to provide indirect retention for the removable partial dentures and to transfer the forces through the long axis of the abutment tooth. Materials and methods: the rest seats were scanned with *Dental Wings® Model DW-IO-001* Intraoral Scan (IOS) and were analyzed the bucco-lingual distance, the mesio-distal distance, thickness and angle formed by the occlusal support and the vertical part of the minor connector. Results: seventeen rest seats were observed and grouped according to teeth groups. Bucco-Lingual (BL) distance of the oclusal rest seats prepared present correct values, excluding canines. The Mesio-Distal (MD) distance is correctly done only in canines and superior premolars. In terms of thicknesses, no rest seat preparation was done according to the guidelines, being more shallow. Only the angle of the rest support surface with the tooth axial wall in inferior premolars was correctly done (<90°). Conclusions: the methodology used in this research to analyse the rest seat dimensions enables us to obtain results with high metric precision. Special care must be taken when supervising students in order to improve clinical results.

1 INTRODUCTION

Rest seats are dental preparations made on a tooth, or a restoration, in order to receive occlusal, lingual or cingular rests. (Driscoll et al. 2017) This rest seats contribute to the support of the dental prosthesis, avoid occlusal interference, reduce the prominence of the rests and also prevent the incidence of lateral harmful forces to the periodontal structures. (Davenport et al. 2001).

The rests are one of the components of a removable partial denture whose main function is to transfer forces through the long axis of the abutment tooth, thus having specific shape and size to prevent support fractures. (Sato et al. 2003) In addition, it can provide indirect retention for the prosthesis keeping it stable. (Rice et al. 2011).

The forces transmitted from the prosthesis to an abutment tooth are directed apically down the long axis of the tooth so that stress can be absorbed by the fibers of the periodontal ligament without damaging it or the supporting bone. (Phoenix, Cagna, and DeFreest 2008).

An oclusal rest seat should comply with some general parameters described in the literature: spoon-saucer shape; minimum 2–2,5 mm wide bucco-lingually and occupy approximately ½ of the tooth from cusp tip to cusp tip; mesio-distally dimension between one-third and one-half of the tooth crown; and thickness should be approximately 1,5 mm. The angle formed by the occlusal support and the vertical part of the minor connector that contacts the interproximal surface, should be less than 90 degrees. (Phoenix, Cagna, and DeFreest 2008) (Carr and Brown 2011).

The preparation of an anterior tooth to receive a cingular rest seat should be: a slightly rounded V form prepared on the lingual surface with the apex to incisal at the junction of the gingival third and the middle third of the tooth. (Carr and Brown 2011).

The ideal dimensions of the preparation for cingular rests are: 2.5 to 3 mm mesio-distal length; 2 mm wide vestibular-lingual and inciso-apical depth a minimum of 1.5 mm. (Carr and Brown 2011) (Nagayassu et al. 2005).

The aim of this study was to quantify the reduction of rest seats performed by dental students.

2 MATERIALS AND METHODS

Rest seats were randomly chosen within a convenience sample of patients within the Removable Prosthodontics Unit of the University Dental Clinic. Rests were prepared by students in the final year of the DMD course, that had previously lessons/instructions (theoretical and hands-on on teeth models) on how to prepare them. The clinical procedure was supervised by a clinical Professor.

The rest seats scan was done with *Dental Wings® Model DW-IO-001* intraoral scan (IOS). The scanning process was done in accordance with the scanner manufacturer's guidelines and instruction manuals. Two scans were made: before and after rest seats preparation.

All scans were exported in STL format, which is compatible with most 3D modeling software.

Geomagic Control X® software was used for the 3D analysis of tooth dimensions, as seen on Figure 1. The variables analysed were: buccolingual (BL) distance, mesio-distal (MD) distance, rest depth and angle of the rest support surface with the tooth axial wall.

Seventeen rest seats were observed and grouped according to teeth groups (canines, premolar and molars). The results of the analysis of the dimensions mentioned in the material and methods section are presented in Table 1.

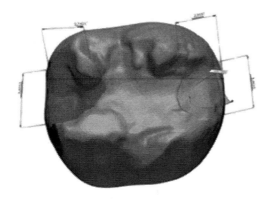

Figure 1. 3D reconstruction of the occlusal rest seat scanned with Dental Wings IOS.

Table 1. Dimensions of the prepared rest seats. (BL: buccal-lingual; MD: mesio-distal).

Rest seat	BL	MD	Thickness	Angle
Canine (superior)	2,7 (31,5%)	2,8 (36,4%)	0,8	NA
Premolar (superior)	2,7 (29,3%)	2,2 (32,9%)	0,7	92,5
2nd Molar (superior)	3,4 (29,9%)	2,4 (24,5%)	0,8	90,9
Premolar (inferior)	2,7 (38%)	2,1 (28%)	0,5	85,4
2nd Molar (inferior)	3,6 (37,9%)	3,0 (28,7%)	0,8	110

Cells with grey shadow represent incorrect values. NA: non aplicable.

The bucco-lingual (BL) distance of the oclusal rest seats prepared present correct values, according to the guidelines taught in the Removable Prosthodontics. Concerning to canines, the value is superior to the intended.

The mesio-distal (MD) distance is correctly done only in canines and superior premolars. The second molars and inferior premolar present values lower than the guidelines.

In terms of thicknesses, no rest seat preparation was done according to the guidelines, being the rest seats more shallow.

Also, the angle of the rest support surface with the tooth axial wall is predominantly not according to the guidelines, being over 90°. Only the angle in inferior premolars was correctly done (<90°). Results obtained with superior premolars and superior second molars were close to the guidelines, but the angle of inferior second molars largely exceed the guidelines.

3 DISCUSSION

Literature presents guidelines for rest seat preparations. This guidelines were determined according to the thickness of tooth enamel, mechanical properties of the seats and biomechanical characteristics of the prosthetic rehabilitation. The noncompliance of this factors may lead to the failure of the prosthetic rehabilitation or even compromise the survival of tooth structures. Special care must be taken on dental education to obtain success in this clinical procedures. (Carr and Brown 2011) (Phoenix, Cagna, and DeFreest 2008).

In this study we intended to evaluate students preparations of this rest seats. Concerning to thickness, the values found may be related to the fact that students are more inexperienced and, in consequence, more careful doing teeth reduction, trying not to reach dentin.

In the angle the discrepancy of the values may also be related to the student's inexperience, and lack of visual notion in the preparation of this particular issue.

4 CONCLUSIONS

Within the limits of this preliminary research we may conclude that: – the methodology used in this research to analyse the rest seat dimensions enables us to obtain results with high metric precision; – special care must be taken when supervising students doing preparations of thickness and support surface of the rest seats, in order to improve clinical results.

REFERENCES

Carr, Alan B, and David T Brown. 2011. *McCracken's Removable Partial Prostodontics.*

Davenport, J.C., R.M. Basker, J.R. Heath, J.P. Ralph, P-O. Glantz, and P. Hammond. 2001. "Tooth Preparation." *British Dental Journal* 190 (6):288–94.

Driscoll, Carl F, Martin A Freilich, Albert D Guckes, Kent L Knoernschild, Thomas J Mcgarry, Gary Goldstein, Charles Goodacre, et al. 2017. "The Glossary of Prosthodontic Terms." *The Journal of Prosthetic Dentistry-Ninth Edition* 117 (55):1–105. https://doi.org/10.1016/j.prosdent.2016.12.001.

Nagayassu, Marcos Paulo, Júlio Tadashi Murakami, Lafayette Nogueira Junior, Carlos Augusto Pavanelli, and Eduardo Shigueyuki Uemura. 2005. "A Clinical Study of the Fit of Cast Cingulum Rests for Removable Partial Denture." *Cienc Odontol Bras* 8 (3):22–28.

Phoenix, Rodney D., David R. Cagna, and Charles F. DeFreest. 2008. *Stewart's Clinical Removable Partial Prosthodontics.* 4th Editio.

Rice, J.A., C.D. Lynch, R. Mcandrew, and P.J. Milward. 2011. "Tooth Preparation for Rest Seats for Cobalt-Chromium Removable Partial Dentures Completed by General Dental Practitioners." *Journal of Oral Rehabilitation* 38 (1):72–78. https://doi.org/10.1111/j.1365-2842.2010.02130.x.

Sato, Yuuji, Nobuaki Shindoi, Katsunori Koretake, and Ryuji Hosokawa. 2003. "The Effect of Occlusal Rest Size and Shape on Yield Strength." *Journal of Prosthetic Dentistry* 89 (5):503–7. https://doi.org/10.1016/S0022-3913(03)52739-6.

Biodental Engineering V – Belinha et al. (Eds)
© 2019 Taylor & Francis Group, London, ISBN 978-0-367-21087-8

Hyaluronic acid vs chlorhexidine in mandibular molar extractions

A.A. Martins, B. Leitão, T. Borges, M. Pereira & A. Correia
Instituto de Ciências da Saúde, Universidade Católica Portuguesa, Viseu, Portugal

R. Figueiredo
Department of Oral Surgery, Faculty of Odontology, University of Barcelona, Spain

ABSTRACT: The search for an ideal antimicrobial agent has been studied in several health areas. Chlorhexidine has been widely used in the post-surgical period and is currently considered the gold standard.

The search for new agents has highlighted hyaluronic acid in several areas of medicine, and good results have already been obtained in dentistry, particularly in the area of periodontology. The aim of this research was to do a comparative evaluation of the single intra-alveolar application of hyaluronic acid gel 0.2% vs. chlorhexidine gel 0.2%, in the postoperative period of mandibular molar extractions. Within the limitations of this study, particularly the size of the sample, it was verified that hyaluronic acid seems to present more favorable results concerning extra-oral edema.

1 INTRODUCTION

The search for an ideal antimicrobial agent has been studied in several health areas. Chlorhexidine has been widely used in the post-surgical period and is currently considered the gold standard. The action of antiseptic substances, such as chlorhexidine, is recommended in protocols of several fields of medicine, namely in dentistry, due to its good bactericidal and bacteriostatic performance. Its properties of low toxicity, easy access, low cost and broad spectrum of action are characteristics that make chlorhexidine the most used antiseptic in the area of dentistry. (Rubio-Palau et al., 2015, Singh et al., 2014) Currently, research on other therapeutic alternatives has been increasingly targeted. An example of this research is the application of hyaluronic acid in dental medicine.

The hyaluronic acid has a great anti-inflammatory capacity through molecular mechanisms of tissue repair and healing, besides the capacity of activation of inflammatory cells, being, in this way able to trigger an immune response. (Dahiya and Kamal, 2013)

The search for new agents has highlighted hyaluronic acid in several areas of medicine, and good results have already been obtained in dentistry, particularly in the area of periodontology. (Cheng et al., 2008, Rubio-Palau et al., 2015) The aim of this research was to do a comparative evaluation of the single intra-alveolar application of hyaluronic acid gel 0.2% vs. chlorhexidine gel 0.2%, in the postoperative period of mandibular molar extractions.

2 MATERIALS AND METHODS

Randomized, double-blinded, controlled clinical trial with current reference substance. The target population of this study comprised all the patients of the Oral Surgery Unit observed in the University Dental Clinic of *Universidade Católica Portuguesa* in Viseu. The patients were selected according to inclusion and exclusion criteria (Table 1).

The study was conducted during the 2016/2017 school year, with approval of the Bioethics Institute of the Portuguese Catholic University—Porto. The sample was calculated using G.Power software: alpha value 0.05, statistical power 80%. The result was 74 (37/group). The sample obtained to date included 33 patients so the results were considered preliminary. The patients were randomly assigned in 2 groups: 19 in group 1, with an intra-alveolar application of hyaluronic acid gel (0.2%) and 14 in group 2 with an intra-alveolar application of chlorhexidine gel (0.2%), after the exodontia. The study comprised 2 clinical times: T0 – clinical data record and exodontia; T1 – postoperative evaluation of the variables: pain at 3 and 8 days, need for ibuprofen intake, occurrence of dry alveolitis, halitosis, hemorrhage, hematoma, trismus and extra-oral edema. Statistical analysis was performed in the SPSS software

Table 1. Inclusion and exclusion criteria.

Inclusion	Exclusion
– Voluntary patients of the University Clinic of the Portuguese Catholic University of Viseu, who completed and signed the informed consent term; – Patients with indication of unitary extraction of mandibular molars;	– Patients classified as ASA III or higher; – Hypersensitivity to any substance used in the design of this study (0.2% hyaluronic acid gel or 0.2% chlorhexidine gel, ibuprofen, Supramid); – Acute or chronic infectious pathology at the moment of exodontia (apical abscesses, cysts or granulomas); – Diabetic or immunode pressed patients; – Patients who take analgesic, anti-inflammatory, antiaggregant or chronic anticoagulant medication; – Pregnant and/or breastfeeding women; – Patients who have or have had therapy with oral or injectable bisphosphonates; – Operating time greater than 45 minutes;

(v.24) through descriptive and inferential statistical tests (Mann-Whitney test and Fisher's exact test).

Null hypothesis: no difference in clinical occurrences in the postoperative period of mandibular molar extractions after the application of hyaluronic acid vs clorhexidine gel.

3 APPLICATION OF THE EXPERIMENTAL PROTOCOL IN THE UNIVERSITY CLINIC MATERIALS AND METHODS

3.1 T0 (day of extraction)

After the selection of the patient and formal verification of the inclusion and exclusion criteria and obtaining written informed consent, the following procedures were performed in T0 (day of the extraction): completion of individual patient identification card, review of clinical history, operative planning and procedure described in the following paragraphs.

Once the anesthetic technique was performed (the anesthetic used was ARTINIBSA (72 mg/1.8 ml + 0.018 mg/1.8 ml) in 1.8 ml cartridges supplied by: Laboratorios Inibsa SA, SINTRA BUSINESS PARK, Zona Industrial da Abrunheira, Edificio

1–2ºI, 2710-089 Sintra—Portugal)) periodontal fibers involving the tooth were discontinued, dislocation of the tooth using levers, dislocation and avulsion with levers and forceps, and alveolar curettage.

Fill the dental alveolus with the gel prepared by the research assistant, randomly assigned to each patient using the surgical curette.

Surgical wound closure using through cross stitch with a Supramid wire, 4/0 SMI in commercial boxes of 12 threads each (lot 160501, valid until 2021/05), provided by ANTÃO Medical, Rua da industria, lote 5, Lugar da Póvoa, Travanca, 3720-571 Travanca OAZ—Portugal. On top of the suture was applied the remaining gel and performed compression for 15 minutes with sterile gauze.

Prescription of 20 ibuprofen 600 mg tablets with the recommended dosage of 1 tablet every 12 hours, as long as there was pain. The patient was instructed to bring the surplus tablets for T1 quantification (postoperative control day).

Explanation of the postoperative instructions, namely general care and expectations after extraction and specifically: do not chew or spit in the first 12 hours, do not use any local antiseptic up to T1, do not perform analgesic, anti-inflammatory or antibiotic medication that is not prescribed in T0.

Patients were also advised to contact the University Dental Clinic if there were any unexpected postoperative complications. In the event of any complication, the patient was examined by the principal investigator, the group to which he or she belonged and the indicated medical therapy was applied, regardless of whether or not to compromise the inclusion of the patient in this study, always safeguarding the patient's physical integrity. All the procedures performed were supervised by Oral Surgery Clinical Professors.

3.2 T0 (Postoperative evaluation consultation)

The postoperative evaluation of the selected variables and suture removal was performed at the postoperative control visit (T1), 8 days after surgery. In this consultation, the following variables were recorded: dry alveolitis, halitosis, hematoma, hemorrhage, trismus, and extra-oral edema; quantification of pain 3 and 8 days after surgery and the quantified need for ibuprofen 600 mg;

Binary categorical variables: dry alveolitis, halitosis, hematoma, hemorrhage, trismus, extraoral edema, presence of suture, presence of plaque in the suture and bleeding on removal of the suture were parameters assessed clinically and/or questioned to the patient and duly registered in T1 by the operator. The need to take ibuprofen 600 mg (discrete quantitative variable) was evaluated by questioning the patient.

The quantification of the continuous quantitative variable postoperative pain was done through a calibrated analogue visual scale of 100 mm at 3 and 8 days, respectively. It was explained to the patient that it was a calibrated scale in which the left end corresponded to "no pain" and the opposite end corresponded to "worst pain imaginable" and the patient was then asked to mark the pain felt at 3 and 8 days. At last it was measured on the scale and recorded the value of pain.

All patients who did not attend the control visit as well as patients who did not comply with the postoperative indications provided were excluded and reported in the results. During all these procedures no collection of biological material was performed.

4 RESULTS

This study had a population of 105 patients but only 33 were included (12 male and 21 female). The remaining 72 patients were excluded from the study according to the inclusion and exclusion criteria (Table 2).

Table 3 shows the age distribution of the sample. The mean age was 46.67 years, with a standard deviation of 20.177 years. The age range varies between 16 and 86 years.

Since the mean age of patients is 46.76, most of the extracted teeth were wisdom teeth as

Table 2. Sample and reasons for exclusion.

	Frequency	Percentage
Included	33	31,4%
Excluded for not attending the postoperative control appointment	10	9,5%
Excluded for not following postoperative therapeutic regimen	6	5,7%
Excluded by taking drugs that are included in the exclusion criteria	8	7,6%
Excluded due to presence of acute/chronic apical pathology at the moment of extraction	10	9,5%
Excluded for exceeding set operating time	13	12,4%
Excluded due to multiple extractions	12	11,4%
Excluded due to the need to prescribe other drugs than the ones on protocols	11	10,5%
Excluded for being underage	2	1,9%
Total	105	100%

Table 3. Distribution of patient ages.

	N	Minimum	Maximum	Average	Standard deviation
Age	33	16	86	46,76	20,177
Valid N* (listwise)	33				

*N = number of patients.

Table 4. Tooth extracted.

Tooth	Frequency	Percentage
36	5	15,2%
37	5	15,2%
38	9	27,3%
46	1	3,0%
47	3	9,1%
48	10	30,3%
Total	33	100%

Table 5. Inferential statistics related to the null hypothesis established.

Variable	H0: no impact of hyaluronic acid gel comparing with clorhexidine gel
Occurrence of dry alveolitis	0,424
Occurrence of halitosis	1,000
Occurrence of hemorrhage	0,024
Occurrence of hematoma	0,067
Occurrence trismus	0,056
Occurrence extra-oral edema	1,000
Pain at 3 days	0,170
Pain at 8 days	0,840
Need for ibuprofen intake	0,326
	(p < 0,05)

described in the Table 3, according to the FDI classification.

Analyzing the statistical inference, we can see tha there was no statistically significant difference for all variables analyzed except for the occurrence of extra-oral edema (Table 5). For this variable, there is statistical evidence ($p = 0.024$) that the applied substance influences the occurrence of this complication. No adverse reactions were verified in relation to the substances used.

The application of hyaluronic acid, besides the physical barrier that establishes against the bacteria and its action in the extracellular matrix has the capacity to induce the formation of granulation tissue inhibiting the inflammation. This ability can be attributed to the action that hyaluronic acid has on bacterial hyaluronidases, deactivating them, and to the normalization of the macro-aggregation of proteoglycans of the connective tissue, being through these actions that an anti-edema effect is created. (Cortivo et al., 1986, Dahiya and Kamal, 2013, Gocmen et al., 2015, Gontiya and Galgali, 2012, Salwowska et al., 2016, Sapna and Vandana, 2011).

5 CONCLUSIONS

Within the limitations of this study, the results obtained show no statistically significant difference between the substances, considering the concentrations used, in the variables under analysis except for the occurrence of extra-oral edema. For this variable the results suggest that hyaluronic acid is superior to chlorhexidine reducing the occurrence of this postoperative complication. There was no adverse reaction to any of the gels

The 0.2% hyaluronic acid gel presented as a viable alternative to 0.2% chlorhexidine gel, currently considered the gold standard for topical application after exodontia.

In order for the results of this work to be published and validated, the sample will, of course, have to reach the values calculated and exposed previously. The authors intend to complete the study over the next year, continuing the established protocol.

The commercial and clinical implications of the results will be important in the development of products for intraoral topical application in post-surgical periods in the fields of oral surgery, periodontics, implantology as well as in the establishment of clinical protocols aimed at optimizing the postoperative period by reducing complications and morbidity of patients.

REFERENCES

Cheng, R.H., Leung, W.K. & Corbet, E.F. 2008. Non-surgical periodontal therapy with adjunctive chlorhexidine use in adults with down syndrome: a prospective case series. *J Periodontol*, 79, 379–85.

Cortivo, R., De Galateo, A., Haddad, M., Caberlotto, M. & Abatangelo, G. 1986. [Glycosaminoglycans in human normal gingiva and in periodontosis: biochemical and histological observations]. *G Stomatol Ortognatodonzia*, 5, 69–72.

Dahiya, P. & Kamal, R. 2013. Hyaluronic Acid: a boon in periodontal therapy. *N Am J Med Sci*, 5, 309–15.

Gocmen, G., Gonul, O., Oktay, N.S., Yarat, A. & Goker, K. 2015. The antioxidant and anti-inflammatory efficiency of hyaluronic acid after third molar extraction. *J Craniomaxillofac Surg*, 43, 1033–7.

Gontiya, G. & Galgali, S.R. 2012. Effect of hyaluronan on periodontitis: A clinical and histological study. *J Indian Soc Periodontol*, 16, 184–92.

Rubio-Palau, J., Garcia-Linares, J., Hueto-Madrid, J.A., Gonzalez-Lagunas, J., Raspall-Martin, G. & Mareque-Bueno, J. 2015. Effect of intra-alveolar placement of 0.2% chlorhexidine bioadhesive gel on the incidence of alveolar osteitis following the extraction of mandibular third molars. A double-blind randomized clinical trial. *Med Oral Patol Oral Cir Bucal*, 20, e117–22.

Salwowska, N.M., Bebenek, K.A., Zadlo, D.A. & Wcislo-Dziadecka, D.L. 2016. Physiochemical properties and application of hyaluronic acid: a systematic review. *J Cosmet Dermatol*, 15, 520–526.

Sapna, N. & Vandana, K.L. 2011. Evaluation of hyaluronan gel (Gengigel((R))) as a topical applicant in the treatment of gingivitis. *J Investig Clin Dent*, 2, 162–70.

Singh, H., Kapoor, P., Dhillon, J. & Kaur, M. 2014. Evaluation of three different concentrations of Chlorhexidine for their substantivity to human dentin. *Indian J Dent*, 5, 199–201.

Biodental Engineering V – Belinha et al. (Eds)
© 2019 Taylor & Francis Group, London, ISBN 978-0-367-21087-8

Research of oral health information by patients of a University dental clinic

H. Costa
Institute of Health Sciences, Universidade Católica Portuguesa, Viseu, Portugal
Health Sciences Research Centre—Faculty of Health Sciences, Beira Interior University, Covilhã, Portugal

B. Oliveira, A. Oliveira & A. Correia
Centre for Interdisciplinary Research in Health (CIIS), Institute of Health Sciences,
Universidade Católica Portuguesa, Viseu, Portugal

ABSTRACT: The World Wide Web is a big repository of information, where generic information is mixed with health information. Health information seekers are increasing in the Internet, looking for information related to general health and also oral health. As so, the aim of this study was to determine the use of the Internet by patients in a university dental clinic to obtain information about their oral health needs and treatment. A questionnaire (adapted from Riordáin, 2009) (1) was applied to patients of the University Dental Clinic of the *Universidade Católica Portuguesa*. The sample consisted of 100 individuals. It was found that 50% of patients had access to the Internet daily, but only 43% of patients sought or had a family member or friend who sought out their oral condition. Of the patients surveyed, 64% are familiar with the use of the Internet in their daily lives and approximately 1 in 2 (36 in 64 patients) use the Internet to research their oral health condition. The internet seems to represent a tool for obtaining relevant information. The dentist/patient doctor relationship has changed since the onset of the internet.

1 INTRODUCTION

In recent years, technological evolution has led to a profound transformation that has guided to an exponential growth in the speed and quantity of information available and access to it. If television was, until a decade ago, the main vehicle of information transmission, today, the Internet has reached a potential that was unimaginable a few years ago. In Portugal, the coverage of last generation mobile networks available is higher than the European average.

The health area is perhaps the area where the most available information has been developed, television programs are dedicated to this theme, apps are produced to monitor and provide information related to health, and on the Internet there are numerous websites and blogs dedicated to health. Obviously, this will not be unrelated to the fact that health has become one of man's main concerns.

There is some evidence of the relationship between the disease in the individual and the search for information on the Internet by him or his relatives. (2) The strong motivation to search for information on the Internet on certain diseases has led to the formation of groups with different pathologies with common interests that share their experiences and all the information related to the disease. (2,3)

The Dentist/patient relationship is not alien to all this evolution and the relationship has been changing over the last few years. The patient nowadays has access to a lot of information, however accessing this information does not always have the capacity to filter, leading to a misinformation that could generate conflicts between the health professional and the patient. (4) Much of the available information is not subject to any review by experts. In this way, misinformation is much more likely than the actual understanding of the facts. (3) The "informed" patient ultimately contributes more accurately to the final decision regarding some procedure proposed by the Dentist and, in some way, will oblige the Dentist to be constantly updated and more available for making more shared decisions. (5) Although the Internet is unlikely to supplant the role of the doctor, it clearly already plays an important role in obtaining health information. It represents a source with unprecedented diversity of information and, because it is private, it becomes particularly important and relevant to many young people. (6)

The main objective of this study was to determine the level of Internet use by patients who are attending a University Dental Clinic to obtain information about their oral health condition, as well as the possible treatment to be performed.

Another aim of the study was to investigate the interest in doing dental consultations online, as well as in dental care in other countries, "dental tourism", since some studies point to an increase in this type of tourism.

2 MATERIALS AND METHODS

A questionnaire (adapted from Riordaine, 2009) (1) was applied to patients from the University Dental Clinic of the *Universidade Católica Portuguesa* in Viseu, Portugal. The number was randomly assigned to 145 patients during the period between March 17, 2017 and April 7, 2018. Patients participating in the study agreed to participate in it. The invitation was made by 14 questions: 12 multiple choice and 2 short answer. The accomplishment of a questionnaire adapted to the patients of the university clinic focused on the following questions: specialty of the consultation; age and gender of the patient; level of education [ISCED classification (7)]; if it was her first time attending the university dental clinic; Internet access (home, work and or public place); reason for the consultation; use of the Internet on a day-to-day basis; Internet search about the dental condition and, if yes, which search engines were used; in the case of a negative answer, if any family or friend did the patient research; Reasons for getting information about your health (improve knowledge about health status or treatment, reduce anxiety, accept the problem, try other medicines or alternative treatments, look for people with similar problems or follow the same treatment); quality of the information obtained; resorting to the Internet to search for information about the health problem or dental problems and treatment; if the patient would consider the possibility of consulting a Dentist on the Internet; if the patient would accept to do dental tourism. The completed questionnaire is attached. The questionnaires answered were saved and a descriptive statistics performed with Excel®Microsoft software.

3 RESULTS

After obtaining all the questionnaires, the sample had a total of 145 respondents, and the questionnaires were all accepted for the study. The mean age of the patients was 45.6 years, with a range between 12 and 88 years. A significant number of respondents completed the questionnaire: 82 female patients and 63 male patients. The level of education was registed mainly in the form of tertiary education [ISCED levels 5–8 (40,0%)], followed by primary education [ISCED levels 1–2 (33,8%)] and, finally, secondary education [ISCED levels 3–4 (24,1%)].

Figure 1 represents the categorization level of patients' education. Of the questionnaires validated for the study, 95 (65,5%) were described as not being the first time attending the university clinic, but 50 (34,5%) answered that they were new patients in the clinic. According to the total of respondents, 13,1% (n = 14) of the patients attended the clinic in the areas of prosthodontics and occlusion; 31,7% (n = 28) of the patients attended the clinic in the area of periodontology; 30,3% (n = 27) of the patients attended the clinic in the dentistry area; 15,2% (n = 19) of the patients attended the clinic in the area of surgery; 3,4% (n = 5) of the patients attended the clinic in the endodontic area; and 6,2% (n = 7) of the patients attended the clinic because of a control visit. Table 1 represents the categorization of consultation reasons.

Most of the patients interviewed use the Internet on a daily basis (60,7%), but only 39,3% (n = 57) do not use the Internet. Of the patients who have daily access to the Internet, most (37,2%) have access at home, at work and in a public place, however 21% have only access at home, 9,7% have access at home and at work, 8,3% access at home and in a public place and 1,4% have access only at work.

Figure 2 shows the ways in which respondents access the Internet. Table 2 represents the reasons

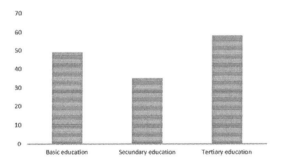

Figure 1. Categorization level of patients' education.

Table 1. Categorization of consultation reasons.

Clinic area	Condition	N	%
Prosthodontics and occlusion	Prosthesis' adjustment	6	4,1%
	Prosthesis' confection	9	6,2%
	Occlusal problems	4	2,8%
Periodontology	Periodontal disease	7	4,8%
	Ultrasonic scaling	39	26,9%
Dentistry	Dental cavity	14	9,7%
	Dental fracture	6	4,1%
	Toothache	24	16,6%
Surgery	Dental extraction	22	15,2%
Endodontic	Devitalization	5	3,4%
Control visit	Control visit	9	6,2%

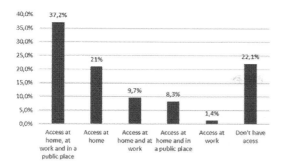

Figure 2. Ways in which respondents access the Internet.

Table 2. Reasons why patients searched the Internet, taking into account the percentage of patients who have daily access to the Internet (n = 88).

Condition	N	%
Improve knowledge about health status or treatment	23	26,1%
Reduce anxiety	6	6,8%
Try alternative medicines or treatment options	3	3,4%
Improve knowledge about health status or treatment and reduce anxiety	9	10,2%
Improve knowledge about health status or treatment and reduce anxiety and help to accept problems	1	1,1%
Improve knowledge about health status or treatment, reduce anxiety and try alternative medicines or treatment options	1	1,1%
Improve knowledge about health status or treatment, try alternative medicines or treatment options, and seek other people with similar problems or follow the same treatment	1	1,1%
Improve knowledge about health status or treatment and try alternative medicines or treatment options	1	1,1%

why patients searched the Internet, taking into account the percentage of patients who have daily access to the Internet (n = 88). Of the patients interviewed, 71 (49,0%) did not inquire about their oral health condition and don't have access to the Internet; 21,0% have access to the Internet, but do not research about their oral health; 27,0% conducted a survey and only 3,0% of the respondents obtained information through a family member or friend who searched the Internet. Figure 3 shows whether or not patients researched their oral condition or procedure and whether or not they had daily access to the Internet. Given the percentage of respondents with daily access to the Internet (60,7%), Google was the search engine most used

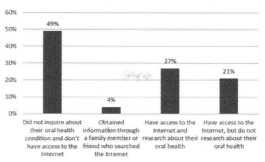

Figure 3. Whether or not patients researched their oral condition or procedure and whether or not they had daily access to the Internet.

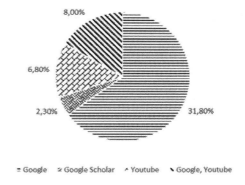

Figure 4. Categorization of search engines.

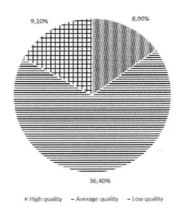

Figure 5. Quality of the information obtained by the patients.

by patients (31,8%) and 36,4% of patients using the Internet daily considered that information obtained was of average quality, 9,1% considered that the quality was low and 8,0% considered it to be high. Figures 4 and 5 represent the categorization of search engines and the quality of the information.

Forty-six (52,3%) of the patients who searched for information about their oral condition/ procedure via the Internet, would consider using it again, and only 28,3% would consult a Dentist on the Internet.

Patients when asked about the possibility of dental tourism, 71,7% were against, 22,1% agreed and 6,2% had no opinion.

4 DISCUSSION

With the increasing evolution and dissemination of telecommunication facilities and the ease of access to new technologies in both family, social and professional environments, we are now living in an increasingly interconnected world in which ordinary people have access to a panoply of daily information available for its own interpretation and judgment.

This raises the question that more and more patients entering the dental office are previously informed about their possible problem and what treatment they need. (8,9) This presents a challenge for the Dentist who must be up-to-date on the most innovative procedures but must be, also, prepared to receive and deal with these possible "misinformed" patients. (10) The amount of information available on the internet leads us to the question of the quality of the same. With this study, an effort was made to obtain a representative sample of the population that uses a university dental clinic. However, due to several factors, such as the compatibility of the timetables for the surveys and the reduced number of patients in the university clinic during the study period (March 17, 2017 and April 7, 2018), the sample obtained is lower than desired. This study has the peculiarity of having been carried out in a university dental clinic, with its own particularities, such as education levels and social and economic status of patients. Of the patients surveyed, 60,7% are familiar with the use of the Internet in their daily lives, which show us that even with a high mean age, almost everyone uses the Internet nowadays. Of the patients who have access to the Internet, more than 23,0% have researched to improve their knowledge about health status or treatment. With the increasing diversity of information available on the Internet, obtaining knowledge from patients is possible. However, not all patients are able to recognize and distinguish credible and scientific information from misinformation that may mislead the patient. (11)

In a study by Riordain and McCreary, 37% of patients showed interest in consulting a Dentist on the Internet. (1) A minor percentage responded affirmatively to the same question in our study, as can be seen from the analysis in Figure 6. At the end of the questionnaire, patients were asked to comment on the reasons why they would consult a Dentist on the Internet. However, none of the patients interviewed did so, so it makes it impossible for us to state the reasons chosen by each patient to answer the question. In the same article mentioned above, the patients who answered not to consult a Dentist on the internet mentioned as main reasons the lack of personal contact and the lack of trust associated with it. (1) The availability of information on the Internet by dental clinics has promoted an increased interest in combining vacations with some dental treatments, so the orientation of patients by health professionals regarding legal and ethical issues is fundamental. (1)

Recently, in a study by Kovacs and Szocska, it has been statistically proven that Hungary is one of the countries that receives patients from all over Europe, mainly from countries such as Germany, Austria and the United Kingdom. (12) According to the study, 70% of the patients surveyed said they did not want to experience dental tourism and only 23 patients said they were curious. Seven patients were in doubt whether they would experiment with treatments outside their country.

5 CONCLUSION

Online research of information by patients about the state of their oral health is a reality. It is beneficial for patients to improve their knowledge of their oral health status. However, this type of research entails some dangers, such as obtaining unreliable information or misinterpretation of it. Regarding the online consultation of a Dentist, the majority of patients do not show interest, demonstrating, in this way, that they value direct personal contact. (1) The current ease of travel around the world makes it quicker to carry out "dental tourism", so both Dentists and competent authorities must be aware of this phenomenon and create conditions so that treatments are carried out with the utmost clinical and ethical rigor.

REFERENCES

[1] Ní Ríordáin R, McCreary C. Dental patients' use of the Internet. Br Dent J [Internet]. 2009;207(12):583–6. Available from: http://dx.doi.org/10.1038/sj.bdj.2009.1137

[2] Berger M, Wagner TH, Baker LC. Internet use and stigmatized illness. Soc Sci Med [Internet]. 2005 Oct 1 [cited 2018 Apr 9];61(8):1821–7. Available from: https://www.sciencedirect.com/science/article/pii/S0277953605001206?via%3Dihub.

[3] Ziebland S. The importance of being expert: the quest for cancer information on the Inter-

net. Soc Sci Med [Internet]. 2004 Nov 1 [cited 2018 Apr 9];59(9):1783–93. Available from: https://www.sciencedirect.com/science/article/pii/S0277953604000784?via%3Dihub.

[4] Hardey M. Doctor in the house: the Internet as a source of lay health knowledge and the challenge to expertise. Sociol Heal Illn [Internet]. 1999;21(6):820–35. Available from: http://doi.wiley.com/10.1111/1467-9566.00185.

[5] Henwood F, Wyatt S, Hart A, Smith J. "Ignorance is bliss sometimes": Constraints on the emergence of the "informed patient" in the changing landscapes of health information. Sociol Heal Illn. 2003;25(6):589–607.

[6] Gray NJ, Klein JD, Noyce PR, Sesselberg TS, Cantrill JA. Health information-seeking behaviour in adolescence: the place of the internet. Soc Sci Med [Internet]. 2005 Apr 1 [cited 2018 Apr 9];60(7):1467–78. Available from: https://www.sciencedirect.com/science/article/pii/S0277953604003934?via%3Dihub.

[7] Eurostat. The EU in the world 2015. 2015. 154 p.

[8] Mattheos N. The Internet and the oral healthcare professionals: potential and challenges of a new era. Int J Dent Hyg. 2007;5(3):151–7.

[9] McMullan M. Patients using the Internet to obtain health information: How this affects the patient-health professional relationship. Patient Educ Couns. 2006;63(1–2):24–8.

[10] Harris CE, Chestnutt IG. CE Harris IG Chestnutt. Int J Dent Hyg. 2005;3:70–3.

[11] Balatsoukas P, Kennedy CM, Buchan I, Powell J, Ainsworth J. The role of social network technologies in online health promotion: A narrative review of theoretical and empirical factors influencing intervention effectiveness. J Med Internet Res. 2015;17(6):e141.

[12] Kovacs E, Szocska G. Vacation for your teeth' – Dental tourists in Hungary from the perspective of Hungarian dentists. Br Dent J [Internet]. 2013;215(8):415–8. Available from: http://dx.doi.org/10.1038/sj.bdj.2013.995.

Biodental Engineering V – Belinha et al. (Eds)
© 2019 Taylor & Francis Group, London, ISBN 978-0-367-21087-8

Effect of bleaching on microleakage of class V composite resin restorations – in vitro study

Tânia Pereira, A. Azevedo, M. Vasconcelos, Pedro Mesquita & Maria T. Carvalho
Faculty of Dental Medicine, Porto University, Portugal

Carlos F. Almeida
Institute of Health Sciences, Portuguese Catholic University, Viseu, Portugal

ABSTRACT: The purpose of this study is to evaluate the effect of bleaching on microleakage of class V resin composite restorations, both occlusal and gingival margins of enamel. One hundred and twenty-eight class V restorations were performed on buccal and lingual surfaces of 64 premolars. Half of them were restored with Synergy D6 and the other one with Filtek Supreme XTE. In all of them, 5th generation adhesive XP Bond, Dentsply® was used. The teeth were submitted to thermal cycling and then divided into three groups: Group I – no bleaching, group II – bleaching with 38% hydrogen peroxide and group III – bleaching with 10% carbamide peroxide. Immersion was performed with 2% methylene blue dye and microleakage was measured according to ISO standards. Data was analyzed using the chi-square test. When composite restorations were submitted to bleaching, microleakage was only statistically significant on the gingival walls of buccal ($\rho < 0.009$) and lingual surfaces ($\rho < 0.002$). Bleaching with 38% hydrogen peroxide and 10% carbamide peroxide may increase microleakage on the gingival wall of class V resin composite restorations.

Keywords: tooth bleaching, dental leakage, composite dental resin, dental restoration

1 INTRODUCTION

Teeth whitening is a procedure that has developed during the last decades, and, is considered a conservative technique, as well as, one of the first choices for discolored teeth. (1). This popularity is due to be easy to use, accessible to the majority of the population compared to other aesthetic procedures and it has a good cost-benefit relationship. (2)

Dental whitening systems are not designed to lighten restorative materials. However, these materials may become a substrate of the bleaching treatment on account of his proximity to the areas to be lightened. There are several studies that had investigated the effect of bleaching products on resin composites, analyzing its porosity, roughness, micro and nanohardness after bleaching. (3, 4) However, few studies had analyzed the effect of bleaching agents on the adhesive interface tooth/restoration, laying out results still very controversial. (5–8) New restorative materials are constantly introduced in the market, improving resin composites with new features. It is necessary to continuously update the scientific literature on the performance of these materials under different conditions that they are submitted to.

The aim of this experimental in vitro study is to evaluate the relationship between 6 experimental groups: three bleaching procedures distributed by 2 resin composites: Synergy D6 and Filtek Supreme XTE) with different levels of microleakage observed at 4 different environments: occlusal, gingival margins, buccal and lingual surfaces.

2 METHODOLOGY

2.1 *Preparation of class V composite resin restorations*

Sixty-four intact premolars were selected. On each tooth, two standardized Class V cavities (buccal and lingual) were prepared by a single operator, with dimensions of $2 \times 2 \times 3$ mm (height $\times$ depth $\times$ length).

The cavity preparation was carried out in the center of the buccal and lingual surface of each tooth with all margins in enamel. The cavities were prepared with diamond cylindrical burs and the cavities walls were finished with a carbide bur. All the features determined by ISO 3823-1:1997 (E), clause 5.3.2.4. (9)

The cavities were etched with 36% phosphoric acid (DeTrey Conditioner 36, DENTSPLY DeTrey,

Konstanz, Germany) and the adhesive (XP Bond DENTSPLY DeTrey, Konstanz, Germany) was applied according to the manufactures' instructions.

Sixty four cavities of the 128 to be restored, were filled with a nanohibrid resin composite (Synergy D6, Coltène/Whaledent AG, Altstatten, Switzerland) and the remaining 64 with a nanoparticulate resin composite (Filtek Supreme XTE, 3M ESPE, St. Paul, USA) alternating the type of resin composite within the buccal and lingual cavities. It was choosen shade A2 for both resin composites which were placed in one layer.

The specimens were light cured with a light-emitting diode (bluephase ® C8, Ivoclar Vivadent AG, Schaan, Liechtenstein) according to the manufactures' instructions. The output of the curing unit was measured with a radiometer (bluephase radiometer, Ivoclar Vivadent AG, Schaan, Liechtenstein) to ensure a minimal value of light intensity, 700 mW/cm^2 throughout all the experiment.

The restorations were finished and polished with aluminum oxide flexible discs (Sof-Lex, 3M ESPE, St. Paul, USA). Then, the teeth were submitted to thermocycling: 500 cycles in water between 5°C and 55°C with an exposure to each bath that during 20 seconds. The time between baths was 5–10 seconds.

The storage, disinfection, cavity preparation and thermalcycling of the specimens were carried out according to ISO/TS 11405: 2003 (E). (10).

2.2 *Whitening procedures*

The teeth were divided in three groups in a similar proportion, each one with half of the teeth restored with Filtek Supreme XTE on the buccal surface and Synergy D6 on the lingual surface and the other half the opposite (Table 1).

Group I – No bleaching treatment: The teeth were not exposed to bleaching products. They were stored in distilled water at 37°C until microleakage testing.

Group II – Hydrogen peroxide 38% (Opalescence Xtra Boost, Ultradent Products Inc, South Jordan, USA).

A layer of 0.5–1 mm thickness (Fig. 1) for 15 minutes was applied, agitating every 5 minutes. Four applications per session were performed. Between each application the product was removed with a gauze. At the end of each session, the whitening product was removed and washed with running water for one minute. Three sessions were realized, each one spaced by three days.

Group III – Carbamide Peroxide 10% (Opalescence PF 10%, Ultradent Products Inc, South Jordan, USA).

The product was applied for 8 hours per day for a period of 14 days on the restoration (Fig. 2).

Table 1. Distribution of the restorations according to the different whitening procedures.

	N° of teeth	N° of restorations	N° of restorations with Synergy®D6	N° of restorations with Filtek™ Supreme XTE
No bleaching	21	42	21 (B = 10; L = 11)	21 (B = 11; L = 10)
Bleaching with 38% hydrogen peroxide	22	44	22 (B = 11; L = 11)	22 (B = 11; L = 11)
Bleaching with 10% carbamide peroxide	21	42	21 (B = 11; L = 10)	21 (B = 10; L = 11)
Total	64	128	64 (B = 32; L = 32)	64 (B = 32; L = 32)

Abbreviations: B – restorations performed on the buccal surface; L – restorations performed on the lingual surface; N° – number.

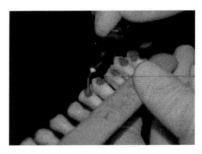

Figure 1. Hidrogen peroxide 38%.

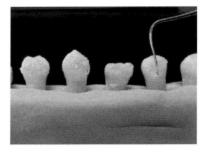

Figure 2. Carbamide peroxide 10%.

After each application, the gel was removed with a gauze and the teeth were cleaned with a tooth brush for 1 min with running water.

Silicon trays were created (Putty, regular set, Aquasil, DENTSPLY DeTrey, Konstanz, Germany) to guarantee the stabilization of samples throughout the whitening procedures. During the whitening treatment, the teeth were kept in a moisture environment at 37°C. The period between whitening treatments, the specimens were stored in distilled water at 37°C. The distilled water was renewed after each application of the whitening agent.

2.3 Preparation of the samples after bleaching

After the bleaching protocol was completed, the teeth were coated with a nail polish except 1 mm diameter ring surrounding the restorations. Each group was stored in a container with a buffered solution of 2% methylene blue dye, where they were immersed for 24 hours at 23°C.

Each tooth was washed, oriented and encased in a transparent epoxy self-curing resin (Epofix Kit, Struers, Ballerup Denmark) (Fig. 3), in order to be sectioned buccolingually in the middle of the restorations.

A low speed diamond saw (TAAB 0.30 nm thick, Crinding Wheel Institute, Ohio, USA) build-up on a hard tissue microtome (Accutom, Struers, Ballerup, Denmark) without refrigeration was employed to cut the specimens. This cut created two test specimens per tooth (Fig. 4), each one with two restorations (Filtek supreme XTE and Synergy D6,) that will be evaluatated under a macroscopic glass. Since the occlusal and gingival wall was measured on each restoration, a total of 8 measurements per tooth were taken. For the purpose of statistical analysis, we selected the highest microleakage measurement between the two test specimens for every existing dental restoration.

2.4 Microleakage evaluation criteria

The microleakage was then assessed using a macroscopic lens (Makroskop Wild, model M420, SA Heerbrug Wild, Heerbrugg, Switzerland) at a 20× magnification. The digital images were obtained through the program Qwin Leica Meteor II Image Light Setup (Leica Imaging Systems, Cambridge, UK) and recorded.

The extent of dye infiltration along the interface tooth/restoration was measured separately for the occlusal and gingival margins, according to ISO/TS 11405:2003 (E) with a scale from 0 to 3:

0-no microleakage; 1-dye penetration into the enamel part of the cavity walls; 2-dye penetration into the dentin part of the cavity wall but not including the pulpal floor of the cavity; 3-dye penetration including the pulpal floor of the cavity. (10).

Microleakage was evaluated according to the 6 groups: Synergy D6 with no bleaching; Synergy D6 with 38% hydrogen peroxide; Synergy D6 with 10% carbamide peroxide; Filtek Supreme XTE with no bleaching; Filtek Supreme XTE with 38% hydrogen peroxide and Filtek Supreme XTE with 10% carbamide peroxide, in 4 different environments: the occlusal and gingival margins and the buccal and lingual surfaces.

2.5 Statistical analysis

To assess the accuracy of the measurement method, Kappa test was applied with 5%. Significance.

The assessment of the relationship between the experimental groups and the respective materials used (independent variables) and the buccal and lingual infiltration (dependent variable) was performed applying the Pearson Chi-square test. It was assumed as significant a value of $\rho < 0.05$.

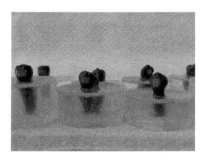

Figure 3. Teeth emerged in a epoxy self-curing resin (Epoxy Kit®).

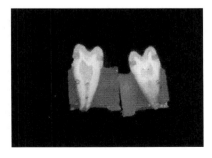

Figure 4. Example of obtaining 2 slides for observation after cutting.

Table 2. Kapa test for precision evaluation in the determination of microleakage.

Symmetrical measurements				
	Value	Asymp. Std. Error[a]	Approx. T[b]	Approx. Sig.
Measure of agreement	Kappa 0.962	0.038	8.898	0.000
Number of valid cases	40			

a. Not assuming the null hypothesis;
b. Using the standard asymptotic error assuming the null hypothesis.

The minimum level of significance (ρ) was adjusted for the number of measurements of infiltration obtained (buccal and lingual infiltration).

3 RESULTS

Analysis of occlusal margin infiltration, on the buccal and lingual surfaces, according to the type of dental whitening procedure and the type of resin composite.

The sample consisted of 128 surfaces observed of which one was excluded. Therefore, the final sample consisted of 127 occlusal surfaces.

It was found that, on the buccal and lingual surfaces, there were no statistically significant differences on the infiltration level ($\rho > 0.27$ and $\rho > 0.36$ respectively), considering the different whitening procedures and the two types of composite resin used.

Analysis of gingival margin infiltration, on the buccal and lingual surfaces, according to the type of dental whitening procedure and the type of resin composite.

As in the previous sample, there were 128 surface observations, of which two were excluded, obtaining a final sample of 126 gingival surface

On the buccal surfaces, there were statistically significant differences on the infiltration levels ($\rho < 0.02$), considering the various whitening procedures and the different types of composite resin used with a high strength of association (Phi = 0,7) and a statistically significancy ($\rho < 0.009$). Thus, it can be stated that the resin composite Synergy D6, when not subjected to bleaching (group I) tends to cause infiltration predominantly in the enamel, and the same resin submitted to bleaching with 10% carbamide peroxide (group III) tends to originate infiltration into the dentin.

On the lingual surface, according to the chi-square test, the results also demonstrate the existence of statistically significant differences on the infiltration level of the gingival margin ($\rho < 0.002$) with an excellent strength of association (Phi = 0,8) and also a statistically significancy ($\rho < 0.002$). It was found that the resin composite Synergy D6, when submitted to bleaching with hydrogen peroxide at 38% (group II), predominantly caused infiltration in the enamel. The resin composite Filtek Supreme XTE tends to induce infiltration into dentin, when submitted to 10% carbamide peroxide (group III) and to the axial wall of the cavity when submitted to bleaching with hydrogen peroxide at 38% (group II). We also observed that the latter composite, when not subjected to bleaching (group I), doesn't tend to cause infiltration.

Different results of microleakage were verified when considering the occlusal and gingival walls of the restorations. The resin composites, when submitted to two different whitening methods have statistically significant differences on infiltration only on the gingival walls of the restorations~

4 DISCUSSION

The major concern for oral health professionals is the outcome of post-operative sensitivity, marginal discoloration and secondary caries after bleaching treatments. (11)

The results of this study show that restorations carried out with Synergy D6 and Filtek Supreme XTE, when subjected to bleaching with 10% carbamide peroxide and 38% hydrogen peroxide can be infiltrated.

One major disadvantage of carrying out in vitro studies is the fact that one cannot fully reproduce in vivo conditions. The samples used in this study were stored in distilled water throughout the experiment. In a literature review, in 2009, Attin et al, verified that all studies that had evaluated the microhardness of enamel after bleaching using human saliva medium did not produce differences in microhardness compared to the baseline. (12) This may indicate that there is a complete recovery of microhardness of enamel surface after bleaching. So, the desmineralizing effect of bleaching products may be offset by the remineralizing and buffering effect of saliva. It would be interesting to verify if there would be a reduction of microleakage replacing the distilled water recommended by ISO protocol, by human saliva or artificial saliva.

In this study there was only significant microleakage on the gingival margin of the restorations which can possibly be explained by the thickness of enamel present. It is known that the cusp tips and incisal edges have greater enamel thickness which gradually becomes thinner at the cervical margin. (13) As the restorations were applied on class V cavities, the occlusal wall of the cavity has a thicker layer of enamel than the gingival wall. In other words, the gingival wall of the cavity has a higher proportion of dentin compared to the occlusal wall. The adhesion to dentin is more complex than to enamel due to the high organic content of this tissue and because of its tubular architecture. Therefore, the greater the thickness of enamel, the more predictable and more effective adhesion will be. (14) Another aspect to consider is the enamel rods orientation. In the cervical area of a tooth, the orientation of its prisms is irregular. (15) According to Berkovitz, the enamel rods just above the cervical margin, reach the surface at a 90 degree angle and this decreases as we approach the occlusal surface. (13) Tagami & Shimada, 2003, showed that the adhesive force was superior on the surface perpendicular to the prisms (which corresponds to the axial wall on a class V enamel restoration) than parallel to the surface (which corresponds to the gingival wall on a class V restoration and on a lesser extent to the occlusal wall). (16) Therefore it is expected that the adhesive strength on the gingival wall will be lower than that observed in an occlusal wall.

In our study we observed, in general, greater infiltration on the gingival margin of the lingual surfaces than on the buccal surfaces of the different restorations submitted to bleaching. This might have two explanations.

According to Ferraris & Muñoz in 2006, the thickness of the buccal enamel is greater than the lingual. (17) Thus, a reduced thickness of the lingual enamel, which can compromise the restorations bond strength, might lead to an adhesive interface more susceptible to bleaching products. The other theory refers to the shape of the cavities. Approximately 41% of the teeth used were inferior premolars. The anatomy of the superior premolars is quite different, specially the inclination of the tooth and the lingual surface. The lower premolars have a lingual inclination of the crown and the lingual surface is narrower and shorter compared to the lingual surface of the upper premolars. Despite the fact that standardized cavities were performed, these anatomical features may have conditioned the conformation of the lingual cavities, which may have influenced the polymerization shrinkage of the composite resin. According to Kubo et al, 1995, (18) the shape of the cavity is a factor that may influence microleakage. Also Hakimeg et al, found that the class V cavities with parallel walls had greater mechanical resistance to displacement of the restorations compared to those who had divergent walls ("V" cavity). (11) In this study, there were different results of microleakage between the two types of composite resin.

In group I (no bleaching), on the buccal surface, restored with Synergy D6, microleakage into the enamel of the cavity wall revealed to be a statistically significant result. On the lingual surface the resin Filtek Supreme XTE, didn't reach any statistically significant infiltration.

Polymerization shrinkage may have been the factor that contributed for these differences. Theoretically, the higher the inorganic filler load in the resin composite, the lower the polymerization contraction and therefore, the lower microleakage. (19) According to the manufacturers' technical product profile, Synergy D6 has a superior inorganic filler volume and weight than Filtek Supreme XTE. However, sometimes the manufacturers values are overestimated, as verified with Synergy D6 in the study of Leprince et al in 2010. (20) These differences may occur because some manufacturers calculate the fraction of inorganic filler load before the sialanization process while others include it in the final percentage. (21)

Leprince et al found that the morphology of the Filtek Supreme XT (previous version of Filtek Supreme XTE) filler load is spherical with clusters of particles of various sizes. As for Synergy D6 the opposite was observed, very irregular particles. These authors found that Filtek Supreme XT had high flexural strength despite being visible large agglomeration areas in this composite resin. They suggested that the morphology of the particles may be the explanation for this mechanical property and for its better modulus of elasticity. (20) The results of our research suggest that Synergy D6 has higher polymerization shrinkage than Filtek Supreme XTE because it presented statistically significant results of microleakage without undergoing any bleaching procedures. It would be interesting to study the differences of polymerization shrinkage of these resins since, the physical and mechanical properties may be partially related to the nature of the particles existing beyond the percentage of filler content. (20)

It was expected that 38% hydrogen peroxide would cause a greater influence on microleakage than 10% carbamide peroxide In the literature, many authors consider that the higher the concentration of hydrogen peroxide is, the bigger are the changes on the enamel. (22) However, this pattern was only seen with Filtek Supreme XTE. The differences between the various whitening products of various brands are not fully studied and clarified, since its effect probably depends not only on the concentration of hydrogen peroxide but also on the time of application and its other constituents. Schiavoni et al, in 2006, tried to explain the fact that there was greater demineralization caused by 10%carbamide peroxide than 16%, based on the viscosity of the products. The 10% agent presented a lower viscosity which would have probably allowed it to spread deeper into the enamel. (22) On the other hand, it would be interesting to quantify the carbopol (thickener) present on both products used because some studies have reported that this agent may contribute for a greater number of changes observed on the enamel surface. (23)

5 CONCLUSION

This study demonstrates that bleaching with either 10% carbamide peroxi 10% de or 38% hydrogen peroxide can increase the microleakage of the gingival margin of both resin composite restorations. Based on these results, we suggest that after bleaching agents application, it is advisable to replace the pre-existing restorations or at least seal its gingival margin with a low viscosity composite. (24) Currently we can verify that there is still a lack of standardization of the experimental methods and materials on the tooth whitening field, which often leads to controversial conclusions. For that reason, further studies are needed to clarify this area of scientific knowledge.

REFERENCES

Attin, T., Hannig, C., Wiegand, A. & Attin, R. 2004. Effect of bleaching on restorative materials and restorations—a systematic review. Dent Mater, 20, 852–61.

Attin, T., Schmidlin, P.R., Wegehaupt, F. & Wiegand, A. 2009. Influence of study design on the impact of bleaching agents on dental enamel microhardness: a review. Dent Mater, 25, 143–57.

Azer, S.S., Machado, C., Sanchez, E. & Rashid, R. 2009. Effect of home bleaching systems on enamel nanohardness and elastic modulus. J Dent, 37, 185–90.

B, B. 2004. Anatomia, embriologia e histologia bucal, Artmed.

Beun, S., Glorieux, T., Devaux, J., Vreven, J. & Leloup, G. 2007. Characterization of nanofilled compared to universal and microfilled composites. Dent Mater, 23, 51–9.

Crawford, P.J., Whittaker, D.K. & Owen, G.M. 1987. The influence of enamel prism orientation on leakage of resin-bonded restorations. J Oral Rehabil, 14, 283–9.

Hakimeh, S., Vaidyanathan, J., Houpt, M.L., Vaidyanathan, T.K. & Von Hagen, S. 2000. Microleakage of compomer class V restorations: effect of load cycling, thermal cycling, and cavity shape differences. J Prosthet Dent, 83, 194–203.

Klukowska, M.A., White, D.J., Gibb, R.D., Garcia-Godoy, F., Garcia-Godoy, C. & Duschner, H. 2008. The effects of high concentration tooth whitening bleaches on microleakage of Class V composite restorations. J Clin Dent, 19, 14–7.

Leprince, J., Palin, W.M., Mullier, T., Devaux, J., Vreven, J. & Leloup, G. 2010. Investigating filler morphology and mechanical properties of new low-shrinkage resin composite types. J Oral Rehabil, 37, 364–76.

Lopes, G.C., Baratieri, L.N., De Andrada, M.A. & Vieira, L.C. 2002. Dental adhesion: present state of the art and future perspectives. Quintessence Int, 33, 213–24.

Ontiveros, J.C. & Paravina, R.D. 2009. Color change of vital teeth exposed to bleaching performed with and without supplementary light. J Dent, 37, 840–7.

Phillips., A.K. 2003. Science of dental materials.

Ramos, R.P., Chinelatti, M.A., Chimello, D.T. & Dibb, R.G. 2002. Assessing microleakage in resin composite restorations rebonded with a surface sealant and three low-viscosity resin systems. Quintessence Int, 33, 450–6.

Rodrigues, J.A., Marchi, G.M., Ambrosano, G.M., Heymann, H.O. & Pimenta, L.A. 2005. Microhardness evaluation of in situ vital bleaching on human dental enamel using a novel study design. Dent Mater, 21, 1059–67.

Sartori N, J.S., Filho A, Arcari G. 2009. Effect of dental bleaching on the microleakage of class V composite restorations. Rev odonto ciênc.

Schiavoni, R.J., Turssi, C.P., Rodrigues, A.L., Jr., Serra, M.C., Pecora, J.D. & Froner, I.C. 2006. Effect of bleaching agents on enamel permeability. Am J Dent, 19, 313–6.

Shahabi, S., Ebrahimpour, L. & Walsh, L.J. 2008. Microleakage of composite resin restorations in cervical cavities prepared by Er,Cr:YSGG laser radiation. Aust Dent J, 53, 172–5.

Shimada, Y. & Tagami, J. 2003. Effects of regional enamel and prism orientation on resin bonding. Oper Dent, 28, 20–7.

Ulukapi, H., Benderli, Y. & Ulukapi, I. 2003. Effect of pre- and postoperative bleaching on marginal leakage of amalgam and composite restorations. Quintessence Int, 34, 505–8.

White, D.J., Duschner, H. & Pioch, T. 2008. Effect of bleaching treatments on microleakage of Class I restorations. J Clin Dent, 19, 33–6.

Yazici, A.R., Keles, A., Tuncer, D. & Baseren, M. 2010. Effect of prerestorative home-bleaching on microleakage of self-etch adhesives. J Esthet Restor Dent, 22, 186–92.

Biodental Engineering V – Belinha et al. (Eds)
© 2019 Taylor & Francis Group, London, ISBN 978-0-367-21087-8

Influence of the Er,Cr:YSGG laser and radial firing tips on the push-out bond strength of glass fiber posts

A.I. Araújo, M. Martins, J.C. Reis Campos, A. Barros & A. Azevedo
Faculty of Dental Medicine, Porto University, Portugal

T. Oliveira
Faculty of Dental Medicine, Conservative Dentistry, Porto University, Portugal

ABSTRACT: As the presence of smear layer created by the post-space preparation is known to compromise the post adhesion to the dentin, the aim of this study was to use Radial Firing Tips and the Er,Cr:YSGG laser prior post cementation and test the push-out bonding strengths compared to a conventional strategy. Forty human incisors were submitted to endodontic treatments and regular post-space preparation. In Group 1, the fiber post space was treated with sodium hypochlorite (5.25%). In Group 2, the fiber post space was treated with Er,Cr:YSGG laser. After post cementation 3 root slices (coronal, medium and apical) were obtained from each sample and subjected to push out tests. For both groups the mean push-out strength increased from coronal to apical. Although the bonding strength mean values were not significantly different from the Group 1, all laser-treated specimens have shown higher push out resistance in all root sections.

1 INTRODUCTION

Due to a significant loss of tooth structure in endodontically treated teeth, both teeth and root fractures are frequently observed turning their restoration a controversial item of debate.

It is generally accepted that the dentin of vital teeth is far more resistant than dentin submitted to an endodontic treatment as it became more brittle due to structural changes such as dehydration and collagen bond breakage (Carter et al., 1983, Helfer et al., 1972, Rivera and Yamauchi, 1993, Sedgley and Messer, 1992).

On the other hand, the amount of remaining hard tissue and restoration technique seems to be preponderant in the occurrence of radicular fractures (Swanson and Madison, 1987). Therefore, if the remaining tooth structure is not sufficient to retain the restorative material, one can preconize the selection and use of a post and core build-up system (Tian et al., 2012).

The post selection should be taken accordingly several physical properties (e.g. similarity to dentine, adherence and biocompatibility to the tooth structure, among others), in order to effectively absorb most of the masticatory forces (Fernandes et al., 2003). Though, the remaining tooth structure and functional requirements are decisive factors in order to choose the most adequate one (Faria et al., 2011).

Glass fiber posts are considered to be the gold-standard posts as, generally, they are made of unidirectional fibers enclosed in a resin matrix becoming more flexible than traditional metallic posts. Accordingly, their elasticity module is considered to be similar to dentin, decreasing the probability of root fractures, namely in anterior teeth (Schwartz and Robbins, 2004).

The post adhesion mechanism the root canal wall is essentially micromechanical, mediated by a resin-based cement, based on the hybridization of a demineralized root surface and resin tags (Topcu et al., 2010). However, the majority of studies addressing long-term outcomes report that the major factor related to failures is the breakage of the dentin-cement bonding interface (Hayashi et al., 2005, Mayhew et al., 2000, Nagase et al., 2011).

Therefore, chemical irrigation is recommended after endodontic and post-space preparation, in order effectively remove organic tissue, inorganic debris and the smear layer from the root canal walls (Baumgartner and Cuenin, 1992, Katsuumi et al., 1986). Such task is usually performed with sodium hypochlorite (NaOCl), EDTA, chlorhexidine, citric acid, phosphoric acid—or their combinations—increasing the post micromechanical retention (Calt and Serper, 2002, Hayashi et al., 2005, Serafino et al., 2004).

However, it has been demonstrated that these irrigation solutions are not completely able to render the root canal system free of debris and smear layer and up-to-date there no consensus regarding the best irrigation regimen to adopt (Fedorowicz et al., 2012).

The use of the Er,Cr:YSGG laser ($\lambda = 2780$ nm) has been lately reported as an effective adjunct method for both deep root canal disinfection and smear layer removal (Ehsani et al., 2013, Franzen et al., 2009, Martins et al., 2014).

Due to its high absorption coefficient in water and in the OH- groups of hydroxyapatite, it has been showing superior ability to remove the smear layer through cavitation effects (Blanken and Verdaasdonk, 2009, De Moor et al., 2009) and positive changes the dentin morphology (Franzen et al., 2009), resulting in a better adaptation of resin-based sealers to the root canal walls (Ozer and Basaran, 2013, Varella and Pileggi, 2007). Such findings are consistent with the idea that the Er,Cr:YSGG laser root canal post-space treatment may also lead to greater retention of glass fiber posts (Nagase et al., 2011).

In addition, specially designed Radial Firing Tips (RFT) were developed to minimize the risks of irradiation beyond the root apex allowing an uniform coverage and energy distribution along the main root canal and enhancing the effects towards the root canal walls (Gordon et al., 2007, Schoop et al., 2009).

2 MATERIALS AND METHODS

Forty (n = 40) superior human incisors were selected and stored in distilled water within 6 months after extraction. The specimens were extracted due to periodontal and/or prosthetic reasons and their inclusion criteria were: (1) existence of one single permeable root canal, (2) straight or slightly curved canal (<10–15°), (3) absence of any restoration, caries or detectable root cracks and (4) absence of previous endodontic treatment, posts or crowns.

All teeth were radiographed to identify root canal irregularities and to evaluate the root integrity and morphology. All the calculi and debris from the root surfaces were removed using an ultrasonic hand-piece (GC1-KAVO®, Germany). Finally, all teeth were de-coronated 1 mm coronal to the cement-enamel junction using a diamond saw (Gebr, Brasseler, GmbH&Co – Komet Dental, Germany).

Endodontic Treatment: Endodontic access was performed using a Peeso drill mounted on a low-speed hand-piece under water-cooling. A K-Flexofile® ISO #10 (Maillefer-Dentsply, Switzerland) was used to ensure patency through all canal length.

All specimens were endodontically prepared up to the working length (set 1 mm from the apex) using a reciprocation technique with Wave-One® Primary files ISO#25.08 (Maillefer-Dentsply, Switzerland). Irrigation was intermittently performed with 3 ml of 3% NaOCl between each file penetration, using a side-vented endodontic syringe (Monoject 30G, Kendal, Tyco, USA).

Afterwards, each canal was dried with Wave-One® Primary paper points (Maillefer-Dentsply, Switzerland) and filled with a single, tapered gutta-percha technique, Wave-One® Primary gutta-percha (Maillefer-Dentsply, Switzerland), a resin-based cement (TopSeal, Dentsply, Switzerland) and vertical compaction.

Post space preparation: The coronal gutta percha was removed and the post space calibrated with specific drills (Rebilda® Post System, Voco) leaving 4 mm of apical sealing. All specimens were prepared by a single operator (A.A.).

The specimens were then divided in two groups: Group 1 (G1, n = 20): the post space was chemically prepared accordingly the manufacturer's instructions (Rebilda DC®, Voco GmBH, Germany). Group 2 (G2, n = 20): the post space was irradiated with a 2780 nm Er,Cr:YSGG laser (Waterlase MD, Biolase, USA), using 320 µm radial firing tips with 17 mm length (RFT3, Endolase tip, Biolase, USA) and the following parameters: 1.25 W, 50 Hz, 140 µs, 24% water and 34% air. Irradiation was performed at the speed of 2 mm.s-1 in a vertical movement from apical to coronal. The irradiation protocol was repeated twice for each specimen. The same tip was used for two specimens.

Post cementation: All root canals were dried with paper points (Maillefer-Dentsply, Switzerland). Prior cementation each fiber post was transversely cut with a diamond disk in order to be 3 mm from the root coronal surface. Each post was cleaned with 70% ethyl alcohol, dried with air and cemented according to the manufacturer's instructions. The adhesive system was applied with microbrushes for 20 seconds. A uniform cement layer was applied to the root canal (Rebilda DC®, Voco GmBH, Germany) from apical to coronal and the fiber post was inserted into the respective root canal. Light-polymerization occurred for 40 seconds and the remaining 3 mm of the post outside the root canal was used to standardize light's distance during polymerization.

Push-out tests: 7 days after post cementation all specimens were included in a self-curing acrylic block (Vertex®, Dental B.V., Netherlands), with the aid of a pre-manufactured cylindrical metallic cast.

20 acrylic cylinders for both G1 and G2 specimens were obtained, with the roots submerged until the cervical edge. The cylinders were sectioned perpendicularly to the long axis of the root with a cutting machine (Isomet 1000 Precision Saw-Buehle, Germany) under constant cooling.

Each root produced 3 discs, spaced by 1.5 mm between them, and with 1 mm thickness each. Each disk was labelled as belonging from the cervical, middle and apical portion. The thickness of each disc was digitally confirmed and measured with 0.01 mm precision (Digimatic calliper, Mitutoyo, Tokyo, Japan).

Push-out tests were performed using a universal testing machine (Instron Corp. 4502, USA), at a speed of 0,5 mm/minute. Each disc was placed on a platform with a central opening, with the apical surface facing upwards. A metal spike (0,8 mm in diameter) was used to apply extrusion forces in coronal direction directly on each disk until the post has registered any movement. The maximum value of failure was recorded in Newtons (N) and converted to MPa according to the following formula: De-bond Stress (Mpa) = De-Bond Force (N) / Area (A).

As all posts were tapered, the area of displacement was calculated by the following formula: $A = \pi(D + d)\sqrt{(D - d)2 + h2}$. "D" and "d" are respectively the largest and smallest diameter of the post, whereas "h" is the height of the slice. The largest and smallest diameter of each post was measured using an optical microscope with 20:1 magnification (Travelling Microscope, Mitutoyo, Tokyo, Japan).

Statistical analysis: Statistical analysis was performed using a statistical significance of p = 0,05 (IBM SPSS®, V.21). Normality of variables was assessed through the Kolmogorov-Smirnov test, whereas the Levène test was used to assess data homogeneity. The independent t-student test compared the control group (G1) and test group (G2) within the same region of the roots (cervical, middle and apical).

The Pearson's analysis of linear correlations was added to legitimize the use of MANOVA, which turned out not to be applicable. Therefore, the ANOVA test for repeated measures was selected to assess the existence of differences in the three regions (cervical, middle and apical) considering separately the two groups (G1 and G2).

3 RESULTS

Table 1 shows the mean value and standard deviation of the push-out tests in the three regions of the root (cervical, middle and apical) for both experimental groups (G1 and G2). It can be observed that the average bond strength in the cervical, middle and apical regions was higher in G2 than in G1. However, no significant statistically differences were found between the two groups (t-student, p > 0,05).

Through the ANOVA test the existence of statistical differences in the three regions within each

Table 1. Means and standard deviations (in MPa) of push-out bond strength in three regions of the root for the two experimental groups.

	Control Group (G1)	Test Group (G2)
Cervical	$6.15 \pm 6,30$	$6,68 \pm 3,83$
Middle	$7,75 \pm 4,10$	$10,15 \pm 6,24$
Apical	$10,23 \pm 5,25$	$11,31 \pm 8,00$

group was evaluated. In G1, the apical region has shown a significant higher resistance to extrusion than cervical region ($P < 0.05$). In any case did not show statistically significant differences.

Comparing the three regions of G2 it was found that apical region has higher resistance to extrusion forces than cervical region ($P < 0.01$), with no statistically significant differences.

4 DISCUSSION

It is generally accepted that teeth submitted to endodontic treatments may demonstrate weakened dentinal structure. Therefore, posts are commonly used to support several rehabilitation techniques (Dimitriu et al., 2009), and distinct post-systems have been used during the past years (e.g. metal, carbon fiber, glass fiber, etc) (Topcu et al., 2010).

Glass fiber posts have an elasticity modulus more resembling to dentine if compared with metal posts. As consequence, teeth restored with glass fiber posts have been presenting significantly lower incidence of fractures than those restored with metal posts (Qing et al., 2007).

It can be understood that the guta-percha removal and post space preparation performed by rotary drills induce heavy deposition of smear layer and such fact may negatively influence the bonding strength between post, cement and dentin In fact, it has been identified that the major cause related to the failure of glass fiber posts is the adhesion failure between cement and dentin. (Akgungor and Akkayan, 2006, Monticelli et al., 2003).

Erbium lasers have been found capable of removing root canal filling materials (Tachinami and Katsuumi, 2010). In addition, the Er,Cr:YSGG laser has gained prominence in endodontics as safety concerns and efficacy issues in endodontics have been successfully addressed (Peeters and Mooduto, 2013, Schoop et al., 2009, Varella and Pileggi, 2007) along with promising clinical results using Radial Firing Tips (Martins et al., 2014, Martins et al., 2013).

Moreover, the mechanisms and effectiveness of this wavelength in removing debris and smear layer through cavitational effects (De Moor et al., 2009, De Moor et al., 2010) are consistent with observed morphologic modifications that increased dentinal permeability (Silva et al., 2010). As consequence, it was demonstrated that higher dentinal permeability created by Er,Cr:YSGG laser irradiation could positively influence adhesion of glass ionomer cements (Garbui et al., 2013).

As regards to the adhesion strength of resin-based cements to dentin, Shafiei et al. reported that, when used at low fluencies, the Er,CrYSGG laser (0.75 W/37.5 mJ/20 Hz/140 µs) did not adversely influence the bonding ability of both etch-and-rinse and the self-etch cements (Shafiei et al., 2013). By it's turn Beer et al., reported that etching with phosphoric acid after laser preparation should be avoided as laser preparation creates a surface texture that positively influence the morphology and stability of the resin-dentin interface (Beer et al., 2012).

In conformity with the idea that self-etching primers seem to be less affected by dentin irradiation with Er,Cr:YSGG laser (Carvalho et al., 2011), the surface treatment with Er,Cr:YSGG laser irradiation (1.5 W/50 mJ/30 Hz/140 µs) prior to bonding with a self-etching adhesive system has proved to significantly increase microtensile bonding strength to eroded dentin (Ramos et al., 2015).

Moreover, in order to evaluate the effect of the Er,Cr:YSGG laser on push-out bond strength of RealSeal Self-Etch sealer, Ehsani et al. reported that using RFT3 (1.5 W/75 mJ/20 Hz/140 µs, 15% water, 15% air, moving at 2 mm/sec in apico-coronal direction), no significant differences were found between push-out bond strength of root canal fillings compared to irrigation with EDTA+NaOCl (Ehsani et al., 2013).

By it's turn, Nagase et al. has compared the bond strength of fiber posts (Angelus, Paraná, Brazil) cemented with a total-etch adhesive (Scotch Bond Multipurpose, 3M/ESPE, Brazil) and a resin cement (RelyX ARC, 3M/ESPE, Brazil), in laser-treated root canals either with Nd:YAG laser, Er,Cr:YSGG laser or both. Evaluation of retention forces were performed prior post cementation. The Er,Cr:YSGG laser-assisted endodontic treatment (0.75 W/37.5 mJ/20 Hz) proved not to interfere with post cementation (Nagase et al., 2011).

In this study, we have hypothesized the possibility of irradiate dentin using the Er,Cr:YSGG laser and Radial Firing Tips with low energy and high frequency (RFT3, 1.25 W/25 mJ/50 Hz/140 µs, 24% water and 34% air) to remove smear layer produced during post-space preparation, increasing dentin permeability and adhesion ability with a uniform pattern.

Mohammadi et al. has reported that the pre-treatment of the main root canal with laser Er.Cr:YSGG laser may increase the bond strength glass fiber posts to the root (Mohammadi et al., 2013). These findings are in partial agreement with our results as for the laser-assisted group (G2) higher mean values for push-out resistance were measured. However, in this study, these differences were not statistically significant when compared to the control group (G1) (P > 0.05).

The same group of researchers also found that the bonding strength was not affected accordingly to the root region (cervical, middle, and apical) (Mohammadi et al., 2013). However, our findings suggest that different values of resistance can be found along the root canal, independently of the protocol adopted, with decreasing bonding strengths from apical to coronal.

Given the potential that Er,Cr:YSGG laser has to alter the morphology of dentin, baring the dentinal tubules, it appears to present a positive influence on the bond strength between posts, sealer and the root canal surface (Ghiggi et al., 2010, Yamada et al., 2004).

5 CONCLUSIONS

The results presented in this study indicates that, despite not being statistically significant compared to the manufacturer's standard protocol, the adjunctive Er,Cr:YSGG laser treatment of the post-space prior cementation increased the bonding strength of glass fiber posts within the entire root length. These results may be attributed to the laser capacity for smear layer removal and modification of dentin morphology, resulting in higher adhesive bonding strength and push-out resistance of glass fiber posts. Further clinical studies may confirm whether this can be considered clinically relevant for the long-term stability of crown restorations.

REFERENCES

Akgungor, G. & Akkayan, B. 2006. Influence of dentin bonding agents and polymerization modes on the bond strength between translucent fiber posts and three dentin regions within a post space. *J Prosthet Dent*, 95, 368–78.

Baumgartner, J.C. & Cuenin, P.R. 1992. Efficacy of several concentrations of sodium hypochlorite for root canal irrigation. *J Endod*, 18, 605–12.

Beer, F., Buchmair, A., Korpert, W., Marvastian, L., Wernisch, J. & Moritz, A. 2012. Morphology of resin-dentin interfaces after Er,Cr:YSGG laser and acid etching preparation and application of different bonding systems. *Lasers Med Sci*, 27, 835–41.

Blanken, J.W. & Verdaasdonk, R.M. 2009. [Laser treatment in root canals. Effective by explosive vapour bubbles]. *Ned Tijdschr Tandheelkd*, 116, 355–60.

Calt, S. & Serper, A. 2002. Time-dependent effects of EDTA on dentin structures. *J Endod*, 28, 17–9.

Carter, J.M., Sorensen, S.E., Johnson, R.R., Teitelbaum, R.L. & Levine, M.S. 1983. Punch shear testing of extracted vital and endodontically treated teeth. *J Biomech,* 16, 841–8.

Carvalho, A.O., Reis, A.F., De Oliveira, M.T., De Freitas, P.C., Aranha, A.C., Eduardo CDE, P. & Giannini, M. 2011. Bond strength of adhesive systems to Er,Cr:YSGG laser-irradiated dentin. *Photomed Laser Surg,* 29, 747–52.

De Moor, R.J.. Blanken, J., Meire, M. & Verdaasdonk, R. 2009. Laser induced explosive vapor and cavitation resulting in effective irrigation of the root canal. Part 2: evaluation of the efficacy. *Lasers Surg Med,* 41, 520–3.

De Moor, R.J., Meire, M., Goharkhay, K., Moritz, A. & Vanobbergen, J. 2010. Efficacy of ultrasonic versus laser-activated irrigation to remove artificially placed dentin debris plugs. *J Endod,* 36, 1580–3.

Dimitriu, B., Varlan, C., Suciu, I., Varlan, V. & Bodnar, D. 2009. Current considerations concerning endodontically treated teeth: alteration of hard dental tissues and biomechanical properties following endodontic therapy. *J Med Life,* 2, 60–5.

Ehsani, S., Bolhari, B., Etemadi, A., Ghorbanzadeh, A., Sabet, Y. & Nosrat, A. 2013. The effect of Er,Cr:YSGG laser irradiation on the push-out bond strength of RealSeal self-etch sealer. *Photomed Laser Surg,* 31, 578–85.

Faria, A.C., Rodrigues, R.C., De Almeida Antunes, R.P., De Mattos MDA, G. & Ribeiro, R.F. 2011. Endodontically treated teeth: characteristics and considerations to restore them. *J Prosthodont Res,* 55, 69–74.

Fedorowicz, Z., Nasser, M., Sequeira-Byron, P., De Souza, R.F., Carter, B. & Heft, M. 2012. Irrigants for non-surgical root canal treatment in mature permanent teeth. *Cochrane Database Syst Rev,* CD008948.

Fernandes, A.S., Shetty, S. & Coutinho, I. 2003. Factors determining post selection: a literature review. *J Prosthet Dent,* 90, 556–62.

Franzen, R., Esteves-Oliveira, M., Meister, J., Wallerang, A., Vanweersch, L., Lampert, F. & Gutknecht, N. 2009. Decontamination of deep dentin by means of erbium, chromium:yttrium-scandium-gallium-garnet laser irradiation. *Lasers Med Sci,* 24, 75–80.

Garbui, B.U., De Azevedo, C.S., Zezell, D.M., Aranha, A.C. & Matos, A.B. 2013. Er,Cr:YSGG laser dentine conditioning improves adhesion of a glass ionomer cement. *Photomed Laser Surg,* 31, 453–60.

Ghiggi, P.C., Dall Agnol, R.J., Burnett, L.H., Jr., Borges, G.A. & Spohr, A.M. 2010. Effect of the Nd:YAG and the Er:YAG laser on the adhesive-dentin interface: a scanning electron microscopy study. *Photomed Laser Surg,* 28, 195–200.

Gordon, W., Atabakhsh, V.A., Meza, F., Doms, A., Nissan, R., Rizoiu, I. & Stevens, R.H. 2007. The antimicrobial efficacy of the erbium, chromium:yttrium-scandium-gallium-garnet laser with radial emitting tips on root canal dentin walls infected with Enterococcus faecalis. *J Am Dent Assoc,* 138, 992–1002.

Hayashi, M., Takahashi, Y., Hirai, M., Iwami, Y., Imazato, S. & Ebisu, S. 2005. Effect of endodontic irrigation on bonding of resin cement to radicular dentin. *Eur J Oral Sci,* 113, 70–6.

Helfer, A.R., Melnick, S. & Schilder, H. 1972. Determination of the moisture content of vital and pulpless teeth. *Oral Surg Oral Med Oral Pathol,* 34, 661–70.

Katsuumi, I., Tsuzuki, T. & Nakamura, Y. 1986. [Scanning electron microscopy of the effects of decalcifying agents on root canal dentin]. *Shigaku,* 74, 1109–118.

Martins, M.R., Carvalho, M.F., Pina-Vaz, I., Capelas, J.A., Martins, M.A. & Gutknecht, N. 2014. Outcome of Er,Cr:YSGG laser-assisted treatment of teeth with apical periodontitis: a blind randomized clinical trial. *Photomed Laser Surg,* 32, 3–9.

Martins, M.R., Carvalho, M.F., Vaz, I.P., Capelas, J.A., Martins, M.A. & Gutknecht, N. 2013. Efficacy of Er,Cr:YSGG laser with endodontical radial firing tips on the outcome of endodontic treatment: blind randomized controlled clinical trial with six-month evaluation. *Lasers Med Sci,* 28, 1049–55.

Mayhew, J.T., Windchy, A.M., Goldsmith, L.J. & Gettleman, L. 2000. Effect of root canal sealers and irrigation agents on retention of preformed posts luted with a resin cement. *J Endod,* 26, 341–4.

Mohammadi, N., Savadi Oskoee, S., Abed Kahnamoui, M., Bahari, M., Kimyai, S. & Rikhtegaran, S. 2013. Effect of Er,Cr:YSGG pretreatment on bond strength of fiber posts to root canal dentin using a self-adhesive resin cement. *Lasers Med Sci,* 28, 65–9.

Monticelli, F., Grandini, S., Goracci, C. & Ferrari, M. 2003. Clinical behavior of translucent-fiber posts: a 2-year prospective study. *Int J Prosthodont,* 16, 593–6.

Nagase, D.Y., De Freitas, P.M., Morimoto, S., Oda, M. & Vieira, G.F. 2011. Influence of laser irradiation on fiber post retention. *Lasers Med Sci,* 26, 377–80.

Ozer, S.Y. & Basaran, E. 2013. Evaluation of microleakage of root canal fillings irradiated with different output powers of erbium, chromium:yttrium-scandium-gallium-garnet laser. *Aust Endod J,* 39, 8–14.

Peeters, H.H. & Mooduto, L. 2013. Radiographic examination of apical extrusion of root canal irrigants during cavitation induced by Er,Cr:YSGG laser irradiation: an in vivo study. *Clin Oral Investig,* 17, 2105–12.

Qing, H., Zhu, Z., Chao, Y. & Zhang, W. 2007. In vitro evaluation of the fracture resistance of anterior endodontically treated teeth restored with glass fiber and zircon posts. *J Prosthet Dent,* 97, 93–8.

Ramos, T.M., Ramos-Oliveira, T.M., De Freitas, P.M., Azambuja, N., Jr., Esteves-Oliveira, M., Gutknecht, N. & De Paula Eduardo, C. 2015. Effects of Er:YAG and Er,Cr:YSGG laser irradiation on the adhesion to eroded dentin. *Lasers Med Sci,* 30, 17–26.

Rivera, E.M. & Yamauchi, M. 1993. Site comparisons of dentine collagen cross-links from extracted human teeth. *Arch Oral Biol,* 38, 541–6.

Schoop, U., Barylyak, A., Goharkhay, K., Beer, F., Wernisch, J., Georgopoulos, A., Sperr, W. & Moritz, A. 2009. The impact of an erbium, chromium:yttrium-scandium-gallium-garnet laser with radial-firing tips on endodontic treatment. *Lasers Med Sci,* 24, 59–65.

Schwartz, R.S. & Robbins, J.W. 2004. Post placement and restoration of endodontically treated teeth: a literature review. *J Endod,* 30, 289–301.

Sedgley, C.M. & Messer, H.H. 1992. Are endodontically treated teeth more brittle? *J Endod,* 18, 332–5.

Serafino, C., Gallina, G., Cumbo, E. & Ferrari, M. 2004. Surface debris of canal walls after post space preparation in endodontically treated teeth: a scanning electron microscopic study. *Oral Surg Oral Med Oral Pathol Oral Radiol Endod,* 97, 381–7.

Shafiei, F., Fekrazad, R., Kiomarsi, N. & Shafiei, E. 2013. Bond strength of two resin cements to dentin after disinfection pretreatment: effects of Er,Cr:YSGG laser compared with chemical antibacterial agent. *Photomed Laser Surg,* 31, 206–11.

Silva, A.C., Guglielmi, C., Meneguzzo, D.T., Aranha, A.C., Bombana, A.C. & De Paula Eduardo, C. 2010. Analysis of permeability and morphology of root canal dentin after Er,Cr:YSGG laser irradiation. *Photomed Laser Surg,* 28, 103–8.

Swanson, K. & Madison, S. 1987. An evaluation of coronal microleakage in endodontically treated teeth. Part I. Time periods. *J Endod,* 13, 56–9.

Tachinami, H. & Katsuumi, I. 2010. Removal of root canal filling materials using Er:YAG laser irradiation. *Dent Mater J,* 29, 246–52.

Tian, Y., Mu, Y., Setzer, F.C., Lu, H., Qu, T. & Yu, Q. 2012. Failure of fiber posts after cementation with different adhesives with or without silanization investigated by pullout tests and scanning electron microscopy. *J Endod,* 38, 1279–82.

Topcu, F.T., Erdemir, U., Sahinkesen, G., Mumcu, E., Yildiz, E. & Uslan, I. 2010. Push-out bond strengths of two fiber post types bonded with different dentin bonding agents. *J Biomed Mater Res B Appl Biomater,* 93, 359–66.

Varella, C.H. & Pileggi, R. 2007. Obturation of root canal system treated by Cr,Er:YSGG laser irradiation. *J Endod,* 33, 1091–3.

Yamada, M.K., Uo, M., Ohkawa, S., Akasaka, T. & Watari, F. 2004. Three-dimensional topographic scanning electron microscope and Raman spectroscopic analyses of the irradiation effect on teeth by Nd:YAG, Er: YAG, and CO(2) lasers. *J Biomed Mater Res B Appl Biomater,* 71, 7–15.

Biodental Engineering V – Belinha et al. (Eds)
© 2019 Taylor & Francis Group, London, ISBN 978-0-367-21087-8

Trigeminal nerve – interdisciplinarity between the areas of dentistry and audiology

Fernanda Gentil
Clínica ORL—Dr. Eurico Almeida, Widex, Escola Superior de Saúde—I.P. Porto, Portugal

J.C. Reis Campos
Faculty of Dental Medicine, Porto University, Portugal

Marco Parente, C.F. Santos, Bruno Areias & R.M. Natal Jorge
Institute of Mechanical Engineering and Industrial Management (INEGI), Porto, Portugal

ABSTRACT: The trigeminal nerve is the most important nerve for the sensory and motor innervation of the oral system. A detailed knowledge of the trigeminal nerve is very important in the diagnosis and possible treatment of any type of orofacial or temporomandibular joint pain.

1 INTRODUCTION

Trigeminal nerve (fifth cranial nerve) is a mixed sensory/motor nerve and the mostly responsible for mastication, sensory innervation of the face, teeth, gums, and the anterior two thirds of the tongue. It also has contributions in terms of innervation of the tensor veli palatine, soft palate, extrinsic laryngeal muscle, mylohyoid and part of the digastric, retraction of the tongue and for opening the Eustachian tube. Considered the largest skull nerve, afferent and efferent characteristics. Innervates structures of the oral cavity and the face. The human face has two trigeminal nerves, one on each side. Every nerve is divided into three branches that transmit sensations of pain and touch of the face, mouth and teeth to the brain. Many experts say that is one of the most unbearable pain to humans. It is estimated that 1 in 15.000 people suffering from trigeminal neuralgia. About of 45.000 people suffer from trigeminal neuralgia in the United States. It is known that the disease affects about 1 million people worldwide. The trigeminal neuralgia is twice more common in women than in men. It is more common in people over 50 years of age. The trigeminal neuralgia is a long-term condition – a chronic illness that usually will gradually worse. The pain usually does not occur during sleep. 4.1% of patients with unilateral trigeminal neuralgia has a family history and 17% of those with bilateral trigeminal have relatives with this disorder (Eijden & Langenbach 2015).

The trigeminal neuralgia occurs if the blood vessels are pressing on the root of the trigeminal nerve, conducting pain signals. Pressure on this nerve may be caused by a tumor or multiple sclerosis, physical damage by a dental or surgical procedure, or infection, or also by family history, once the formation of blood vessels is inherited.

2 ANATOMY AND PHYSIOLOGY

The trigeminal nerve has three divisions (Kamel & Toland 2001):

- Ophthalmic;
- Maxillary;
- Mandibular branches (Figure 1).

2.1 Ophthalmic nerve

The ophthalmic nerve is the first division of the trigeminal nerve (Figure 2). It comes out of the upper end of the trigeminal ganglion, from inside the cranial cavity to the orbits by the superior orbital fissure. Is uniquely sensitive and it is the smallest of the 3 branches. Before projecting through the superior orbital fissure (apparent cranial origin), emits the meningeal branch that innervates the dura.

After passing through the superior orbital fissure is divided into three sensitives branches:

- Lacrimal;
- Frontal;
- Nasociliary nerves.

The ophthalmic nerve is an afferent nerve, that conveys sensory information from the:

- Scalp,
- Forehead,
- Upper parts of the sinuses,

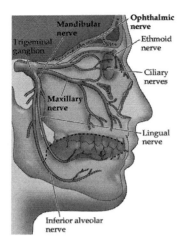

Figure 1. Branches of trigeminal nerve (from: Neuroscience, 2004, Third Edition).

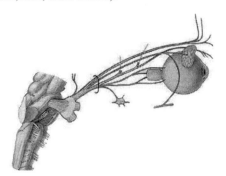

Figure 2. Ophtalmic nerve. (from: https://pt.slideshare.net/LucasStolfoMaculan/trigemeo).

- Upper eyelid,
- Nasal mucosa,
- Bulb,
- Lacrimal gland,
- External nose.

2.2 Maxillary nerve

The maxillary nerve transmits sensory information from the:

- Lower eyelid and associated mucous membranes;
- Middle part of the sinuses;
- Nasal cavity and middle part of the nose;
- Cheeks;
- Upper lip;
- Some of the teeth of the upper jaw and associated mucous membranes;
- Roof of the mouth.

This nerve comes to the pterygopalatine fossa where emits another collateral branch, the zygomatic nerve (Figure 3). It is responsible for relaying postganglionic fibers to the lacrimal gland.

The branches of the maxillary nerve are the:

- Zygomatic;
- Infraorbital;
- Superior alveolar branches;
- Pterygopalatine nerves.

2.3 Mandibular nerve

The mandibular division is the only part of the trigeminal nerve that has both sensory and motor functions (Figure 4).

It communicates sensory information from the:

- Part of the auricle of the ear;
- Lower part of the mouth and the associated mucous membranes;
- Front and middle parts of the tongue;
- Teeth of the lower jaw and the associated mucous membranes;
- Lower lip;
- Chin.

It also stimulates movement of the muscles in the jaw and some of the muscles within the inner ear.

It runs through the foramen oval dividing into six branches:

- Deep temporal;
- Masseteric;
- Buccal;
- Lateral and medial pterygoid;

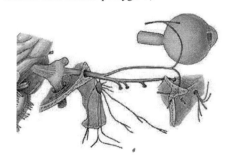

Figure 3. Maxillary nerve. (from: https://pt.slideshare.net/LucasStolfoMaculan/trigemeo).

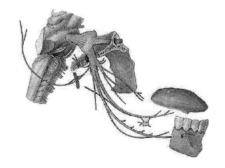

Figure 4. Mandibular nerve. (from: https://pt.slideshare.net/LucasStolfoMaculan/trigemeo).

- Meningeal;
- Auriculotemporal (this innervates the ear).

The tensor veli palatine and tensor tympani are branches of the medial pterygoid nerve.

3 TRIGEMINAL NERVE LESIONS

Trigeminal neuralgia is a neuropathic pain sudden and abrupt of the face. Often felt like a shock or shot along the course of the affected nerve. The pain usually involves the lower part of the face and jaw, but the symptoms can appear near the nose, ears, eyes or lips.

The crisis may last a few seconds to minutes. The episodes can last days, weeks, months, or more. 97% of patients experience pain only on one side of the face, while 3% are affected on both sides. Sudden attacks of pain, which are triggered by touching the face, chew, talk or brushing your teeth. There may be tingling or numbness in the face before the pain develop.

The cause of trigeminal neuralgia is usually idiopathic, but can also be caused by structural disease. A blood vessel pressed against the root of the trigeminal nerve or vascular compression on the sensory root in the proximal part. The secondary causes can include: multiple sclerosis (due to demyelination of the nerve, usually appears in later stages of the disease); trigeminal nerve root infiltration by malignant neoplasia or amyloidosis; herpes zoster involving the optic nerve trigeminal branch; skull base abnormalities and tumors (Selby, G. 1984). A tumor presses against the trigeminal nerve, but this is a rare cause.

Trigeminal neuropathy is less common than facial palsy. More associated with Sjögren syndrome, systemic lupus erythematosus or others neuropathies.

Patients with purely sensory dysfunction of trigeminal nerve present numbness over the ipsilateral face. This numbness depends on which branches of the trigeminal nerve are involved. Involvement of the motor branch causes difficulty chewing and deviation of the jaw to the contralateral side when opening the mouth.

This neuralgia can be by nerve injury as a dental procedure, surgery or infection.

The ear receives sensation fibers from cranial nerves trigeminal and facial and others as IX and X. These nerves have long courses in the head and face, which is why so many diseases can cause ear pain. This pain can be secondary from dental causes (Ely et al. 2008).

4 DIAGNOSIS

The diagnosis of trigeminal neuralgia is mostly based on the description of the pain by the patient.

There are 3 main criteria to characterize the trigeminal neuralgia:

- Type – the related pain is sudden, brief, similar to an electric shock;
- Location – you can verify whether it is even of trigeminal neuralgia from the parts of the face that are affected by pain;
- Triggers – this pain is usually caused by external stimulation or by simple actions such as eating, talking or exposed to the breeze and the wind.

The diagnosis is essentially clinical, however, if there are neurological deficit associated with trigeminal neuralgia, must be ordered imaging studies. Neuroimaging tests, like MRI and CT, should always be requested to dispose of routine structural lesions, being useful for the determination of secondary causes of trigeminal neuralgia (Scully 2013).

The differential diagnosis of trigeminal neuralgia includes:

- Facial neuralgia;
- Herpes zoster compromising the optical nerve trigeminal branch;
- Facial pain consequent neoplastic processes of the face;
- Facial pain associated with the temporomandibular joint arthropathy;
- Glossopharyngeal and vagus nerves neuralgia; pain consequent to dental affections;
- Paget's disease;
- Acromegaly;
- Temporal arteritis.

The clinical examination of the trigeminal nerve includes the sensory, motor and corneal reflex tests (Preston & Shapiro 2013).

In the sensory test, ask the patient to close their eyes and evaluate the tactile sensory of the face by the three divisions of the trigeminal nerve.

In the motor test, the movement of the mouth and mandible are evaluated, to check the medial and lateral pterygoid muscles.

In the test for corneal reflex, is required the ophthalmic branch and temporal and zygomatic branches of the facial nerve.

5 TREATMENT

Drug therapy is considered the first-line treatment. Surgical treatment should only be considered when the patient does not respond to systemic medication. The most commonly used medication for the trigeminal neuralgia begin with the use of anticonvulsants and antispasmodics (Bagheri et al. 2004). These medications decrease or block the pain signals sent to the brain. The normal painkillers such as Tylenol (Acetaminophen) do not relieve the pain of trigeminal neuralgia, which is why doctors prescribe anticonvulsant medication. Sometimes, the anticonvulsants are beginning to lose effectiveness over time. If this occurs, the doctor may increase the dosage or switching to another anticonvulsant (Lawal et al. 2012).

Only a doctor can tell you what the most appropriate medicine for your case, as well as the correct dosage and duration of treatment. Mindfulness and relaxation techniques, such as yoga or meditation, can also help to relax nearby muscles and ease pain.

Some cares are important such to eat nourishing and liquid meals, avoiding spicy, hot or cold food, or things such as caffeine, citrus fruits and bananas.

The trigeminal nerve surgeries have two objectives: stop a vein or artery is pressed against the trigeminal nerve and damage to the trigeminal nerve so that the signs of pain stop.

There are a number of percutaneous procedures that can offer some help temporarily, by inserting a needle or thin tube through the cheek and into the trigeminal nerve. They're carried out using X-rays, heavily sedated or under general anaesthetic.

The surgical treatments as percutaneous procedures in gasser ganglion include (Gronseth et al. 2008):

- Glycerol injections – the glycerol is injected around the gasser ganglion, in the three main branches of the trigeminal nerve.
- Microvascular decompression – Microvascular decompression is only dealing with the etiology of the disease, while the radio balloon compression and rizolisis with glycerol treat the symptoms (Nordqvist 2017).
- Gamma Knife – More recently, there is a new modality of treatment of trigeminal neuralgia through radiosurgery, targeting the gasser ganglion, but the effectiveness and limitations of this procedure have not yet been established. In surgery by Gamma Knife, a focused radiation aimed at the root of the trigeminal in the posterior fossa (Raval et al. 2014). A year after the surgery by Gamma Knife, 69% of patients remain pain-free and without additional medication. After 3 years, 52% still without pain. Pain relief may occur after a month of the surgery. The side effects include sensory complications in 6% that can develop over a period of up to 6 months, facial numbness at 9–37%, which improves over time, and paresthesias in 6–13%. The quality of life improves in 88%. The main drawback of Gamma Knife surgery is cost.

These procedures work by intentionally damaging the trigeminal nerve, which is thought to disrupt the pain signals travelling along it. The pain returns usually in a few years or a few months. Sometimes these procedures don't work at all. The major side effect of these procedures is numbness of the face. These procedures also carry a risk of other complications, including bleeding, facial bruising, eye problems and impaired hearing on the affected side. Very rarely, it can cause stroke.

6 CONCLUSIONS

Living with trigeminal neuralgia make the quality of life significantly affected.

The emotional tension of living with trigeminal neuralgia can lead to psychological problems, such as depression or even suicide in the extreme cases.

Even when no pain, the person lives in fear of the pain returning.

The aim of this paper is to summarize the anatomical knowledge of the trigeminal nerve and its branches, and to show the clinical usefulness of such information in applying anesthesia in the region of the maxilla. Although the upper teeth and midface regions are the most commonly affected areas, trigeminal neuralgia can trigger pain in the ear. A correct diagnosis between ear pain and trigeminal neuralgia is very important since it will correspond to different treatments.

REFERENCES

Bagheri, SC et al. 2004. Diagnosis and treatment of patients with trigeminal neuralgia. *Journal of the American Dental Association*. 135 (12): 1713–1717.

Eijden, T.M., Langenbach, G.E.J. 2015. Anatomy of the trigeminal nerve. Pocket Dentistry.

Ely, J.W., Hansen, M.R., Clark, E.C. 2008. Diagnosis of Ear Pain. *Am Fam Physician*. University of Iowa Carver College of Medicine, Iowa City, Iowa, 77(5): 621–628.

Gronseth, G., Cruccu, G., Alksne, J., Argoff, C., Brainin, M., Burchiel, K., Nurmikko, T., Zakrzewska, J.M. 2008. Practice Parameter: The diagnostic evaluation and treatment of trigeminal neuralgia (an evidence-based review), *Neurology* 71(15): 1183–90.

Hinojosa, A.Q. 2012. *Schmidek, and Sweet: Operative Neurosurgical Techniques Indications, Methods and Results*, 6th Edition, (2): 2329–2382.

Kamel, H.A.M., Toland J. 2001. Trigeminal Nerve Anatomy Illustrated Using Examples of Abnormalities. American Journal of Roentgenology 176: 247–251.

Lawal, A.O., Adisa, A.O., Akinyamoju, A.O., Kolude, B. 2012. Management of Trigeminal Neuralgia using Amitriptyline and Pregablin combination Therapy. *Afr. J. Biomed. Res*. (15), 201–203.

Nordqvist, C. 2017. Trigeminal neuralgia: Symptoms, causes, and treatment. Medical News today. https://www.medicalnewstoday.com.

Preston, D.C., Shapiro, B.E. 2013. Differential diagnosis of facial weakness in Electromyography and Neuromuscular Disorders (Third Edition).

Raval, A.B., Salluzzo, J., Dvorak, T., Price, L.L., Mignano, J.E., Wu, J.K. 2014. Salvage Gamma Knife Radiosurgery after failed management of bilateral trigeminal neuralgia. Surg Neurol Int., 5: 160.

Scully, C. 2013. Trigeminal and other neuralgias in Oral and Maxillofacial Medicine (Third Edition).

Selby, G. 1984. Diseases of the fifth cranial nerve. In: Dyck PF, Thomas PK, Lambert EH, eds. Peripheral neuropathy. 2nd ed. Philadelphia: W.B. Saunders:1224–65.

Biodental Engineering V – Belinha et al. (Eds)
© 2019 Taylor & Francis Group, London, ISBN 978-0-367-21087-8

Facial nerve—a clinical and anatomical review

Fernanda Gentil
Clínica ORL—Dr. Eurico Almeida, Widex, Escola Superior de Saúde—I.P. Porto, Portugal

J.C. Reis Campos
Faculty of Dental Medicine, Porto University, Portugal

Marco Parente, C.F. Santos, Bruno Areias & R.M. Natal Jorge
Institute of Mechanical Engineering and Industrial Management (INEGI), Porto, Portugal

ABSTRACT   The information that pass through the facial nerve allows the expression of our smile, joy or sadness, the "facial expression". The face is the mark of our individuality. The facial nerve is responsible for innervation of the face muscles, like the previous two-thirds of the tongue and secretion of salivary and tears glands. The aim of this work is to remember the anatomy and physiology of the facial nerve, pathology and possible treatments of facial paralysis.

1 INTRODUCTION

Facial palsy deserves a very special treatment, because it leads to great difficulties for patients to express themselves naturally, and to accept their disfigured face. This condition generates anguish, social networking and professional difficulties, requiring immediate medical treatment Facial palsy refers to the interruption of the motor information to the facial muscles. For the patient, the main complaints are related to the difficulty in closing the eyes, and when smiling. Other symptoms commonly referred include reductions or alterations in taste, dizziness, pain or discomfort, sinusitis, headache, numbness of the tongue, hypersensitivity to noises, dryness of the eye, and difficulty in chewing. Immediate care of the patient is important, since the wallerian degeneration occurs within 24–72 hours after the onset of paralysis (Myckatyn & Mackinnon 2004).

Crossing a path of more or less 35 mm within a bony canal, the facial nerve is subject to the action of compressive and infections, which can disrupt the nervous influx blocking its functions.

Risk factors for a bad facial motility recovery include the age of 59 years, diabetes and hypertension. It is less common before age 15 or after age 60.

The prognosis of Bell's palsy is usually good, with about 90% of full recovery after 1 month. There is a higher incidence, 3 times more, in pregnant women. The lifetime risk is 1 in 60. The recurrence rate is approximately 10%. Patients with diabetes have 5 times more likely to develop the disease. The most frequent location of the lesion is the foramen meatal (Glass & Tzafetta 2014). Bell's palsy usually begins without warning and progresses fast.

2 ANATOMY AND PHYSIOLOGY

The facial nerve emerges from the pons of the brainstem, and goes to the face, neck, salivary glands and external ear.

The facial nerve is a mixed nerve, being 80% of it motor fibers to the face (Toulgoat et al. 2013). The facial nerve and the VIII pair (auditory nerve) enter the inner ear canal, the middle ear and mastoid and emerge from the base of the skull, splitting into two branches which are distributed on the face and neck. This nerve performs basically four functions:

a. Motor – controls the muscles of the face and neck.
b. Sensitive – responsible for the external ear sensitivity.
c. Secretory – the secretory fibers control the lacrimal gland, the mucous membranes of the nose and mouth, and the submandibular and sublingual salivary glands
d. Sensory – tasting fibers of the anterior 2/3 of the tongue.

The facial nerve exits the cerebellum and has two courses, a intratemporal and extratemporal.

2.1 *Intratemporal course of facial nerve*

A intratemporal course through the petrosal portion of the temporal bone from the internal auditory meatus to the stylomastoid foramen, is divided into 3 segments (Figure 1):

a. Labyrinthine segment (2.5–6 mm) – extends from the internal auditory meatus to the genicu-

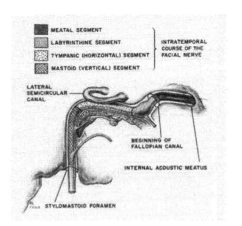

Figure 1. Intratemporal course of facial nerve (from: www.entusa.com/images/Facial%20Nerve%20Intratemporal%20-%20750.jpg).

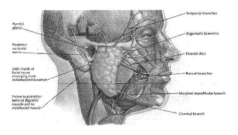

Figure 2. Extratemporal facial nerve ramifications (Frank H. Netter, "Netter's Atlas of Human Anatomy", 2014).

late ganglion. Here, the large superficial petrosal nerve leaves to take parasympathetic fibers to the lacrimal glands.
b. Tympanic segment (8–11 mm) – starts next to the geniculate ganglion where does a curvature of 40° to 80° (1st knee), to the lateral semicircular canal, through the tympanic cavity. A branch out of this segment, to innervates the stapedius muscle.
c. Mastoid segment (9–12 mm) – the nerve makes a 90° curvature (2nd knee) and goes down to the stylomastoid foramen, inside the mastoid, where it exits of the temporal bone to the parotid gland (Esslen 1977).

2.2 Extratemporal course of facial nerve

In the parotid gland, the nerve divides in two branches: temporal-zygomatic and cervico-facial. The temporal-zygomatic is divided into the temporal and the zygomatic. The cervico-facial into three branches: buccal, mandibular and cervical (Figure 2).

3 FACIAL PARALYSIS TYPES

The facial nerve can be injured at any level along its course. If the injury occurs before nerve exit the brain stem is known by central facial paralysis. If the lesion reaches the nerve after the departure of the brainstem occurs a peripheral facial paralysis.

3.1 Central facial paralysis

This type of the paralysis is caused most often by a stroke. Only the facial muscles under her eyelids, muscles of the middle and lower third of the contralateral nerve lesion hemiface, are paralyzed. The eye closes and the forehead moves, as the muscles responsible for these movements receive cortical bilateral denervation.

3.2 Peripheral facial paralysis

The patient with peripheral facial paralysis cannot wrinkle forehead, does not close the eye, does not open the nostrils and mouth strayed to the side. All muscles of facial expression are paralyzed. The face is sad, inexpressive and the twisted smile. The most common causes are: Bell'palsy, facial trauma, trauma by otologic surgery or of the parotid gland, Ramsay Hunt syndrome (Worme et al. 2013), acute or chronic otitis media, Lyme disease, tumors, Melkerson-Rosenthal syndrome, bilateral paralysis and congenital facial paralysis (Jain et al. 2006). Injury to the geniculate ganglion and proximal to this region can lead to decreased lacrimation. If the damage is proximal to the nerve of stapedius can result in hyperacusis in the affected ear (Gordin et al. 2015).

4 DIAGNOSIS TECHNIQUES

To characterize the degree of facial paralysis, the House-Brackman Facial Nerve Grading System is the most used (House & Brackman 1985). This scale present six grades, being Grade I the normal function; Grade II, slight dysfunction (at rest there are normal symmetry and tonus and in the motion the forehead has moderate to good function, the eye has complete closure with minimum effort and the mouth has slight asymmetry); Grade III, moderate dysfunction (at rest too normal symmetry and tonus but in the motion, the forehead has slight to moderate movement, the eye only has complete closure with effort, the mouth is slightly weak with maximum effort); Grade IV, moderate to severe dysfunction, the gross has obvious weakness and/or disfiguring asymmetry (at rest, yet normal symmetry but without motion of the forehead, the eye has incomplete closure, the mouth is asymmetric with maximum effort); Grade V, severe dysfunction (there are asymmetry at rest, no motion for the forehead, the eye has incomplete closure and the mouth has slight movement); Grade VI – Total Paralysis (without movement).

Diagnostic techniques include the anamnesis (start and duration of the paralysis, family history, other symptoms associated) evaluation of motor function of the facial muscles (facial assessment at rest and motion, eye movement, nose, mouth, cheeks), audiometric examination (tonal and vocal audiogram, acoustic stapedius reflex, electrophysiological tests) and imaging.

The neurological signs diagnosed as Bell's palsy are seen in Figure 3.

It is, still, possible to do simple tests that allow to check the location of the injury site in the path of the facial nerve, to advance in the most correct solution. The tests include (Kawamoto & Ikeda 2002):

a. The Shirmer test – evaluates the function of greater superficial petrosal nerve and the amount of tearing. Place a filter paper in both lower eyelids. After 3 to 5 minutes compare the roles. A difference of more than 25% of the affected side (least amount of wet paper) indicates a lesion in the geniculate ganglion or the amount of this.
b. Acoustic stapedius reflex – evaluates the stapedius branch of the facial nerve. The absence of reflexes may indicate the lesion before of this branch.
c. Taste evaluation – sensations from the anterior two-thirds of the tongue (innervated by chorda tympani). Placement of small amount of salt, sugar or lemon juice on his tongue. The loss of taste can indicate the amount of damage before of the chorda tympani.
d. Test of Blatt – evaluates the integrity of the salivary glands. On catheterize the channels of Wharton bilaterally and salivary flow measurements after 5 minutes; a difference of over 25% indicates a supra-cordal injury.

To help the diagnosis and treatment of the patient some tests can be used, such as Hilger test, nerve excitability test, maximum stimulation test, electroneuronography, electromyography and others (Tomás & Gomes 1998).

Hilger test consists in stimulating the facial nerve next to your emergency in the stylomastoid foramen with a low-current electrical stimulator electrode and increases from 0 to 10 mA, first on the normal side and then on the injured side. It is looking for minimum current intensity allowing a contraction of the muscles of the face. Use as interpretation the comparison of the both facial sides. It is a subjective, inexpensive and an easy to do test.

The electroneuronography technique was referred to for the first time in 1973 by Esslen, keeping your utility and still today (Esslen 1977). The principle is based on the evaluation of the latency and amplitude of nerve conduction using skin electrodes. It is an objective electrophysiological technique, which records a compound muscle action potential, by stimulation of the facial nerve and that allows for comparison with the normal side, knowing the percentage of injured fibers of the the paralyzed side. The prognosis depends on the percentage of the injured fibers. The electroneuronographic study should be done two to three days after the paralysis and repeated periodically until about the 12th day after the onset of paralysis for a better prognosis. Nerve wallerian degeneration completed in eight to ten days, it is in this period that can predict the percentage of fibers that remain and which would degenerate sequels, makes no sense to repeat the test after the 14th day after the initiation the injury.

The electromyography test consists of the register of electrical muscle activity through a needle inserted into the muscle or a surface electrode (Cramer & Kartush 1991). This test has your utility from the 14th day of the onset of paralysis, since the potential of indicating degeneration fibrillation appear only to 10 to 20 days after the onset of injury. It has an incontestable interest in the medium and long term recovery.

5 TREATMENT

The aim of treatment in Bell's palsy is to reestablish symmetry in facial look and movements of facial muscles, for desired facial expressions. Most of the facial paralysis has a favorable evolution. Many of them recover spontaneously without any treatment. Others, however, require medical treatment, physiotherapy of the face or surgical treatment.

5.1 *Medical treatment*

In cases of paralysis linked to idiopathic or viric cause, the drug treatment should include a medicine steroid-antiviral (Sullivan et al. 2007). Corticosteroids have been recommended as a treatment for Bell's palsy for reducing edema, enhancing cranial nerve VII regeneration, and improving motor function (Bracken et al. 1990).

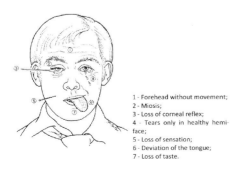

1 - Forehead without movement;
2 - Miosis;
3 - Loss of corneal reflex;
4 - Tears only in healthy hemiface;
5 - Loss of sensation;
6 - Deviation of the tongue;
7 - Loss of taste.

Figure 3. Neuronal signals diagnosed as Bell's palsy.

Antibiotics are indicated in cases of facial paralysis secondary to acute otitis media. The treatment requires special attention to the cornea, suggesting baths with salt water, or drops, keeping the eye wet. Vitamins B12, B6 and zinc seem to help in the recovery of the nerve.

The most common benign tumor is acoustic neuroma and the most common malignant tumor is the mucoepidermoid carcinoma and the adenoid cystic carcinoma of the parotid gland. The prognosis about the paralysis by tumors is always bad, even after rehabilitation techniques.

The Melkerson-Rosenthal syndrome, that is a rare disease, consists of a triad of symptoms: recurrent orofacial edema, facial paralysis and fissured tongue, recurrent possibly with headache and usually begins on the second day of life. The prognosis in this case is not good (Cirpaciu et al. 2014).

5.2 *Physioterapy of the face*

This procedure used in the treatment of facial paralysis consists of massage therapy for relaxation in hemiface not compromised, stimulating massage therapy on hemiface paralyzed, cryotherapy (cold treatment) and kinesitherapy. Facial massage with your fingertips in a circular motion to stimulate blood flow and maintain muscle tone, prevents nerve atrophy during recovery from paralysis.

Both the use of heat as the cryotherapy is indicated as a therapeutic resource on facial paralysis. Cryotherapy has as main goal the stimulation for obtaining of muscle contraction, flaccid paralysis phase during 15 minutes approximately. On the other hand, the heat applied through infra-red lamp or hot pockets provides muscle relaxation in the hypertonia.

Biofeedback therapies, and of several exercises (as raising eyebrows, wrinkling forehead, wrinkling his nose and lips, blow, smile, move the jaw forward and to the side) are too recommended (Finsterer 2008).

5.3 *Surgical treatment*

The facial nerve decompression, is recommended in patients with Bell's palsy or in cases of herpes zoster if a patient develop into a total paralysis within two weeks with proper therapy and when in the electroneuronography the percentage degeneration of the fibers is higher than 90%, and in cases of traumatic injuries. Myringotomy in cases of the acute otitis media.

6 CONCLUSIONS

The study of facial nerve becomes extremely complex for your anatomy and pathophysiology. Despite the diagnostic tests present some limitations are of particular interest in guiding therapy, prognosis and recovery of facial nerve paralysis. A good knowledge of facial nerve anatomy is very important to avoid its inadvertent injury during procedures such as maxillofacial and other related with the oral cavity (Myckatyn & Mackinnon, 2004).

The study of facial paralysis continues to grow. Artificial nerve graft channels will be manufactured from biological and synthetic materials, such as silicone, polyamide, collagen, and polylactide, with biodegradable polymers to restore the injured nerve.

REFERENCES

Bracken, M.B., Shepard, M.J., Collins, W.F., et al. 1990. A randomized, controlled trial of methylprednisolone or naloxone in the treatment of acute spinal-cord injury. Results of the Second National Acute Spinal Cord Injury Study. *N Engl J Med*; 322: 1405–1411.

Cirpaciu, D., Goanta, C.M., Cirpaciu, M.D. 2014. Recurrences of Bell's palsy. *J Med Life*. 7 Spec No. 3:68–77.

Cramer, H.B., Kartush, J.M. 1991. Testing facial nerve function. *Otolaryngologic Clinics of Nort America*, 24: 555–570.

Esslen, E. 1977. *The Acute Facial Palsies*. Springer-Verlag Berlin Heidelberg New York.

Finsterer, J. 2008. Management of peripheral facial nerve palsy. *Eur Arch Otorhinolaryngol*. 265(7): 743–752.

Glass, G.E., Tzafetta, K. 2014. Bell's palsy: a summary of current evidence and referral algorithm. *Fam Pract*. Dec31(6): 631–42.

Gordin, E., Lee, T.S., Ducic, Y., Arnaoutakis, D. 2015. Facial Nerve Trauma: Evaluation and Considerations in Management. Craniomaxillofac Trauma Reconstr. 8(1): 1–13.

House, J.W., Brackman, D.E. 1985. House Brackman facial nerve grading system. *Otolaryngol. Head Neck Surg*, (93): 146–147.

Jain, V., Deshmukh, A., Gollomp, S. 2006. Bilateral facial paralysis: case presentation and discussion of differential diagnosis. *J Gen In-tern Med*. Jul 21(7): C7–10.

Kawamoto, H., Ikeda, M. 2002. Evaluation of greater petrosal nerve function in patients with acute peripheral facial paralysis: comparison of soft palate electrogustometry and Schirmer's tear test. Acta Otolaryngol Suppl. (546): 110–5.

Myckatyn, T.M., Mackinnon, S.E. 2004. A review of facial nerve anatomy. *Semin Plast Surg*, 18(1): 5–12.

Sullivan, F.M., Swan, I.R., Donnan, P.T., et al. 2007. Early treatment with prednisolone or acyclovir in Bell's palsy. *N Engl J Med*; 357: 1598–1607.

Tomás, L.G., Gomes, A. 1998. O nervo facial e os testes electrofisiológicos: A Electroneuronografia, *Rev. Port. ORL*, 36 (4): 287–298.

Toulgoat, F., Sarrazin, J.L., Benoudiba, F., et al. 2013. Facial nerve: from anatomy to pathology. *Diagn Interv Imaging*. Oct 94(10): 1033–42.

Worme, M., Chada, R., Lavallee, L. 2013. An unexpected case of Ramsay Hunt syndrome: case report and literature review. *BMC Res Notes*. Aug 286: 337.

Biodental Engineering V – Belinha et al. (Eds)
© 2019 Taylor & Francis Group, London, ISBN 978-0-367-21087-8

Prenatal ultrasound features in a case of Arnold Chiari malformation

B. Fernandes, I. Côrte-Real & P. Vaz
Faculty of Dental Medicine, University of Porto, Porto, Portugal

R. Nogueira
CGC Genetics—Laboratory of Pathology, Porto, Portugal
Life and Health Sciences Research Institute (ICVS), School of Health Sciences (ECS), University of Minho, Braga, Portugal

F. Valente
Prenatal Diagnosis Unit, CHVNGE Hospital, Vila Nova de Gaia, Portugal

A.C. Braga
Department of Production and Systems Engineering, University of Minho, Braga, Portugal

ABSTRACT: Chiari malformations comprises a group of brain diseases in which mainly the cerebellum is the structure affected. The prenatal diagnosis by ultrasound through identification of specific sonographic signs is already described. However, as some pediatric cases reported in literature are associated with craniofacial anomalies, the fetal face study performed on this clinical case intend to screen the same and to contribute for a more routinely application of the fetal face assessment on this type of cases to promote a more earlier prenatal diagnosis.

1 INTRODUCTION

Chiari malformations (CM's) is a disorder of embryological development (Ball et al. 1995) that presents a variation in the configuration of the cerebellum and brainstem at the craniovertebral junction (Susman et al. 1989). Normally, the cerebellum and part of the brainstem are above the foramen magnum, but on this clinical condition the referred structures, both or only one, is projected into the upper medullary canal across the foramen magnum. This herniation of cerebellum can occur on the presence of an alteration of the skull development, when part of the skull is smaller than normal or when it is deformed. Consequently the functions of the cerebellum and of the brainstem are compromised by compression and the flow of cerebrospinal fluid, that surrounds and protects the brain and spinal cord, is blocked (Susman et al. 1989). For diagnosis purposes can be classified four clinical types. In Type I cerebellar displacement are typical but hydrocephalus and syringomyelia are variable. In type II usually there are myelomeningocele and severe hydrocephalus. In type III the same features of type II are observed but associated with occipito-cervical encephalocele. In type IV there is severe hypoplasia or cerebellar aplasia associated with a small size of the posterior fossa (Ball et al. 1995). A few reports described cases of these malformations associated with craniofacial disorders (Lee et al. 2003, Tubbs & Oakes 2006, Hopkins & Haines

2003). The aim of this study in presenting a clinical case of a Chiari malformation is to emphasize to the relevance of an earlier prenatal ultrasound diagnosis on this type of pathological entity and to the possible importance of the fetal facial study for it.

2 CASE REPORT

A 34-year-old Caucasian woman, healthy, was monitored at Prenatal Diagnosis Unit of Centro Hospitalar de Vila Nova de Gaia/Espinho for a single spontaneous pregnancy. For performing a two-dimensional ultrasound examination was used the GE E8 Voluson® (GE Medical Systems, Tiefenbach, Zipf, Austria) system with an abdominal transducer. All images were processed in Astraia® software (version 1.23.0, Astraia GMBH, Munich, Germany). In accordance with legal norms, the written consent was obtained to perform karyotype study, medical interruption of gestation and post-mortem examination.

Further the routine ultrasound assessment a more detailed ultrasound examination of the fetal face on the second trimester was proposed and performed after informed consent. This case report was included in a study group for determining the growth patterns of different facial structures and detecting potential anomalies that could support an early prenatal diagnosis of facial anomalies, either alone or associated with congenital conditions.

The mentioned study group was approved by the ethics committee of the Dental Medicine Faculty of the University of Porto and authorized by the Portuguese Data Protection Authority. The first trimester screening did not identified any alterations or development restrictions. However, the second trimester screening detected the presence of myelomeningocele and indirect sonographic signs (Nicolaides et al. 1986) of the anomaly described by Campbell et al., respectively the "lemon signal" (Fig. 1) due to an angulation at the level of the metopic suture giving to the cranial contour the appearance of a lemon, and the "banana signal" (Fig. 2) caused by the displacement of the cerebellum toward the posterior fossa giving it the appearance of a banana.

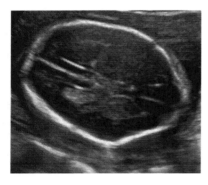

Figure 1. Two-dimensional ultrasound at second trimester. Axial view of fetal head showing the lemon sign.

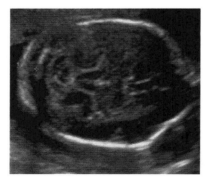

Figure 2. Two-dimensional ultrasound at second trimester. Axial view of fetal head showing the banana sign.

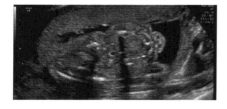

Figure 3. Two-dimensional ultrasound at second trimester. Axial view of the fetal face showing the measurements of maxilla bone.

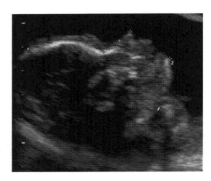

Figure 4. Two-dimensional ultrasound at second trimester. Midsagittal view of the fetal face showing the measurements of nasal bone.

The midsagittal and axial plane were obtained for face evaluation only once during gestation (Figs. 3–4). Despite of this type of condition can be associated with other craniofacial anomalies the ultrasound evaluation did not detected any type of alterations on this structures.

3 CONCLUSIONS

The fetal face screening by ultrasound should be accomplished regularly for a better knowledge of its normal development in order to detect early and subtle anomalies that can contribute for a more accurate diagnosis. The clinical presented case prove the importance of ultrasound evaluation in the early prenatal diagnosis of this pathology. In suspicion of this condition, other ecographic features relative to craniofacial structure should be also assessed in order to make a more detailed and adequate diagnosis and prognosis.

REFERENCES

Ball, W.S. Jr., Crone, K.R. 1995. Chiari I malformation: from Dr Chiari to MR imaging. *Radiology* 195(3): 602–4.
Hopkins, T.E., Haines, S.J. 2003. Rapid development of Chiari I malformation in an infant with Seckel syndrome and craniosynostosis. Case report and review of the literature. *J Neurosurg* 98(5): 1113–5.
Lee, J., Hida, K., Seki, T., Kitamura, J., Iwasaki, Y. 2003. Pierre-Robin syndrome associated with Chiari type I malformation. *Childs Nerv Syst* 19(5–6): 380–3.
Nicolaides, K.H., Campbell, S., Gabbe, S.G., Guidetti, R. 1986. Ultrasound screening for spina bifida: cranial and cerebellar signs. *Lancet* 2(8498): 72–4.
Susman, J., Jones, C., Wheatley, D. 1989. Arnold-Chiari malformation: a diagnostic challenge. *Am Fam Physician* 39(3): 207–11.
Tubbs, R.S., Oakes, W.J. 2006. Chiari I malformation, caudal regression syndrome, and Pierre Robin Syndrome: a previously unreported combination. *Childs Nerv Syst* 22(11): 1507–8.

Biodental Engineering V – Belinha et al. (Eds)
© 2019 Taylor & Francis Group, London, ISBN 978-0-367-21087-8

Relevance of facial features in ultrasound diagnosis of Holoprosencephaly

B. Fernandes, I. Côrte-Real, P. Mesquita, M.H. Figueiral & P. Vaz
Faculty of Dental Medicine, University of Porto, Porto, Portugal

F. Valente
Prenatal Diagnosis Unit, CHVNGE Hospital, Vila Nova de Gaia, Portugal

ABSTRACT: Holoprosencephaly is a brain pathology, with a significant phenotypic variability, that is characterized by forebrain and face development alterations. Prenatal diagnosis for this type of condition is relevant because the main features, included the facial ones, can be detected earlier and may support decisions concerning the management of the pregnancy, for the severe forms, or, may afford an early treatment plan for the less forms. In the case reported the ultrasound study of the fetal face detected the presence of an orofacial cleft that together with the identification of the typical brain defect of holoprosencephaly contribute for the final diagnosis. Therefore with this case is intended to highlight for the main facial features prevalent on this situations detectible by ultrasound evaluation and for the relevance of this type of screening to an earlier prenatal diagnosis.

1 INTRODUCTION

Holoprosencephaly (HPE) is a rare brain malformation that affects the forebrain and the face and often the extremities. This malformation occurs between the 18th and the 28th day of gestation and results from incomplete division of the forebrain. The estimated prevalence is 1/16,000 live births and 1/250 conceptions. Clinically it can be classified into three classic forms of increasing severity, respectively, lobar, semi-lobar and alobar HPE. A lighter subtype designated as an interhemispheric midline variant or syntelencephaly is also described. The less severe forms are called microforms and are characterized by midline defects, without the typical brain defect of HPE (Chaudhari et al. 2012). Severe forms (especially in the presence of a chromosomal abnormality) are often fatal and mortality is related to the severity of cerebral malformation and associated defects (Dubourg et al. 2007).

Patients with HPE have a wide variety of manifestations, including delayed development, instability in body temperature control, heart rate and respiration, epilepsy, and eating difficulties. In addition to the above, endocrine disorders such as diabetes insipidus, adrenal hypoplasia, hypogonadism, thyroid hypoplasia and growth hormone deficiency are also common (Dubourg et al. 2007).

Regarding aetiology, until the date, are described seven genes involved in HPE: *Sonic hedgehog* (*SHH*), *ZIC2, SIX 3, TGIF, PTCH, GLI2* and *TDGF1*. Currently, molecular diagnosis, by genomic

sequencing and allele quantification, can be performed for the four major genes, SHH, ZIC2, SIX3 and TGIF respectively. However, it is estimated that in about 70% of cases the molecular basis of the disease remains unknown, which makes suggestive the existence of several other responsible genes or even environmental factors. The multifactorial origin assigned, resulting from the interaction of genetic and/or environmental factors (like maternal diabetes), has even been proposed to explain the wide clinical variability of HPE (Dubourg et al. 2007).

In these clinical situations the treatment is symptomatic and requires a multidisciplinary approach. The prognosis depends on the associated medical and neurological complications and their severity (Chaudhari et al. 2012).

The description of the present clinical case of HPE have as purpose to emphasize the characteristic facial alterations that can be detected by prenatal ultrasound and that consequently contributes for a more precise diagnosis.

2 CASE REPORT

A single spontaneous pregnancy of a healthy Caucasian woman was followed at Prenatal Diagnosis Unit of Centro Hospitalar de Vila Nova de Gaia/ Espinho. A two-dimensional ultrasound evaluation was preconized using the GE E8 Voluson® (GE Medical Systems, Tiefenbach, Zipf, Austria) system with an abdominal transducer. For processing the images was used the Astraia® software (version 1.23.0, Astraia GMBH, Munich, Germany). Besides the routine ultrasound evaluation a more detailed ultrasound examination of the fetal face on the second trimester was proposed and performed after informed consent. This case report was integrated into a study group for determining the growth patterns of different facial structures and detecting potential anomalies that could support an early prenatal diagnosis of facial anomalies, either alone or associated with congenital conditions. The referred study group was approved by the ethics committee of the Dental Medicine Faculty of the University of Porto and authorized by the Portuguese Data Protection Authority. The midsagittal and axial plane were obtained for face evaluation only once during gestation (Figs. 1–2).

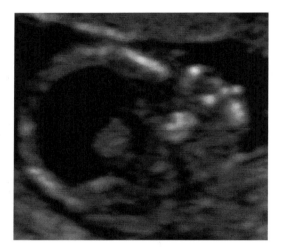

Figure 1. Two-dimensional ultrasound at second trimester. Midsagittal view of fetal face.

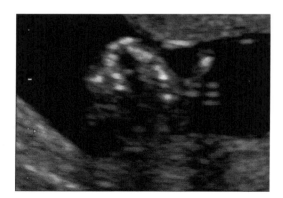

Figure 2. Two-dimensional ultrasound at second trimester. Axial view of fetal face showing the presence of a bilateral orofacial cleft.

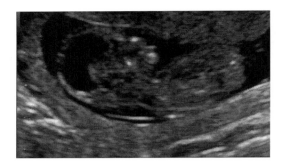

Figure 3. Two-dimensional ultrasound at second trimester. Midsagittal view of the fetus showing HPE and cystic hygroma.

Genetic counselling was performed and, after informed consent, was decided to medically interrupt the pregnancy and to proceed with a postmortem examination due to the diagnosis made.

Prenatal screening on the first trimester did not identify any anomalies or growth restrictions. Although the ultrasound study on second trimester revealed the presence of HPE, cystic hygroma, in Figure 3, and detected, during the face evaluation,çpçl. the presence of a bilateral orofacial cleft.

In these clinical cases, it is import the fetal face study for detecting the main facial features that can be observed, that can include cyclopean, proboscis, premaxilla agenesis, medial or bilateral cleft of the palate, hypotelorism or single upper central incisor, among others. These latter defects in the midline can occur without cerebral malformations in the so-called microforms (Chaudhari et al. 2012).

3 CONCLUSIONS

The fetal face evaluation by ultrasound should be achieved routinely in order to detect early and subtle anomalies that can contribute for a more accurate diagnosis.

This clinical case presentation wished-for to call the attention of the main facial features prevailing on this type of pathology, which can be identified by ultrasound evaluation and how the imaging can be crucial to an earlier prenatal diagnosis.

REFERENCES

Chaudhari, H.D., Thakkar, G., Darji, P., Khokhani, P. 2012. Prenatal ultrasound diagnosis of holoprosencephaly and associated anomalies. *BMJ Case Rep.*

Dubourg, C., Bendavid, C., Pasquier, L., Henry, C., Odent, S., David, V. 2007. Holoprosencephaly. *Orphanet J Rare Dis* 2: 8.

Orthodontic stainless steel wire and nickel release

S. Castro, M.J. Ponces, J.D. Lopes, M. Vasconcelos, J.C. Reis Campos & C. Pollmann
Faculty of Dental Medicine, University of Porto, Porto, Portugal

ABSTRACT: The release of nickel was not necessarily proportional to the alloy's nickel content. Stainless steel has 8% in his content, however, this biocompatibility may be altered with possible differences in salivary pH and presence of fluoride. The analysis of the corrosion products was carried out for the nickel ion using the spectrophotometers GBC 932 Scientific Equipment PTY, model 932 and Unican, model 939 for each sample as a function of pH (4 and 6,75)/time/ppm fluoride ion (1500 and 22600 ppm). The condition with the longest immersion time at pH 4 was the only one that presented an outcome for the Ni ion above the sensitivity limit of the technique Considering the drawbacks of this in vitro study the results lead to conclude that lowering pH and increasing the immersion time are the most corrosive conditions.

1 INTRODUCTION

The biocompatibility of orthodontic wires occurs when oral tissues do not experience any toxic, irritating, inflammatory, allergic, mutagenic, or carcinogenetic effects, after being in contact with the wires (Kao, 2007). In orthodontics, nickel is a commonly used metal because it is a component of superelastic shape-memory wires, as well as stainless stell (SS) and other alloys in different percentages. However, nickel is the most common metal to cause contact dermatitis and it is responsible for the most cases of allergic reactions. It is estimated that 4,5% to 28,5% of the population have hypersensitivity to this metal, with higher prevalence in females (Rahilly, 2003). The release of nickel was not necessarily proportional to the alloy's nickel content. Stainless steel has 8% in his content but its crystalline network binds to the nickel ions, making them unavailable to react (Yan, 2010). However, this biocompatibility may be altered with possible differences in quantity and quality of saliva, salivary pH, plaque, amount of protein in saliva, physical and chemical properties of food and liquids, general and oral health and presence of fluoride (Yonekura 2004, Gursoy 2005, Sfondrini 2010, Krishnan 2011, Castro 2014).

2 MATERIAL AND METHODS

The analysis of the corrosion products was carried out for the nickel ion. Table 1 displays the assignment used for each sample as a function of pH/time/ppm fluoride ion. Each sample corresponds to a set of stainless steel springs, elaborated according to the method described in the work of Castro S.M. (2015), immersed in artificial saliva with pH 4 or 6.75, in the presence or not of fluoride. The springs were placed in Falcon tubes containing 5 mL of artificial saliva.

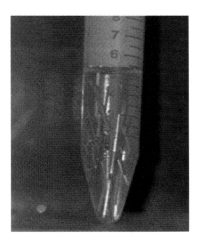

Figure 1. Falcon tube with springs.

Table 1. Sample as a function of pH/time/ppm fluoride ion.

Sample	Material	pH	Immersion time
SS-control	Saliva	4	5 months
SSpH4t3	SS	4	3 months
SS-pH6,75t3	SS	6,75	3 months
SS-pH4t5	SS	4	5 months
SS-ph6,75t5	SS	6,75	5 months
SS-pH4–1500	SS1500ppmF	4	30 min.
SS-pH4–22600	SS22600ppmF	4	5 min.

The amount of saliva used is in accordance with ISO 10993, 0.2 g wire for each 1 mL of saliva (ISO, 1999). The number of springs per sample was 8, as each spring corresponded to a weight of 0.121 grams (Fig. 1).

Table 2. Sample as a function of pH/time/ppm fluoride ion.

Spectrophotometer analysis parameters	Instrumental parameters
Lamp current (mA)	4,0
Wavelength (nm)	232,0
Slit width	0,2
Flame Control Parameters	
Flame type	Air-Acetylene
Oxidant flow	10,0
Fuel flow (l/min)	2,0

Table 3. Results of the nickel ion research.

Sample	Ni Ion (Mg/L)
SS-control	<0,083
SSpH4t3	<0,083
SS-pH6,75t3	<0,083
SS-pH4t5	<0,215
SS-ph6,75t5	<0,083
SS-pH4–1500	<0,083
SS-pH4–22600	<0,083

Two saliva samples at pH 4 and 6.75 were used as controls. Samples were placed in an oven at 37°C in a wet atmosphere containing 5% CO_2 (EHRET®-BIOFASE 2-IP 20 DIN 40050), in the Laboratory for Bone Metabolism and Regeneration of the Faculty of dental Medicine of University of Porto. Completed the immersion time for each sample, the nickel ion research was performed in the Department of Chemistry of Faculty of Engineering of University of Porto, using the spectrophotometers GBC 932 Scientific Equipment PTY, model 932 and Unican, model 939, whose parameters are shown in Table 2.

3 RESULTS

The results of the nickel ion research are shown in Table 3, with the assignment used for each sample as a function of pH/time/ppm fluoride ion.

The condition with the longest immersion time at pH 4 was the only one that presented an outcome for the Ni ion above the sensitivity limit of the technique.

4 DISCUSSION

Although according to Eliades & Athanasiou (2007), the concentration of nickel found in the blood of patients under orthodontic treatment was not different from patients not submitted to orthodontic treatment. The possible deleterious effects of nickel concentration associated with orthodontic treatment will be more correlated with local concentrations than systemic presence.

The choice of nickel ion was in accordance with the method reported by several other studies related to stainless steel ion liberation, considered as reading parameter of the corrosive phenomenon (Kao 2007, Rahilly 2003, Sfrondrini 2010, Gursoy 2005). It was verified that only the most theoretically aggressive condition presented values above the threshold limits of the technique. Regarding the fluoride factor, the results were below the sensitivity of the technique. This outcome can be explained perhaps by the shorter times employed, which are consistent with the clinical practice.

5 CONCLUSIONS

Considering the drawbacks of this in vitro study the results lead to conclude that lowering pH and increasing the immersion time are the most corrosive conditions.

REFERENCES

Castro S.M. & Moreira R. & Braga A.C. & Ferreira A.P. & Poll-mann M.C. 2015. Effect of activation and preactivation on the mechanical behaviour and neutral position of stainless steel and beta-titanium T-Loop. *Korean J Orthod*, 45: 198–208.

Castro S.M. & Ponces M.J. & Lopes J.D. & Vasconcelos M. & Pollmann M.C.F. 2014. Orthodontic wires and its corrosion- The pecif case of stainless stell and beta-titanium. *Journal of Dental Sciences*, 20: 1–7.

Eliades T. & Athanasiou A.E. 2007. In vivo aging ofor-thodontic alloys: implications for corrosion potential, nickel release, and biocompatibility. *Angle Orthod*, 72: 222–237.

Gursoy S. & Acar A.G. & Sesen C. 2005. Comparison of metal release from new and recycled bracket-archwire combinations. *Angle Orthod*, 75: 92–4.

Kao, C.T. 2007. The cytotoxicity of orthodontic metal bracket immersion media. *Eur J Orthod*, 29: 198–203.

Krishnan V. 2011. Development and evaluation of two PVD-coated titanium orthodontic archwires for fluoride-induced corrosion protection. Acta Biomaterialia, 7: 1913–1927.

Rahilly G. & Price N. 2003. Nickel allergy and orthodontics. *J. Orthod*, 30: 171–4.

Sfondrini M.F. 2010. Nickel release from new conventional stainless steel recycled, and nickel-free orthodontic bracket: an in vitro study. *Am J Orthod* 137: 809–15.

Yang K. & Ren Y. 2010. Nickel-free austenitic stainless stells for medical applications. *Sci. Technol. Adv. Mater*, 11: 141–154.

Yonekura Y. 2004. In vitro corrosion characteristics of commercially available orthodontic wire. *Dental Mater Journal* 23: 197–202.

Biodental Engineering V – Belinha et al. (Eds)
© 2019 Taylor & Francis Group, London, ISBN 978-0-367-21087-8

Influence of thermocycling and colorants in the color of a bis-acryl composite resin—in vitro study

M.G.F. de Macedo
Faculty of Dental Medicine, University of Porto, Portugal

C.A.M. Volpato
Department of Dentistry, Federal University of Santa Catarina, Brazil

B.A.P.C. Henriques
Department of Engineering, Federal University of Santa Catarina, Brazil

P.C. Vaz
Department of Prosthodontics, Faculty of Dental Medicine, University of Porto, Portugal

F.S. Silva
Department of Mechanical Engineering, University of Minho, Portugal

C.F.C.L. Silva
Department of Prosthodontics, Faculty of Dental Medicine, University of Porto, Portugal

ABSTRACT: The aim of this study was to evaluate the color stability of the bis-acryl composite resin employed for the manufacturing of the short and long-term provisional prosthesis. For this, the bis-acryl resin was polished with different particle sizes, and the disks were aged in a thermocycler for 20, 100 and 200 cycles. Other disks, polished and unpolished, were immersed in the colorants beverages (green tea, red wine and coffee with sugar) for 24 hours, one week and one month. All groups and times were measured by a spectrophotometer and with the L*a*b* coordinates, the color ($\Delta E00$), lightness ($\Delta L'$), chroma ($\Delta C'$) and hue ($\Delta H'$) differences were calculated using the CIEDE2000 formula. The results showed that the unpolished group presented the greatest color differences after 200 cycles (3.73), as well as after 1 month of immersion in red wine (8.57) and coffee (5.48) ($P < 0.001$). Although the polished groups presented a statistically similar behavior, these groups showed higher staining with increasing immersion time.

1 INTRODUCTION

The success of oral rehabilitation is influenced by tissue health, adequate occlusion pattern and satisfactory esthetics. For success to be achieved, several clinical and laboratory steps must be respected throughout the treatment. One of them is the transition phase, in which the patient remains with provisional prostheses while awaiting the definitive pros-thesis [1]. Provisional prostheses are usually employed soon after dental preparation, allowing the pulp protection of vital teeth, aesthetics, function and comfort [2].

Traditionally, polymethylmethacrylate (PMMA) resins have been the most widely used materials for the manufacture of provisional prostheses. More recently, bis-acryl composite resins have been the material of choice for manufacturing provisional pros-theses and mock-ups. This is due to their easy

handling, reduction of clinical time, repair capacity, low polymerization contraction, reduced exothermic reaction and polishing possibility [3,4].

However, high cost, low creep resistance and chromatic instability have been cited as disadvantages of these materials. These limitations become more evident when provisional prostheses remain for longer periods of time in the oral cavity, especially in relation to their chromatic instability, which may result in surface staining, compromising the quality and longevity of the restorations.

Color change in provisional prostheses is related to extrinsic and intrinsic factors, which are most often associated. Degree of polymerization, sorption capacity, chemical reactivity with the oral environment, resin composition, inclusion of air bubbles, surface roughness, as well as oral hygiene are some of the variables related to this problem

[4,5]. Besides that, when the patient often consumes food or beverages that have coloring agents in their composition, the resin staining may become even more evident [6,7,8].

Several studies have been conducted to simulate the color change in acrylic and bis-acrylic composite resins by immersion of the resin samples in artificial saliva, coffee, coffee with sugar, tea, red wine, cola-based soft drinks, grape juice, curry, saffron, cranberry solution or chlorhexidine [1,3,5,7,8,9,10,11,12]. Accelerated aging methods employing thermocycling or ultraviolet (UV) rays have also been employed with or without coloring solutions [3,5,6,7,11,12].

On the other hand, the authors suggest techniques of surface finishing and polishing, as well as the use of surface sealants, to minimize color changes [6,10,11]. Smoother surfaces, resulting from the use of these techniques, reduce bacterial plaque accumulation, minimizing water infiltration, as well as retention of pigments from diet [7]. In addition, this is a practical and accessible procedure to the dentist, which can result in better performance and clinical time of provisional restoration. In this way, this study evaluated the color stability of the bis-acryl composite resin, polished or not, and submitted to thermal aging and colorants.

2 MATERIALS AND METHODS

Eighty bis-acryl composite resin disks (Protemp 4, 3M ESPE, USA) were made from a metal matrix with a 12-mm diameter and a 2-mm thickness and divided into 4 groups: no polishing (NP), polishing with 3-μm sized particles (3P), polishing with 3-μm and 1-μm (1P) and polishing with 3-μm, 1-μm and 0.5-μm sized particles (05P). Twenty disks (5 from each group) were thermocycled for 20, 100 and 200 cycles in artificial saliva, with 20 seconds of immersion for each temperature (5°C and +55°C). The other 60 disks were immersed in the colorants beverages (green tea, red wine and coffee with sugar) for 24 hours, one week and one month. During the immersion period, the disks were kept in plastic bottles, in a dark place, at room temperature.

The disks were positioned on the white background (standard calibration tile with CIE L*=93.84, a*=−1.48, b*=3.76) and measured three times at their center by a spectrophotometer (CM-2600d, Konica Minolta, Japan), before and after thermocycling and immersion times. The color (ΔE00), lightness (ΔL′), chroma (ΔC′) and hue (ΔH′) differences were calculated using the CIEDE2000 formula according to the following equation:

$$\Delta E_{00} = \left[\left(\frac{\Delta L'}{K_L S_L} \right)^2 + \left(\frac{\Delta C'}{K_C S_C} \right)^2 + \left(\frac{\Delta H'}{K_H S_H} \right)^2 \right. $$
$$\left. + R_T \left(\frac{\Delta C'}{K_C S_C} \right) \left(\frac{\Delta H'}{K_H S_H} \right) \right]^{\frac{1}{2}}$$

where ΔL′, ΔC′ and ΔH′ are differences in lightness, chroma and hue; RT is a rotation function that explains the interaction between chroma and hue in the blue region; SL, SC and SH are weighting functions and KL, KC and KH are parametric factors adjusted for 1. The color differences (ΔE00) in all the conditions tested were studied by statistical analysis with 3-way ANOVA. The lightness (ΔL′), chroma (ΔC′) and hue (ΔH′) differences were analyzed by re-peated measures ANOVA. Multiple comparisons were made by the Tukey's test ($\alpha = 0.05$).

3 RESULTS

When the disks were submitted to thermocycling, the color differences (ΔE00) became more evident as the cycles increased. The largest color differences were observed in the unpolished group (3.73), although all polished groups presented differences close to 3ΔE00 for 200 cycles (Table 1). Both groups and aging were significant statistically (P = 0.02 and P < 0.001, respectively). For all groups, the color difference (ΔE00) found is mainly related to the decrease in chroma (ΔC′) and the increase in hue (ΔH′) (P < 0.001).

Table 1. Means of the color differences (ΔE00) between the groups (ST, 3P, 1P, 05P), according to the number of thermocycles (20, 100, 200 cycles), colorants (tea, wine and coffee) and the immersion times (24 hours, 1 week and 1 month).

	NP	3P	1P	05P
Non-thermocycled	0.45	0.96	1.20	1.44
20 cycles	1.83	1.95	2.44	3.18
100 cycles	2.88	2.95	2.45	3.26
200 cycles	3.73	3.12	3.40	3.38
Tea – 24 hours	1.49	0.65	0.77	1.17
Tea – 1 week	2.16	0.69	0.86	1.32
Tea – 1 month	2.20	0.83	0.99	1.68
Wine – 24 hours	3.79	1.35	1.69	1.97
Wine – 1 week	5.72	3.22	2.52	2.79
Wine – 1 month	8.57	3.27	4.49	3.63
Coffee – 24 hours	5.04	2.87	3.24	3.01
Coffee – 1 week	5.51	3.73	3.24	3.23
Coffee – 1 month	5.48	4.22	3.43	3.32

The NP group immersed in red wine showed the greatest color changes (8.57ΔE00) (P < 0.001), followed by coffee with sugar (5.48ΔE00) (Table 1). Both the groups, colorants and time employed were statistically significant (P < 0.001). However, according to Tukey's test, the polished groups showed similar behavior. The immersion time also presented statistically divergent behaviors. When the ΔL', ΔC' and ΔH' were evaluated, it was observed the reduction of lightness (L'), increase of hue (H'), and little change in chroma (C'), confirming that the use of colorants changes these colorimetric parameters, especially after prolonged immersion times.

4 DISCUSSION

The results found in this study demonstrated that the polished surfaces were more resistant to pigmentation than unpolished surfaces, especially when the bis-acryl composite resin was immersed in coloring beverages. This finding reinforces the need for adequate polishing prior to the installation of provisional prostheses, since these restorations will be submitted to different foods and beverages during the useful life, besides the possibility of remaining in function by prolonged clinical times [10,11].

To simulate the longevity of this material, accelerated aging tests were employed. The aging of the samples in artificial saliva contributed to the chemical degradation of bis-acryl composite resin. The most evident chromatic difference was found in the NP group (3.73ΔE00), although the polished groups also showed color changes close to 3ΔE00 after the thermal cycling. These changes were more evident as the cycles increased. If more thermal cycles had been per-formed, probably more striking color changes could be found.

The coloring beverages selected for this study are part of the diet of many patients. It is important to know the chromatic effects of materials susceptible to staiting after the use of these beverages and how to minimize those effects. The staining occurs due to the ability of the bis-acryl composite resin in absorbing pigments present in beverages and foods. Some studies found important color changes when red wine and coffee were used [7,8], in agreement with the results of the present study. According to Gujjari et al. [9], less polar dyes and water-soluble polyphenols (such as the tannin present in the coffee) are deposited in the spaces formed as a function of the polymerization contraction, promoting staining. Moreover, for Gujjari et al., the intensity of the staining also depends on the time in which the coloring agent remains in contact with the surface of the resin.

This study also presented limitations. Longer thermocycling times and the association of oral hygiene agents should also be investigated to simulate ex-tended times of clinical use, as well as to correlate the potential of hygiene habits in reducing material staining.

5 CONCLUSIONS

Bis-acryl composite resin is a material subject to staining. Polishing minimizes this problem, as well as reducing the consumption of colorants such as red wine and coffee.

REFERENCES

[1] Givens E.J., Neiva G., Yaman P., Dennison J.B. 2008. Marginal adaptation and color stability of four provisional materials. J Prosthodont 17(2): 97–101.

[2] Burns D.R., Beck D.A., Nelson S.K. 2003. A review of selected dental literature on contemporary provisional fixed prosthodontic treatment: report of the Committee on Research in Fixed Prosthodontics of the Academy of Fixed Prosthodontics. J Prosthet Dent 90(5): 474–97.

[3] Sham A.S.K., Chu F.C.S., Chai J., Chow T.W. 2004. Color stability of provisional prosthodontic materials. J Prosthet Dent 91(5): 447–52.

[4] Patras M., Naka O., Doukoudakis S., Pissiotis A. 2012. Management of provisional restorations' deficiencies: a literature review. J Esthet Restor Dent 24(1): 26–38.

[5] Haselton D.R., Diaz-Arnold A.M., Dawson D.V. 2005. Color stability of provisional crown and fixed partial denture resins. J Prosthet Dent 93(1): 70–5.

[6] Doray P.G., Li D., Powers J.M. 2001. Color stability of provisional restorative materials after accelerated aging. J Prosthodont 10(4): 212–6.

[7] Rutkunas V., Sabaliauskas V., Mizutani H. 2010. Effects of different food colorants and polishing techniques on color stability of provisional prosthetic materials. Dent Mater J 29(2): 167–76.

[8] Gupta G., Gupta T. 2011. Evaluation of the effect of various beverages and food material on the color stability of provisional materials – An in vitro study. J Conserv Dent 14(3): 287–92.

[9] Gujjari A.K., Bhatnagar V.M., Bsavaraju R.M. 2013. Color stability and flexural strength of poly (methylmethacrylate) and bis-acrylic composite based provisional crown and bridge auto-polymerizing resins exposed to beverages and food dye: an in study. Indian J Dent Res 24(2): 172–7.

[10] Köroglu A., Sahin O., Dede D.O., Yilmaz B. 2016. Effect of different surface treatment methods on the surface roughness and color stability of interim prosthodontic materials. J Pros-thet Dent 115(4): 447–55.

[11] Guler A.U., Kurt S., Kulunk T. 2005. Effects of various fin-ishing procedures on the staining of provisional restorative materials. J Prosthet Dent 93(5): 453–8.

[12] Turgut S., Bagis B., Ayaz E.A., Ulusoy K.U., Altintas SH, Korkmaz FM et al. 2013. Discoloration of provisional resto-rations after oral rinses. Int J Med Sci 10(11): 1503–9.

Biodental Engineering V – Belinha et al. (Eds)
© 2019 Taylor & Francis Group, London, ISBN 978-0-367-21087-8

Flexible prosthesis in polyamide: Literature revision

R.F.A. da Costa, M.H. Figueiral, M. Sampaio-Fernandes, S. Oliveira & J.C. Reis Campos
Faculty of Dental Medicine, University of Porto (FMDUP), Porto, Portugal

ABSTRACT: Flexible polyamide dentures are currently used as an alternative to conventional prostheses due to its aesthetic and functional characteristics. However, despite the growing popularity of this material in recent years, there is a very limited knowledge about their clinical performance in long-term rehabilitations, including an absence of evident guidelines for their use. The main aim of this literature revision was to find reports of recent advances in polyamide prostheses, with the intention to provide objective information about their design, along with indications and contraindications of their use.

According to the current removable prosthodontic principles and the limitations found in this review, dental prostheses produced entirely in polyamides should be used on a provisional basis or in specific cases, such as patients with microstomia or with allergy to other denture base materials. If the rigidity of the denture is ensured by the inclusion of metal, the polyamide denture can be used in a wider number of clinical situations. Conducting further follow-up studies to assess the effectiveness of these dentures are indispensable to evaluate their clinical performance, understand their limitations and directions, thus being able to outline guidelines for their use and ensuring an adequate clinical performance.

1 INTRODUCTION

Conventional removable dentures have been used for decades in the rehabilitation of partially or totally edentulous patients, with the objective of restoring the function and aesthetics previously lost (Singh K, 2011).

The materials currently used for the confection of these prostheses – metal alloys and acrylic resins, as any material in dentistry, present some limitations associated with their use, not being suitable for all clinical situations (Fueki K, 2014). Alternative materials have been researched to overcome these limitations, and the flexible prosthesis has gained popularity in recent years (Fueki K, 2014).

Amongst the various materials available to produce flexible prosthesis, polyamide is the most frequently used, as it has been since the 50's, until now, being widely used in U.S.A and Japan (Singh K, 2011).

Flexible prosthesis in polyamide have advantageous characteristics, like the reduced or null risk of allergic reactions due to the absence of monomer in its constitution, high flexibility which allows to produce lighter and thinner prosthesis, improving the level of comfort reported by patients, and lastly, the aesthetic features that allow the reproduction of the underlying mucosa color, attending to the aesthetic demands of the patients (Fueki K, 2014).

However, despite this material being extensively used in some countries, there aren't currently enough clinical trials or follow up studies on its clinical performance, coupled with insufficient information on how to properly use this material (Fueki K, 2014). The inappropriate use of flexible resins follows, resulting in clinical failure due to the arbitrary confection of the dentures and its use in inadequate clinical situations (Fueki K, 2014).

This fact, coupled with the inherent limitations of the flexible resins, such as higher rate of discoloration, roughness of the polished surface, difficulties in relining or repairing, and the most concerning one, the higher risk of bone resorption, results in the necessity of performing additional research in how to properly use this material (Yoda N, 2012).

The purpose of this literature revision was to ascertain developments in the field of the flexible dentures in polyamide, with the intent of providing a set of indications of clinical situations in which this material can be used as well as where the necessary care in the confection and design of the prosthesis so as to increase the clinical success of oral rehabilitation.

2 MATERIALS AND METHODS

The research of scientific articles for this literature revision was performed on the online platform Pubmed. The key words used were "denture", "nylon", "polyamide", "flexible denture" and "thermoplastic resin". Exclusion criteria restricted articles with more than 16 years and that weren't related with flexible dentures in polyamide. From a total of 175 articles obtained with the selection criteria, 115 were excluded (90 after reading the title, 15 after reading the abstract and 10 after reading the article). With an additional 6 articles deemed worthy when reading the other articles, this literature revision was based on a total of 66 articles.

3 DISCUSSION

The mechanical and physical properties of polyamide dentures have been mentioned in several studies and were compared with the most common material used in removable prosthesis, the polimethilmetacrylate (PMMA). Through the employed studies, it was demonstrated that the polyamide dentures possessed inferior mechanical properties when compared with conventional dentures, possessing lower values of flexural strength and flexural modulus, which could result in permanent deformation of the base of the prosthesis or lack of rigidity, respectively, which could lead to an higher risk of bone resorption (Hamanaka I, 2011). Additionally, the polyamide dentures have a higher surface roughness, due to its low melting temperature, which results in difficulties in the finishing and polishing phases (Abuzar MA, et al, 2010). In consequence, the polyamide dentures have higher discoloration rates when contacting with drinks such as coffee, tea or wine, and a higher accumulation of bacterial plaque, which can harm the health of hard and periodontal tissues. It is also important to mention that between the different brands of polyamide resin, it has been shown that the brand Lucitone FRS presents superior mechanical characteristics (flexural strength, flexural modulus) in comparison with the brand Valplast (Takahashi Y, 2012). Unfortunately, other brands have not been compared.

Thus, it is considered that the polyamide dentures need a considerably higher level of maintenance when compared with the conventional PMMA dentures, regardless of the brand of choice (Iwata Y, 2016).

Considering the general inferior mechanical and physical properties of the polyamides dentures, their use has to be restricted to very specific and limited situations. However, these clinical situations are not well delineated due to the lack of information and investigation regarding flexible dentures (Fueki K, 2014).

Nonetheless, there are some general guidelines that we should have in mind when utilizing flexible dentures in polyamide, the majority being provided by the Japanese Prosthodontic Society.

The flexible dentures in polyamide can be built entirely in flexible resin or in conjecture with metal infrastructures, as a major connector and metallic oclusal rests (Fueki K, 2014). But regardless of the material chosen, we have to remember the design principles of partial dentures and movements performed by the dentures when subjected to masticatory forces, so that the configuration and extension of denture it is designed correctly, ensuring its correct behavior (Fueki K, 2014).

The analysis of the limitations of each clinical situation will guide us trough what is the best for each case. The following factors should exclude the use of a denture build entirely in polyamide (Dhiman, 2009) (Fueki K, 2014):

- Reduced number of natural teeth
- Unstable occlusion, which could result in fracture of resin clasps or residual ridge resorption
- Absent molar support
- Insufficient inter-arch space for the placement of acrylic teeth (< 4 mm)
- Prominent residual alveolar ridges, which do not allow the placement of teeth for lack of labial space
- Flaccid alveolar ridges, offering poor soft tissue support
- Reduced or excessive clinical crown undercuts, resulting in inadequate shape and thickness of the resin clasps.

In the presence of such factors, to use a polyamide denture, an hybrid denture has to be built, incorporating metal elements that secure the rigidity of denture (metallic major connector) (Yoda N, 2012), and prevent the "sinking" and horizontal rotation of the denture that can traumatize the marginal gingiva and cause excessive mobility of the pillar teeth (metallic oclusal rests) (Fueki K, 2014).

In conclusion, the JPS recommends that dentures built entirely in polyamide by the brand Valplast, should only be used to rehabilitate small edentulous spaces, e.g. one or two missing incisor, additionally recommending the inclusion of a metallic oclusal rest when replacing a missing molar (Fueki K, 2014). As for the brand Lucitone FRS, the JPS states that it can be used to replace one missing incisor or premolar that's not exposed to high masticatory loads (Fueki K, 2014). The inclusion of a metal infrastructure expands the clinical situations where the polyamide denture may be used (Fueki K, 2014).

4 CONCLUSION

Despite the popularity of the polyamide flexible dentures, some caution should be taken into account, bearing in mind the current inferior mechanical and physical properties of these dentures when compared to conventional resin PMMA, which could lead to worst performance and a greater risk of failure. The most concerning disadvantages of polyamides is the imminent risk of bone resorption due to the reduced rigidity of these materials.

Taking into account the current prosthetic institutions, prostheses manufactured entirely in polyamide should only be used on a provisional basis and in accordance with the situations mentioned above. If metallic infrastructures are included, as a major connector or metallic oclusal rests, these prostheses can be used in a large number of situations, combining the best of both worlds. Regardless of the format used, it is recommended to perform regular appointments, taking into account the reduced information available about the clinical behavior of these prostheses.

Additional clinical trials, thorough follow-up studies and in vitro research of physical and mechanical properties of this material, are necessary to allow the documentation of specific prosthetic principles for safe and effective use of flexible prostheses.

REFERENCES

Abuzar MA, Bellur S, Duong N, Kim BB, Lu P, Palfreyman N, et al. Evaluating surface roughness of a polyamide denture base material in comparison with poly (methyl methacrylate). Journal of oral science. 2010;52(4):577–81.

Dhiman RK, Roy Chowdhury SK. Midline fractures in single maxillary complete acrylic vs flexible dentures. Medical Journal Armed Forces India. 2009;65(2):141-5.

Fueki K, Ohkubo C, Yatabe M, Arakawa I, Arita M, Ino S, et al. Clinical application of removable partial dentures using thermoplastic resin-part I: definition and indication of non-metal clasp dentures. Journal of prosthodontic research. 2014;58(1):3–10.

Hamanaka I, Takahashi Y, Shimizu H. Mechanical properties of injection-molded thermoplastic denture base resins. Acta odontologica Scandinavica. 2011;69(2):75–9.

Hundal M, Madan R. Comparative clinical evaluation of removable partial dentures made of two different materials in Kennedy Applegate class II partially edentulous situation. Medical journal, Armed Forces India. 2015;71(Suppl 2):S306–12.

Iwata Y. Assessment of clasp design and flexural properties of acrylic denture base materials for use in non-metal clasp dentures. Journal of prosthodontic research. 2016.

Singh K, Aeran H, Kumar N, Gupta N. Flexible thermoplastic denture base materials for aesthetical removable partial denture framework. Journal of clinical and diagnostic research: JCDR. 2013;7(10):2372–3.

Takahashi Y, Hamanaka I, Shimizu H. Effect of thermal shock on mechanical properties of injection-molded thermoplastic denture base resins. Acta odontologica Scandinavica. 2012;70(4):297–302.

Yoda N, Watanabe M, Suenaga H, Kobari H, Hamada T, Sasaki K. Biomechanical Investigation of the "Non-clasp Denture" Based on the Load Exerted on Abutment Teeth and under the Denture Base. Annals of Japan Prosthodontic Society. 2012;4(2):183–92.

Biodental Engineering V – Belinha et al. (Eds)
© 2019 Taylor & Francis Group, London, ISBN 978-0-367-21087-8

Application of chitosan in dentistry—a review

J.M.S. Gomes
Institute of Science and Innovation in Mechanical and Industrial Engineering (INEGI), Porto, Portugal

J. Belinha
Department of Mechanical Engineering, School of Engineering, Polytechnic of Porto (ISEP), Porto, Portugal

R.M. Natal Jorge
Department of Mechanical Engineering, Faculty of Engineering, University of Porto (FEUP), Porto, Portugal

ABSTRACT: Present tissue engineering strategies are mainly focused on repairing and regenerating the architecture of tissues, such as bone by transplantation of scaffolds functionalized with cells or growth factors. In the recent decades, much attention has been given to chitosan, a biocompatible, biodegradable and non-toxic biomaterial that has been used in several biomedical fields. Chitosan-based scaffolds have been regarded as suited candidates for the construction of bone grafts and barrier membranes with application in dentistry. They trigger a minimal foreign body response, promote cell growth and proliferation. In addition, chitosan-based scaffolds have mucoadhesive and antibacterial properties. In this work, a literature survey is performed regarding chitosan applications in dentistry and its importance in this clinical field.

1 BONE

The structural scaffold of our body is the skeleton, and the bones that constitute it are key elements for locomotion, antigravity support, life-sustaining functions, and protection of viscera (Graber, Vanarsdall, Vig, & Huang, 2017; Walsh, 2018). Bone tissue is a specialized form of highly vascularized connective tissue which main components are collagen and calcium phosphate (Q. Li, Ma, & Gao, 2015). Bone is divided in cortical and trabecular tissues. The first is a hard and outer layer that surrounds the marrow space, while the latter resembles a honeycomb-like network of interspersed plates and rods, occupying a larger surface area (Clarke, 2008; Walsh, 2018). The cellular component of the bone includes osteoblasts, osteoclasts and osteocytes, each one of them with specific functions. Osteoblasts are responsible for forming bone by synthesizing the organic matrix, which is mainly type I collagen, and for giving bone resistance and tensile forces. On the other hand, osteoclasts, that derive from the monocyte/macrophage cell line, locally degrade the bone matrix during the resorption process. Osteocytes are localized between the bone matrix and are terminally differentiated osteoblasts that convert mechanical loading into biomechanical stimulus (Feng & McDonald, 2011).

As a living organ and a dynamic structure, bone is in constant adaptation to its surrounding environment and in constant remodeling, so its microstructure can be maintained. This process is regulated by central and local pathways and it happens because of homeostatic damage and physical trauma (Graber et al., 2017; Walsh, 2018). The remodeling process extends throughout life not only as an adaptation to changing biomechanical forces but also to remove old and damaged bone and replace it with new and mechanically stronger bone (Clarke, 2008).

2 BONE DISORDERS

Bone is the second most commonly transplanted tissue in the world, with an estimated 1.5 million grafts being placed in the United States every year, making it a billion-dollar industry. By 2020, it is expected that the incidence of bone disorders doubles, being aged and obese populations the main concern (Levengood & Zhang, 2014). Epidemiologic data show that worldwide bone and tooth loss are substantial health problems, having an estimated cost in the United States of $5–6 billion per year for the surgical treatments (Ibrahim, El-Hawary, Butler, & Mostafa, 2014).

Periodontal disease is characterized by an exaggerated immune response caused by a microbial community. The development of a chronic inflammation, tissue destruction and damage of the epithelial barrier are caused by a deregulated immune response. The increase of the permeability of the tissue enables further infiltration of the bacteria, which leads to a magnified inflammatory response (Gjoseva et al., 2018; Popa, Ghica, & Dinu-Pîrvu, 2013). Antimicrobial agents are used in cases of moderate and severe periodontal disease as a suppression or, if possible, eradication method of bacteria (Ikinci et al., 2002). This inflammatory disease affects several structures, such as gingiva and alveolar bone. It is considered a major burden for health care systems since it is the leading cause of tooth loss worldwide, surpassing caries. It prevails in approximately 50% of adults, being that 10–30% presents severe forms of the disease (Schröder et al., 2005; Zhang et al., 2006).

A bone defect can result from systemic and dental disorders. Considering periodontal diseases, bone resorption leads, for most cases, to bone repair (Ezoddini-Ardakani, Navab Azam, Yassaei, Fatehi, & Rouhi, 2011). These defects can result from different situations such as trauma, infection or tumor resection. Segmental mandibular defects are an example and they can be treated using a non-vascularized bone graft. Consequently, patient's basic activities such as eating and communicating might be affected (Fan et al., 2014). When the defect reaches a critical size, an intervention is needed because the physiological path of the regeneration process does not occur (Levengood & Zhang, 2014).

3 REPAIR STRATEGIES

There are different strategies that can be implemented to help the healing process of bone. They include bone grafts, bone substitute materials, growth factors and metalwork to stabilize the bone (Turnbull et al., 2017). The conventional methods used for bone repair are autografts and allografts, which can be used in cases of bone defects created by tumors, traumas or diseases (Park et al., 2013). Autografts are still considered the gold standard in the range of repair strategies. However, their use requires a second surgery to harvest the graft from the patient, leading to donor site morbidity, mismatch in size, infection and prolonged pain following surgery (Q. Li et al., 2015; Turnbull et al., 2017). Contrarily to autografts, allografts are harvested from cadavers, which can possibly cause an immune reaction and infection transmission (Ezoddini-Ardakani et al., 2011; Levengood & Zhang, 2014). As for metal grafts, even though they have a good mechanical strength, they may also be the cause of stress shielding, infections and chronic pain (Q. Li et al., 2015).

Nowadays, in dentistry, most of the damaged tissues are replaced with biocompatible materials that do not fulfil all the needs and do not match the behavior of the original tissue. These disadvantages led to unsatisfactory results, which directed the focus to the development of materials with optimal characteristics (Zandparsa, 2014). Thus, bone tissue engineering has emerged as a tool that provides promising alternative approaches to autografts and allografts by introducing the use of synthetic grafts to guide bone tissue regeneration (Levengood & Zhang, 2014).

Scaffolds used in bone tissue engineering must possess a set of specific characteristics. An ideal three-dimensional scaffold must be biocompatible, biodegradable and the mechanical properties of the material must be coincident with those of the tissue that is being replaced (Turnbull et al., 2017). It should also support the movement, proliferation and differentiation of cells (Zhang et al., 2006). Porosity is another important characteristic of these scaffolds since it will allow the permeation and adaptation of nutrients and cells that intervene in the bone regeneration process (Shirosaki et al., 2009).

When an inflammatory process takes place, the goal becomes to repair the damaged tissues with periodontal therapy, which can promote the regeneration of ligaments such as the periodontal ligament (Zhang et al., 2006). With this therapy, one can also use bone-substituting materials that enhance the process of bone regeneration in periodontal defects. These include materials such as bone powder or calcium phosphate ceramic. They have emerged from the need of finding alternatives with a more similar structure to bone than other materials. However, there are some disadvantages: bone resorption, immune response, low biodegradability, and poor adaptation. To overcome the drawbacks of these bone-substituting materials, biodegradable polymers and ceramics combined with collagen started being used (Jeong Park et al., 2000).

When it is necessary to prevent the migration of gingival epithelial cells into a bone defect, one can use barrier membranes to protect the affected area. These structures can promote the growth of progenitor bone and periodontal ligament cells. They must possess some specific characteristics, such as mechanical stability, optimal porosity and biodegradability so a second surgery is avoided (Norowski Jr et al., 2015; Shirosaki et al., 2009).

In the selection process of the material to be used for the tissue engineering approach, polymers, either natural or synthetic, are often chosen. They can be used as single constituents of the scaffold but also combined with, for example, bioceramics or bioglasses to overcome their limitations (Horst, Chavez, Jheon, Desai, & Klein, 2012). It is possible to customize the degradation rate and the mechanical properties to a certain extent depending on the application. However, polymers are often associated with low mechanical strength and shape retention failure (Z. Li, Ramay, Hauch, Xiao, & Zhang, 2005). They often have biofunctional molecules on the surface that will promote cell attachment and differentiation (Horst et al., 2012). Besides natural polymers, bone repairing scaffolds can also be constructed using synthetic polymers. The most commonly used are polylactic acid (PLA), polyglycolic acid (PGA) and polycaprolactone (PCL). Even though they are biocompatible and non-toxic, they present an insufficient cell adhesion. Also, they lack functional groups at their surfaces, which are hydrophobic, thus hindering the cell growth in a three-dimensional architecture (Galler, D'Souza, Hartgerink, & Schmalz, 2011; Z. Li et al., 2005). There are some concerns regarding the degradation products of these polymers, which by reducing the local pH can accelerate the degradation rate and cause an inflammatory response (Maitz, 2015).

The interest in finding new and improved materials for bone repair in dentistry, that help overcoming some of the previously mentioned disadvantages, have increased in recent years (Horst et al., 2012). One of these promising materials is chitosan. Hence, its properties and its different ways of being used will be described in the next section.

4   CHITOSAN

Many synthetic and natural materials can be used for the construction of bone-repairing and bone-regenerating scaffolds. One of these natural materials is chitosan that has been extensively studied and characterized and, thus, considered as a viable option for bone tissue engineering.

Chitosan is a natural polysaccharide obtained from chitin, the second most abundant polymer found in nature. It can be found in the exoskeleton of insects, crustaceans and fungi (Dash, Chiellini, Ottenbrite, & Chiellini, 2011; Q. Li et al., 2015). Chitosan is composed of glucosamine and N-acetylglucosamine units linked in a $\beta(1–4)$ manner. The ratio between these two units will determine the degree of deacetylation. When it reaches about 50%, chitin becomes soluble in aqueous acidic media, originating chitosan (Di Martino, Sittinger, & Risbud, 2005; Rinaudo, 2006). When the degree of deacetylation increases, the viscosity of chitosan also increases, which will influence biological influences, such as osteogenesis enhancement. Furthermore, the degree of deacetylation influences the degradation rate of chitosan. Highly deacetylated structures degrade more slowly and may last for months in vivo (Dash et al., 2011; Di Martino et al., 2005).

There is a set of properties that a biomaterial must possess to be considered optimal for a specific biomedical application. Several of these properties can be found in chitosan, such as biodegradability, biocompatibility, non-antigenicity and non-toxicity (Z. Li et al., 2005; Shirosaki et al., 2009). Particularly, chitosan's biocompatibility may primarily be associated with its similarity to glycosaminoglycans present in the extracellular matrix (ECM) (Park et al., 2013). Furthermore, it can be processed in a variety of three-dimensional forms, it evokes minimal foreign-body response and its hydrophilic surface promotes cell adhesion and proliferation (Levengood & Zhang, 2014). Depending on the tissue where it is going to be applied and the final goal of the application itself, chitosan can be reproduced in many forms, such as hydrogels, films, sponges, and powders (Rinaudo, 2006).

Concerning bone tissue engineering, chitosan has been widely studied to evaluate the possibility of using it as a bone substitute or as a drug delivery system. It has been shown that chitosan on itself is not sufficient to induce rapid bone regeneration at the initial phase of bone healing. One of the reasons for this is that chitosan is mechanically unstable and weak, and it may be unable to maintain a predefined shape for transplantation under physiological conditions as a result of swelling (Maurício et al., 2011).

To overcome this disadvantage, chitosan can be associated to other materials, such as calcium phosphate, calcium sulfate, hydroxyapatite, and other natural polymers. Furthermore, growth factors can be seeded on chitosan scaffolds which will stimulate their activity and improve bone-forming efficacy (Lee et al., 2002; Turnbull et al., 2017). Also, chitosan scaffolds have been proven to be osteoconductive, enhancers of bone formation and promoters of cell growth (Dash et al., 2011; Z. Li et al., 2005). Chitosan has been used as a drug delivery system for the treatment of dental and gingival pathologies because of its mucoadhesive and antibacterial properties (Di Martino et al., 2005).

5   REPAIR STRATEGIES USING CHITOSAN

Despite having a set of properties that make it a widely used biomaterial for biomedical applications, chitosan has a low mechanical strength. For this, many researchers choose to develop scaffolds where chitosan is the base material and then combine it with bioactive polymers, inorganic ceramics or proteins. This will also affect and even enhance the tissue regenerative efficacy (Lee et al., 2002). In this section, it will be shortly described some studies that used chitosan for bone repair and regeneration in dentistry.

Gjoseva et al. developed sodium tripolyphosphate/chitosan microparticles that work as carriers of an antimicrobial and anti-inflammatory drug called doxycycline. The microparticles were administered in a local intrapocket infusion manner for treatment and controlled delivery of the drug. Additionally, the microparticles were coated with ethyl cellulose to retard the release of the highly soluble drug since chitosan has a high degree of swelling. The study showed that the microparticles were able to interact with elements of the immune system, causing specific biological responses, and that they were not cytotoxic (Gjoseva et al., 2018).

Zhang et al. have studied the behaviour of a gene-activated chitosan/collagen scaffold cultured with human periodontal ligament cells (HPLCs). The scaffolds were combined with plasmid and virus encoding the human transforming growth factor-β1, which can up-regulate the production of components of the ECM, including collagen. The study has shown that the composite scaffolds have better cytocompatibility than pure chitosan/collagen scaffolds since HPLCs recruited surrounding tissues to grow in the scaffold after it was implanted *in vivo*. For this, the researchers believe that these composite scaffolds are good candidates in periodontal tissue engineering (Zhang et al., 2006).

Also considering chitosan combined with other materials, Park et al. developed chitosan-based scaffolds to be used as bone grafts with three different formulations: pure chitosan, chitosan/alginate and chitosan/chondroitin 4-sulfate, being the last two anionic polymers. The scaffolds were coated with a layer of apatite to enhance bone ingrowth and their bonding ability. Additionally, they were seeded with mouse bone marrow stromal cells and the influence of the apatite coating was measured. In terms of cell spreading, proliferation and osteogenic differentiation, the coating was proven to enhance the cell activity on the scaffolds. All scaffolds were then mechanically evaluated by measurement of their compressive modulus, which proved to be higher in the composite scaffolds than in the pure chitosan ones. This lead to the conclusion that adding alginate or chondroitin 4-sulfate increases the mechanical strength of the scaffolds, which will make them more suitable for bone tissue engineering (Park et al., 2013).

In another study, Lee et al. projected bone substitutes in the form of porous chitosan scaffolds, as well as porous polylactic acid/chitosan scaffolds to improve the mechanical stability. By loading them with platelet-derived growth factor-BB, a promoter of periodontal tissue regeneration, they worked as drug delivery devices that could shorten the therapeutic period. Before inserting the scaffolds in a craniotomy defect in rats, they were cultured with rat calvarial osteoblasts. The obtained results showed that the controlled release of PDGF-BB from the scaffolds significantly promoted bone healing and regeneration. Additionally, these scaffolds promoted cell attachment and cell migration through their porous matrices (Lee et al., 2002).

Considering the bioadhesion and permeability of chitosan, Ikinci et al. developed gels and films of chitosan with different molecular weights. These structures were loaded with chlorhexidine gluconate, a drug used to fight oral microbial species, such as *porphyromonas gingivalis*, which is an aggressive pathogen that leads to periodontal destruction in humans. The results showed the antimicrobial activity of chitosan and chlorhexidine, as well as the bioadhesion property of chitosan. This constitutes an important feature because it will contribute for the retention of the drug in the periodontal pocket and also for the prolonged release of the drug (Ikinci et al., 2002).

Ezoddini-Ardakani and co-workers conducted a study in which they evaluated the efficacy on bone healing of chitosan powder used to fill a dental socket after tooth extraction. The mean density of regenerated bone was assessed ten weeks after the surgeries took place. After comparing with untreated sockets, it was concluded that chitosan supported the proliferation of osteoblastic cells considering the rate of bone formation and the speed of bone regeneration in the dental cavities (Ezoddini-Ardakani et al., 2011).

Since commercially available barrier membranes degrade rapidly and in an unpredictable manner, Norowski et al. attempted to make chitosan nanofibrous membranes with an extended degradation time. The scaffolds were cross-linked with genipin, which has been shown to increase the biocompatibility and decrease the inflammatory response. The results of this study demonstrated that the crosslinking improved the mechanical properties and prolonged the degradation time of the membranes, not affecting the cytocompatibility. Therefore, the cross-linked chitosan membranes may be considered as a good option for guided bone regeneration (Norowski Jr et al., 2015).

6 CONCLUSIONS

It is very important to develop good biodegradable and biocompatible scaffolds that can fulfill their roles as temporary matrices. This aspect will enable the success of therapies that may also consist of cell and growth factors transplantation. The efficacy of chitosan has already been proven but there is still space for improvements that turn it into a preferable material when it comes to bone repair in dentistry.

ACKNOWLEDGEMENTS

The authors truly acknowledge the funding provided by Ministério da Ciência, Tecnologia e Ensino Superior—Fundação para a Ciência e a Tecnologia (Portugal) by project funding MIT-EXPL/ISF/0084/2017. Additionally, the authors gratefully acknowledge the funding of Project NORTE-01-0145-FEDER-000022—SciTech—Science and Technology for Competitive and Sustainable Industries, cofinanced by Programa Operacional Regional do Norte (NORTE2020), through Fundo Europeu de Desenvolvimento Regional (FEDER).

REFERENCES

Clarke, B. (2008). Normal bone anatomy and physiology. *Clinical Journal of the American Society of Nephrology*, 131–139. https://doi.org/10.2215/CJN.04151206.

Dash, M., Chiellini, F., Ottenbrite, R. M., & Chiellini, E. (2011). Chitosan—A versatile semi-synthetic polymer in biomedical applications. *Progress in Polymer Science (Oxford)*, *36*(8), 981–1014. https://doi.org/10.1016/j.progpolymsci.2011.02.001.

Di Martino, A., Sittinger, M., & Risbud, M. V. (2005). Chitosan: A versatile biopolymer for orthopaedic tissue-engineering. *Biomaterials*, *26*(30), 5983–5990. https://doi.org/10.1016/j.biomaterials.2005.03.016.

Ezoddini-Ardakani, F., Navab Azam, A., Yassaei, S., Fatehi, F., & Rouhi, G. (2011). Effects of chitosan on dental bone repair. *Health*, *3*(4), 200–205. https://doi.org/10.4236/health.2011.34036.

Fan, J., Park, H., Lee, M. K., Bezouglaia, O., Fartash, A., Kim, J., … Lee, M. (2014). Adipose-Derived Stem Cells and BMP-2 Delivery in Chitosan-Based 3D Constructs to Enhance Bone Regeneration in a Rat Mandibular Defect Model. *Tissue Engineering Part A*, *20*(15–16), 2169–2179. https://doi.org/10.1089/ten.tea.2013.0523.

Feng, X., & McDonald, J. M. (2011). Disorders of Bone Remodeling. *Annual Review of Pathology: Mechanisms of Disease*, *6*(1), 121–145. https://doi.org/10.1146/annurev-pathol-011110-130203.

Galler, K. M., D'Souza, R. N., Hartgerink, J. D., & Schmalz, G. (2011). Scaffolds for Dental Pulp Tissue Engineering. *Advances in Dental Research*, *23*(3), 333–339. https://doi.org/10.1177/0022034511405326.

Gjoseva, S., Geskovski, N., Sazdovska, S. D., Popeski-Dimovski, R., Petruševski, G., Mladenovska, K., & Goracinova, K. (2018). Design and biological response of doxycycline loaded chitosan microparticles for periodontal disease treatment. *Carbohydrate Polymers*, *186*, 260–272. https://doi.org/10.1016/j.carbpol.2018.01.043.

Graber, L. W., Vanarsdall, R. L., Vig, K. W. L., & Huang, G. J. (2017). *Orthodontics: Current principles and techniques* (Sixth edit). St. Louis, Missouri: Elsevier. Retrieved from https://books.google.pt/books?hl=pt-PT&lr=&id=N0SwDAAAQBAJ&oi=fnd&pg=PA99&dq=bone+physiology&ots=uVNc4oc2Uh&sig=o2FS9 sJVlOIBjqXergFV6dOeM8U&redir_esc=y#v=onepage&q=bone physiology&f=false.

Horst, O. V., Chavez, M. G., Jheon, A. H., Desai, T., & Klein, O. D. (2012). Stem Cell and Biomaterials Research in Dental Tissue Engineering and Regeneration. *Dental Clinics of North America*, *56*(3), 495–520. https://doi.org/10.1016/j.cden.2012.05.009.

Ibrahim, F. M., El-Hawary, Y. M., Butler, I. S., & Mostafa, S. I. (2014). Bone repair stimulation in rat mandible by new chitosan silver(i) complexes. *International Journal of Polymeric Materials and Polymeric Biomaterials*, *63*(16), 846–858. https://doi.org/10.1080/00914037.2014.886222.

Ikinci, G., Şenel, S., Akincibay, H., Kaş, S., Erciş, S., Wilson, C. G., & Hincal, A. A. (2002). Effect of chitosan on a periodontal pathogen Porphyromonas gingivalis. *International Journal of Pharmaceutics*, *235*(1–2), 121–127. https://doi.org/10.1016/S0378-5173(01)00974-7.

Jeong Park, Y., Moo Lee, Y., Nae Park, S., Yoon Sheen, S., Pyoung Chung, C., & Lee, S. J. (2000). Platelet derived growth factor releasing chitosan sponge for periodontal bone regeneration. *Biomaterials*, *21*(2), 153–159. https://doi.org/10.1016/S0142-9612(99)00143-X.

Lee, J. Y., Nam, S. H., Im, S. Y., Park, Y. J., Lee, Y. M., Seol, Y. J., … Lee, S. J. (2002). Enhanced bone formation by controlled growth factor delivery from chitosan-based biomaterials. *Journal of Controlled Release*, *78*(1–3), 187–197. https://doi.org/10.1016/S0168-3659(01)00498-9.

Levengood, S. K. L., & Zhang, M. (2014). Chitosan-based scaffolds for bone tissue engineering. *Journal of Materials Chemistry B*, *2*(21), 3161–3184. https://doi.org/10.1039/c4tb00027 g.

Li, Q., Ma, L., & Gao, C. (2015). Biomaterials for in situ tissue regeneration: development and perspectives. *J. Mater. Chem. B*, *3*(46), 8921–8938. https://doi.org/10.1039/C5TB01863C.

Li, Z., Ramay, H. R., Hauch, K. D., Xiao, D., & Zhang, M. (2005). Chitosan-alginate hybrid scaffolds for bone tissue engineering. *Biomaterials*, *26*(18), 3919–3928. https://doi.org/10.1016/j.biomaterials.2004.09.062.

Maitz, M. F. (2015). Applications of synthetic polymers in clinical medicine. *Biosurface and Biotribology*, *1*(3), 161–176. https://doi.org/10.1016/j.bsbt.2015.08.002.

Maurício, A. C., Gärtner, A., Armada-da-Silva, P., Amado, S., Pereira, T., Veloso, A. P., … Geuna, S. (2011). Cellular systems and biomaterials for nerve regeneration in neurotmesis injuries. *Biomaterials Applications for Nanomedicine*, 415–440.

Norowski Jr, P. A., Fujiwara, T., Clem, W. C., Adatrow, P. C., Eckstein, E. C., Haggard, W. O., & Bumgardner, J. D. (2015). Novel naturally crosslinked electrospun nanofibrous chitosan mats for guided bone regeneration membranes: material characterization and cytocompatibility. *Journal of Tissue Engineering and Regenerative Medicine*, (9), 577–583. https://doi.org/10.1002/term.1648.

Park, H., Choi, B., Nguyen, J., Fan, J., Shafi, S., Klokkevold, P., & Lee, M. (2013). Anionic carbohydrate-containing chitosan scaffolds for bone regeneration. *Carbohydrate Polymers*, *97*(2), 587–596. https://doi.org/10.1016/j.carbpol.2013.05.023.

Popa, L., Ghica, M. V., & Dinu-Pîrvu, C. (2013). Periodontal Chitosan-gels designed for improved local intra-pocket drug delivery. *Farmacia*, *61*(2), 240–250.

Rinaudo, M. (2006). Chitin and chitosan: Properties and applications. *Progress in Polymer Science (Oxford)*, *31*(7), 603–632. https://doi.org/10.1016/j.progpolymsci.2006.06.001.

Schröder, N. W. J., Meister, D., Wolff, V., Christan, C., Kaner, D., Haban, V., ... Schumann, R. R. (2005). Chronic periodontal disease is associated with single-nucleotide polymorphisms of the human TLR-4 gene. *Genes and Immunity*, *6*(5), 448–451. https://doi.org/10.1038/sj.gene.6364221.

Shirosaki, Y., Tsuru, K., Hayakawa, S., Osaka, A., Lopes, M. A., Santos, J. D., ... Fernandes, M. H. (2009). Physical, chemical and in vitro biological profile of chitosan hybrid membrane as a function of organosiloxane concentration. *Acta Biomaterialia*, *5*(1), 346–355. https://doi.org/10.1016/j.actbio.2008.07.022.

Turnbull, G., Clarke, J., Picard, F., Riches, P., Jia, L., Han, F., ... Shu, W. (2017). 3D bioactive composite scaffolds for bone tissue engineering. *Bioactive Materials*, 1–37. https://doi.org/10.1016/j.bioactmat.2017.10.001.

Walsh, J. S. (2018). Normal bone physiology, remodelling and its hormonal regulation. *Surgery (United Kingdom)*, *36*(1), 1–6. https://doi.org/10.1016/j.mpsur.2017.10.006.

Zandparsa, R. (2014). Latest biomaterials and technology in dentistry. *Dental Clinics of North America*, *58*(1), 113–134. https://doi.org/10.1016/j.cden.2013.09.011.

Zhang, Y., Cheng, X., Wang, J., Wang, Y., Shi, B., Huang, C., ... Liu, T. (2006). Novel chitosan/collagen scaffold containing transforming growth factor-$\beta 1$ DNA for periodontal tissue engineering. *Biochemical and Biophysical Research Communications*, *344*(1), 362–369. https://doi.org/10.1016/j.bbrc.2006.03.106.

Biodental Engineering V – Belinha et al. (Eds)
© 2019 Taylor & Francis Group, London, ISBN 978-0-367-21087-8

Computational simulation of the vestibular system using a meshless particle method

C.F. Santos & Marco Parente
Institute of Science and Innovation in Mechanical and Industrial Engineering (INEGI), Unit of Design and Experimental Validation, Porto, Portugal

J. Belinha
Department of Mechanical Engineering, School of Engineering, Polytechnic of Porto (ISEP), Porto, Portugal

R.M. Natal Jorge
Department of Mechanical Engineering, Faculty of Engineering, University of Porto (FEUP), Porto, Portugal

Fernanda Gentil
Clínica ORL—Dr. Eurico Almeida e Escola Superior de Saúde—P. Porto, Portugal

ABSTRACT: Vestibular rehabilitation is the most used therapy in cases of unbalance diagnosis. The vertigo symptoms are commonly related with inner ear diseases, affecting 20%-30% of the world population (von Brevern & Neuhauser, 2011). Its prevalence is higher in elders. In this work, a three-dimensional model of the semi-circular canal of the vestibular system, containing the fluids that promote body balance, will be used. The Smoothed-Particle Hydrodynamics (SPH) method, a meshless particle method, will be the discrete numerical technique used to simulate the fluid behaviour. In the SPH the discretization is represented by particles with constant mass (G.R. Liu & Liu, 2003). The obtained results allow to understand the behaviour of the vestibular structures during the rehabilitation manoeuvres.

1 THE VESTIBULAR SYSTEM

1.1 *Introduction*

The human body is a biomechanical mechanism structured in several sensory parts, connected in several different ways with the purpose of keeping the body alive. One of the most sensory components is the tiny inner ear. The posterior part of the inner ear is the main responsible of our sense of gait and posture, and it is known as vestibular system.

The balance comes from the vestibular system. The main structure of this system is the three semi-circular canals, placed orthogonally and linked to each other (Broglio, Sosnoff, Rosengren, & McShane, 2009). Each ear has its own canals, therefore each individual have six semi-circular canals, which work coordinated in the balance task. In Figure 1 there is a representation of one semi-circular canal.

The structure of the canal comprise a membranous labyrinth embraced by a bony labyrinth with the same shape. The membranous labyrinth is full of fluid called endolymph, which promotes the human movement. Moreover, a fluid called perilymph take place between both labyrinths (Davis, Xue, Peterson, & Grant, 2007). The complex and detailed structure of the vestibular system is not completed without mentioning the cupula and the macula of the ear. These structures are the ones with the sensory hair cells, responsible for sending signals to the brain, signalling the physical movement. The sensory cells exhibit a constant discharge of neurotransmitters that are modified by the direction of cupula deflection (Wolfe, 2012). Regarding the macula placed in the saccule and the utricle, which are the adjacent structures of the semi-circular canals, it is a membranous structure composed by a gel layer that contains calcium carbonate crystals called otoconia. The mass of the otolithic membrane allows the macula to be sensitive to gravity and linear acceleration.

The vestibular system, from the functional point of view, has three main functions: it corrects any inadvertent movement of the body centre of mass and its balance position on its support base (feet) to avoid the fall; it provides an accurate perception

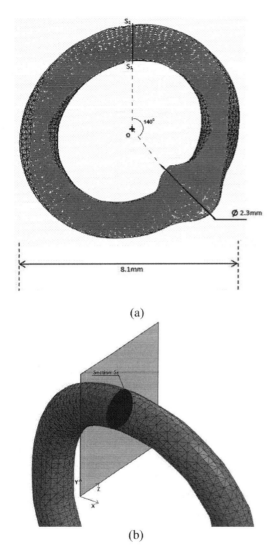

Figure 1. (a) Model of the semi—circular canal. (b) Section of the canal analyzed.

of the position of the body in its surroundings and the perception of the direction and acceleration movements; and, finally, it controls the eyes' movement for the maintenance of one clear visual field when the individual, the surroundings, or both, are in movement (Hall, n.d.).

Balance corresponds to the stabilization of the body and vision, resulting from the integration of the information transmitted by three sensorial afferents: vestibular, visual and proprioceptive. The vestibular system permanently participates in the adaptation of reactions, determining the head position in the space relatively to the fundamental posture, as in relation to the displacement (Hall, n.d.; Herdman, 2013).

1.2 Inner ear diseases and rehabilitation

Some vestibular conditions could influence the performance of the vestibular system. There are several external factors that could change the behaviour of complete the mechanism. The quality of life of someone suffering from the main symptom caused by vestibular disorders (vertigo), decrease significantly.

Vertigo and dizziness are the main symptoms occurring when the vestibular system is affected or when the information coming from all systems related to balance and gait, do not match; which could happen for several reasons and in recurrent episodes.

The common complaint of the patients is the perception of a spinning motion and, sometimes, could also happen an impression of displacement of the environment to the individual or an intensive sensation of rotation inside the head (Taylor & Goodkin, 2011), as described by the patients. This symptom is often associated with nausea and vomiting, which could lead to complications in standing or walking (Karatas, 2008). Other incapacitating symptoms like blurred vision, difficulty speaking and hearing loss may also occur (Strupp et al., 2011).

Vertigo affects approximately 20%–30% of the world population (von Brevern & Neuhauser, 2011), mainly elders and it's prevalence is twice higher in women (Neuhauser & Lempert, 2009).

The literature shows that 85% of balance conditions could be related with inner ear disorders (Gámiz & Lopez-Escamez). Individuals with symptoms like vertigo and dizziness have a higher risk of falls and depression. Therefore, the development of methods to help the decrease these symptoms is a priority.

The main therapy method used when severe crises of dizziness and unbalance problems occur is the vestibular rehabilitation, due the positive results showed with this method, evaluated mainly by the patient feedback (Obrist, 2007).

The vestibular rehabilitation exercises stimulate the brain to use visual clues and proprioceptive alternatives to keep balance and gait. There are evidence that improve nystagmus, control postural dizziness and all other symptoms vertigo, which makes it the definitive treatment for most patients (Kerrigan, Costigan, Blatt, Mathiason, & Domroese, 2013). The exercises progression is guided by both patient symptoms and related physio-pathological mechanisms.

Techniques used in vestibular rehabilitation therapy are based on both precise, individual diagnosis of lesions and follow-up of condition progress. Specific methods include manoeuvres aiming at dislodging or repositioning otoliths, habituation, adaptation or substitution exercises. Non-specific methods consist generally in rehabilitating overall endurance, and strengthening specific muscle groups so as to sustain posture and gait (Obrist, 2007).

The main disadvantage of the reported methodology is the empirical character of the process. Due to the reduced dimensions of the vestibular system, the computational numerical methods seem to be an opportunity to perform a biomechanical study of such important structure to the human sense of balance.

The aim of the present work is to achieve a procedure to be applied in the vestibular rehabilitation in order to obtain improved results from the patient's perspective. In this work, a meshless particle method – the smooth particle method – was the computational tool selected to simulate the rehabilitation process.

2 PARTICLE METHODS IN BIOMECHANICS

The numerical computational simulation is a powerful tool in the biological field. Finite Element Method (FEM), as applied in engineering, is a computational tool for performing virtual mechanical analyses. It includes the use of mesh generation techniques for dividing a complex problem into small elements.

Simulation methods for fluid/structure interaction with FEM have been gradually developed.

Additionally, other complemental numerical procedure, known as meshless methods allow to obtain solution fields (displacements, stresses, strain, etc.) with an extra smoothness and accuracy.

Both numerical approaches are very useful to, for example, predict the rupture of biological tissues and the remodelling process of biological materials. Furthermore, recent works show that the combination of medical imaging techniques (CAT scan and MRI) with meshless methods is more efficient than using the FEM (Wong, Wang, Zhang, Liu, & Shi, 2010) (Chen et al., 2010).

Meshless methods present several advantages used in biological simulation, as the re-meshing flexibility and natural efficiency. It allows to deal with the large distortions of soft materials (tendons, internal organs, skin, muscles, etc.) and, simultaneously, permits to simulate explicitly fluid flow (the respiration, the hemodynamics, the swallow, the endolymph, etc.).

Doweidar et al. (Doweidar, Calvo, Alfaro, Groenenboom, & Doblaré, 2010) have several works in the biomechanical field, showing that meshless methods own some advantages over the FEM, mainly in biomechanical conditions dealing with large strains, such as the human lateral collateral ligament and the human knee joint simulations. Additionally, Zhang et al. (Zhang, Wittek, Joldes, Jin, & Miller, 2014) extended a meshless method to the nonlinear explicit dynamic analysis of the brain tissue response. The results obtained by Zang et al. confirmed the accuracy of meshless methods with nonlinear hyperelastic biomaterials. Similarly, other authors using meshless methods to simulate brain damage (Marques, Belinha, Dinis, & Natal Jorge, 2018).

Regarding hemodynamic, meshless methods have been widely used with encouraging results.

In the literature, several research works show the reliability of meshless methods when applied to simulate the motion of a deformable red blood cell in flowing blood plasma (Tsubota, Wada, & Yamaguchi, 2006) or to study the effect of red blood cells on the primary thrombus formation (Mori et al., 2008).

Computational prediction of bone tissue remodelling is other branch of computational biomechanical in which meshless methods proved to possess clear advantages (Doblaré et al., 2005).

Liew et al. back in 2002, published the first work dealing with bone structures and using meshless methods (Liew, Wu, & Ng, 2002). Then, other authors applied meshless methods to simulate the bone tissue remodelling process with success (Lee, Chen, Zeng, Eskandarian, & Oskard, 2007) (Taddei, Pani, Zovatto, Tonti, & Viceconti, 2008). A new bone tissue remodelling algorithm relying on the meshless method accuracy was recently presented by Belinha and co-workers (Belinha, Natal Jorge, & Dinis, 2012) (Belinha, Dinis, & Natal Jorge, 2013).

Meshless methods were also used to simulate the non-linear behaviour of biological materials like the cupula in the ear (Santos, Belinha, Gentil, Parente, & Jorge, 2017). Due to the iterative nature of this kind of problems, the precision and smoothness of the stress/strain field is essential to achieve stable solutions. Belinha and co-workers have developed and presented non-linear elastoplastic constitutive models (Moreira, Belinha, Dinis, & Jorge, 2016) to reproduce the biomechanical behaviour of bone structures (Tavares, Belinha, Dinis, & Natal Jorge, 2015) and atherosclerotic plaque tissue (Belinha, Dinis, & Natal, 2014).

Another examples of meshless formulation are meshless particle methods, such as the smoothed-particle hydrodynamics (SPH), which is a computational method used for fluid flow simulation. It is based in the Lagrangian method, in which the particle mass is constant and the background lattice is attached to the material and background lattice deform with the it.

The SPH method works by dividing a continuous field into a set of discrete sample points, called particles. These particles have a spatial distance, over which their properties are "smoothed" by a kernel function. The particles as identified with some characteristics like mass, position, velocity, etc., but particles can also carry estimated physical properties depending of the problem, like mass-density, temperature and pressure.

These variables are in the form of partial differential equations, but it is not always possible to obtain an analytical solution for that problems. In order to provide a better result, an approximation function (kernel function) is applied to produce a set of ordinary differential equations. The kernel function helps to ensure the stability of the numerical solution (Lobovský & Křen, 2007).

Through the years, this method has been applied to problems with reduced mesh deformations, such as metal structures (Hopkins, 2012).

SPH was first developed to simulate astrophysical fluid dynamics. Then, it has been successfully applied to a vast range of problems, as fluid flows. It was developed by Gingold and Monaghan (1977) and Lucy (1977).

This method has some advantages over grid-based techniques because it integrate complex physical effects into the SPH formalism in an easier way (G.R. Liu & Liu, 2003; Monaghan, 2005).

During 1995, Liu and co-workers (W.K. Liu, Jun, Li, Adee, & Belytschko, 1995), proposed a reproducing kernel particle method which improves the accuracy of SPH calculation.

Over the years SPH method has been optimized and despite its new improvement, which increases its efficiency, SPH still possesses some disadvantages, such as the high computation time of the simulation.

3 VESTIBULAR NUMERICAL MODEL

The model shown in the Figure 1 represent the SCC full of fluid. The green dots inside the channel are the particles made with the Smoothed Particle Hydrodynamic (SPH) method and represent the endolymph.

The boundary conditions imposed in the model are the displacement obtained from the accelerometer data and the interaction between both structures. The material properties used in the canal and the endolymph was obtained from the literature.

The fluid flow shown in Figure 2 corresponds to the section S_1 represented in Figure 1b) in two different instants of the simulation.

The velocity profiles obtained with the performed simulation are shown in Figure 2.

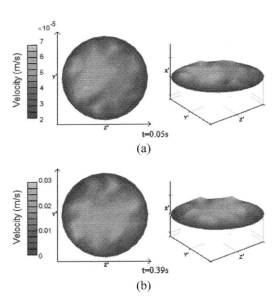

Figure 2. Fluid Velocity in Section S1 in two different moments (a)instant t = 0.05 s (b) instant t = 0.39 s.

The vestibular system model built in within the scope of this work aimed to be the first step to validate or enhance the rehabilitation process. In order to improve all the process, several computational simulations of the rehabilitation will be performed, aiming to fully understand the phenomenon and to provide suggestions and recommendations to improve the actual therapy. Furthermore, the full simulation of the balance procedures will allow a close study of the mechanical behaviour of the vestibular system. The fluidmechanics of the semicircular canals is another portion of the vestibular system that requires more research.

Additionally, the development of one specific tool capable to help audiologists in their daily activities and treatments is an important improvement in this clinical/scientific field.

ACKNOWLEDGEMENTS

The authors acknowledge the funding by Ministério da Ciência, Tecnologia e Ensino Superior– Fundacão para a Ciência e a Tecnologia, Portugal and POCH—Programa Operacional Capital Humano by Fundo Social Europeu and MCTES under research grants SFRH/BD/108292/2015, IF/00159/2014 and by project funding MIT-EXPL/ISF/0084/2017. Additionally, the authors acknowledge the funding of Project NORTE-01-0145-FEDER-000022-SciTech cofinanced by Programa Operacional Regional do

Norte (NORTE2020), through Fundo Europeu de Desenvolvimento Regional (FEDER).

REFERENCES

Belinha, J., Dinis, L.M.J.S., & Natal Jorge, R.M. (2013). A meshless microscale bone tissue trabecular remodelling analysis considering a new anisotropic bone tissue material law. *Computer Methods in Biomechanics and Biomedical Engineering*, *16*(11), 1170–84. https://doi.org/10.1080/10255842.2012.654783.

Belinha, J., Dinis, L., & Natal, R. (2014). The meshless simulation of the atherosclerotic plaque tissue using an elasto-plastic model. In T.D.R. Isabel Ramos, João Manuel R.S. Tavares, José Alberto Duarte, Maria Emília Costa, Olívia Pinho, Maria Helena Figueiral, R.M. Natal Jorge, Sofia Brandão, Teresa Mascarenhas (Ed.), *BioMedWomen* (1st ed., p. 10). CRC Press—Taylor & Francis Group.

Belinha, J., Natal Jorge, R.M., & Dinis, L.M.J.S. (2012). Bone tissue remodelling analysis considering a radial point interpolator meshless method. *Engineering Analysis with Boundary Elements*, *36*(11), 1660–1670. https://doi.org/10.1016/j.enganabound.2012.05.009.

Broglio, S.P., Sosnoff, J.J., Rosengren, K.S., & McShane, K. (2009). A comparison of balance performance: computerized dynamic posturography and a random motion platform. *Archives of Physical Medicine and Rehabilitation*, *90*(1), 145–50. https://doi.org/10.1016/j.apmr.2008.06.025.

Chen, G., Schmutz, B., Epari, D., Rathnayaka, K., Ibrahim, S., Schuetz, M.A., & Pearcy, M.J. (2010). A new approach for assigning bone material properties from CT images into finite element models. *Journal of Biomechanics*, *43*(5), 1011–1015. https://doi.org/10.1016/j.jbiomech.2009.10.040.

Davis, J.L., Xue, J., Peterson, E.H., & Grant, J.W. (2007). Layer thickness and curvature effects on otoconial membrane deformation in the utricle of the red-ear slider turtle: static and modal analysis. *Journal of Vestibular Research/: Equilibrium & Orientation*, *17*(4), 145–62. Retrieved from http://www.pubmedcentral.nih.gov/articlerender.fcgi?artid=2442736&tool=pmcentrez&rendertype=abstract.

Doblaré, M., Cueto, E., Calvo, B., Martínez, M.A., Garcia, J.M., & Cegoñino, J. (2005). On the employ of meshless methods in biomechanics. *Computer Methods in Applied Mechanics and Engineering*, *194*(6–8), 801–821. https://doi.org/10.1016/j.cma.2004.06.031.

Doweidar, M.H., Calvo, B., Alfaro, I., Groenenboom, P., & Doblaré, M. (2010). A comparison of implicit and explicit natural element methods in large strains problems: Application to soft biological tissues modeling. *Computer Methods in Applied Mechanics and Engineering*, *199*(25–28), 1691–1700. https://doi.org/10.1016/j.cma.2010.01.022.

Gámiz, M.J., & Lopez-Escamez, J.A. Health-related quality of life in patients over sixty years old with benign paroxysmal positional vertigo. *Gerontology*, *50*(2), 82–6. https://doi.org/10.1159/000075558.

Hall, J.E. (John E. (n.d.). *Guyton and Hall textbook of medical physiology*.

Herdman, S.J. (2013). *Vestibular rehabilitation. Current opinion in neurology* (Vol. 26). https://doi.org/10.1097/WCO.0b013e32835c5ec4.

Hopkins, P.F. (2012). A General Class of Lagrangian Smoothed Particle Hydrodynamics Methods and Implications for Fluid Mixing Problems, *0*(October).

Karatas, M. (2008). Central Vertigo and Dizziness. *The Neurologist*, *14*(6), 355–364. https://doi.org/10.1097/NRL.0b013e31817533a3.

Kerrigan, M.a, Costigan, M.F., Blatt, K.J., Mathiason, M. a, & Domroese, M.E. (2013). Prevalence of benign paroxysmal positional vertigo in the young adult population. *PM & R/: The Journal of Injury, Function, and Rehabilitation*, *5*(9), 778–85. https://doi.org/10.1016/j.pmrj.2013.05.010

Lee, J.D., Chen, Y., Zeng, X., Eskandarian, A., & Oskard, M. (2007). Modeling and simulation of osteoporosis and fracture of trabecular bone by meshless method. *International Journal of Engineering Science*, *45*(2–8), 329–338. https://doi.org/10.1016/j.ijengsci.2007.03.007.

Liew, K.M., Wu, H.Y., & Ng, T.Y. (2002). Meshless method for modeling of human proximal femur: treatment of nonconvex boundaries and stress analysis. *Computational Mechanics*, *28*(5), 390–400. https://doi.org/10.1007/s00466-002-0303-5.

Liu, G.R., & Liu, M.B. (2003). *Smoothed Particle Hydrodynamics*. WORLD SCIENTIFIC. https://doi.org/10.1142/5340.

Liu, W.K., Jun, S., Li, S., Adee, J., & Belytschko, T. (1995). Reproducing kernel particle methods for structural dynamics. *International Journal for Numerical Methods in Engineering*, *38*(10), 1655–1679. https://doi.org/10.1002/nme.1620381005.

Lobovský, L., & Křen, J. (2007). Smoothed particle hydrodynamics modelling of fluids and solids. *Applied and Computational Mechanics*, *1*, 521–530.

Marques, M., Belinha, J., Dinis, L.M.J., & Natal Jorge, R. (2018). A brain impact stress analysis using advanced discretization meshless techniques. *Proceedings of the Institution of Mechanical Engineers, Part H: Journal of Engineering in Medicine*, *232*(3), 257–270. https://doi.org/10.1177/0954411917751559.

Monaghan, J.J. (2005). Smoothed particle hydrodynamics. *Reports on Progress in Physics*, *68*(8), 1703–1759. https://doi.org/10.1088/0034-4885/68/8/R01.

Moreira, S.F., Belinha, J., Dinis, L.M.J.S., & Jorge, R.M.N. (2016). The anisotropic elasto-plastic analysis using a natural neighbour RPIM version. *Journal of the Brazilian Society of Mechanical Sciences and Engineering*, 1–23. https://doi.org/10.1007/s40430-016-0603-x.

Mori, D., Yano, K., Tsubota, K., Ishikawa, T., Wada, S., & Yamaguchi, T. (2008). Computational study on effect of red blood cells on primary thrombus formation. *Thrombosis Research*, *123*(1), 114–21. https://doi.org/10.1016/j.thromres.2008.03.006.

Neuhauser, H.K., & Lempert, T. (2009). Vertigo: epidemiologic aspects. *Seminars in Neurology*, *29*(5), 473–81. https://doi.org/10.1055/s-0029-1241043.

Obrist, D. (2007). Fluidmechanics of semicircular canals – revisited. *Zeitschrift Für Angewandte Mathematik Und Physik*, *59*(3), 475–497. https://doi.org/10.1007/s00033-007-6037-7.

Santos, C.F., Belinha, J., Gentil, F., Parente, M., & Jorge, R.N. (2017). An alternative 3D numerical method to study the biomechanical behaviour of the human inner ear semicircular canal. *Acta of Bioengineering and Biomechanics*, *19*(1), 3–15. Retrieved from http://www.ncbi.nlm.nih.gov/pubmed/28552920.

Strupp, M., Thurtell, M.J., Shaikh, A.G., Brandt, T., Zee, D.S., & Leigh, R.J. (2011). Pharmacotherapy of vestibular and ocular motor disorders, including nystagmus. *Journal of Neurology*, *258*(7), 1207–1222. https://doi.org/10.1007/s00415-011-5999-8.

Taddei, F., Pani, M., Zovatto, L., Tonti, E., & Viceconti, M. (2008). A new meshless approach for subject-specific strain prediction in long bones: Evaluation of accuracy. *Clinical Biomechanics (Bristol, Avon)*, *23*(9), 1192–9. https://doi.org/10.1016/j.clinbiomech.2008.06.009.

Tavares, C.S.S., Belinha, J., Dinis, L.M.J.S., & Natal Jorge, R.M. (2015). The elasto-plastic response of the bone tissue due to the insertion of dental implants. *Procedia Engineering*, *110*, 37–44. https://doi.org/10.1016/j.proeng.2015.07.007.

Taylor, J., & Goodkin, H.P. (2011). Dizziness and vertigo in the adolescent. *Otolaryngologic Clinics of North America*, *44*(2), 309–21, vii–viii. https://doi.org/10.1016/j.otc.2011.01.004.

Tsubota, K., Wada, S., & Yamaguchi, T. (2006). Particle method for computer simulation of red blood cell motion in blood flow. *Computer Methods and Programs in Biomedicine*, *83*(2), 139–46. https://doi.org/10.1016/j.cmpb.2006.06.005.

von Brevern, M., & Neuhauser, H. (2011). Epidemiological evidence for a link between vertigo and migraine. *Journal of Vestibular Research : Equilibrium & Orientation*, *21*(6), 299–304. https://doi.org/10.3233/VES-2011-0423.

Wolfe, J.M. (2012). *Sensation & perception*. Sinauer Associates.

Wong, K.C.L., Wang, L., Zhang, H., Liu, H., & Shi, P. (2010). Meshfree implementation of individualized active cardiac dynamics. *Computerized Medical Imaging and Graphics*, *34*(1), 91–103. https://doi.org/10.1016/j.compmedimag.2009.05.002.

Zhang, G.Y., Wittek, A., Joldes, G.R., Jin, X., & Miller, K. (2014). A three-dimensional nonlinear meshfree algorithm for simulating mechanical responses of soft tissue. *Engineering Analysis with Boundary Elements*, *42*, 60–66. https://doi.org/10.1016/j.enganabound.2013.08.014.

Biodental Engineering V – Belinha et al. (Eds)
© 2019 Taylor & Francis Group, London, ISBN 978-0-367-21087-8

Using meshless methods to simulate the free vibrations of the cupula under pathological conditions

C.F. Santos & Marco Parente
Institute of Science and Innovation in Mechanical and Industrial Engineering (INEGI), Unit of Design and Experimental Validation, Porto, Portugal

J. Belinha
Department of Mechanical Engineering, School of Engineering, Polytechnic of Porto (ISEP), Porto, Portugal

R.M. Natal Jorge
Department of Mechanical Engineering, Faculty of Engineering, University of Porto (FEUP), Porto, Portugal

Fernanda Gentil
Clínica ORL—Dr. Eurico Almeida e Escola Superior de Saúde—P. Porto, Portugal

ABSTRACT: Each canal of the vestibular system of the inner ear is composed of a circular path of continuum fluid. Inside each semicircular canal, it is possible to find a cupula, a gelatinous body containing sensory hair cells, and the focus of this work. One of the causes of vestibular disorders is the abnormal concentration of otoconia particles near the cupula. The accurate determination of the natural frequency (first vibration frequency) of the cupula would allow to know which external frequency could be induce to stimulate externally the cupula. Thus, theoretically, the resonance effect would induce physical vibration to the cupula and disperse the otoconia particles, reducing the vertigo symptoms. Hence, in this wok, two-dimensional and three-dimensional geometrical models of the cupula were constructed. Then, a free vibration analysis was performed using three distinct numerical techniques, the Finite Element Method (FEM), and two meshless methods: the Radial Point Interpolation Meshless Method (RPIM) and the Natural Neighbour Radial Point Interpolation Method (NNRPIM).

1 THE INNER EAR SENSOR

1.1 Cupula introduction

The main sensory structure of the human body is the cupula (Figure 1a)) of the inner ear. In fact, there are six cupulas in each human being, three in each ear. The cupula is placed in the ampullar part of each semicircular canal (SCC).

The SCC is the main structure of the vestibular system responsible for the balance function. These three SCC in each ear are positioned in three orthogonal planes and they are sensitive to angular (rotational) acceleration (Jaeger, Takagi, & Haslwanter, 2002; Wu et al., 2011). Each canal is comprised of a circular path of continuous fluid, interrupted at the ampulla, where the sensory epithelium is placed. The hair cells of the ampulla rest on a tuft of blood vessels, nerve fibers, and supporting tissue called the cupula. Endolymph surround all the structures forming the cupula (Figure 1b).

The sensory hair cells exhibit constant discharge of neurotransmitters that are modified by the direction of cupula deflection. This output signal has origin in the velocity of head rotation. This is the reason why these cells are called "rate sensor" in engineering terms. Also, there are other conditions that could influence the signal rate, such some vestibular disorders.

Saccule and utricle are the structures of the vestibular system, placed near the SCC, sensitive to the linear accelerations. Both structures are constituted by a macula layer where some calcium carbonate particles, which have an important role in the balance function are placed. This particles, known as otoconia, could detach from the macula and get lost in the SCC, which could lead to vertigo symptoms. Cupulolithiasis, represented in Figure 1c), is a vestibular condition when the otoconia get attached to the cupula inducing a false sensation of movement, leading to dizziness

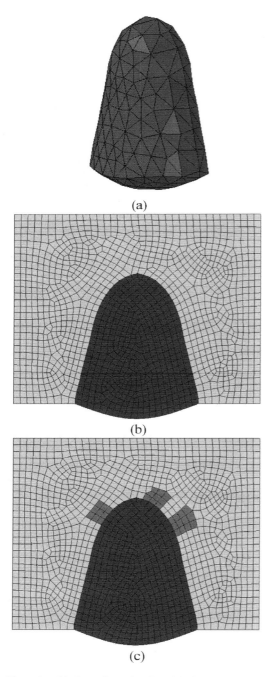

Figure 1. (a) Three dimensional model of the cupula. (b) Two-dimensional model of the cupula with fluid. (c) Two-dimensional model of the cupula with fluid and otoconia.

episodes. There are some rehabilitation manoeuvres that can be performed to solve the described problem. However, such manoeuvres do not always work. The symptoms of vertigo are severe and incapacitating, reducing the quality of life of patients.

Due to the extremely reduced dimensions of the vestibular system, computational models could represent an important tool to study these biological system. The outputs could allow to improve the empirical methodologies applied today.

Thus, the present work aims to obtain the natural free vibration of a general cupula of the inner ear using three advanced discretization techniques: the finite element model (FEM) and two distinct meshless methods.

1.2 Numerical methods

Today, numerical methods are being used to simulate an extensive variety of physical, chemical and biological phenomenon. The finite element method (FEM) is a well-known discretization technique applied widely in engineering as a computational analysis tool. It includes the use of mesh generation techniques for dividing a complex problem into small elements.

This method can be used in many scientific fields, including biomechanics, due to its high flexibility and efficiency. Depending on the formulation in which it is applied, FEM allows the analysis of displacements, stresses, velocities, etc. Therefore, it is important to know the basic concepts of FEM in order to obtain best results with the model and the simulations (Reddy, 2006).

The analysis performed with FEM involve some steps, such as defining the domain and discretise it in small elements, this task is known as meshing. After defining the mesh in the domain it is necessary to attribute properties to the materials. After that step, it is important to define the distribution of displacement in each element. The displacement functions define the deformation inside each element. The difference between this deformation and the initial state of the model and the material properties define the stress distribution. Other important parameters that must be defined are the essential and natural boundary conditions of the model. After all the conditions defined, it is possible obtain all the mechanical results related with the model.

The discretization technique is the one of main steps of the procedure that can influence and affect the final result. Furthermore, it represents a heavy pre-processing cost, especially if a uniform mesh is intended.

In the last decades, meshless methods (Nguyen, Rabczuk, Bordas, & Duflot, 2008) have been under strong development and are continuously extending their application field. This approach allows a more flexible discretization, which will lead to a competitive and alternative numerical method in computational mechanical analysis, due to the efficiency and accuracy of their discretization formulation (T.Belytschko,Y.Krongauz,D.Organ,M. Fleming, 1996).

Meshless methods allow to discretize the domain based in a cloud of nodes (Belinha, 2014; Belinha, Araújo, Ferreira, Dinis, & Natal Jorge, 2016; GU, 2005; Nguyen et al., 2008; T. Belytschko, Y. Krongauz, D. Organ, M. Fleming, 1996), instead of the rigid element model used in FEM. In the early years, the solution of partial differential equations was the main focus of interest (T. Belytschko, Y. Krongauz, D. Organ, M. Fleming, 1996). However, today, meshless methods are applied in several scientific fields, included biomechanics (Belinha, 2014).

Meshless methods can be divided in classes or sub-classes; being the "not-truly meshless methods" or "truly meshless methods" (Belinha, 2014) one of the most used classifications.

A meshless method is considered "not-truly" when a support mesh is used to perform the numerical integration of the integro-differential equations ruling the studied physical phenomenon.

On the other hand, "truly" meshless methods only require a cloud of nodes to discretize the problem domain. In this approach, the influence domain, integration points, shape functions and other necessary mathematical constructions are obtained directly from the nodal spatial coordinates.

In the present work, two distinct meshless methods will be compared with FEM: the radial point interpolation method and the natural neighbour radial point interpolation method.

The Radial Point Interpolation Method (RPIM) is an interpolator meshless method where the nodal connectivity is enforced using influence-domains. To solve the integro-differential equations governing the physical phenomenon, the RPIM uses a background cloud of integration points, constructed using integration cells and the Gauss-Legendre quadrature rule.

The other meshless method used is the natural neighbour radial point interpolation method (NNRPIM), which is a truly meshless method (Belinha, 2014). NNPRIM uses the Voronoï diagram to define the background distribution of integration points in order to solve the integro-differential equations governing the physical phenomenon.

Both the FEM and the meshless methods use weak formulations because a differential equation (strong formulation) may shows solutions which are not exactly differentiable. Alternatively, a weak formulation allows to find such solutions. In the next section, some examples of meshless methods successfully applied in the biomechanics field will be presented.

2 MESHLESS METHODS IN BIOMECHANICS

One of the advantage of meshless methods over FEM are the efficiency in the re-meshing process, which in biomechanics structures could be the key to a reliable final result (Ho, Tsou, Green, & Fels, 2014; Z. ElZahab, E. Divo, 2009).

The re-meshing flexibility is one of the advantages of the meshless methods, which allows to deal with the large distortions of soft materials, as the the constituents of the human body, like tendons, internal organs, skin, muscles, etc.; and, simultaneously, permits to simulate explicitly fluid flow (the respiration, the hemodynamic, the swallow, the endolymph, the urine, etc).

Further advantages of the meshless methods are the possibility to obtain robust solution fields (displacements, stresses, strain, etc.) with an extra smoothness and a superior accuracy. These numerical properties are useful to predict the nonlinear material behaviour of such biological tissues and the remodelling process of such biomaterials. Additionally, there are some recent works showing that the combination of medical imaging techniques like computerized axial tomography (CAT) scan and Magnetic Resonance Imaging (MRI), with meshless methods is more efficient than using the FEM (Wong, Wang, Zhang, Liu, & Shi, 2010) (Chen et al., 2010).

Regarding the specific case of biomechanics, the Doweidar et al. work showed (Doweidar, Calvo, Alfaro, Groenenboom, & Doblaré, 2010) a simulation of the human lateral collateral ligament and the human knee joint, which provided support of the clear advantages of the meshless methods over the FEM, especially in biomechanical problems dealing with large strains. Additionally, Zhang et al. (Zhang, Wittek, Joldes, Jin, & Miller, 2014) obtained results which confirmed the accuracy of meshless methods to deal with highly demanding nonlinear hyperelastic biomaterials, such as the nonlinear explicit dynamic analysis of the brain tissues.

Furthermore, meshless methods are frequently used to simulate hemodynamics, as the motion of a deformable red blood cell in flowing blood plasma (Tsubota, Wada, & Yamaguchi, 2006) or to study the effect of red blood cells on the primary thrombus formation (Mori et al., 2008).

Bone tissue remodelling simulation is another popular computational biomechanical field in which meshless methods proved to possess clear advantages (Doblaré et al., 2005). It started during 2002, when, Liew et al. published the first work dealing with bone structures and using meshless methods (Liew, Wu, & Ng, 2002). Then, several other authors applied meshless methods to simulate the bone tissue remodelling process with success (Lee, Chen, Zeng, Eskandarian, & Oskard, 2007) (Taddei, Pani, Zovatto, Tonti, & Viceconti, 2008). A new bone tissue remodelling algorithm relying on the meshless method accuracy was recently presented by Belinha and co-workers (Belinha, Natal Jorge, & Dinis, 2012) (Belinha, Dinis, & Natal Jorge, 2013). The proposed methodology was capable to obtain numerical solutions very close with the clinical X-ray images of natural bones (Belinha et al., 2012) (Belinha et al., 2013) (Belinha, Dinis, & Natal Jorge, 2015) and natural bones with implants (Belinha, Dinis, & Jorge, 2015) (Belinha, Dinis, & Natal Jorge, 2016), and it is applied also to predict the bone biological behaviour in dental biomechanics (Moreira, Belinha, Dinis, & Jorge, 2014) (Duarte, Andrade, Dinis, Jorge, & Belinha, 2015) (C.S.S. Tavares, Belinha, Dinis, & Natal Jorge, 2015) (C.S. Tavares, Belinha, Dinis, & Natal, 2014). Also another constitutive elasto-plastic models was developed to reproduce the bone structures behaviour (Moreira, Belinha, Dinis, & Jorge, 2016) (C.S.S. Tavares et al., 2015) and atherosclerotic plaque tissue (Belinha, Dinis, & Natal, 2014). Another interesting application of meshless methods is the simulation of the inner ear structure described in the introduction of the present work, the cupula and their surrounding fluid, the endolymph; which are some fundamental parts of the vestibular system, which plays an important role in vertigo.

3 RESULTS AND DISCUSSION

The three methodologies previously described were applied to the model described in Figure 1(b) and the vibration modes and vibration frequencies were obtained and presented in Figure 2.

Notice that, Figure 2 shows two different views of the three dimensional cupula (view Oxz and Oyz). In each view, the first and second vibration modes and the respective vibration frequencies are presented. The simulations of the different situations shown in Figure 1 were performed with four different meshes. The results permitted to understand that the meshless formulations (RPIM and NNRPIM) allowed to achieve higher convergence rates than FEM.

Regarding the NNRPIM, two distinct formulations were used: the first degree influence cell NNRPIM formulation (NNRPIMv1) and the second degree influence-cell NNRPIM (NNPRIMv2)

The obtained results have shown that the three techniques are capable to achieve similar results regarding the natural frequencies of the cupula. It was also possible to observe that, regardless the

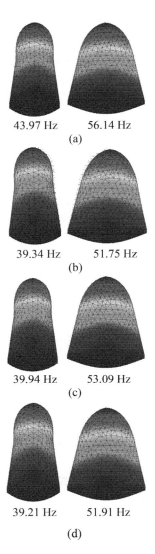

Figure 2. First two modes and natural frequencies of the three-dimensional cupula with different methods (a) FEM. (b) RPIM (c) NNRPIM_1 (d) NNRPIM_2.

advanced discretization technique used, the solutions obtained using the 2D model were very close with the 3D solutions.

To conclude, this work opens a new research branch in the computational analysis of the vestibular system. Since theoretically, the resonance phenomena will force the cupula to vibrate, and consequently to the detachment of the otoconia particles from the cupula, reducing the vertigo symptoms. This could be achieved with non-invasive way, such as listening to music.

ACKNOWLEDGEMENTS

The authors acknowledge the funding by Ministério da Ciência, Tecnologia e Ensino Superior–Fundacão para a Ciência e a Tecnologia, Portugal and POCH—Programa Operacional Capital Humano by Fundo Social Europeu and MCTES under research grants SFRH/BD/108292/2015, IF/00159/2014 and by project funding MIT-EXPL/ISF/0084/2017. Additionally, the authors acknowledge the funding of Project NORTE-01-0145-FEDER-000022-SciTech cofinanced by Programa Operacional Regional do Norte (NORTE2020), through Fundo Europeu de Desenvolvimento Regional (FEDER).

REFERENCES

Belinha, J. (2014). *Meshless Methods in Biomechanics – Bone Tissue Remodelling Analysis*. (J.M.R.S. Tavares & R.M. Natal Jorge, Eds.) (Vol.16). Lecture Notes in Computational Vision and Biomechanics, Springer Netherlands.

Belinha, J., Araújo, A.L., Ferreira, A.J.M., Dinis, L.M.J.S., & Natal Jorge, R.M. (2016). The analysis of laminated plates using distinct advanced discretization meshless techniques. *Composite Structures*, *143*, 165–179. https://doi.org/10.1016/j.compstruct.2016.02.021.

Belinha, J., Dinis, L.M.J.S., & Jorge, R.M.N. (2015). The Mandible Remodeling Induced By Dental Implants: a Meshless Approach. *Journal of Mechanics in Medicine and Biology*, *15*(4), 1550059. https://doi.org/10.1142/S0219519415500591.

Belinha, J., Dinis, L.M.J.S., & Natal Jorge, R.M. (2013). A meshless microscale bone tissue trabecular remodelling analysis considering a new anisotropic bone tissue material law. *Computer Methods in Biomechanics and Biomedical Engineering*, *16*(11), 1170–84. https://doi.org/10.1080/10255842.2012.654783.

Belinha, J., Dinis, L.M.J.S., & Natal Jorge, R.M. (2015). The meshless methods in the bone tissue remodelling analysis. *Procedia Engineering*, *110*, 51–58. https://doi.org/10.1016/j.proeng.2015.07.009.

Belinha, J., Dinis, L.M.J.S., & Natal Jorge, R.M. (2016). The analysis of the bone remodelling around femoral stems: A meshless approach. *Mathematics and Computers in Simulation*, *121*, 64–94. https://doi.org/10.1016/j.matcom.2015.09.002.

Belinha, J., Dinis, L., & Natal, R. (2014). The meshless simulation of the atherosclerotic plaque tissue using an elasto-plastic model. In T.D.R. Isabel Ramos, João Manuel R.S. Tavares, José Alberto Duarte, Maria Emília Costa, Olívia Pinho, Maria Helena Figueiral, R.M. Natal Jorge, Sofia Brandão, Teresa Mascarenhas (Ed.), *BioMedWomen* (1st ed., p. 10). CRC Press—Taylor & Francis Group.

Belinha, J., Natal Jorge, R.M., & Dinis, L.M.J.S. (2012). Bone tissue remodelling analysis considering a radial point interpolator meshless method. *Engineering Analysis with Boundary Elements*, *36*(11), 1660–1670. https://doi.org/10.1016/j.enganabound.2012.05.009.

Belytschko, T., Y. Krongauz, D. Organ, M. Fleming, P.K. (1996). Meshless methods: An overview and recent developments. *Computer Methods in Applied Mechanics and Engineering*, *139*(1–4), 3–47. https://doi.org/10.1016/S0045-7825(96)01078-X.

Chen, G., Schmutz, B., Epari, D., Rathnayaka, K., Ibrahim, S., Schuetz, M.A., & Pearcy, M.J. (2010). A new approach for assigning bone material properties from CT images into finite element models. *Journal of Biomechanics*, *43*(5), 1011–1015. https://doi.org/10.1016/j.jbiomech.2009.10.040.

Doblaré, M., Cueto, E., Calvo, B., Martínez, M.A., Garcia, J.M., & Cegoñino, J. (2005). On the employ of meshless methods in biomechanics. *Computer Methods in Applied Mechanics and Engineering*, *194*(6–8), 801–821. https://doi.org/10.1016/j.cma.2004.06.031.

Doweidar, M.H., Calvo, B., Alfaro, I., Groenenboom, P., & Doblaré, M. (2010). A comparison of implicit and explicit natural element methods in large strains problems: Application to soft biological tissues modeling. *Computer Methods in Applied Mechanics and Engineering*, *199*(25–28), 1691–1700. https://doi.org/10.1016/j.cma.2010.01.022.

Duarte, H.M.S., Andrade, J.R., Dinis, L.M.J.S., Jorge, R.M.N., & Belinha, J. (2015). Numerical analysis of dental implants using a new advanced discretization technique. *Mechanics of Advanced Materials and Structures*, *23*(4), 467–479. https://doi.org/10.1080/15376494.2014.987410.

Gu, Y.T. (2005). Meshfree Methods and their comparisons. *International Journal of Computational Methods*, *2*(4), 477–515. https://doi.org/10.1142/S0219876205000673.

Ho, A.K., Tsou, L., Green, S., & Fels, S. (2014). A 3D swallowing simulation using smoothed particle hydrodynamics. *Computer Methods in Biomechanics and Biomedical Engineering: Imaging & Visualization*, *2*(4), 237–244. https://doi.org/10.1080/21681163.2013.862862.

Jaeger, R., Takagi, A., & Haslwanter, T. (2002). Modeling the relation between head orientations and otolith responses in humans. *Hearing Research*, *173*(1–2), 29–42. https://doi.org/10.1016/S0378-5955(02)00485-9.

Lee, J.D., Chen, Y., Zeng, X., Eskandarian, A., & Oskard, M. (2007). Modeling and simulation of osteoporosis and fracture of trabecular bone by meshless method. *International Journal of Engineering Science*, *45*(2–8), 329–338. https://doi.org/10.1016/j.ijengsci.2007.03.007.

Liew, K.M., Wu, H.Y., & Ng, T.Y. (2002). Meshless method for modeling of human proximal femur: treatment of nonconvex boundaries and stress analysis. *Computational Mechanics*, *28*(5), 390–400. https://doi.org/10.1007/s00466-002-0303-5.

Moreira, S.F., Belinha, J., Dinis, L.M.J.S., & Jorge, R.M.N. (2014). A Global Numerical Analysis of the "Central Incisor/Local Maxillary Bone" System using a Meshless Method. *MCB: Molecular & Cellular Biomechanics*, *11*(3), 151–184. https://doi.org/10.3970/mcb.2014.011.151.

Moreira, S.F., Belinha, J., Dinis, L.M.J.S., & Jorge, R.M.N. (2016). The anisotropic elasto-plastic analysis using a natural neighbour RPIM version. *Journal of the Brazilian Society of Mechanical Sciences and Engineering*, 1–23. https://doi.org/10.1007/s40430-016-0603-x.

Mori, D., Yano, K., Tsubota, K., Ishikawa, T., Wada, S., & Yamaguchi, T. (2008). Computational study on effect of red blood cells on primary thrombus formation. *Thrombosis Research*, *123*(1), 114–21. https://doi.org/10.1016/j.thromres.2008.03.006.

Nguyen, V.P., Rabczuk, T., Bordas, S., & Duflot, M. (2008). Meshless methods: A review and computer implementation aspects. *Mathematics and Computers in Simulation*, *79*(3), 763–813. https://doi.org/10.1016/j.matcom.2008.01.003.

Reddy, J.N. (Junuthula N. (2006). *An introduction to the finite element method*. McGraw-Hill Higher Education.

Taddei, F., Pani, M., Zovatto, L., Tonti, E., & Viceconti, M. (2008). A new meshless approach for subject-specific strain prediction in long bones: Evaluation of accuracy. *Clinical Biomechanics (Bristol, Avon)*, *23*(9), 1192–9. https://doi.org/10.1016/j.clinbiomech.2008.06.009.

Tavares, C.S., Belinha, J., Dinis, L., & Natal, R. (2014). The biomechanical response of a restored tooth due to bruxism: a mesh- less approach. In T.D.R. Isabel Ramos, João Manuel R.S. Tavares, José Alberto Duarte, Maria Emília Costa, Olívia Pinho, Maria Helena Figueiral, R.M. Natal Jorge, Sofia Brandão, Teresa Mascarenhas (Ed.), *BioMedWomen* (p. 7). CRC Press—Taylor & Francis Group.

Tavares, C.S.S., Belinha, J., Dinis, L.M.J.S., & Natal Jorge, R.M. (2015). The elasto-plastic response of the bone tissue due to the insertion of dental implants. *Procedia Engineering*, *110*, 37–44. https://doi.org/10.1016/j.proeng.2015.07.007.

Tsubota, K., Wada, S., & Yamaguchi, T. (2006). Particle method for computer simulation of red blood cell motion in blood flow. *Computer Methods and Programs in Biomedicine*, *83*(2), 139–46. https://doi.org/10.1016/j.cmpb.2006.06.005.

Wong, K.C.L., Wang, L., Zhang, H., Liu, H., & Shi, P. (2010). Meshfree implementation of individualized active cardiac dynamics. *Computerized Medical Imaging and Graphics*, *34*(1), 91–103. https://doi.org/10.1016/j.compmedimag.2009.05.002.

Wu, C., Hua, C., Yang, L., Dai, P., Zhang, T., & Wang, K. (2011). Dynamic analysis of fluid-structure interaction of endolymph and cupula in the lateral semicircular canal of inner ear. *Journal of Hydrodynamics, Ser. B*, *23*(6), 777–783. https://doi.org/10.1016/S1001-6058(10)60176-X.

Zahab, Z.El., E. Divo, A.J.K. (2009). A localized collocation meshless method (LCMM) for incompressible flows CFD modeling with applications to transient hemodynamics. *Engineering Analysis with Boundary Elements*, *33*(8–9), 1045–1061. https://doi.org/10.1016/J.ENGANABOUND.2009.03.006.

Zhang, G.Y., Wittek, A., Joldes, G.R., Jin, X., & Miller, K. (2014). A three-dimensional nonlinear meshfree algorithm for simulating mechanical responses of soft tissue. *Engineering Analysis with Boundary Elements*, *42*, 60–66. https://doi.org/10.1016/j.enganabound.2013.08.014.

Biodental Engineering V – Belinha et al. (Eds)
© 2019 Taylor & Francis Group, London, ISBN 978-0-367-21087-8

Development of an image processing based algorithm to define trabecular bone mechanical properties using the fabric tensor concept

M. Marques
Institute of Mechanical Engineering and Industrial Management (INEGI), Porto, Portugal

J. Belinha
Department of Mechanical Engineering, School of Engineering, Polytechnic of Porto (ISEP), Porto, Portugal

R.M. Natal Jorge
Department of Mechanical Engineering, Faculty of Engineering, University of Porto (FEUP), Porto, Portugal

A.F. Oliveira
Institute of Biomedical Sciences Abel Salazar, University of Porto (ICBAS), Porto, Portugal

ABSTRACT: Bone is as structure that is extensively studied. Many studies attempt to understand the mechanical behaviour of bone tissue. One key factor to fully understand and predict its structural response is the accurate determination of its mechanical properties. As the bone morphology changes (resulting from bone adaptation to external loads), bone tissue mechanical properties change as well. Therefore, its estimation is a never-ending challenging task. In this work, it was developed a methodology that allows, using medical images of micro-CT, to define the mechanical properties of trabecular bone, based on its morphological structure. This methodology uses the fabric tensor concept and a phenomenological material law to estimate the mechanical properties. The developed methodology as overall error of 2% upon the detection of trabecular bone material principal direction.

1 INTRODUCTION

Bone is a structure mainly defined by bone matrix and by bone cells, which are responsible for the production and resorption of the bone matrix itself. This resorption/production process is known as bone remodelling and it allows the replacement of old bone matrix by a newer one [1]. Bone remodelling is progressive and it is induced to fulfil and optimize the specific physiological function of structural support by adapting the bone morphology to any new external loads [2]–[4]. The concept that strain/stress induces bone remodelling was firstly reported by Wolff in 1886 [5]. Later in 1892, Wolff found that the orientation of trabecular bone coincides with the direction of the stress trajectories. Later, bone started to be classified in distinct hierarchical structures, constituted of many scale levels with specific interactions and with very complex architectures [6]. Bone hierarchy can be defined has having a macro-scale structure (whole bone) and micro-scale structure (single osteon, cortical bone functional unit, and single trabecula). Some authors also classify bone with different structural levels from the macroscale to sub-nanoscale (hydroxyapatite crystals, components of the inorganic phase of bone and TC molecules) [7]–[9]. Bone has different functional requirements at different scales and, in order to analyse the equivalent mechanical behaviour of bone material, it is necessary to investigate the mechanical properties of its components and the structural relationships between them at different scales [10]–[11]. For example, at the macroscale and microscale, bone, due to its different functional requirements, has different densities and corresponding mechanical properties. In order to study the remodelling process of bone tissue, some authors developed models that considered bone as an isotropic material. Such assumption is a simplistic approach on the behaviour of trabecular bone, disregarding the importance of structural orientation of individual trabeculae in the remodelling process [12]–[15]. Other authors developed models that couple material density and orientation, allowing to assume an orthotropic behaviour [16]–[19]. This approaches lead to multiscale remodelling models that not only avoids any a priori assumption on material but also take into account the trabecular architecture features, by using information from more than one hierarchical bone scale. This multiscale models also enable the possibility of modelling actual biological features considering mechanobiological models that consider both biological and mechanical factors based on bone cell activity [20]–[23]. Some authors, started to characterize bone mechanical properties, considering and encoding the material orientation and orthotropic behaviour, but at the same time overcoming the problems that could result from the highly heterogeneous medium, by using the fabric tensor concept, **A** [24], [25].

1.1 Fabric tensor

A fabric tensor is a symmetric second rank tensor that characterizes the arrangement of a multiphase material, where is encoded the orientation and orthotropic behaviour of the material. Cowin, 1985, developed a relation between the fourth rank elasticity tensor C_{ijkl}, and a fabric tensor **A**. The results obtained by Cowin, 1985shows that an ellipsoid may be associated with the varieties of material symmetries observed in many natural materials [26].

Fabric tensors can be obtained using mechanical based methods or morphologic-based methods. The mechanical based methods directly calculate the fabric tensors from mechanical properties obtained through mechanical experiments. The fabric tensor in these cases is calculated using numerical simulations. Morphologic-based methods use the interface between phases of the material to estimate the fabric tensors. For the bone case, using micro-CT (at the microscale) or a CT (at the macroscale), it is possible to obtain information of the changes of phase of bone material. Thus, morphologic-based techniques are frequently used when the fabric tensor is applied to bone tissue.

Most of the fabric tensors proposed obtained using morphologic-based methods are usually computed, first, with an orientation distribution function (ODF), which is estimated from an orientation-dependent feature of interest. Afterwards, the fabric tensor is approximated by the ODF.

One of the most popular morphologic-based methods in trabecular bone research is the mean intercept length (*MIL*) tensor, developed by Whitehouse, 1974 [27]. It is considered a golden standard since it exists a large amount of works that sustenance its appropriateness to predict mechanical properties of trabecular bone [27]–[31]. This method implementation is efficient in the spatial and in frequency domains. One characteristic that makes this tensor wide popular is the fact that it shares the same eigenvectors, when used in binary images, with the *MIL* methodology, enabling the compare of methodologies [32].

1.1.1 Mean interception length tensor

Mean Intercept Length tensor is usually computed by defining a family of parallel lines to a specified direction τ. The number of intersections, $C(\tau)$, between lines and the interface between both phases is counted. *MIL* is a function of τ (an angle increment), and computed as a reason between the summation of the length of traced lines, h, with the number of intersections $C(\tau)$, as represented in equation (1)

$$MIL(\tau) = \frac{h}{C(\tau)} \tag{1}$$

This calculus defines the orientation-dependent feature, describing the orientation distribution function (ODF) of *MIL*. Researchers found that for many types of materials, in particularly bone trabeculae, when disposing the ODF data on a polar plot and fitting in it an ellipse, the ellipse parameters could be correlated with the material principal directions [33]. With this, in 2D the *MIL* fabric tensor, **A**, could be computed as a 2×2 matrix that represents the estimated ellipse. The objective of this work was to develop a fabric tensor algorithm capable to provide enough information to estimate the mechanical properties of trabecular bone using a region of interest of medical images. The developed methodology aims to be part of a low-cost and efficient multiscale methodology, with which it will be possible to study the bone remodelling process. This work focus on the methodology used to acquire de ODF data

2 METHODOLOGY

The presented work was developed using MATLAB 2016b. In this process, two types of images were considered: clinical and benchmark images. The clinical image was obtained by selecting a square Region Of Interest (ROI) from a set of cuboid micro-CTs. The benchmark images were created using MATLAB 2016b, with the objective of creating images with a well-known material principal direction. The defined images were analysed with the developed algorithm, which is capable of processing the image and acquire data, which can be fitted to an ellipse using *MIL* methodology. Thus, the algorithm allows to acquire parameters to define a fabric tensor, which possesses a close relation with the bone mechanical properties. In this the work, it is investigated the performance of the developed algorithm, by testing different benchmark images with well-known principal material direction.

2.1 Mean intercept length development

The *MIL* methodology was developed using image processing methodologies. The first step of the algorithm is the binarization of the input ROI image, I_{ROI}, using the Otsu methodology [34], with the purpose of defining I_{ROIBW}, image type represented in Figure 1c. The second step was the construction an image, $I_{pl}\tau$, with $\tau = 0°$, with the same size of I_{ROI}, containing a set of parallel and horizontal lines, as represented in Figure 3a. These images represent the family of parallel lines for the specified direction $\tau = 0°$. Counting the interceptions $I_{pl}0$ with the pixels representing the change of phase of material in I_{ROIBW}, was possible to obtain the orientation-dependent feature (ODF), in this case for the specified direction $\tau = 0°$.

Rotating $I_{pl}\tau$ in the interval $\tau = [0,180]$ degrees, with a specific angle increment τ, and counting the interception of $I_{pl}\tau$ with the pixels representing the change of phase of material in I_{ROIBW}, it was possible to obtain the ODF for τ for that I_{ROIBW}. The data for the interval $\tau = [180,360]$ is a repetition of the $\tau = [0,180]$ data, since the ODF only depends on the orientation and not on the direction.

Multiplying the I_{ROIBW} with each one of the $I_{pl}\tau$, it was possible to obtain figure I_{Rxpl} where the white pixels exist only where $I_{pl}\tau$ white pixels are coincident with the white pixels of the I_{ROIBW}, as illustrated in Figure 2a. Filtering I_{Rxpl}, it was possible to acquire an *image, Ifiltered$_{Rxpl}$* with white pixels only present in the changes of phase of the material, represented in image I_{ROI}. This allows to acquire an image type that can be represented by Figure 2b. The number of white pixels represent the number of intersections, $C(\tau)$, between lines with direction τ and the interface between phases of the material represented by I_{ROI}. The number of white pixel in

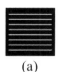
(a)

(b)

(c)

Figure 1. In this figure are presented the I_{ROIBW} used in this work: a): Benchmark Image 1, $\beta = 0°$; b): Benchmark Image 2, $\beta = 45°$; c): Trabecular Bone Binary ROI

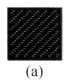
(a)
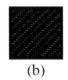
(b)

Figure 2. a): Image type of I_{Rxpl}, where the white pixels represent $I_{ROIBW} \cap I_{pl}\tau$; b): Image type of *Ifiltered$_{Rxpl}$*.

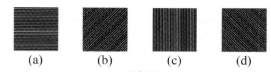

Figure 3. Images of parallel lines rotation $I_{pl}\tau$ with an angle increment of 45°, within the interval $o\tau = [0,135]$, being the image for $\tau = 180$, a repetition of Figure 3a.

each $I_{pl}\tau$ represents the length of traced lines, h, required to calculate the $MIL(\tau)$ as explained previously in this section.

2.2 Ellipse fitting

Using the ODF data it is possible to fit to it an ellipse. This ellipse parameters, as mentioned in the literature, can be use to define the mechanics properties of the trabecular bone [26]–[31]. In order to fit an ellipse to the acquired ODF data, it was used the methodology developed by Andrew et al. [35]. This fitting allows to acquire a set of ellipse parameters: the major axis length β_{max}, the major axis length β_{min} and the major axis angle θ. In this work, the main focus will be to β, since it is the parameter that defines the I_{ROI} principal direction. This method has the particularity that it is ellipse-specific. Therefore, it will always return an ellipse. Additionally, it can be solved naturally by a generalized Eigen system, proving to be extremely robust, efficient and easy to implement [35].

2.3 Mechanical properties formulation

Using the information from the fitted ellipse and the average apparent density of the binary image I_{ROIBW}, it was possible to define I_{ROIBW} homogenized orthotropic mechanical properties. The average apparent density, ρ_{app} was obtained using the number of white pixels α_w, and black pixels α_b, of I_{ROIBW} and assuming the cortical bone as having an apparent density of 2.1 g/cm^3, equation (2). Using ρ_{app} and the phenomenological material law defined by Belinha 2012, [36], the axial Young's modulus E_{axial} can be defined. To define the transverse elastic modulus E_{transv} it was used the relation between β_{min}, β_{max} and E_{axial} as shown in equation (3). Poisson's coefficient, υ, was calculated according the mixture theory using the relation between I_{ROIBW}, α_w and α_b, as represented in equation (4). The shear modulus, G, was expeditiously calculated using equation (5)

$$\rho_{app} = \left(\frac{\alpha_w}{\alpha_b}\right) \times \rho_{app}^{cortical} \qquad (2)$$

$$E_{transv} = \frac{(\|\beta_{\min}\| E_{axial})}{\|\beta_{\max}\|} \quad (3)$$

$$\upsilon = \frac{0.0(\alpha_b) + 0.3(\alpha_w)}{\alpha_t} \quad (4)$$

$$G = \frac{E_{axial}}{2(1+\upsilon)} \quad (5)$$

3 RESULTS

In this section are illustrated some results obtained using the medical image and the benchmark images. The medical image was acquired using cuboid bone micro-CT DICOM, from which it was selected a ROI possessing a perceptible material orientation. The two benchmarks images were created using MATLAB, where one of them has a material direction of $\tau = 0°$, Figure 1a, and the other one, Figure 1b, has a material direction of $\tau = 45°$. To test the behaviour of the developed methodology were created five $I_{pl}\tau$ with $\tau = [0°, 45°, 90°, 135°, 180°]$, Figure 3 that represent the *MIL* parallel lines family for $\tau = [0°, 45°, 90°, 135°, 180°]$. The increment of the orientation, τ, was defined as 45° to simplify the visualization of the following images. In Figure 4, Figure 5, Figure 6, are represented for each tested image, the five $I_{pl}\tau$ where are represented the family of parallel lines, the red pixels R_{px}, the I_{ROIBW}, the dark blue pixels DB_{px}, and the interceptions between $Ifiltered_{Rxpl}$ and $I_{pl}\tau$, the cyan blue pixels CB_{px}.

For the case of the benchmark with the principal direction of $\tau = 0°$, Figure 1a, can be notice on Figure 4 that the number of CB_{px} is lower at the $\tau = 0°$, the principal material direction of the image, and higher at $\tau = 90°$, the perpendicular direction of the principal material direction of the image. For the benchmark image, with $\beta = 45°$, Figure 1a, it can be notice on Figure 5, that the number of CB_{px}, is lower at $\tau = 0° \wedge \tau = 225°$, the preferential direction of the image, and higher at its perpendicular direction. For the medical ROI image, as can be notice in Figure 6, the number of CB_{px} visually do not changes significantly for different τ. In Figure 7a, Figure 7b and Figure 7c, the red dots represent the acquired ODF data for the used figures, Figure 1a, Figure 1b and Figure 1c, respectively. Using the acquired data and the ellipse fitting algorithm, it was possible to fit an ellipse to the ODF data, the solid blue lines present in Figure 7a, Figure 7b and Figure 7c. It is notorious that the ellipses represents the preferential direction of the respective I_{ROIBW} figure, since $\beta_{\max}$ is align with the principal material direction of each figure. Even in Figure 1c, where, apparently, the number of CB_{px} do not changed

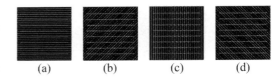

Figure 4. Grid Lines Rotation Interceptions of Figure 1a.

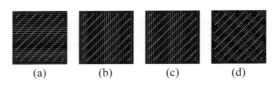

Figure 5. Grid Lines Rotation Interceptions of Figure 1b.

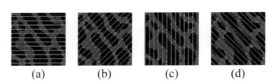

Figure 6. Grid Lines Rotation Interceptions of Figure 1c.

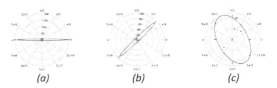

Figure 7. a): ODF Data, red points, and filled ellipse from Figure 1a, with $\beta = 0°$; b): ODF Data, red points, and filled ellipse from Figure 1b, with $\beta = 45°$; c): ODF Data, red points, and filled ellipse from Figure 1c, with $\beta = 130°$.

significantly for different τ, it is notorious by the ODF data, the red point, and the fitted ellipse $\beta_{\max}$ that the I_{ROI} has a principal direction.

3.1 *Analysing image rotation*

In order to verify the stability of the developed algorithm, some tests were executed, in which the input images were rotated. Afterwards, it was verified if β was coincident with the imposed rotation of the image. It was used a rotation of 20°, 40°, 60°, 80°, 100°, 120°, 140°, 160°, 180° always relative to the initial image.

In Figure 8 are presented the errors for each input image, when comparing the acquired β and the β that should have been obtained. As

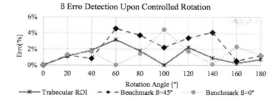

Figure 8. β Error detection upon controlled rotation. Errors for trabecular ROI, and for the two created Benchmarks.

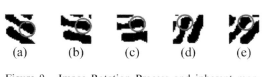

Figure 9. Image Rotation Process and inherent morphologic change. a) 20°; b) 40°; c) 60°; d) 100°; e) 120°.

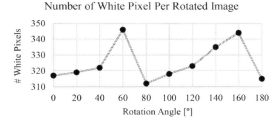

Figure 10. Number of White Pixel Per Rotated Image.

an illustrating example, looking to the original tabular binary ROI image, Figure 1c, it has a $\beta = 130°$. Adding to this value the imposed rotation 20°, it is acquired a supposed $\beta = 150°$, but applying the developed methodology to the figure, it is obtained a $\beta = 152°$, that represents an error of 1%. For the three analysed images, an average error of 2% is verified. This value can be explained by the process used to rotate the input, that result in slight different images, as can be seen in Figure 9. In these images the red circle marks the same region in different rotation images, where the pixel information changes. This variation results in different β because this methodology is intimately related with the number of white pixels in the image. As Figure 10 shows, the image rotation leads to significant variations on the number of white pixels.

4 CONCLUSIONS

The current work allows the definition of a fabric tensor using 2D images of micro-CT scans. Using the data of the orientation distribution function, and using the methodology defined by Andrew et al. [35], it was possible to approximate the orientation distribution to a ellipse function. As described by Moreno et al. [33], this ellipse function can be used to define the mechanical properties of trabecular bone by means of a 2×2 matrix (second order tensor) representing estimated ellipse. This work focus on the methodology used to acquire de ODF data. It is necessary to refer that the developed algorithm is sensible to some input parameters, such as the angular increment applied to the family of parallel lines. Using a lower angle increment allows to create a higher number of images, resulting in more ODF data. Also the threshold image processing tools used was automatic, which can lead to some variability in results. The variability described in the image rotation test is not to be of major concern, since in a real use the input images will not be rotated. In the future, this methodology could integrate a formulation to allow the definition of the mechanical proprieties of ROI. In addition, this methodology could be further developed to 3D.

ACKNOWLEDGEMENTS

The authors truly acknowledge the funding provided by Ministério da Ciência, Tecnologia e Ensino Superior—Fundação para a Ciência e a Tecnologia (Portugal), under Grants SFRH/BD/110047/2015 and by project funding MIT-EXPL/ISF/0084/2017. Additionally, the authors gratefully acknowledge the funding of Project NORTE-01-0145-FEDER-000022—SciTech—Science and Technology for Competitive and Sustainable Industries, cofinanced by Programa Operacional Regional do Norte (NORTE2020), through Fundo Europeu de Desenvolvimento Regional (FEDER).

REFERENCES

[1] X. Feng and J.M. McDonald, "Disorders of bone remodeling," *Annu. Rev. Pathol.*, vol. 6, pp. 121–45, Jan. 2011.
[2] G.E. Wnek and G.L. Bowlin, *Encyclopedia of Biomaterials and Biomedical Engineering*, no. April. New York: Informa Healthcare USA, 2008.
[3] D.R. Carter, M.C. Van Der Meulen, and G.S. Beaupré, "Mechanical factors in bone growth and development," *Bone*, vol. 18, no. 1 Suppl, p. 5S–10S, Jan. 1996.

[4] V.C. Mow, A. Ratcliffe, and A.R. Poole, "Cartilage and diarthrodial joints as paradigms for hierarchical materials and structures.," *Biomaterials*, vol. 13, no. 2, pp. 67–97, 1992.

[5] J. Wolff, "The Law of Bone Remodelling," *Journal of Anatomy*, 1986. [Online]. Available: http://www.springer.com/us/book/9783642710339. [Accessed: 25-Mar-2015].

[6] S.V. Dorozhkin, "Nanosized and nanocrystalline calcium orthophosphates," *Acta Biomater.*, vol. 6, no. 3, pp. 715–734, Mar. 2010.

[7] E. Lucchinetti, "Composite Models of Bone Properties," in *Bone Mechanics Handbook, Second Edition*, CRC Press, 2001, pp. 12–1-12–19.

[8] E. Hamed and I. Jasiuk, "Elastic modeling of bone at nanostructural level," *Mater. Sci. Eng. R Reports*, vol. 73, no. 3–4, pp. 27–49, 2012.

[9] A. Barkaoui, B. Tlili, A. Vercher-Martínez, and R. Hambli, "A multiscale modelling of bone ultrastructure elastic proprieties using finite elements simulation and neural network method," *Comput. Methods Programs Biomed.*, vol. 134, pp. 69–78, 2016.

[10] S. Weiner and W. Traub, "Bone structure: from angstroms to microns.," *FASEB J.*, vol. 6, no. 3, pp. 879–85, Feb. 1992.

[11] W.J. Landis, "The strength of a calcified tissue depends in part on the molecular structure and organization of its constituent mineral crystals in their organic matrix," *Bone*, vol. 16, no. 5, pp. 533–544, 1995.

[12] R.T. Hart, D.T. Davy, and K.G. Heiple, "A Computational Method for Stress Analysis of Adaptive Elastic Materials With a View Toward Applications in Strain-Induced Bone Remodeling," *J. Biomech. Eng.*, vol. 106, no. 4, p. 342, 1984.

[13] R. Huiskes, H. Weinans, and M. Dalstra, "Adaptive bone remodeling and biomechanical design considerations for noncemented total hip arthroplasty.," *Orthopedics*, vol. 12, no. 9, pp. 1255–1267, 1989.

[14] D.R. Carter, D.P. Fyhrie, and R.T. Whalen, "Trabecular bone density and loading history: Regulation of connective tissue biology by mechanical energy," *J. Biomech.*, vol. 20, no. 8, pp. 785–794, Jan. 1987.

[15] G.S. Beaupré, T.E. Orr, and D.R. Carter, "An approach for time-dependent bone modeling and remodeling-theoretical development," *J. Orthop. Res.*, vol. 8, no. 5, pp. 651–661, Sep. 1990.

[16] C.R. Jacobs, J.C. Simo, G.S. Beaupré, and D.R. Carter, "Adaptive bone remodeling incorporating simultaneous density and anisotropy considerations," *J. Biomech.*, vol. 30, no. 6, pp. 603–613, 1997.

[17] P. Fernandes, J.M. Guedes, and H. Rodrigues, "Topology optimization of three-dimensional linear elastic structures with a constraint on 'perimeter,'" *Comput. Struct.*, vol. 73, no. 6, pp. 583–594, 1999.

[18] M. Doblaré and J.M. García, "Application of an anisotropic bone-remodelling model based on a damage-repair theory to the analysis of the proximal femur before and after total hip replacement," *J. Biomech.*, vol. 34, no. 9, pp. 1157–1170, 2001.

[19] M. Doblaré and J.M. García, "Anisotropic bone remodelling model based on a continuum damage-repair theory," *J. Biomech.*, vol. 35, no. 1, pp. 1–17, 2002.

[20] J.M. García-Aznar, T. Rueberg, and M. Doblare, "A bone remodelling model coupling microdamage growth and repair by 3D BMU-activity," *Biomech. Model. Mechanobiol.*, vol. 4, no. 2–3, pp. 147–167, 2005.

[21] S.J. Hazelwood, R. Bruce Martin, M.M. Rashid, and J.J. Rodrigo, "A mechanistic model for internal bone remodeling exhibits different dynamic responses in disuse and overload," *J. Biomech.*, vol. 34, no. 3, pp. 299–308, 2001.

[22] D. Taylor and T.C. Lee, "Microdamage and mechanical behaviour: predicting failure and remodelling in compact bone," *J. Anat.*, vol. 203, no. 2, pp. 203–211, Aug. 2003.

[23] C.J. Hernandez, G.S. Beaupré, and D.R. Carter, "A model of mechanobiologic and metabolic influences on bone adaptation.," *J. Rehabil. Res. Dev.*, vol. 37, no. 2, pp. 235–244, 2000.

[24] J. Hazrati Marangalou, K. Ito, and B. van Rietbergen, "A novel approach to estimate trabecular bone anisotropy from stress tensors," *Biomech. Model. Mechanobiol.*, vol. 14, no. 1, pp. 39–48, Jan. 2015.

[25] R. Moreno, Ö. Smedby, and D.H. Pahr, "Prediction of apparent trabecular bone stiffness through fourth-order fabric tensors," *Biomech. Model. Mechanobiol.*, vol. 15, no. 4, pp. 831–844, Aug. 2016.

[26] S.C. Cowin, "The relationship between the elasticity tensor and the fabric tensor," *Mech. Mater.*, vol. 4, no. 2, pp. 137–147, 1985.

[27] W.J. Whitehouse, "The quantitative morphology of anisotropic trabecular bone," *J. Microsc.*, vol. 101, no. 2, pp. 153–168, 1974.

[28] S.C. Cowin and S.B. Doty, *Tissue Mechanics*. Springer Science, 2007.

[29] K. Mizuno, M. Matsukawa, T. Otani, M. Takada, I. Mano, and T. Tsujimoto, "Effects of structural anisotropy of cancellous bone on speed of ultrasonic fast waves in the bovine femur," *IEEE Trans. Ultrason. Ferroelectr. Freq. Control*, vol. 55, no. 7, pp. 1480–1487, Jul. 2008.

[30] A. Odgaard, "Three-dimensional methods for quantification of cancellous bone architecture," *Bone*, vol. 20, no. 4, pp. 315–328, 1997.

[31] P.K. Zysset, "A review of morphology–elasticity relationships in human trabecular bone: theories and experiments," *J. Biomech.*, vol. 36, no. 10, pp. 1469–1485, 2003.

[32] R. Moreno, M. Borga, and O. Smedby, "Generalizing the mean intercept length tensor for gray-level images," *Med. Phys.*, vol. 39, no. 7, p. 4599, 2012.

[33] R. Moreno, M. Borga, and O. Smedby, "Techniques for Computing Fabric Tensors – A Review," in *Mathematics and Visualization*, vol. 5, no. 12, 2014, pp. 271–292.

[34] N. Otsu, "A Threshold Selection Method from Gray-Level Histograms," *IEEE Trans. Syst. Man. Cybern.*, vol. 9, no. 1, pp. 62–66, Jan. 1979.

[35] W. Andrew *et al.*, "Direct Least Squares Fitting of Ellipses," pp. 253–257, 1996.

[36] J. Belinha, R.M.N. Jorge, and L.M.J.S. Dinis, "A meshless microscale bone tissue trabecular remodelling analysis considering a new anisotropic bone tissue material law," *Comput. Methods Biomech. Biomed. Engin.*, vol. 5842, no. August 2012, pp. 1–15, Jan. 2012.

Biodental Engineering V – Belinha et al. (Eds)
© 2019 Taylor & Francis Group, London, ISBN 978-0-367-21087-8

A homogenization multiscale procedure for trabecular bone tissue using meshless methods

M. Marques
Institute of Science and Innovation in Mechanical and Industrial Engineering (INEGI), Porto, Portugal

J. Belinha
Department of Mechanical Engineering, School of Engineering, Polytechnic of Porto (ISEP), Porto, Portugal

R.M. Natal Jorge
Department of Mechanical Engineering, Faculty of Engineering, University of Porto (FEUP), Porto, Portugal

A.F. Oliveira
Institute of Biomedical Sciences Abel Salazar, University of Porto (ICBAS), Porto, Portugal

ABSTRACT: Multiscale techniques are being used to study the behaviour of heterogeneous anatomical structures, such as bones. It is known that multiscale techniques usually use highly discretized Representative Volume Elements (RVEs), leading to high computational costs. In this works, it is analysed a methodology that allows to obtain from a heterogeneous RVE (representing trabecular bone tissue highly heterogeneous medium) the homogenized orthotropic material properties. The resulting material property and direction are strongly correlated with the RVE's apparent density and trabeculae orientation, respectively. This was analysed with an advanced discretization meshless method, the Radial Point Interpolation Method (RPIM), and with the Finite Element Method (FEM). In the end, several elasto-static analysis were performed using heterogeneous RVEs and an equivalent solid patch with homogenized orthotropic material properties. It was found that both analyses provide similar results. However, the heterogeneous RVE demands a much higher computational power than the homogenous counterpart. Such results demonstrate the potential of the proposed technique in multiscale analysis.

1 INTRODUCTION

Discrete numerical methods were introduced to orthopaedic biomechanics in 1972 to evaluate mechanical stresses in human bones. The use of this discrete numerical methods, an innovative technology at the time, allowed to start studying and analysing, *in silico*, the behaviour of materials and structures. Bone is a mineralized biological structure, which can be classified in different hierarchical structures. Such structures represent distinct scale levels with specific interactions and with very complex architectures [1]. Bone adapts its morphology, inducing changes in its mechanical properties. Such dynamic behaviour aims to optimize its specific physiological function—the body's structural support [2], [3]. Many researchers addressed the study of bone mechanical behaviour by developing

analytical and numerical models, using a broad range of advanced constitutive models, such as multiscale [4]–[8] and homogenization techniques [9], [10], combine with diverse discrete numerical approaches, such as finite element methods or meshless methods. This allows to describe the mechanical behaviour of bone at a certain scale level, or in a set of scales. Bone remodelling is a progressive biological process that occurs to renew bone and to adapt the bone morphology to any new external loads. This process is highly studied, *in vivo* and *in silico*.

The concept that bone remodelling process could be induced by strain/stress applied to the bone was firstly reported in 1886 by Wolff [11]. Wolff reported that the direction of the applied loads directly influences the direction of the trabeculae in bone tissue, adapting it to existing external load. Such concept is known as the Wolff's law.

1.1 Discrete numerical techniques

Today, FEM is the most popular discrete numerical method [12]. Nevertheless, the literature reports other numerical methods, such as meshless methods. The first developed meshless method dated form 1977, where Gingold and Monaghan proposed the smoothed-particle hydrodynamics (SPH) [13]. Since then, several other meshless techniques have been developed, such as the Natural Neighbour Radial Point Interpolation Method (NNRPIM) [14], that is based on the combination of the natural neighbour concept with the radial point interpolators [15], [16], and the Natural Radial Element Method (NREM) [17] that combines the simplicity of low-order finite elements connectivity with the geometric flexibility of meshless methods.

When compared with FEM, meshless methods follow a very distinct discretization procedure. For instances, to discretize problem domain, meshless methods do not use elements to establish the nodal/element connectivity. In meshless methods, the problem domain is discretized using a unstructured node set in which the nodes can be regularly or irregularly distributed. In meshless methods, the nodal discretization just requires the spatial coordinates of the nodes and, possibly, its individually material properties. How each node interacts with its neighbour, is obtained using geometrical and mathematical constructions, allowing to define the 'influence domain' concept, the equivalent to the 'element' concept in the finite element methods.

One of the oldest meshless methods ever developed is the Smoothed-Particle Hydrodynamics method (SPH) [13]. Firstly developed for astronomy, the SPH is in the origin of the Reproducing Kernel Particle Method (RKPM) [18]. Another worthmentioning meshless method is the meshless local Petrov-Galerkin method (MLPG) [19], an important meshless method initially developed to solve linear and nonlinear potential problems. Afterwards, Oñate and co-workers developed a new meshless method, the Finite Point Method (FPM) [20]–[22].

The Radial Basis Function Method (RBFM) [23], [24] is distinct from the previous mentioned meshless methods since it uses the radial basis functions to approximate the variable fields within the entire domain or in small domains. This method was initially used to approximate multidimensional data [25] and later it was used to solve differential equations [26], [27].

Meshless methods can be divided in two classes, approximation meshless method (using shape functions without the delta Kronecker property) and interpolation methods (using shape functions possessing the delta Kronecker property). The lack of the delta Kronecker property hinders the direct imposition of the essential and natural boundary conditions, which have to be enforced by computational expensive numeric techniques, such as the Lagrange multipliers [28]. In order to avoid the above mentioned difficulty, several interpolation meshless methods were developed, such as: the Point Interpolation Method (PIM) [29]; the Point Assembly Method (PAM) [30]; the Radial Point Interpolation Method (RPIM) [15], [16]; the Meshless Finite Element Method (MFEM) [31]; the Natural Neighbour Finite Element Method (NNFEM) [32]; the Natural Element Method (NEM) [33], [34] the Natural Neighbour Radial Point Interpolation Method (NNRPIM) [14], [28], [35] and; the Natural Radial Element Method (NREM) [17], [36], [37]. In meshless methods using weak formulation (such as the Galerkin weak form), it is mandatory the construction of a background integration mesh. However, in fact, the use of a background mesh for integration purposes, contradicts the "meshless" term. Thus, only meshless methods capable to construct the background integration mesh (completely) dependent on the nodal distribution are called truly meshless methods, because they allow to directly define the spatial position and the integration weight of all integration points only using the spatial positions of the nodes [38].

In this work, it is used the RPIM. The RPIM is an interpolator meshless method that uses the influence domain concept (the influence domain is a set of neighbour nodes surrounding an integration point) to force the nodal connectivity. In the RPIM, these set of nodes are found using a radial search. Overlapping the influence-domains of each node allows to obtain the nodal connectivity [15], [17]–[19], [39], [40]. RPIM has the ability to use local influence-domains, instead of global influence-domains, permitting to generate sparse and banded stiffness matrices. This feature becomes an advantage in the biomechanical analysis, since it is possible to analyse extremely irregular meshes and convex boundaries [41].

Meshless methods require the construction of a background grid of integration points that are used to integrate the integro-differential equations ruling the studied physical phenomenon.

To obtain the integration mesh it is necessary to select an integration scheme, that in meshless methods, generally, is obtained using a background grid, in which each grid-cell is filled with integration points via the Gauss-Legendre quadrature rule [38]. RPIM shape functions are obtained using the Radial Point Interpolators (RPI), combined with the radial basis functions with polynomial basis functions [38].

1.2 Homogenization technique

The presented homogenization technique allows to define the anisotropic mechanical proprieties of the trabecular bone, a highly heterogeneous material. This homogenization technique uses the fabric tensor concept. The fabric tensor, a symmetric second rank tensor that characterizes the arrangement of a multiphase material [42], can be obtained by two techniques: (1) the mechanical based techniques and (2) the morphologic-based techniques, that uses the interface between phases of the material to estimate the fabric tensor. For bone cases using micro-CT or a CT it is possible to more easily obtain information regarding the phase change. Thus, morphologic-based techniques are more frequently used when fabric tensor are applied to bone tissue.

The main objective of this work is to evaluate the behaviour of the developed methodology. This was achieved by creating two RVEs. One with a homogenized geometry defined with the mechanical properties obtained using the developed multiscale methodology, and one with a heterogeneous geometrical model representative of the trabecular bone, defined with mechanical properties obtained in the literature. For comparison purposes, the stress analysis of both models was performed using two different numerical methods, the RPIM and de FEM.

2 METHODOLOGY

In order to verify the efficiency of the developed methodology, it was performed a numerical analysis, using FEM and the RPIM, assuming two distinct models: (1) a homogenized RVE, represented in Figure 1a, with the homogenized anisotropic mechanical properties obtained using the developed multiscale homogenization methodology, and (2) a heterogeneous RVE, Figure 1b, with mechanical properties obtained from the literature.

Concerning the RPIM formulation, it was assumed one integration point per each integration sub-cell, a constant polynomial basis and the multi-quadrics RBF (MQ-RBF). Concerning the MQ-RBF shape parameters c and p, in this work, these parameters were defined as 0,0001 and 0,9999, respectively.

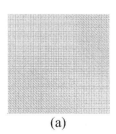 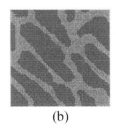

Figure 1. a) figure representing the homogenous RVE; b) figure representing the heterogeneous RVE.

The results of the two numerical examples were compared using the homogenized von Mises effective stress field.

The boundary conditions used in this numerical study are represented in Figure 2. It was imposed a displacement of $0.1 \times L$ to all the nodes at the top layer of the RVE, where $y = L$, being L the dimension of the RVE, as demonstrated in Figure 2. The nodes with $x = 0$ and $x = L$ were constrained on O_x direction, $u = 0$, and the nodes at $y = 0$ and $y = L$, were constrained on O_y direction, $v = 0$, as represented in Figure 2.

For the case of the realistic trabecular RVE (the heterogeneous RVE), the initial RVE represented in Figure 1b was repeated 2×2 and 3×3, allowing to have two additional models. For the homogenous RVE, it was also created a 2×2 model repetition.

The mechanical properties considered in this work for each RVE are presented in the Table 1 and Table 2. Therefore, Table 1 represent the mechanical properties of the homogenous RVE, which were acquired using the developed multiscale homogenization methodology. In Table 2 are shown the mechanical properties that were considered for the

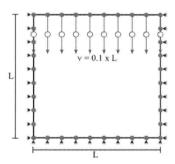

Figure 2. Boundary conditions applied to all RVEs.

Table 1. Homogenous RVE mechanical properties.

E_{axial} [MPa]	4488,548
E_{transv} [MPa]	2520,426
G [MPa]	10066,1
θ [Degrees]	56
v	0,3

Table 2. Heterogeneous RVE mechanical properties.

Trabecular bone		Void space	
$E[MPa]$	11600	$E[MPa]$	100
v	0,36	v	0,459

realistic trabecular RVEs. For this case, the models were defined by two materials, one representing the trabecular bone itself, defined as isotropic, and other material representing the void space existent between trabeculae, characteristic of the trabecular bone [43]. To simulate the void material (and make sure that it would not significantly interfere with the global structural response of the RVE), the Young's modulus of the void material was assumed much lower than the Young's modulus of the trabecular bone.

3 RESULTS

Regardless the level of the discretization or the used numerical method (FEM or RPIM), the results from the homogeneous RVEs were very similar, as can be seen in Figure 3a and Figure 3b. In these figures, it is also perceptible the preferential orientation of the material, which was obtained using the developed methodology. Concerning the comparison between the two numerical methods (observing, for instances, images with the same RVE, such as Figure 3a and Figure 3b), it is perceptible that meshless methods are capable to produce smother stress fields. Regarding the heterogeneous RVE, the results obtained with FEM are slightly different from the ones obtained with RPIM, dissimilarities that are inherent to the differences between both formulations.

To better compare the results between the RVEs and the numerical methods, it was used a homogenized stress variable, σ_{eff}^h. This variable, that summarizes the RVE's von Mises effective stress field in an average scalar, is shown in equation (1), being n_Q the number of integration points discretizing the problem domain not belonging to its physical boundary.

FEM integration mesh is constructed differently from the RPIM, resulting in a different special position for the integration points of both formulations. In Figure 4, some integration meshes are presented: the integration mesh of the homogenized RVE model for the FEM (Figure 3a) and for the RPIM (Figure 3b) and the integration mesh of the heterogeneous RVE model for the FEM (Figure 3c) and for the RPIM (Figure 3d). The blue points of Figure 4 represent the integration points that will be included to calculate σ_{eff}^h and in red are shown the integration points that will be excluded from equation (1). This process excludes 2% of the integration points forming the integration mesh. This was done to avoid the stress concentrations that appear near the domain boundary, as can be seen in Figure 3.

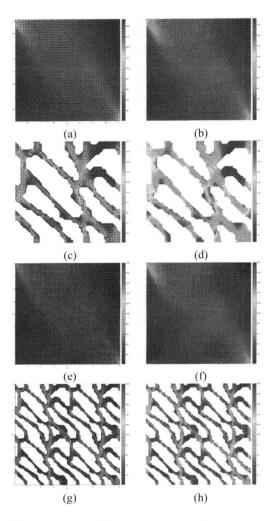

Figure 3. a): von Mises stress map for the homogeneous RVE using FEM; b) von Mises stress map for the homogeneous RVE using RPIM; c) von Mises stress map for the heterogenous RVE using FEM; d) von Mises stress map for the heterogenous RVE using RPIM; e) von Mises stress map for the homogeneous RVE repetition using FEM; f) von Mises stress map for the homogeneous RVE repetition using RPIM; g) von Mises stress map for the heterogenous RVE repetition using FEM; h) von Mises stress map for the heterogenous RVE repetition using RPIM.

$$\sigma_{eff}^h = \frac{1}{n_Q} \sum_{i=1}^{n_Q} \sigma(x_i)_{eff} \qquad (1)$$

The results for the homogenized von Mises effective stress, σ_{eff}^h obtained for each analysed

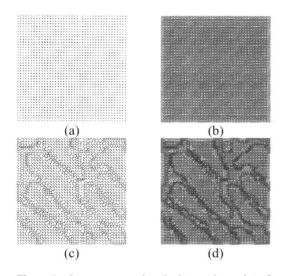

Figure 4. Image representing the integration point of the used models. a) Homogenous RVE with FEM formulation. b) Homogenous RVE with RPIM formulation. c) Heterogeneous RVE with FEM formulation. d) Heterogeneous RVE with RPIM formulation.

RVE, using both FEM and RPIM methodologies are summarized in Figure 5.

Analysing Figure 5, it is notorious that for the considered heterogeneous RVEs, as the model detail increases, the σ_{eff}^h decreases. As expected, the results from both analysed homogeneous models, the results are almost coincident.

One of the main goals of this work was to achieve a low-cost and efficient homogenization technique. Thus, in order to understand the computational efficiency of the proposed methodology, a computational cost study was performed.

In Figure 6 is shown computational cost of each structural analysis for both heterogeneous and homogenous RVEs. In this graphic, only the computational cost of the 1×1 homogeneous model is shown, because, as seen in Figure 5, it provides very similar result compared to the 2×2, and to the 3×3 heterogeneous model. Comparing the computational time to perform an elasto-static analysis, the analysis of the heterogeneous RVE takes 4164s to finish and the homogeneous RVE only requires $4 - 10$ s. However, despite the significant difference, both analyses provide very similar σ_{eff}^h.

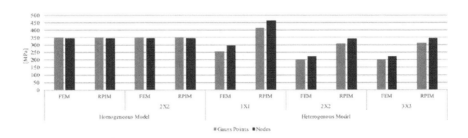

Figure 5. Effective stress σ_{eff}^h for homogeneous model: FEM 1×1; RPIM 1×1; FEM 2×2; RPIM 2×2 and for heterogeneous models: FEM 1×1; RPIM 1×1; FEM 2×2 RPIM 2×2 and FEM 3×3; RPIM 3×3.

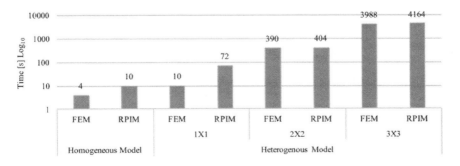

Figure 6. Computational cost (in seconds) of each analysis.

4 CONCLUSIONS

The objective of this work was to evaluate a developed methodology where was used the fabric tensor concept and a material law, that together were able to define the mechanical properties of a micro-CT trabecular square ROI without any a-priory knowledge.

The developed methodology was evaluated by studying and comparing the behaviour of a homogeneous.

This homogenization technique was capable to produce results that are comparable with results obtained using a non homogenized methodology. However the proposed methodology is much more efficient. Comparing the numerical methods, FEM integration mesh is constructed differently from the RPIM. This result in a slight different spatial position of the two methods' integration points, and so, in slightly different results.

Analysing the results obtained with the heterogeneous RVEs, it is perceptible that, as the model detail increases (the detail is governed by the number of repetitions: the 1×1 RVE has a lower detail than the 3×3 RVE), the obtained σ_{eff}^{h} decreases, and converge, in the case of the RPIM methodology, for the results obtained using the homogenized RVE. This shows that the homogenization methodology is capable to obtain accurate results, and also capable to obtain the homogenized anisotropic material properties of a trabecular patch.

Comparing the FEM and the RPIM results, it is notorious that in the case of the homogeneous RVEs', the results are very similar. However, analysing the results obtained with the heterogeneous RVEs, are notorious some differences, that could be explain by locking effects in the FEM

Being one of the objectives of this homogenization technique to achieve a low-cost and efficient homogenization technique, a computational cost study was performed. In this comparison study, it was perceptible the high efficient of the developed methodology, showing a very low computational time. Thus, due to this efficiency, novel multiscale frameworks can be developed combining the proposed methodology with classical numerical approaches. This proposed homogenization methodology shows that is possible to reduce the cost of the multiscale analysis.

ACKNOWLEDGEMENTS

The authors truly acknowledge the funding provided by Ministério da Ciência, Tecnologia e Ensino Superior—Fundação para a Ciência e a Tecnologia (Portugal), under Grants SFRH/ BD/110047/2015 and by project funding MIT-EXPL/ISF/0084/2017. Additionally, the authors gratefully acknowledge the funding of Project NORTE-01-0145-FEDER-000022—SciTech—Science and Technology for Competitive and Sustainable Industries, cofinanced by Programa Operacional Regional do Norte (NORTE2020), through Fundo Europeu de Desenvolvimento Regional (FEDER).

REFERENCES

[1] S.V. Dorozhkin, "Nanosized and nanocrystalline calcium orthophosphates," *Acta Biomater.*, vol. 6, no. 3, pp. 715–734, Mar. 2010.

[2] D.R. Carter, M.C. Van Der Meulen, and G.S. Beaupré, "Mechanical factors in bone growth and development," *Bone*, vol. 18, no. 1 Suppl, p. 5S–10S, Jan. 1996.

[3] V.C. Mow, A. Ratcliffe, and A.R. Poole, "Cartilage and diarthrodial joints as paradigms for hierarchical materials and structures," *Biomaterials*, vol. 13, no. 2, pp. 67–97, 1992.

[4] A. Barkaoui, B. Tlili, A. Vercher-Martínez, and R. Hambli, "A multiscale modelling of bone ultrastructure elastic proprieties using finite elements simulation and neural network method," *Comput. Methods Programs Biomed.*, vol. 134, pp. 69–78, 2016.

[5] J. Martínez-Reina, J. Domínguez, and J.M. García-Aznar, "Effect of porosity and mineral content on the elastic constants of cortical bone: A multiscale approach," *Biomech. Model. Mechanobiol.*, vol. 10, no. 3, pp. 309–322, Jun. 2011.

[6] E. Hamed, Y. Lee, and I. Jasiuk, "Multiscale modeling of elastic properties of cortical bone," *Acta Mech.*, vol. 213, no. 1–2, pp. 131–154, Aug. 2010.

[7] Y.J. Yoon and S.C. Cowin, "An estimate of anisotropic poroelastic constants of an osteon," *Biomech. Model. Mechanobiol.*, vol. 7, no. 1, pp. 13–26, Feb. 2008.

[8] Y.J. Yoon and S.C. Cowin, "The estimated elastic constants for a single bone osteonal lamella," *Biomech. Model. Mechanobiol.*, vol. 7, no. 1, pp. 1–11, Feb. 2008.

[9] J. Hazrati Marangalou, K. Ito, and B. van Rietbergen, "A novel approach to estimate trabecular bone anisotropy from stress tensors," *Biomech. Model. Mechanobiol.*, vol. 14, no. 1, pp. 39–48, Jan. 2015.

[10] R. Moreno, Ö. Smedby, and D.H. Pahr, "Prediction of apparent trabecular bone stiffness through fourth-order fabric tensors," *Biomech. Model. Mechanobiol.*, vol. 15, no. 4, pp. 831–844, Aug. 2016.

[11] J. Wolff, "The Law of Bone Remodelling," *Journal of Anatomy*, 1986. [Online]. Available: http://www.springer.com/us/book/9783642710339. [Accessed: 25-Mar-2015].

[12] O.C. Zienkiewicz and R.L. Taylor, *The Finite Element Method*, 4th ed. London: McGraw-Hill, 1994.

[13] R.A. Gingold and J.J. Monaghan, "Smooth particle hydrodynamics: theory and application to non-spherical stars," *Mon. Not. R. Astron. Soc.*, vol. 181, pp. 375–389, 1977.

[14] L.M.J.S. Dinis, R.M. Natal Jorge, and J. Belinha, "Analysis of 3D solids using the natural neighbour radial point interpolation method," *Comput. Methods Appl. Mech. Eng.*, vol. 196, no. 13–16, pp. 2009–2028, Mar. 2007.

[15] J.G. Wang and G.R. Liu, "A point interpolation meshless method based on radial basis functions," *Int. J. Numer. Methods Eng.*, vol. 54, no. 11, pp. 1623–1648, Aug. 2002.

[16] J.G. Wang and G.R. Liu, "On the optimal shape parameters of radial basis functions used for 2-D meshless methods," *Comput. Methods Appl. Mech. Eng.*, vol. 191, no. 23–24, pp. 2611–2630, Mar. 2002.

[17] J. Belinha, L.M.J.S. Dinis, and R.M.N. Jorge, "The natural radial element method," *Int. J. Numer. Methods Eng.*, vol. 93, no. 12, pp. 1286–1313, Mar. 2013.

[18] W.K. Liu, S. Jun, and Y.F. Zhang, "Reproducing kernel particle methods," *Int. J. Numer. Methods Fluids*, vol. 20, no. 8–9, pp. 1081–1106, Apr. 1995.

[19] S.N. Atluri and T. Zhu, "A new Meshless Local Petrov-Galerkin (MLPG) approach in computational mechanics," *Comput. Mech.*, vol. 22, no. 2, pp. 117–127, Aug. 1998.

[20] E. Oñate, S. Idelsohn, O.C. Zienkiewicz, and R.L. Taylor, "A Finite Point Method in Computational Mechanics—Applications to Convective Transport and Fluid Flow," *Int. J. Numer. Methods Eng.*, vol. 39, no. 22, pp. 3839–3866, Nov. 1996.

[21] E. Oñate, S. Idelsohn, O.C. Zienkiewicz, R.L. Taylor, and C. Sacco, "A stabilized finite point method for analysis of fluid mechanics problems," *Comput. Methods Appl. Mech. Eng.*, vol. 139, no. 1–4, pp. 315–346, Dec. 1996.

[22] E. Oñate, F. Perazzo, and J. Miquel, "A finite point method for elasticity problems," *Comput. Struct.*, vol. 79, no. 22–25, pp. 2151–2163, Sep. 2001.

[23] E.J. Kansa, "Multiquadrics-A scattered data approximation scheme with applications to computational fluid-dynamics-II solutions to parabolic, hyperbolic and elliptic partial differential equations," *Comput. Math. with Appl.*, vol. 19, no. 8–9, pp. 147–161, Jan. 1990.

[24] E.J. Kansa, "Multiquadrics-A scattered data approximation scheme with applications to computational fluid-dynamics-I surface approximations and partial derivative estimates," *Comput. Math. with Appl.*, vol. 19, no. 8–9, pp. 127–145, Jan. 1990.

[25] R.L. Hardy, "Theory and applications of the multiquadric-biharmonic method 20 years of discovery 1968–1988," *Comput. Math. with Appl.*, vol. 19, no. 8–9, pp. 163–208, Jan. 1990.

[26] A.J.M. Ferreira, C.M.C. Roque, and P.A.L.S. Martins, "Radial basis functions and higher-order shear deformation theories in the analysis of laminated composite beams and plates," *Compos. Struct.*, vol. 66, no. 1–4, pp. 287–293, Oct. 2004.

[27] C.M. Tiago and V.M.A. Leitão, "Application of radial basis functions to linear and nonlinear structural analysis problems," *Comput. Math. with Appl.*, vol. 51, no. 8, pp. 1311–1334, Apr. 2006.

[28] J. Belinha, *Meshless Methods in Biomechanics—Bone Tissue Remodelling Analysis*, Vol.16. Lecture Notes in Computational Vision and Biomechanics, Springer Netherlands, 2014.

[29] G.R. Liu and Y.T. Gu, "A point interpolation method for two-dimensional solids," *Int. J. Numer. Methods Eng.*, vol. 50, no. 4, pp. 937–951, Feb. 2001.

[30] G.R. Liu, "A point assembly method for stress analysis for two-dimensional solids," *Int. J. Solids Struct.*, vol. 39, no. 1, pp. 261–276, Jan. 2002.

[31] S.R. Idelsohn, E. Oñate, N. Calvo, and F. Del Pin, "The meshless finite element method," *Int. J. Numer. Methods Eng.*, vol. 58, no. 6, pp. 893–912, Oct. 2003.

[32] N. Sukumar, B. Moran, A.Y. Semenov, and V.V. Belikov, "Natural neighbour Galerkin methods," *Int. J. Numer. Methods Eng.*, vol. 50, no. 1, pp. 1–27, Jan. 2000.

[33] J. Braun and M. Sambridge, "A numerical method for solving partial differential equations on highly irregular evolving grids," *Nature*, vol. 376, no. 6542, pp. 655–660, Aug. 1995.

[34] N. Sukumar and T. Belytschko, "The natural element method in solid mechanics," *Int. J. Numer. Methods Eng.*, vol. 43, no. 5, pp. 839–887, Nov. 1998.

[35] S. Moreira, J. Belinha, L.M.J.S. Dinis, and R.M. Natal Jorge, "Análise de vigas laminadas utilizando o natural neighbour radial point interpolation method," *Rev. Int. Métodos Numéricos para Cálculo y Diseño en Ing.*, vol. 30, no. 2, pp. 108–120, Feb. 2014.

[36] J. Belinha, L.M.J.S. Dinis, and R.M. Natal Jorge, "Analysis of thick plates by the natural radial element method," *Int. J. Mech. Sci.*, vol. 76, pp. 33–48, Nov. 2013.

[37] J. Belinha, L.M.J.S. Dinis, and R.M.N. Jorge, "Composite laminated plate analysis using the natural radial element method," *Compos. Struct.*, vol. 103, pp. 50–67, Sep. 2013.

[38] J. Belinha, *Meshless Methods in Biomechanics: Bone Tissue Remodelling Analysis*, vol. 2. Dordrecht: Springer Netherlands, 2014.

[39] T. Belytschko, Y.Y. Lu, and L. Gu, "Element-free Galerkin methods," *Int. J.*, vol. 37, no. April 1993, pp. 229–256, Jan. 1994.

[40] V.P. Nguyen, T. Rabczuk, S. Bordas, and M. Duflot, "Meshless methods: A review and computer implementation aspects," *Math. Comput. Simul.*, vol. 79, no. 3, pp. 763–813, Dec. 2008.

[41] J. Belinha, L.M.J.S. Dinis, and R.M.N. Jorge, "The Mandible Remodeling Induced by Dental Implants: A Meshless Approach," *J. Mech. Med. Biol.*, vol. 15, no. 4, p. 1550059, Aug. 2015.

[42] S.C. Cowin, "The relationship between the elasticity tensor and the fabric tensor," *Mech. Mater.*, vol. 4, no. 2, pp. 137–147, 1985.

[43] A.N. Natali, E.L. Carniel, and P.G. Pavan, "Constitutive modelling of inelastic behaviour of cortical bone," *Med. Eng. Phys.*, vol. 30, no. 7, pp. 905–912, Sep. 2008.

Biodental Engineering V – Belinha et al. (Eds)
© 2019 Taylor & Francis Group, London, ISBN 978-0-367-21087-8

Bone remodeling mathematical models using advanced discretization techniques: A review

M.M.A. Peyroteo
Institute of Science and Innovation in Mechanical and Industrial Engineering (INEGI), Porto, Portugal

J. Belinha
Department of Mechanical Engineering, School of Engineering, Polytechnic of Porto (ISEP), Porto, Portugal

L.M.J.S. Dinis & R.M. Natal Jorge
Department of Mechanical Engineering, Faculty of Engineering, University of Porto (FEUP), Porto, Portugal

ABSTRACT: This work presents a brief state of the art regarding bone remodeling models and their combination with numerical methods. The concept of bone remodeling arises from Wolff's law, in which it is suggested a relationship between the mechanical environment and bone's morphology. Since then, several models have tried to reproduce this adaptation process. Remodeling models first took into account only the mechanical component of the process, correlating the apparent density of the bone with its mechanical properties. Later, biochemical models emerged aiming to mathematically describe the dynamic interaction between bone cells and their controlling autocrine and paracrine signaling pathways. Currently, the trend is to create biomechanical models that simultaneously include bone cellular response to biochemical and mechanical stimuli. Therefore, in this work, some of the most relevant bone remodeling models are addressed along with a brief description of the remodeling process. Also, some applications resulting from the combination of these algorithms with distinct numerical techniques, including meshless methods, are presented.

1 STATE OF THE ART

1.1 *Bone remodeling*

Bone has a strong mechanical function, being a key biological structure for movement, support and protection of other organs. However, in order to ensure these functions, bone must be able to adapt its morphology to distinct stimuli (Xiao et al., 2016). Bone thence undergoes a remodeling process, in which new bone tissue is formed or resorbed according to the stimulus (Rucci, 2008). Osteoclasts are the bone cells responsible for resorption and osteoblasts for forming new tissue. There are also osteocytes, which are the mechanical sensor cells, able to detect any changes in the mechanical environment.

Bone remodeling can be classified into two different types, depending on whether it is targeted or not. Targeted bone remodeling occurs in the presence of a non-physiological load. Although the type of the triggering mechanical stimulus (e.g. stress, strain) is still a topic under discussion, several studies show that osteoclasts are highly active in low strain/stress regions, while osteoblasts present high activity levels in high strain/stress regions (Courteix et al., 1998; Fiore et al., 1991; Kiratli et al., 2000). Non targeted remodeling occurs periodically, in which old or damaged tissue is replaced with new material to assure a healthy skeleton. This process has several phases beginning with an activation followed by a resorption phase. At this stage, osteoclasts synthesize a set of electrolytes and degradative enzymes that provide an acid environment conducive to bone resorption (Teitelbaum, 2007). Afterwards, during the reversal phase, bone transitions from resorption to formation, preparing bone's surface and recruiting preosteoblasts (Locklin et al., 1999). Then, bone mass is restored during formation and mineralization phases, thanks to the action of osteoblasts (Kini and Nandeesh, 2012).

Ruling both types of remodeling are a set of bone regulatory factors, such as insulin-like growth factors (IGF) I and II, transforming growth factor-β (TGF-β) superfamily, matrix metalloproteinases

(MMPs), receptor activator of nuclear factor-Kb (RANK) and its cognate partner RANK ligand (RANKL), osteoprotegerin (OPG), fibroblast growth factor-2 (FGF-2) and bone morphogenetic proteins (BMPs). Among these, the RANKL/RANK/OPG system plays a key role in the control of bone resorption. When activated by RANKL, RANK causes differentiation of osteoclasts and promotes their function and survival (Cohen Jr., 2006; Teitelbaum and Ross, 2003; Xiao et al., 2016). However, OPG can bind to RANKL, preventing it from binding to RANK, which leads to an inhibition of osteoclastogenesis (Graves et al., 2011; Simonet et al., 1997). Thus, RANKL/OPG ratio expression ratio is a relevant indication of bone resorption. Regarding bone tissue formation, TGF-β is an important stimulator involved in osteoblastic differentiation and production of bone matrix (Bonewald and Dallas, 1994), as well as FGF-2 (Downey et al., 2009). Moreover, IGF I and II are responsible for controlling the number and function of osteoblasts (Cohick and Clemmons, 1993), as well as mediating the interaction between osteoblasts and osteoclasts (Mohamed, 2008).

Bone remodeling is also influenced by certain hormones. Studies show that estrogen enhances osteoblasts' activity (Ernst et al., 1989). Therefore, when postmenopausal women suffer from estrogen deficiency, bone formation is reduced (Gallagher, 2007). This bone mass loss is even more evident since estrogen deficiency also leads to an expression increase of RANKL and decrease of OPG (Post et al., 2010). Parathyroid hormone (PTH) is also a relevant hormone, being responsible for calcium homeostasis. However, the impact of PTH depends on the method of administration. When administered continuously, PTH causes bone loss, while in intermittent applications it stimulates bone formation (Kramer et al., 2010).

These and many other biological factors, comprise the autocrine and paracrine signalling pathways of bone. Autocrine signalling is composed by factors secreted by osteoclasts and osteoblasts that affect their respective formation. Paracrine signalling reflects the factors secreted by osteoblasts that affect osteoclasts formation and vice versa (Ayati et al., 2010).

1.2 *Remodeling models*

Thanks to experimental works, a deepened knowledge about bone remodeling and its key players was achieved. Consequently, several authors proposed mathematical models potentially capable to reliably reproduce bone remodeling. Those authors were certain of the potential of such mathematical models to obtain faster and equally reliable results as the ones obtained with experimental testing.

Starting with a purely mechanical approach, Cowin and Hegedus (Cowin and Hegedus, 1976) proposed one of the first isotropic models of bone remodeling, known as the "Adaptive Elasticity Model". The authors described the remodeling of cortical bone caused by a strain state alteration, forcing bone to adapt its configuration. Huiskes et al. (Huiskes et al., 1987) proposed some changes to this work, considering strain energy density (SED), instead of strain, as the mechanical stimulus triggering bone remodeling. This has been particularly relevant, since most current models choose to use also the SED field, U, which can be obtained with the following

$$U = \frac{1}{2}\varepsilon_{ij}\sigma_{ij} \tag{1}$$

where ε_{ij} is the strain tensor and σ_{ij} the stress tensor. Also, following the assumption proposed by Carter (Carter, 1984), the existence of a lazy zone is considered, in which only points over and under certain threshold values are able to remodel. However, there are also studies that consider stress level as a stimulus, as presented by Beaupré et al. (Beaupré et al., 1990a) in a time-dependent remodeling model.

Fyhrie and Carter (Fyhrie and Carter, 1986) proposed a distinct approach, presenting the "Self-Optimization" theory, assuming that bone remodeling is ultimately reflected by changes of bone's apparent density. Thus, when mechanical environment is disturbed, trabecular morphology has to adapt, aligning with principal stresses' orientation. Also, using Equation (2), bone's apparent density, ρ, is updated,

$$\rho = A\sigma_{eff}^{\alpha} \tag{2}$$

in which σ_{eff} is the effective stress and A and α are constants.

Then, as computational power increased, mechanical models became more complex, being able to take into account the orthotropy of bone's tissue. So, Jacobs et al. (Jacobs et al., 1997) extended Beaupré's work to include the anisotropic behavior of trabecular bone. Then, Belinha et al. (Belinha et al., 2013) applied this remodeling algorithm but with a new anisotropic material law based on the experimental work of Zioupos et al. (Zioupos et al., 2008). This law stresses the relevance of the apparent density to determine the mechanical properties of both cortical and trabecular bone. Adopting a very distinct approach, Doblaré and García-Aznar (Doblaré and García-Aznar, 2002) considered the use of a remodeling tensor based on the principles of Continuum Damage Mechanics (CDM). This tensor includes data from the apparent density and the fabric tensor, which are respectively associated with the porosity and directionality of the trabeculae.

In a more recent past, a new family of remodeling models has been created—biochemical models. In this type of models, bone mass does not vary due to a mechanical stimulus, but rather due to biochemical changes affecting the autocrine and paracrine signalling pathways of bone. In the literature, Komarova's (Komarova et al., 2003) and Lemaire's (Lemaire et al., 2004) models stand out for their strong influence on current models. Both use differential equations to describe the temporal evolution of the cell density of osteoclasts and osteoblasts, as well as their effect on bone mass. Komarova et al. (Komarova et al., 2003) reproduced single and cyclic remodeling events, analysing the dynamic response of bone cells under healthy and Paget's disease conditions. Lemaire et al. (Lemaire et al., 2004) also considered the communication between osteoclasts and osteoclasts, but included the complete differentiation lineage of these bone cells. In this work, unbalanced bone remodeling was studied due to estrogen and vitamin D deficiency. The main aspect distinguishing these two models is the definition of the remodeling regulatory factors. Lemaire et al. uses receptor binding equations for each regulatory factor (Knauer et al., 1984; Lauffenburger and Linderman, 1996). Equation (3) exemplifies one of these equations,

$$
\begin{array}{c}
p_p \\
\downarrow \quad\quad k_5 \\
P + P_R \rightleftharpoons P_R \cdot P \\
\uparrow \quad\quad k_6 \\
d_p
\end{array}
\tag{3}
$$

where P represents PTH and $P_R \cdot P$ represents the complex formed by PTH and its receptor. Parameters p_p and d_p represent PTH production and destruction flux, respectively. Moreover, k_5 and k_6 are, respectively, the rate of PTH binding and unbinding with its receptor.

On the other hand, Komarova et al. proposes an aggregation of all of these factors into four parameters, according to the type of signalling (i.e. autocrine and paracrine) and the type of bone cell (i.e. osteoclasts and osteoblasts). Thus, the influence of these factors is directly expressed in the equations used to determine the cell density of osteoclasts and osteoblasts, as Equation (4) shows,

$$
dC/dt = \alpha_C C^{g_{CC}} B^{g_{BC}} - \beta_C C
\tag{4}
$$

in which C and B are the cell density of osteoclasts and osteoblasts, respectively. Parameter α_C reflects cell production, while β_C reflects cell removal. The autocrine and paracrine factors of osteoclasts are lumped together in parameters g_{CC} and g_{BC}, respectively. A similar equation is applied to determine the cell density of osteoblasts.

Due to the success of these two approaches, several extensions have been proposed. Pivonka et al. (Pivonka et al., 2008) extended Lemaire's work, using instead activator/repressor Hill functions to describe the action of each bone regulatory factor. This model was then used to study therapeutic strategies for osteoporosis (Pivonka et al., 2010), osteolytic lesions caused by multiple myeloma (Wang et al., 2011) and prostate cancer metastasis (Buenzli et al., 2011). In regards to extensions of Komarova's model, two distinct spatio-temporal models have been created. Ryser et al. (Ryser et al., 2009) replicated the movement of a bone multicellular unit (BMU) during remodeling of a microfracture. Ayati et al. (Ayati et al., 2010) developed a diffusion model with one spatial dimension, adding a second order spatial partial derivative to Komarova's equations. The model was applied to the study of myeloma bone disease.

Recently, some authors have proposed a more complete and realistic approach, developing biomechanical models. Derived from Lemaire's (Lemaire et al., 2004) and Pivonka's (Pivonka et al., 2010) models, multiscale biomechanical approaches have been proposed (Lerebours et al., 2016; Pastrama et al., 2018; Pivonka et al., 2013). After Pivonka's biochemical model (Pivonka et al., 2008), the author extended his work proposing a multiscale homogenisation approach connecting microscopic strains with macroscopic loading (Pivonka et al., 2013), in which the remodeling process is triggered by variations of the SED field. Moreover, the model, included an experimental law correlating bone specific surface and bone porosity. This model was then used to study bone remodeling across the midshaft of a femur, with results very close to experimental observations (Lerebours et al., 2016). In the future, the authors intend to apply this approach in patient specific models to predict bone loss adapted to the age and other specific factors of the patient. Pastrama et al. (Pastrama et al., 2018), also based in Pivonka's work, addressed with more detail the mechanical transduction of osteocytes at vascular and lacunar pores. However, the biomechanical models mentioned above present some limitations, namely their high complexity and number of parameters.

Hambli (Hambli, 2014) also proposed a biomechanical model, but this time based on Komarova's model (Komarova et al., 2003). The author proposed a strain-damage stimulus function to correlate the mechanical environment of bone with the autocrine and paracrine factors. However, the model considers bone as an isotropic homogeneous material, neglecting the orthotropic properties of bone tissue.

157

1.3 *Remodeling and numerical methods*

Several of the models mentioned in previous section were combined with numerical methods, since they are an efficient technique to solve complex mathematical problems. Thus, many of the mechanical remodeling models mentioned previously were combined with the Finite Element Method (FEM) (Beaupré et al., 1990b; Carter et al., 1987; Jacobs et al., 1995; Rossi and Wendling-Mansuy, 2007; Weinans et al., 1992), achieving great success in the field of orthopaedic biomechanics (Huiskes and Chao, 1983; Huiskes and Hollister, 1993). Mostly were applied to the study of bone remodeling of femoral stems after total hip arthroplasty (THA). These works revealed the source of important details and solved relevant problems associated with THA, such as the phenomenon causing the "stress shielding" and the techniques to minimize such effect. Regarding biomechanical models, FEM was also combined with the remodeling algorithms of Hambli, Lerebours et al. and Pastrama et al.

However, FEM has some limitations related with the mesh based interpolation (Nguyen et al., 2008). Thus, since the accuracy of the solution is intimately dependent on the quality of the mesh, this can be a very limiting factor when analysing organic structures such as bone. Therefore, meshless methods appear as an alternative, using only the nodal distribution instead of a mesh. Regarding bone remodeling algorithms, the Natural Neighbour Radial Point Interpolation Method (NNRPIM) has been combined with the mechanologic remodeling algorithm proposed by Belinha et al. (Belinha et al., 2013), studying the adaptation of the trabecular architecture to different mechanical stimuli using bone patches. Other studies focused on obtaining the optimized equilibrium morphology of the calcaneus bone (Belinha et al., 2012), the femur bone with and without a femoral stent (Belinha et al., 2016), natural teeth and dental implants (Belinha et al., 2014). A distinct meshless method was also combined with the mechanologic model of Belinha et al. (Belinha et al., 2013). The Radial Point Interpolation Method (RPIM) was thence applied to the study of femoral bone remodeling (Peyroteo et al., 2018). The combination of RPIM and NNRPIM can be valuable, since they offer higher remeshing flexibility and higher accuracy when compared with FEM. Also, both of them are interpolant meshless methods, which means they possess the Kronecker delta property as FEM does. However, no biochemical or biomechanical models of bone remodeling using meshless methods were found in the literature. Thus, the combination of these methods with more complex remodeling models is still lacking.

2 CONCLUSIONS

In this brief review, some of the most relevant works regarding *in silico* models of bone remodeling have been addressed. When comparing the first theories proposed and the current models, it is possible to conclude that thanks to computational evolution more complete and so more complex models have been presented. Nowadays, the trend is to develop biomechanical models that integrate bone cell dynamics and their response to different mechanical stimuli.

ACKNOWLEDGEMENTS

The authors truly acknowledge the funding provided by Ministério da Ciência, Tecnologia e Ensino Superior—Fundação para a Ciência e a Tecnologia (Portugal), under grants: SFRH/BD/133105/2017 and by project funding MIT-EXPL/ISF/0084/2017. Additionally, the authors gratefully acknowledge the funding of Project NORTE-01-0145-FEDER-000022—SciTech—Science and Technology for Competitive and Sustainable Industries, co-financed by Programa Operacional Regional do Norte (NORTE2020), through Fundo Europeu de Desenvolvimento Regional (FEDER).

REFERENCES

Ayati, B.P., Edwards, C.M., Webb, G.F., Wikswo, J.P., 2010. A mathematical model of bone remodeling dynamics for normal bone cell populations and myeloma bone disease. Biol. Direct 5, 28.

Beaupré, G.S., Orr, T.E., Carter, D.R., 1990a. An approach for time-dependent bone modeling and remodeling. Theoretical development. J. Orthop. Res. 8, 651–61.

Beaupré, G.S., Orr, T.E., Carter, D.R., 1990b. An approach for time-dependent bone modeling and remodeling-application: a preliminary remodeling simulation. J. Orthop. Res. 8, 662–70.

Belinha, J., Dinis, L.M.J.S., Jorge, R.M.N., 2014. The bone tissue remodelling analysis in dentistry using a meshless method, in: Proceedings of the III International Conference on Biodental Engineering. Taylor & Francis Group, Porto, pp. 213–220.

Belinha, J., Dinis, L.M.J.S., Natal Jorge, R.M., 2016. The analysis of the bone remodelling around femoral stems: A meshless approach. Math. Comput. Simul. 121, 64–94.

Belinha, J., Jorge, R.M.N., Dinis, L.M.J.S., 2013. A meshless microscale bone tissue trabecular remodelling analysis considering a new anisotropic bone tissue material law. Comput. Methods Biomech. Biomed. Engin. 16, 1170–1184.

Belinha, J., Jorge, R.M.N., Dinis, L.M.J.S., 2012. Bone tissue remodelling analysis considering a radial point interpolator meshless method. Eng. Anal. Bound. Elem. 36, 1660–1670.

Bonewald, L.F., Dallas, S.L., 1994. Role of active and latent transforming growth factor β in bone formation. J. Cell Biochem. 55, 350–357.

Buenzli, P.R., Pivonka, P., Smith, D.W., 2011. Spatiotemporal structure of cell distribution in cortical Bone Multicellular Units: A mathematical model. Bone 48, 918–926.

Carter, D.R., 1984. Mechanical loading histories and cortical bone remodeling. Calcif. Tissue Int. 36 Suppl 1, S19–24.

Carter, D.R., Fyhrie, D.P., Whalen, R.T., 1987. Trabecular bone density and loading history: regulation of connective tissue biology by mechanical energy. J. Biomech. 20, 735–94.

Cohen Jr., M.M., 2006. The new bone biology: Pathologic, molecular, and clinical correlates. Am. J. Med. Genet. Part A 140, 2646–2706.

Cohick, W.S., Clemmons, D.R., 1993. The Insulin-Like Growth Factors. Annu. Rev. Physiol. 55, 131–153.

Courteix, D., Lespessailles, E., Peres, S.L., Obert, P., Germain, P., Benhamou, C.L., 1998. Effect of physical training on bone mineral density in prepubertal girls: A comparative study between impact-loading and non-impact-loading sports. Osteoporos. Int. 8, 152–158.

Cowin, S.C., Hegedus, D.H., 1976. Bone remodeling I: theory of adaptive elasticity. J. Elast. 6, 313–326.

Doblaré, M., García-Aznar, J.M., 2002. Anisotropic bone remodelling model based on a continuum damage-repair theory. J. Biomech. 35, 1–17.

Downey, M.E., Holliday, L.S., Aguirre, J.I., Wronski, T.J., 2009. In vitro and in vivo evidence for stimulation of bone resorption by an EP4 receptor agonist and basic fibroblast growth factor: Implications for their efficacy as bone anabolic agents. Bone 44, 266–274.

Ernst, M., Heath, J.K., Rodan, G.A., 1989. Estradiol effects on proliferation, messenger ribonucleic acid for collagen and insulin-like growth factor-I, and parathyroid hormone-stimulated adenylate cyclase activity in osteoblastic cells from calvariae and long bones. Endocrinology 125, 825–33.

Fiore, C.E., Cottini, E., Di Salvo, G., Foti, R., Rastagliesi, M., 1991. The effects of muscle-building exercise on forearm bone mineral content and osteoblast activity in drug-free and anabolic steroids sell-administering young men. Bone Miner. 13, 78–83.

Fyhrie, D.P., Carter, D.R., 1986. A unifying principle relating stress to trabecular bone morphology. J. Orthop. Res. 4, 304–317.

Gallagher, J.C., 2007. Effect of early menopause on bone mineral density and fractures. Menopause 14, 567–71.

Graves, D.T., Oates, T., Garlet, G.P., 2011. Review of osteoimmunology and the host response in endodontic and periodontal lesions. J. Oral Microbiol. 3.

Hambli, R., 2014. Connecting mechanics and bone cell activities in the bone remodeling process: an integrated finite element modeling. Front. Bioeng. Biotechnol. 2, 6.

Huiskes, R., Chao, E.Y., 1983. A survey of finite element analysis in orthopedic biomechanics: the first decade. J. Biomech. 16, 385–409.

Huiskes, R., Hollister, S.J., 1993. From structure to process, from organ to cell: recent developments of FE-analysis in orthopaedic biomechanics. J. Biomech. Eng. 115, 520–7.

Huiskes, R., Weinans, H., Grootenboer, H.J., Dalstra, M., Fudala, B., Slooff, T.J., 1987. Adaptive bone-remodeling theory applied to prosthetic-design analysis. J. Biomech. 20, 1135–50.

Jacobs, C.R., Levenston, M.E., Beaupré, G.S., Simo, J.C., Carter, D.R., 1995. Numerical instabilities in bone remodeling simulations: the advantages of a node-based finite element approach. J. Biomech. 28, 449–59.

Jacobs, C.R., Simo, J.C., Beaupre, G.S., Carter, D.R., 1997. Adaptive bone remodeling incorporating simultaneous density and anisotropy considerations. J. Biomech. 30, 603–613.

Kini, U., Nandeesh, B.N., 2012. Physiology of Bone Formation, Remodeling, and Metabolism, in: Radionuclide and Hybrid Bone Imaging. Springer Berlin Heidelberg, Berlin, Heidelberg, pp. 29–57.

Kiratli, B.J., Smith, A.E., Nauenberg, T., Kallfelz, C.F., Perkash, I., 2000. Bone mineral and geometric changes through the femur with immobilization due to spinal cord injury. J. Rehabil. Res. Dev. 37, 225–33.

Knauer, D.J., Wiley, H.S., Cunningham, D.D., 1984. Relationship between epidermal growth factor receptor occupancy and mitogenic response. Quantitative analysis using a steady state model system. J. Biol. Chem. 259, 5623–31.

Komarova, S.V., Smith, R.J., Dixon, S.J., Sims, S.M., Wahl, L.M., 2003. Mathematical model predicts a critical role for osteoclast autocrine regulation in the control of bone remodeling. Bone 33, 206–215.

Kramer, I., Loots, G.G., Studer, A., Keller, H., Kneissel, M., 2010. Parathyroid hormone (PTH)-induced bone gain is blunted in SOST overexpressing and deficient mice. J. Bone Miner. Res. 25, 178–89.

Lauffenburger, D.A., Linderman, J.J., 1996. Receptors: Models for binding, trafficking and signaling.

Lemaire, V., Tobin, F.L., Greller, L.D., Cho, C.R., Suva, L.J., 2004. Modeling the interactions between osteoblast and osteoclast activities in bone remodeling. J. Theor. Biol. 229, 293–309.

Lerebours, C., Buenzli, P.R., Scheiner, S., Pivonka, P., 2016. A multiscale mechanobiological model of bone remodelling predicts site-specific bone loss in the femur during osteoporosis and mechanical disuse. Biomech. Model. Mechanobiol. 15, 43–67.

Locklin, R., Oreffo, R.O., Triffitt, J.T., 1999. Effects of TGFβ and BFGF on the differentiation of human bone marrow stromal fibroblasts. Cell Biol. Int. 23, 185–194.

Mohamed, A.M., 2008. An overview of bone cells and their regulating factors of differentiation. Malaysian J. Med. Sci. 15, 4–12.

Nguyen, V.P., Rabczuk, T., Bordas, S., Duflot, M., 2008. Meshless methods: A review and computer implementation aspects. Math. Comput. Simul. 79, 763–813.

Pastrama, M.-I., Scheiner, S., Pivonka, P., Hellmich, C., 2018. A mathematical multiscale model of bone remodeling, accounting for pore space-specific mechanosensation. Bone 107, 208–221.

Peyroteo, M.M.A., Belinha, J., Vinga, S., Dinis, L.M.J.S., Natal Jorge, R.M., 2018. Mechanical bone remodelling:

Comparative study of distinct numerical approaches. Eng. Anal. Bound. Elem.

Pivonka, P., Buenzli, P.R., Scheiner, S., Hellmich, C., Dunstan, C.R., 2013. The influence of bone surface availability in bone remodelling-A mathematical model including coupled geometrical and biomechanical regulations of bone cells. Eng. Struct. 47, 134–147.

Pivonka, P., Zimak, J., Smith, D.W., Gardiner, B.S., Dunstan, C.R., Sims, N.A., John Martin, T., Mundy, G.R., 2010. Theoretical investigation of the role of the RANK-RANKL-OPG system in bone remodeling. J. Theor. Biol. 262, 306–316.

Pivonka, P., Zimak, J., Smith, D.W., Gardiner, B.S., Dunstan, C.R., Sims, N.A., Martin, T.J., Mundy, G.R., 2008. Model structure and control of bone remodeling: A theoretical study. Bone 43, 249–263.

Post, T.M., Cremers, S.C.L.M., Kerbusch, T., Danhof, M., 2010. Bone Physiology, Disease and Treatment. Clin. Pharmacokinet. 49, 89–118.

Rossi, J.-M., Wendling-Mansuy, S., 2007. A topology optimization based model of bone adaptation. Comput. Methods Biomech. Biomed. Engin. 10, 419–27.

Rucci, N., 2008. Molecular biology of bone remodelling. Clin. Cases Miner. Bone Metab. 5, 49–56.

Ryser, M.D., Nigam, N., Komarova, S. V, 2009. Mathematical Modeling of Spatio-Temporal Dynamics of a Single Bone Multicellular Unit. J. Bone Miner. Res. 24, 860–870.

Simonet, W.S., Lacey, D.L., Dunstan, C.R., Kelley, M., Chang, M.S., Lüthy, R., Nguyen, H.Q., Wooden, S., Bennett, L., Boone, T., Shimamoto, G., DeRose, M., Elliott, R., Colombero, A., Tan, H.L., Trail, G., Sullivan, J., Davy, E., Bucay, N., Renshaw-Gegg, L., Hughes, T.M., Hill, D., Pattison, W., Campbell, P., Sander, S., Van, G., Tarpley, J., Derby, P., Lee, R., Boyle, W.J., 1997. Osteoprotegerin: a novel secreted protein involved in the regulation of bone density. Cell 89, 309–19.

Teitelbaum, S.L., 2007. Osteoclasts: what do they do and how do they do it? Am. J. Pathol. 170, 427–35.

Teitelbaum, S.L., Ross, F.P., 2003. Genetic regulation of osteoclast development and function. Nat. Rev. Genet. 4, 638–649.

Wang, Y., Pivonka, P., Buenzli, P.R., Smith, D.W., Dunstan, C.R., 2011. Computational modeling of interactions between multiple myeloma and the bone microenvironment. PLoS One 6, 14–16.

Weinans, H., Huiskes, R., Grootenboer, H.J., 1992. The behavior of adaptive bone-remodeling simulation models. J. Biomech. 25, 1425–41.

Xiao, W., Wang, Y., Pacios, S., Li, S., Graves, D.T., 2016. Cellular and Molecular Aspects of Bone Remodeling. Front. Oral Biol. 18, 9–16.

Zioupos, P., Cook, R.B., Hutchinson, J.R., 2008. Some basic relationships between density values in cancellous and cortical bone. J. Biomech. 41, 1961–8.

Biodental Engineering V – Belinha et al. (Eds)
© 2019 Taylor & Francis Group, London, ISBN 978-0-367-21087-8

Predicting the trabecular architecture in the vicinity of natural teeth: A comparison between finite elements and meshless methods

M.M.A. Peyroteo
Institute of Mechanical Engineering and Industrial Management (INEGI), Porto, Portugal

J. Belinha
Department of Mechanical Engineering, School of Engineering, Polytechnic of Porto (ISEP), Porto, Portugal

L.M.J.S. Dinis & R.M. Natal Jorge
Department of Mechanical Engineering, Faculty of Engineering, University of Porto (FEUP), Porto, Portugal

ABSTRACT: This work consists in a bone remodeling study applied to the trabecular bone in the vicinity of a natural tooth. Knowing that bone can adapt its morphology according to a certain loading scenario, many mechanologic remodeling models have been proposed, aiming to predict the typical bone's architecture observed in X-ray or micro-CT images. This work applies Belinha's model, further extended by Peyroteo and co-workers, that consists in an optimization process aiming to minimize the strain energy density field. The remodeling process is reflected by changes of bone's mechanical properties and apparent density that are correlated with an experimental law obtained by Zioupos et al. A two-dimensional model of a healthy tooth is the numerical example used in this study. This model is analyzed with distinct numerical techniques: the Finite Element Method (FEM) and two meshless methods—the Radial Point Interpolation Method (RPIM) and the Natural Neighbour Radial Point Interpolation Method (NNRPIM). The use of this mechanologic model applied to a natural tooth revealed a good agreement with results presented in the literature.

1 INTRODUCTION

1.1 *Bone remodeling*

Bone is a biological material highly active and responsive to different internal and external stimuli. Being an important load bearing structure, bone is required to alter its structural organization, resorbing or forming new tissue according to the sensed stimulus (Leblanc et al., 2009; Vico and Alexandre, 1992). So, through a biological process named bone remodeling, bone is able to adapt to different loading conditions (Moroz et al., 2006). Ultimately, this adaptation process is reflected by variations of bone's apparent density and stiffness (Colletti et al., 1989; Lotz et al., 1991).

Bone remodeling was firstly described scientifically by Wolff (Wolff, 1986), suggesting a relation between the stress state and bone's architecture. According to this work, bone is depicted as an optimized structure to certain mechanical requirements. Following Wolff's ideology, Frost (Frost, 1988, 1987) proposed the "mechanostat" theory, suggesting that

bone mass is regulated by the strain state. This study introduces the concept of a "minimum effective strain" (MES) value that leads to remodeling, causing addition or reinforcement of bone's trabeculae (Tyrovola and Odont, 2015). When remodeling finishes, normal strain levels are restored. These works of Wolf (Wolff, 1986) and Frost (Frost, 1987) were preponderant for the development of *in silico* mechanologic bone remodeling models.

1.2 *Mechanologic bone remodeling models*

Cowin and Hegedus (Cowin and Hegedus, 1976; Hegedus and Cowin, 1976) proposed one of the first mechanical models, known as the "Adaptive Elasticity theory". Considering bone remodeling as a thermomechanical phenomenon, the authors suggested a distinction between surface and internal remodeling (H. M. Frost, 1964). Surface remodeling occurred according to a linear function between stress and material resorption or deposition, as introduced by Gjelsvick (Gjelsvik, 1973a, 1973b). In turn, internal remodeling was based on Martin's work (Martin, 1972), in which bone was considered an elastic porous material with a porosity degree dependent on strain levels. Due to a high number of parameters, Huiskes et al. (Huiskes et al., 1987) presented a simplification to this model, using the strain energy density (SED) as the remodelling criterion.

A distinct approach known as "Self-Optimization theory" was also presented (Fyhrie and Carter, 1986). This work proposes an objective function to be optimized in order to predict bone's apparent density distribution. Then, Carter and co-workers (Carter et al., 1989, 1987; Whalen et al., 1988) extended this work to include a fatigue damage accumulation and several loading conditions with distinct load cycles.

Many other bone remodelling mechanologic models have been presented, such as the cell biology model of Hart and Davy (Hart and Davy, 1989), the continuum damage-repair algorithm of Doblaré and García-Aznar (Doblaré and García-Aznar, 2002) and the accumulated damage model of Prendergast and Taylor (Prendergast and Taylor, 1994).

In the past, mechanical models assumed bone as an isotropic material. However, with the improvement of experimental studies, remodelling models became anisotropic, being able to describe the true behaviour of bone. An important anisotropic material law, based on experimental data, was proposed by Zioupos and co-workers (Zioupos et al., 2008), in which the mechanical properties of cortical and trabecular bone are determined with the same phenomenological law.

Many of the remodelling models mentioned above have been combined with the Finite Element Method (FEM) (Beaupré et al., 1990; Carter et al., 1987; Jacobs et al., 1995; Rossi and Wendling-Mansuy, 2007; Weinans et al., 1992) with important relevance in orthopaedics and sports medicine. In the dentistry field, works of Lin and co-workers. (Lin et al., 2009), Mellal and co-workers. (Mellal et al., 2004) and Li and co-workers. (Li et al., 2007) are bone remodeling studies regarding dental implant insertion. Also, FEM has been used to predict mandible bone trabecular architecture in works of Poiate and co-workers and Watzak and co-workers (Poiate et al., 2011; Watzak et al., 2005).

However, there are also important bone remodeling works combined with meshless methods (Doblaré et al., 2005). One of the first meshless studies used the Reproducing Kernel Particle Method (RKPM) to analyze the stress distributions during remodeling of a human proximal femur (Liew et al., 2002). Moreover, Taddei and co-workers (Taddei et al., 2008) proposed a new meshless approach implementing the Cell Method meshless method to predict strain distributions in a femur bone and Lee et and co-workers (Lee et al., 2007) studied osteoporosis applying a meshless method based on the moving least square technique. Another approach was proposed by Belinha et and co-workers (Belinha et al., 2013; J. Belinha et al., 2012), who presented an adaptation of Carter's model (Carter et al., 1987) to meshless methods, namely the Natural Neighbor Radial Point Interpolation Method (NNRPIM). This model has been applied to the dentistry field predicting the equilibrium bone's morphology in natural teeth (Belinha et al., 2014; Moreira et al., 2014) and the response of bone due to the insertion of dental implants (Belinha et al., 2015; Tavares et al., 2015). Belinha's model (Belinha et al., 2013) was then extended by Peyroteo et al (Peyroteo et al., 2018), who combined for the first time the Radial Point Interpolation Method (RPIM) with a bone remodeling algorithm.

This work applies Peyroteo's model (Peyroteo et al., 2018) to study bone remodeling in the vicinity of a natural tooth, comparing the performance of three distinct numerical techniques—the FEM, the RPIM and the NNRPIM.

2 REMODELING ALGORITHM

In this study, a bone remodeling model is applied to the vicinity of a tooth, taking into account its mechanical microenvironment. This study uses the mechanical model proposed by Belinha and co-workers. (Belinha et al., 2013) extended by Peyroteo and co-workers. (Peyroteo et al., 2018).

The implemented algorithm can be briefly divided into five phases as can be depicted in Figure 1.

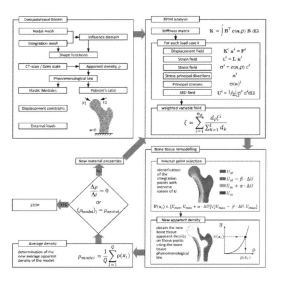

Figure 1. Graphical description of the bone remodelling algorithm (Peyroteo et al., 2018).

In a first phase, the computational model is created, occurring the discretization of the problem's domain and the determination of nodal and integration points, as well as the shape functions. Then, according to the boundary conditions applied to the problem, a two-dimensional plane stress mechanical analysis is conducted. The third phase consists on determining the points to undergo remodeling. In this work, the concept of "lazy zone" is applied, in which only the overloaded and underloaded integration points are chosen to remodel. This choice is made by seriating the strain energy density level, $U(x_I)$, of each integration point, x_I, that is obtained with the following expression

$$U(x_I) = \frac{1}{2}\int_{\Omega_I}\left\{\sigma_{xx}(x_I)\,\sigma_{yy}(x_I)\,\sigma_{xy}(x_I)\right\}\begin{Bmatrix}\varepsilon_{xx}(x_I)\\ \varepsilon_{yy}(x_I)\\ \gamma_{xy}(x_I)\end{Bmatrix}d\Omega_I \quad (1)$$

in which σ is the stress tensor, ε is the strain tensor and Ω_I is the area associated to the integration point, x_I. Then, after having U, it is possible to determine the set of points to undergo remodeling with Equation (2).

$$H(x_I) \in [U_{min}, U_{min} + \alpha \cdot \Delta U[V]U_{max} - \beta \cdot \Delta U, U_{max}] \quad (2)$$

In Equation above, $U_{min} = \min(U) = \min(\mathbf{U})$, $U_{max} = \max(\mathbf{U})$ and $\Delta U = U_{max} - U_{min}$. Parameters α and β are the growth and decay rate of bone mass. Then, remodeling occurs, in which the bone's apparent density of those points is updated according to its mechanical properties. This is attained by applying the experimental law proposed by Zioupos and co-workers (Zioupos et al., 2008), defined by the following expressions

$$E = \begin{cases} \sum_{j=0}^{3} a_j \cdot \rho^j & \text{if } \rho \leq 1.3 g/cm^3 \\ \sum_{j=0}^{3} b_j \cdot \rho^j & \text{if } \rho > 1.3 g/cm^3 \end{cases} \quad (3)$$

$$\sigma_{ult} = \sum_{j=0}^{3} c_j \cdot \rho^j \quad (4)$$

where ρ is the apparent density, E is the elasticity modulus and σ_{ult} is the ultimate compressive or tensile stress. both expressed in MPa. Parameters values of a, b and c can be found in the literature (Jorge Belinha et al., 2012).

The final step is to determine the medium apparent density of the domain under analysis, ρ_{model}, with the following

$$\rho_{model} = \frac{1}{Q}\sum_{I=1}^{Q}\rho(x_I) \quad (5)$$

being Q the total number of integration points. In the following iteration, since some points have altered their apparent density, it is required to update the mechanical properties of these points, before performing another mechanical analysis, using so Equations (2) and (3). The simulation finishes when ρ_{model} stabilizes meaning that an equilibrium bone morphology has been achieved.

3 NUMERICAL SIMULATION

3.1 Computational model

A two-dimensional model of a healthy tooth was used to study bone remodeling in tooth's vicinity, aiming to obtain an equilibrium trabecular morphology. In order to obtain a bone's architecture as similar as possible to the reality, three load cases with different degrees of inclination were applied. Thus, a load of 100 N was applied on the top of the tooth's crown, with 45º, 90º and 135º inclination with the tooth's longitudinal axis. Moreover, the nodes in the base of the model were constrained in the Oy direction, whereas the side nodes were constrained in the Ox direction. The model was discretized with 2463 nodes and 4710 elements, as presented in Figure 2. Also in this figure, is possible to distinguish the presence of three distinct materials—tooth, cortical and trabecular

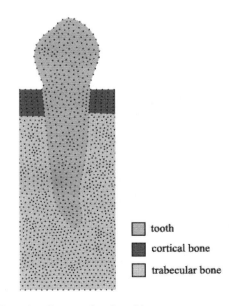

Figure 2. Computational model.

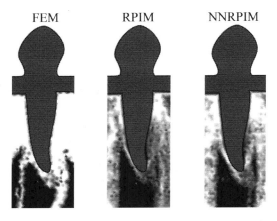

Figure 3. Apparent density distribution for each numerical method. White represents trabecular bone and black is non-bone material.

bone. For the purpose of this study, it was considered that only trabecular bone was able to remodel.

3.2 *Results and discussion*

In Figure 3, the apparent density distribution of trabecular bone obtained for each numerical technique is presented. It is possible to depict that trabeculae form accordingly with the loading scenario imposed in the numerical example, supporting the use of this remodeling model to obtain the equilibrium morphology of bone in the vicinity of a natural tooth.

Moreover, in Figures Figure 4 and Figure 5, the first and second principal stresses are presented, respectively, for the beginning and the end of the simulation. When comparing these maps with bone's apparent density spatial distribution, it is

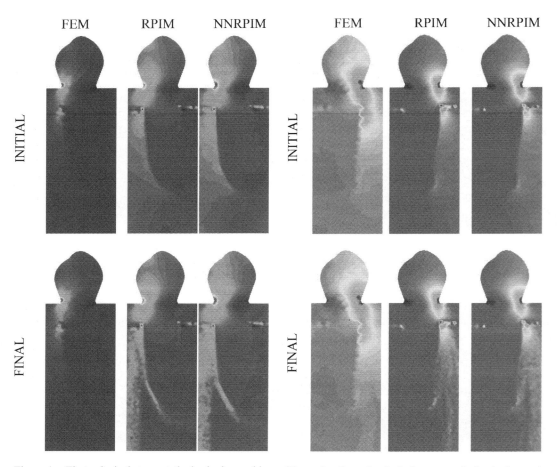

Figure 4. First principal stress at the beginning and in the end of the simulation obtained for each numerical method tested.

Figure 5. Second principal stress at the beginning and in the end of the simulation obtained for each numerical method tested.

possible to notice that bone's trabeculae overlap with zones with high principal stresses.

In regards to the numerical techniques tested, FEM's solution presents better individualized trabeculae, while meshless solutions present a more organic result. To improve the latter results, distinct shape parameters should be tested, as well as distinct schemes of nodal connectivity.

4 CONCLUSIONS

This work applies, for the first time, Peyroteo's model to the dentistry field. The implemented remodeling algorithm proved to be an efficient and accurate approach to obtain the typical morphology of trabecular bone in the vicinity of a natural tooth. The three numerical methods tested were able to produce solutions in agreement with the literature, although FEM's solution was the one presenting better defined trabeculae.

ACKNOWLEDGEMENTS

The authors truly acknowledge the funding provided by Ministério da Ciência, Tecnologia e Ensino Superior—Fundação para a Ciência e a Tecnologia (Portugal), under grants: SFRH/BD/133105/2017 and by project funding MIT-EXPL/ISF/0084/2017. Additionally, the authors gratefully acknowledge the funding of Project NORTE-01-0145-FEDER-000022—SciTech—Science and Technology for Competitive and Sustainable Industries, co-financed by Programa Operacional Regional do Norte (NORTE2020), through Fundo Europeu de Desenvolvimento Regional (FEDER).

REFERENCES

Beaupré, G.S., Orr, T.E., Carter, D.R., 1990. An approach for time-dependent bone modeling and remodeling-application: a preliminary remodeling simulation. J. Orthop. Res. 8, 662–70.

Belinha, J., Dinis, L.M.J.S., Jorge, R.M.N., 2015. The Mandible Remodeling induced by dental implants: A Meshless Approach. J. Mech. Med. Biol. 15, 1550059.

Belinha, J., Dinis, L.M.J.S., Jorge, R.M.N., 2014. The bone tissue remodelling analysis in dentistry using a meshless method, in: Proceedings of the III International Conference on Biodental Engineering. Taylor & Francis Group, Porto, pp. 213–220.

Belinha, J., Jorge, R.M.N., Dinis, L.M.J.S., 2013. A meshless microscale bone tissue trabecular remodelling analysis considering a new anisotropic bone tissue material law. Comput. Methods Biomech. Biomed. Engin. 16, 1170–1184.

Belinha, J., Jorge, R.M.N., Dinis, L.M.J.S., 2012. Bone tissue remodelling analysis considering a radial point interpolator meshless method. Eng. Anal. Bound. Elem. 36, 1660–1670.

Belinha, J., Jorge, R.M.N., Dinis, L.M.J.S., 2012. A meshless microscale bone tissue trabecular remodelling analysis considering a new anisotropic bone tissue material law. Comput. Methods Biomech. Biomed. Engin. 1–15.

Carter, D.R., Fyhrie, D.P., Whalen, R.T., 1987. Trabecular bone density and loading history: regulation of connective tissue biology by mechanical energy. J. Biomech. 20, 785–94.

Carter, D.R., Orr, T.E., Fyhrie, D.P., 1989. Relationships between loading history and femoral cancellous bone architecture. J. Biomech. 22, 231–44.

Colletti, L.A., Edwards, J., Gordon, L., Shary, J., Bell, N.H., 1989. The effects of muscle-building exercise on bone mineral density of the radius, spine, and hip in young men. Calcif. Tissue Int. 45, 12–4.

Cowin, S.C., Hegedus, D.H., 1976. Bone remodeling I: theory of adaptive elasticity. J. Elast. 6, 313–326.

Doblaré, M., Cueto, E., Calvo, B., Martínez, M.A., Garcia, J.M., Cegoñino, J., 2005. On the employ of meshless methods in biomechanics. Comput. Methods Appl. Mech. Eng. 194, 801–821.

Doblaré, M., García-Aznar, J.M., 2002. Anisotropic bone remodelling model based on a continuum damage-repair theory. J. Biomech. 35, 1–17.

Frost, H.M. 1964. Bone remodeling dynamics. Arthritis Rheum. 7, 545–545.

Frost, H.M., 1988. Vital biomechanics: proposed general concepts for skeletal adaptations to mechanical usage. Calcif. Tissue Int. 42, 145–56.

Frost, H.M., 1987. Bone "mass" and the "mechanostat": A proposal. Anat. Rec. 219, 1–9.

Fyhrie, D.P., Carter, D.R., 1986. A unifying principle relating stress to trabecular bone morphology. J. Orthop. Res. 4, 304–317.

Gjelsvik, A., 1973a. Bone remodeling and piezoelectricity—I.J. Biomech. 6, 69–77.

Gjelsvik, A., 1973b. Bone remodeling and piezoelectricity—II.J. Biomech. 6, 187–193.

Hart, R.T., Davy, D.T., 1989. Theories of bone modeling and remodeling, in: Cowin SC (Ed.), Bone Mechanics. CRC Press, Boca Raton, pp. 253–277.

Hegedus, D.H., Cowin, S.C., 1976. Bone remodeling II: small strain adaptive elasticity. J. Elast. 6, 337–352.

Huiskes, R., Weinans, H., Grootenboer, H.J., Dalstra, M., Fudala, B., Slooff, T.J., 1987. Adaptive bone-remodeling theory applied to prosthetic-design analysis. J. Biomech. 20, 1135–50.

Jacobs, C.R., Levenston, M.E., Beaupré, G.S., Simo, J.C., Carter, D.R., 1995. Numerical instabilities in bone remodeling simulations: the advantages of a node-based finite element approach. J. Biomech. 28, 449–59.

Leblanc, A.D., Schneider, V.S., Evans, H.J., Engelbretson, D.A., Krebs, J.M., 2009. Bone mineral loss and recovery after 17 weeks of bed rest. J. Bone Miner. Res. 5, 843–850.

Lee, J.D., Chen, Y., Zeng, X., Eskandarian, A., Oskard, M., 2007. Modeling and simulation of osteoporosis and fracture of trabecular bone by meshless method. Int. J. Eng. Sci. 45, 329–338.

Li, J., Li, H., Shi, L., Fok, A.S.L., Ucer, C., Devlin, H., Horner, K., Silikas, N., 2007. A mathematical model for simulating the bone remodeling process under mechanical stimulus. Dent. Mater. 23, 1073–1078.

Liew, K.M., Wu, H.Y., Ng, T.Y., 2002. Meshless method for modeling of human proximal femur: treatment of nonconvex boundaries and stress analysis. Comput. Mech. 28, 390–400.

Lin, D., Li, Q., Li, W., Swain, M., 2009. Dental implant induced bone remodeling and associated algorithms. J. Mech. Behav. Biomed. Mater. 2, 410–432.

Lotz, J.C., Gerhart, T.N., Hayes, W.C., 1991. Mechanical properties of metaphyseal bone in the proximal femur. J. Biomech. 24, 317–29.

Martin, R.B., 1972. The effects of geometric feedback in the development of osteoporosis. J. Biomech. 5, 447–455.

Mellal, A., Wiskott, H.W.A., Botsis, J., Scherrer, S.S., Belser, U.C., 2004. Stimulating effect of implant loading on surrounding bone. Comparison of three numerical models and validation by in vivo data. Clin. Oral Implants Res. 15, 239–48.

Moreira, S., Belinha, J., Dinis, L.M.J.S., Jorge, R.M.N., 2014. A Global Numerical analysis of the "central incisor/local maxillary bone" system using a meshless method. Mol. Cell. Biomech. 11, 151–84.

Moroz, A., Crane, M.C., Smith, G., Wimpenny, D.I., 2006. Phenomenological model of bone remodeling cycle containing osteocyte regulation loop. Biosystems 84, 183–190.

Peyroteo, M.M.A., Belinha, J., Vinga, S., Dinis, L.M.J.S., Natal Jorge, R.M., 2018. Mechanical bone remodelling: Comparative study of distinct numerical approaches. Eng. Anal. Bound. Elem.

Poiate, I.A.V.P., Vasconcellos, A.B., Mori, M., Poiate, E., 2011. 2D and 3D finite element analysis of central incisor generated by computerized tomography. Comput. Methods Programs Biomed. 104, 292–299.

Prendergast, P.J., Taylor, D., 1994. Prediction of bone adaptation using damage accumulation. J. Biomech. 27, 1067–76.

Rossi, J.-M., Wendling-Mansuy, S., 2007. A topology optimization based model of bone adaptation. Comput. Methods Biomech. Biomed. Engin. 10, 419–27.

Taddei, F., Pani, M., Zovatto, L., Tonti, E., Viceconti, M., 2008. A new meshless approach for subject-specific strain prediction in long bones: Evaluation of accuracy. Clin. Biomech. 23, 1192–1199.

Tavares, C.S.S., Belinha, J., Dinis, L.M.J.S., Jorge, R.M.N., 2015. The Elasto-plastic Response of the Bone Tissue Due to the Insertion of Dental Implants. Procedia Eng. 110, 37–44.

Tyrovola, J.B., Odont, X., 2015. The "Mechanostat Theory" of Frost and the OPG/RANKL/RANK System. J. Cell. Biochem. 116, 2724–2729.

Vico, L., Alexandre, C., 1992. Microgravity and bone adaptation at the tissue level. J. Bone Miner. Res. 7, S445–S447.

Watzak, G., Zechner, W., Ulm, C., Tangl, S., Tepper, G., Watzek, G., 2005. Histologic and histomorphometric analysis of three types of dental implants following 18 months of occlusal loading: a preliminary study in baboons. Clin. Oral Implants Res. 16, 408–416.

Weinans, H., Huiskes, R., Grootenboer, H.J., 1992. The behavior of adaptive bone-remodeling simulation models. J. Biomech. 25, 1425–41.

Whalen, R.T., Carter, D.R., Steele, C.R., 1988. Influence of physical activity on the regulation of bone density. J. Biomech. 21, 825–37.

Wolff, J., 1986. The Law of Bone Remodelling. Springer Berlin Heidelberg, Berlin, Heidelberg.

Zioupos, P., Cook, R.B., Hutchinson, J.R., 2008. Some basic relationships between density values in cancellous and cortical bone. J. Biomech. 41, 1961–8.

Biodental Engineering V – Belinha et al. (Eds)
© 2019 Taylor & Francis Group, London, ISBN 978-0-367-21087-8

Comparing the stress distribution between atrophic maxillary rehabilitation techniques using FEM

K.F. Vargas
Institute of Science and Innovation in Mechanical and Industrial Engineering (INEGI), Porto, Portugal

G.A.R. Caldas
Faculty of Engineering, University of Porto (FEUP), Porto, Portugal

J. Belinha
Department of Mechanical Engineering, School of Engineering, Polytechnic of Porto (ISEP), Porto, Portugal

R.M. Natal Jorge
Department of Mechanical Engineering, Faculty of Engineering, University of Porto (FEUP), Porto, Portugal

P.A.G. Hernandez, A. Ozkomur, R. Smidt, M.M. Naconecy & L.E. Schneider
Faculty of Dentistry, University Lutheran of Brazil, Canoas, RS, Brazil

ABSTRACT: In this study two different surgical techniques for insertion of dental implants were analysed and compared: (1) 4-On-Pillars, a new surgical approach for the insertion of implants in atrophic maxilla; and (2) All-On-4, a well-known technique for the same purpose previously referred. The 2D models were discretised with an element mesh. In order to simulate the surrounding structures, natural and essential boundary conditions were applied to the model. These models were numerically analysed using the Finite Element Method (FEM). The results show different stress distributions between the two techniques studied, being possible to conclude that in the All-On-4 model the distribution was more homogeneous, unlike the 4-On-Pillars model, in which stress distribution was more concentrated.

1 STATE OF THE ART

1.1 *Introduction*

The World Health Organization (WHO) defines health as "a state of complete physical, mental and social well-being and not only the absence of affections and diseases". In the absence of a dental element several functions are compromised, such as masticatory functions, speech, aesthetics, and, above all, the individual's emotional and social behaviour. Rehabilitation of the occlusion/function should restore the lost condition of well-being.

Implant success expectations are around 98%, and, after 15 years, the success rate of this technique is about 90%. Several factors affect the success of a dental implant, such as implant design, remaining bone, surgical technique, among others. Failure of this dental prothesis is associated to an insufficient osseointegration, inadequate biomechanical behaviour of the complex implant/prosthesis/bone

or poor hygiene. Numerous advances have been registered in implantology, both in the materials/implants, in surgical techniques adopted and in the technology used in the studies.

Patients with an edentulous maxilla are rehabilitated, in large part, by a well-known technique called All-On-4®. This is a minimally invasive procedure consisting of replacing all maxillary teeth using only 4 dental implants, which will support a fixed bridge that is screwed to the implants. Maló and colleagues advocated the following distribution: two anterior implants positioned in the lateral incisor regions, one on each side, and two posterior implants in the premolar regions, one on each side, positioned at 30° of inclination in relation to the occlusal plane tangential to the anterior wall of the maxillary sinus (Figure 1(a)) (Malo, Rangert, & Nobre, 2005) (Maló, De Araújo Nobre, Lopes, Francischone, & Rigolizzo, 2012). This configuration allows the rehabilitation of an arch with 12 dental elements, with a distal cantilever in the molar topographies (Dos Santos, Meloto, Bacchi, & Correr-Sobrinho, 2017).

The anterior portion of the pterygoid process of the sphenoid bone consists of a lamina of cortical bone. Thus, this anatomical structure represents an alternative anchorage for posterior implants in atrophic jaws. Through a literature review, it was possible to conclude that pterygoid implants have high success rates, bone loss levels similar to conventional implants, minimal complications and good patient acceptance. Therefore, these are an alternative for the treatment of patients with posterior atrophic maxilla (Candel, Peñarrocha, & Peñarrocha, 2012). Another study demonstrated a cumulative survival rate of 88.2% for placement of pterygoid implants in edentulous jaws (Balshi, Wolfinger, & Balshi, 1999). Thus, a new approach has been proposed called 4-On-Pillars (Figure 1(b)), which corresponds to the insertion of four implants: two in the canine abutments (one on each side) and two in the pterygoid pillars (one on each side). In this proposal, the rehabilitation of the upper arch is complete (14 dental elements), without requiring a cantilever. The authors of this work did not find in the literature documents related to the numerical analysis of this type of surgical technique.

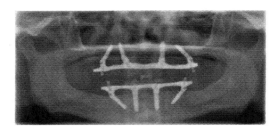

(a)

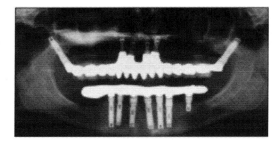

(b)

Figure 1. Orthopantomography of unknown patients representative of: (a) Bimaxillary rehabilitation trough the All-On-4® technique (Maló et al., 2012); and (b) bilateral 4-on-Pillars maxillary implants (Balshi et al., 1999).

1.2 Numerical methods

One of the most popular discrete numerical tool used is the Finite Element Method (FEM) (Zienkiewicz & Taylor, 1994). FEM is recognized and commonly used in many fields of engineering. It is characterized by the problem domain discretization into small elements connected through nodes. Such discretization comprises the creation of the mesh, the elements, their respective nodes and definition of boundary conditions (Geng, Tan, & Liu, 2001) (Alencar et al., 2017).

In the literature, the efficiency of FEM and the recognition of this numerical method as the most adequate tool to predict the biomechanical behaviour of biological structures is acknowledged. Thus, FEM allows to save time; to avoid the use of experimental animals and; to minimize the economic costs of scientific research (Holmes, Grigsby, Goel, & Keller, 1992) (Brunski, 2014) (Bordin, Bergamo, Fardin, Coelho, & Bonfante, 2017).

2 NUMERICAL ANALYSIS

2.1 Geometrical and numerical models

All-On-4® model comprises anterior implants with 4.3 mm of width and 10 mm of length, and posterior implants with 4.3 mm of width and 13 mm of length.

The 4-On-Pillars model consists of anterior implants with 3.5 mm of width and 10 mm of length and posterior implants with 4.3 mm of width and 13 mm of length, as demonstrated in Figure 2.

The element mesh, for both All-On-4® and 4-On-Pillars 2D models developed, are composed by triangular elements (constant strain elements) and it was constructed in FEMAP software version 11.4.1 Free (Siemens®, Munich, Germany). Therefore, the All-On-4® is composed by 7300 elements and 3943 nodes. The 4-On-Pillars model is composed by 7316 elements and 3949 nodes.

After the element mesh definition, the models were exported, to FEMAS—Finite Element and Meshless Analysis Software, which is an academic software capable to perform several kinds of computational mechanics analysis, using both the FEM and meshless methods (more details in cmech.webs.com)

For both models the materials considered were: (1) Titanium implants; and (2) prosthetic bar of chromium-cobalt alloy (Co-Cr). The structure of the prosthetic bar of the All-On-4® model presented a 10 mm distal cantilever. All materials were considered isotropic, homogeneous and linear. The properties of the materials considered are presented in Table 1.

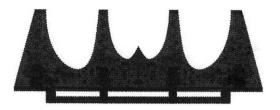

Figure 2. 2D model of the 4-On-Pillars technique.

Table 1. Properties of the materials considered in this article (Duarte, Andrade, Dinis, & Jorge, 2016).

Material	Young's modulus (E) [GPa]	Poisson's ratio (υ)
Cortical bone	13.7	0.3
Trabecular bone	1.37	0.3
Implants	110	0.3
Co-Cr structure	220	0.3

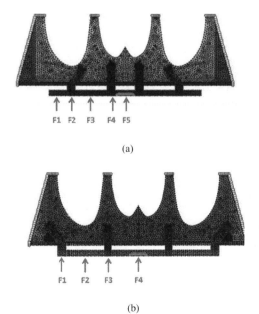

Figure 3. (a) Model All-On-4® with the natural and essential boundary conditions. Nodes marked in green are constrained in Oy and nodes marked in yellow are constrained in Ox and OY; (b) Models 4-On-Pillars with the natural and essential boundary conditions. Nodes marked in green are constrained in Oy and nodes marked in yellow are constrained in Ox and OY.

Then, the same boundary conditions were inserted in both models, demonstrated in Figure 2, in which it is possible to observe that superior

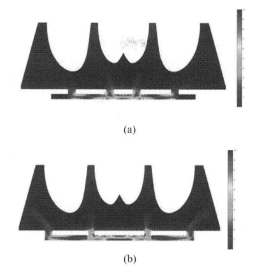

Figure 4. (a) Stress distribution in the All-On-4® model, for load case F5; (b) Stress distribution in the 4-On-Pillars model, for load case F4.

nodes, marked in green, were constrained in y direction, and the lateral nodes, marked in yellow, were constrained in both the Ox and Oy directions.

The All-On-4® model was loaded axially with 1 N loads in 5 different locations: (1) left cantilever; (2) left posterior implant; (3) implant structure; (4) left anterior implant; and (5) structure between anterior implants, as demonstrated in Figure 3(a).

In the 4-On-pillars model what differs is only the absence of the first loading since there is no cantilever in this model, as demonstrated in Figure 3(b).

2.2 Results

According to the methodology described, the following results (shown in Figure 4) were obtained with the main objective of comparing the stress distribution of the 2D All-On-4® and 4-On-Pillars models.

3 CONCLUSIONS

The results show that the All-On-4 model presents a smoother stress distribution, which can potentially induce a more uniform remodelling of the bone tissue.

Furthermore, the 4-On-Pillars model showed a more tapered stress distribution, being the higher density trabecular zones, the ones presenting higher stress concentration.

As for the micro-movement, the 4-On-Pillars model showed lower local vertical displacements on the bar implant, which can lead to a feeling of comfort for the patient.

This work demonstrated the importance of these numerical tools in predicting the structural behaviour of the implant and supporting bone structures, allowing a more efficient design of the distribution of the implants in the dental arch, thus producing a more adequate support for the prosthetic structure.

ACKNOWLEDGEMENTS

The authors acknowledge the support provided by Coordenação de Aperfeiçoamento de Pessoal de Nível Superior (CAPES), process nº 88881.135070/2016-01, of the Ministry of Education (MEC) of Brazil. Furthermore, the authors truly acknowledge the funding provided by Ministério da Ciência, Tecnologia e Ensino Superior—Fundação para a Ciência e a Tecnologia (Portugal) by project funding MIT-EXPL/ISF/0084/2017. Additionally, the authors gratefully acknowledge the funding of Project NORTE-01-0145-FEDER-000022—SciTech—Science and Technology for Competitive and Sustainable Industries, cofinanced by Programa Operacional Regional do Norte (NORTE2020), through Fundo Europeu de Desenvolvimento Regional (FEDER).

REFERENCES

Alencar, M.M., Bastos, L., Verde, L., Moura, W.L. De, Dolores, C., & Soares, V. (2017). FEA of Peri-Implant Stresses in Fixed Partial Denture Prosthese with Cantilevers. *Journal of Prosthodontics*, *26*, 150–155. https://doi.org/10.1111/jopr.12384.

Balshi, T.J., Wolfinger, G.J., & Balshi, S.F. (1999). Analysis of 356 Pterygomaxillary Implants in Edentulous Arches for Fixed Prosthesis Anchorage. *International Journal of Oral & Maxillofacial Implants*, *14*(3), 398–406.

Bordin, D., Bergamo, E.T.P., Fardin, V.P., Coelho, P.G., & Bonfante, A. (2017). Journal of the Mechanical Behavior of Biomedical Materials Fracture strength and probability of survival of narrow and extra-narrow dental implants after fatigue testing : In vitro and in silico analysis. *Journal of the Mechanical Behavior of Biomedical Materials*, *71*(December 2016), 244–249. https://doi.org/10.1016/j.jmbbm.2017.03.022.

Brunski, J.B. (2014). Biomechanical aspects of the optimal number of implants to carry a cross-arch full restoration. *European Journal of Oral Implantology*, *7*, 111–131.

Candel, E., Peñarrocha, D., & Peñarrocha, M. (2012). Rehabilitation of the Atrophic Posterior Maxilla With Pterygoid implants: A Review. *Journal of Oral Implantology*, *38*(1), 461–466.

Dos Santos, M.B.F., Meloto, G.D.O., Bacchi, A., & Correr-Sobrinho, L. (2017). Stress distribution in cylindrical and conical implants under rotational micromovement with different boundary conditions and bone properties : 3-D FEA. *Computer Methods in Biomechanics and Biomedical Engineering*, *20*(8), 893–900. https://doi.org/10.1080/10255842.2017.1309394.

Duarte, H.M.S., Andrade, J.R., Dinis, L.M.J.S., & Jorge, R.M.N. (2016). Numerical analysis of dental implants using a new advanced discretization technique. *Mechanics of Advanced Materials and Structures*, *23*(4), 467–479. https://doi.org/10.1080/15376494.2014.987410.

Geng, J.-P., Tan, K.B.C., & Liu, G.-R. (2001). Application of finite element analysis in implant dentistry: A review of the literature. *J Prosthet Dent*, *85*(6), 585–598. https://doi.org/10.1067/mpr.2001.115251.

Holmes, D.C., Grigsby, W.R., Goel, V.K., & Keller, J.C. (1992). Comparison of Stress Transmission in the IMZ Implant System With Polyoxymethylene or Titanium Intramobile Element : A Finite Element Stress Analysis. *International Journal of Oral & Maxillofacial Implants*, *7*, 450–458.

Maló, P., De Araújo Nobre, M., Lopes, A., Francischone, C., & Rigolizzo, M. (2012). "All-on-4" Immediate-Function Concept for Completely Edentulous Maxillae: A Clinical Report on the Medium (3 Years) and Long-Term (5 Years) Outcomes. *Clinical Implant Dentistry and Related Research*, *14*(SUPPL. 1), 139–150. https://doi.org/10.1111/j.1708-8208.2011.00395.x.

Malo, P., Rangert, B., & Nobre, M. (2005). All-on-4 Immediate-Function Concept with Branemark SystemR Implants for Completely Edentulous Maxillae: A 1-Year Retrospective Clinical Study. *Clinical Implant Dentistry and Related Research*, *7*(s1), s88–s94. https://doi.org/10.1111/j.1708-8208.2005.tb00080.x.

Zienkiewicz, O.C., & Taylor, R.L. (1994). *The finite element method* (4th ed). London: McGraw-Hill.

Biodental Engineering V – Belinha et al. (Eds)
© 2019 Taylor & Francis Group, London, ISBN 978-0-367-21087-8

The numerical analysis of 4-On-Pillars technique using meshless methods

K.F. Vargas
Institute of Science and Innovation in Mechanical and Industrial Engineering (INEGI), Porto, Portugal

G.A.R. Caldas
Faculty of Engineering, University of Porto (FEUP), Porto, Portugal

J. Belinha
Department of Mechanical Engineering, School of Engineering, Polytechnic of Porto (ISEP), Porto, Portugal

R.M. Natal Jorge
Department of Mechanical Engineering, Faculty of Engineering, University of Porto (FEUP), Porto, Portugal

P.A.G. Hernandez, A. Ozkomur, R. Smidt, M.M. Naconecy & L.E. Schneider
Faculty of Dentistry, University Lutheran of Brazil, Canoas, RS, Brazil

ABSTRACT: In this study, a new surgical technique for the insertion of implants in atrophic maxilla (4-On-Pillars) was numerically analysed, using the Finite Element Method (FEM) and a meshless method—the Radial Point Interpolation Method (RPIM). Based on anonymized radiographs, a 2D model was constructed. In order to simulate the surrounding structural environment, natural and essential boundary conditions were calculated and imposed into the model. The results showed distinct stress distribution for the two methods used. It was possible to observe that meshless methods produce smoother stress distribution when compared to FEM.

1 STATE OF THE ART

1.1 Introduction

The reestablishment of occlusion has been one of the most relevant and positive factors in the life of edentulous patients. The absence of teeth compromises masticatory function, temporomandibular joint (TMJ) function, phonation and even, socioeconomic of the individuals involved, affecting the patient's health at different levels. In the literature, is possible to find several articles related to rehabilitation techniques for edentulous jaws. The most traditional technique, called All-On-4, promotes the fixation of the denture prosthesis on four osseointegrated implants.

The maxilla presents its own anatomical characteristics, structures with different bone densities, and the presence of the maxillary sinuses. Such particularities may, in some cases, contraindicate the surgical process. In these cases, previous grafting procedures are performed. Maló and colleagues, promoted a different positioning of the posterior All-On-4 implants, to avoid these grafting procedures. Therefore, the posterior implants were installed at 30° of inclination in relation to the occlusal plane tangential to the anterior wall of the maxillary sinus. Thus, this arrangement of the implants allows a prosthetic rehabilitation from molar to molar with a distal cantilever (Malo, Rangert, & Nobre, 2005) (Maló, De Araújo Nobre, Lopes, Francischone, & Rigolizzo, 2012).

In the literature, alternatively to this configuration, it possible to find an approach where the posterior implants are fixed into the anterior portion of the pterygoid process of the sphenoid bone. This rigid anatomical structure consists of a lamina of cortical bone. (Balshi, Wolfinger, & Balshi, 1999) (Balshi, Wolfinger, Slauch, & Balshi, 2013a) (Balshi, Wolfinger, Slauch, & Balshi, 2013b). With this new technique, called 4-On-Pillars, the implants are inserted on the canine and pterygoid pillars on both sides. In the literature there were no articles related to this innovative technique.

1.2 Numerical methods

One of the most popular numerical tool used is the Finite Element Method (FEM) (Zienkiewicz & Taylor, 1994), which can be used to predict the biomechanical behaviour of implants, prostheses and bone remodelling. FEM is recognized and commonly used in many fields of engineering and science. It is characterized by the problem domain discretization into small elements connected through nodes. Such discretization comprises the creation of the mesh, the elements, their respective nodes and definition of boundary conditions (Geng, Tan, & Liu, 2001) (Alencar et al., 2017). This numerical method allows to solve engineering problems for which it is difficult to obtain an exact analytical solution. Additionally, it allows to save time, minimizing the costs of scientific research. Furthermore, the virtual simulation of biotissue avoids the use of experimental tests in animals. (Holmes, Grigsby, Goel, & Keller, 1992) (Brunski, 2014) (Bordin, Bergamo, Fardin, Coelho, & Bonfante, 2017). However, FEM has some limitations, mostly related to the generation of the element mesh, which represents most of the computational cost of the complete FEM analysis. Therefore, this is a mesh-dependent discretization method and the solution is directly influenced by the element mesh arrangement (C. Tavares, Belinha, Dinis, & Jorge, 2015).

Consequently, meshless methods have been the object of attention and study. These advanced discretization techniques have been applied in several engineering fields, such as solid mechanics, biomechanics and fluid mechanics (J. Belinha, Dinis, & Natal Jorge, 2016)(J Belinha, Dinis, & Jorge, 2015).

1.3 Meshfree advanced discretization techniques

With meshless methods, the problem domain is discretized with an unstructured nodal distribution, so field functions are approximated within an influence-domain, rather than an element. No pre-established relation between the nodes is necessary and influence-domains must overlap each other (C. Tavares et al., 2015).

Meshless methods can be classified as approximation and interpolation, according to the different functions that each one uses in its formulation. The approximation methods present a limitation in the imposition of essential and natural boundary conditions due to the absence of the delta Kronecker property. To solve these problems, the interpolation methods were developed.

In meshless methods the first step is the definition of the geometry of the problem and of the essential and natural boundary conditions. Afterwards, the problem domain is discretized by a nodal set. Then, nodal connectivity must be imposed, through influence-domains. The influence-domains are found by searching a specific number of nodes within a given area, for a 2D problem, or a given volume, for a 3D problem, and can present variable size and shape (Jorge Belinha, 2014). Since in meshless methods there is no elements, the influence-domain is the geometric concept that allows to impose the nodal connectivity. To guarantee the nodal connectivity, these influence-domains can and should overlap each other (J. Tavares & Jorge, 2012). Next, a background integration mesh is created, for RPIM with the use of Gaussian integration meshes being adjusted to the problem domain (Jorge Belinha, 2014). The last step is the determination of the field variables through approximation or interpolation functions, depending on the method used, based on the combination of Radial Basis Functions (RBFs) with polynomial basis functions.

2 NUMERICAL ANALYSIS

2.1 Geometrical and numerical model

The 2D model was developed in the FEMAP software, version 11.4.1 Free (Siemens®, Munich, Germany). It comprises anterior implants with 3.5 mm of width and 10 mm of length, and posterior implants with 4.3 mm of width and 13 mm of length. Thus, simulating the 4-On-Pillars technique, as demonstrated in Figure 1(a).

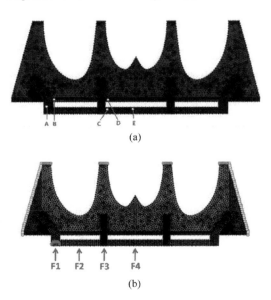

Figure 1. (a) 2D model of the 4-On-Pillars technique with five points marked (A-E), for comparison of stresses; and (b) Models 4-On-Pillars with the natural and essential boundary conditions. Nodes marked in green are constrained in Oy and nodes marked in yellow are constrained in Ox and OY.

The element mesh is composed of triangular elements, with 7316 elements and 3949 nodes.

After the element mesh definition, the models were exported, to FEMAS—Finite Element and Meshless Analysis Software, which is an academic software capable to perform several kinds of computational mechanics analysis, using both the FEM and meshless methods (more details in cmech.webs.com).

Table 1. Properties of the materials considered in this article (Duarte, Andrade, Dinis, & Jorge, 2016).

Material	Young's modulus (E) [GPa]	Poisson's ratio (υ)
Cortical bone	13.7	0.3
Trabecular bone	1.37	0.3
Implants	110	0.3
Co-Cr structure	220	0.3

The materials considered were: (1) Titanium implants; and (2) prosthetic bar of chromium-cobalt alloy (Co-Cr). All materials were considered isotropic, homogeneous and linear. The properties of the materials considered are presented in Table 1.

Then the boundary conditions, demonstrated in Figure 1(b), were defined, in which is possible to observe that superior nodes, marked in green, were constrained in y direction, and the lateral nodes, marked in yellow, were constrained in both the x and y directions.

The model was loaded axially with 1 N loads in 4 different locations: (1) left posterior implant;

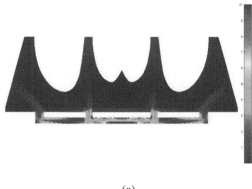

(a)

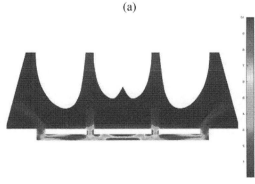

(b)

Figure 2. (a) Stress distribution in the 4-On-Pillars model, for load case F4 and FEM; and (b) Stress distribution in the 4-On-Pillars model, for load case F4 and RPIM.

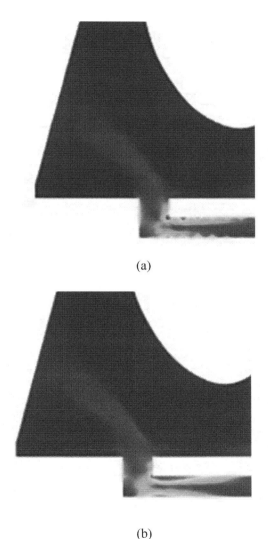

Figure 3. (a) Expanding Figure 2(a); and (b) Expanding Figure 2(b).

173

Table 2. Effective von Mises values for the points of interest, according to the load case applied and the numerical method used.

σef	Method	A	B	C	D	E
F1	FEM	4,17E+00	3,82E-01	3,98E-01	1,85E-01	6,47E-01
	RPIM	1,22E+00	8,98E-01	1,53E+00	8,24E-01	1,41E+00
F2	FEM	2,83E+00	8,95E-01	4,79E-01	6,64E-01	1,40E+00
	RPIM	8,70E-01	6,12E-01	1,01E+00	7,25E-01	9,20E-01
F3	FEM	2,99E+00	8,33E-01	4,06E+00	7,36E-01	8,04E-01
	RPIM	5,10E-01	3,37E-01	5,38E-01	4,83E-01	4,81E-01
F4	FEM	2,12E+00	9,43E-01	7,08E+00	7,71E-01	8,70E+00
	RPIM	1,39E-01	5,69E-02	9,04E-03	1,78E-01	1,66E-02

(2) implant structure; (3) left anterior implant; and (4) structure between anterior implants, as demonstrated in Figure 1(b).

2.2 *Results*

According to the methodology described, the following results (shown in Figure 2 and Figure 3) were obtained for comparative analysis of FEM and RPIM numerical methods.

The values of the von Mises stresses for the points of interest marked in Figure 1(a) (A, B, C, D, E), according to the loads of the forces (F1, F2, F3, F4) and for both numerical methods used, are shown in Table 2.

3 CONCLUSIONS

The results obtained according to the methodology followed in the analysis of the pioneer rehabilitation technique of atrophic maxilla, demonstrated that the meshless method used was able to produce displacements very close to the FEM solution and smoother stress fields when compared to the FEM.

ACKNOWLEDGEMENTS

The authors acknowledge the support provided by Coordenação de Aperfeiçoamento de Pessoal de Nível Superior (CAPES), process n° 88881.135070/2016-01, of the Ministry of Education (MEC) of Brazil. Furthermore, the authors truly acknowledge the funding provided by Ministério da Ciência, Tecnologia e Ensino Superior—Fundação para a Ciência e a Tecnologia (Portugal) by project funding MIT-EXPL/ ISF/0084/2017. Additionally, the authors gratefully acknowledge the funding of Project NORTE-01-0145-FEDER-000022—SciTech—Science and Technology for Competitive and Sustainable

Industries, cofinanced by Programa Operacional Regional do Norte (NORTE2020), through Fundo Europeu de Desenvolvimento Regional (FEDER).

REFERENCES

Alencar, M.M., Bastos, L., Verde, L., Moura, W.L. De, Dolores, C., & Soares, V. (2017). FEA of Peri-Implant Stresses in Fixed Partial Denture Prosthese with Cantilevers. *Journal of Prosthodontics*, 26, 150–155. https://doi.org/10.1111/jopr.12384.

Balshi, T.J., Wolfinger, G.J., & Balshi, S.F. (1999). Analysis of 356 Pterygomaxillary Implants in Edentulous Arches for Fixed Prosthesis Anchorage. *International Journal of Oral & Maxillofacial Implants*, 14(3), 398–406.

Balshi, T.J., Wolfinger, G.J., Slauch, R.W., & Balshi, S.F. (2013a). A retrospective comparison of implants in the pterygomaxillary region: implant placement with two-stage, single-stage, and guided surgery protocols. *The International Journal of Oral & Maxillofacial Implants*, 28(1), 184–9. https://doi.org/10.11607/jomi.2693.

Balshi, T.J., Wolfinger, G.J., Slauch, R.W., & Balshi, S.F. (2013b). Brånemark System Implant Lengths in the Pterygomaxillary Region: Retrospective Comparison. *Implant Dentistry*, 22(6), 610–612. https://doi.org/10.1097/ID.0b013e3182a5d181.

Belinha, J. (2014). Meshless Methods in Biomechanics: Bone Tissue Remodelling Analysis. In *Lecture Notes in Computational Vision and Biomechanics*. Springer. https://doi.org/10.1007/978-3-319-06400-0.

Belinha, J., Dinis, L.M.J.S., & Jorge, R.M.N. (2015). The meshless methods in the bone tissue remodelling analysis. *Procedia Engineering*, 110, 51–58. https://doi.org/10.1016/j.proeng.2015.07.009.

Belinha, J., Dinis, L.M.J.S., & Natal Jorge, R.M. (2016). The analysis of the bone remodelling around femoral stems: A meshless approach. *Mathematics and Computers in Simulation*, 121, 64–94. https://doi.org/10.1016/j.matcom.2015.09.002.

Bordin, D., Bergamo, E.T.P., Fardin, V.P., Coelho, P.G., & Bonfante, A. (2017). Journal of the Mechanical Behavior of Biomedical Materials Fracture strength and probability of survival of narrow and extra-narrow dental implants after fatigue testing : In vitro and in silico analysis. *Journal of the Mechanical Behavior of Biomedical Materials*, *71*(December 2016), 244–249. https://doi.org/10.1016/j.jmbbm.2017.03.022.

Brunski, J.B. (2014). Biomechanical aspects of the optimal number of implants to carry a cross-arch full restoration. *European Journal of Oral Implantology*, *7*, 111–131.

Duarte, H.M.S., Andrade, J.R., Dinis, L.M.J.S., & Jorge, R.M.N. (2016). Numerical analysis of dental implants using a new advanced discretization technique. *Mechanics of Advanced Materials and Structures*, *23*(4), 467–479. https://doi.org/10.1080/15376494.201 4.987410.

Geng, J.-P., Tan, K.B.C., & Liu, G.-R. (2001). Application of finite element analysis in implant dentistry: A review of the literature. *J Prosthet Dent*, *85*(6), 585–598. https://doi.org/10.1067/mpr.2001.115251.

Holmes, D.C., Grigsby, W.R., Goel, V.K., & Keller, J.C. (1992). Comparison of Stress Transmission in the IMZ Implant System With Polyoxymethylene or Titanium Intramobile Element : A Finite Element Stress Analysis. *International Journal of Oral & Maxillofacial Implants*, *7*, 450–458.

Maló, P., De Araújo Nobre, M., Lopes, A., Francischone, C., & Rigolizzo, M. (2012). "All-on-4" Immediate-Function Concept for Completely Edentulous Maxillae: A Clinical Report on the Medium (3 Years) and Long-Term (5 Years) Outcomes. *Clinical Implant Dentistry and Related Research*, *14*(SUPPL. 1), 139–150. https://doi.org/10.1111/j.1708-8208.2011.00395.x.

Malo, P., Rangert, B., & Nobre, M. (2005). All-on-4 Immediate-Function Concept with Branemark SystemR Implants for Completely Edentulous Maxillae: A 1-Year Retrospective Clinical Study. *Clinical Implant Dentistry and Related Research*, *7*(s1), s88–s94. https://doi.org/10.1111/j.1708-8208.2005.tb00080.x.

Tavares, C., Belinha, J., Dinis, L., & Jorge, R.N. (2015). The numerical analysis of a restored tooth using meshless methods. *Proceedings—2015 IEEE 4th Portuguese Meeting on Bioengineering, ENBENG 2015*. https://doi.org/10.1109/ENBENG.2015.7088872.

Tavares, J., & Jorge, N. (Eds.). (2012). Lectures Notes in Computational Vision and Biomechanics.

Zienkiewicz, O.C., & Taylor, R.L. (1994). *The finite element method* (4th ed). London: McGraw-Hill.

Biodental Engineering V – Belinha et al. (Eds)
© 2019 Taylor & Francis Group, London, ISBN 978-0-367-21087-8

Numerical analysis of support structures on an adhesive dental bridge

G.A.R. Caldas
Faculty of Engineering, University of Porto (FEUP), Porto, Portugal

J. Belinha
Department of Mechanical Engineering, School of Engineering, Polytechnic of Porto (ISEP), Porto, Portugal

R.M. Natal Jorge
Department of Mechanical Engineering, Faculty of Engineering, University of Porto (FEUP), Porto, Portugal

ABSTRACT: In this work the support structures of an adhesive dental bridge are analysed. The objective of this article is to test if the abutments teeth can support the resin-bonded bridge, used in dental reconstructions. The study was conducted on a 3D model of a part of maxilla where a tooth was missing. This model was developed through CT scans of an unknown patient. It was used the Finite Element Method (FEM) to study and analyse the results obtained. FEM is a technique that gives the solution of a complex mechanical problem through the discretization of the problem domain into multiple subdomains, called finite elements. Therefore, a complex problem is simplified by splinting the problem domain into smaller and simpler domains. The simple equations that model these finite elements are then assembled into a larger system of equations that models the entire problem. In the analysed case, the stresses measured were not sufficient to damage the abutments teeth that are responsible for supporting the bridge. The resin-bonded bridges appear to be a valid method of dental reconstruction since it does not damage the original teeth of the patient.

1 STATE OF THE ART

1.1 *Introduction*

Oral diseases can have a significant impact on quality of life, compromising functional or aesthetic roles such as chewing and smile. Lost or extracted teeth can cause infections, so it is very important to replace them. Adhesive bridges are a type of fixed prothesis in which the pontic tooth (replaced tooth) is attached to a structure that is cemented on the abutment teeth (adjacent teeth to the space of the missing tooth and that will serve as a support) (Walmsley et al., 2007). With this type of restoration, the replaced teeth are sealed primarily to enamel, and therefore the fixed dental prosthesis is supported by natural teeth. Enamel has to be etched to provide mechanical retention for the resin cement (Lopes et al., 2014).

These bridges can only be used when the abutment teeth are healthy or with very small fillers. This is because when using this method, the load applied on the pontic will be transmitted to the adjacent teeth through the bridge. For this reason, these type of dental restoration is commonly used to replace front teeth that are subjected to smaller masticatory forces.

1.2 *Numerical simulation*

Numerical simulation allows the development of virtual models for the analysis of complex problems with a difficult analytical solution (Magne, 2007).

Today, modern medical imaging is a common tool used in computational mechanics research, since through medical imaging it is possible to obtain detailed three-dimensional (3D) architecture data. In the field of mechanical simulation, this 3D architecture data allows to simulate and study natural phenomena, such as the study of the function and morphology of the human body (Bushberg, Seibert, Leidholdt, Boone, & Goldschmidt, 2003).

One of the most popular numerical tool used is the Finite Element Method (FEM) (Zienkiewicz & Taylor, 1994).

1.3 *Finite element method*

FEM is characterized by the domain discretization into multiple subdomains called finite elements. Thus, a complex problem is simplified by splitting the problem domain into smaller and simpler domains (Geng, Tan, & Liu, 2001).

Each finite element consists of multiple nodes, whose coordinates establish the geometry of the structure to be analysed. In this way, the multiple elements are connected through the nodes, forming a mesh (Trivedi, 2014). The elements cannot overlap each other and cannot present any gap disrupting the model continuum. The process of creating the mesh with its elements and their respective nodes is defined as the discretization step of the process. The type, the arrangement and the total number of elements has impact on the accuracy of the results (Trivedi, 2014). These elements can be irregular and may have different properties, allowing the discretization of structures composed of different materials.

For each one of the finite elements the field variables are interpolated by simple functions, the shape functions. The FEM combined with the theory of elasticity allow to predict several variable fields, such as displacement, strain and stress fields. These solution fields depend on the assumptions made in the modelling of the structure under study, such as the structure geometry, the properties of the materials considered, the essential and natural boundary conditions and, in the case of dentistry, the bone-implant interfaces, for example (Geng et al., 2001).

The solution is obtained after assembling the stiffness matrix of each element (coming from the Galerkin weak formulation) into a global stiffness matrix. The application of boundary conditions and loads in the model leads to a set of equilibrium equations which generally corresponds to the following:

$$Ku = f \qquad (1)$$

where K is the stiffness matrix of the structure, u the displacement vector and f the vector of forces. Through the solution of these equations it is possible to obtain the displacements and the strains/stresses on each node and integration point, respectively, of the model in analysis, as shown in Equations 2, 3 and 4.

$$u = K^{-1}f \qquad (2)$$
$$\varepsilon = Bu \qquad (3)$$
$$\sigma = D\varepsilon \qquad (4)$$

where ε corresponds to the strain vector, B the deformability matrix, σ the stress vector and D the elasticity matrix.

1.4 *Finite element method in oral biomechanics*

FEM was initially developed in the 60's to solve aeronautic problems and was first introduced in dental medicine in the early 1970s (Geng et al., 2001) (Farah, Craig, & Sikarskie, 1973) (Thresher & Saito, 1973). The first works focused on the displacement field and the stress field in human tooth, as a way of studding numerically the transferring of occlusal loads from the tooth into the surrounding structures (Thresher & Saito, 1973) (Farah et al., 1973).

Since the introduction of this numerical method to dental medicine, there have been some publications devoted to the study of dental bridges. Cantilever bridges are the most studied and it is possible to draw two major conclusions: (1) most of the stresses are transmitted to the tooth closest to the pontic, so the maximum von Mises stresses are in the connector between these teeth; and (2) long cantilever bridges are not advisable (Awadalla, Azarbal, Ismail, & El-Ibiari, 1992) (Wang, Lee, Wang, & Chang, 1998) (Zhang et al., 2015) (Eraslan, Sevimay, Usumez, & Eskitascioglu, 2005) (H.-S. Yang, Chung, & Park, 1996). Yang et al. (1996) and Wang et al. (1998) studied the level of bone support, verifying that reduced bone support increases the stress concentration (Wang et al., 1998) (H.-S. Yang et al., 1996). Henyš et al. (2017) studied a mandibular cantilever bridge with six units subjected to fatigue cycles verifying that in an extreme situation of a bite force of 1280 N, the bridge failed in less than one day. As such, it becomes extremely important to consider the dynamic character of bite forces and the fatigue damages, due to excessive biting force, as failure factors of dental bridges (Henyš et al., 2017).

Fixed-fixed bridges have also been subject of investigation. The conclusions obtained when studding these bridges are similar to the ones obtained when studding cantilever bridges: (1) the connectors in fixed partial dentures (FPDs) are the weakest areas and responsible for failure in most cases, once this is the area with highest stress concentration; and (2) the increase of the abutment teeth does not translate into a proportional reduction of stress in the periodontium (Rappelli, Scalise, Procaccini, & Tomasini, 2005) (Mokhtarikhoee, Jannesari, Behroozi, & Mokhtarikhoee, 2008) (Reimann, Żmudzki, & Dobrzański, 2015) (H. Yang, Lang, & Felton, 1999) (Lin, Hsu, & Wu, 2005). Yang et al. (1999) studied fixed-fixed dental bridges with the aim of understanding the effect of different levels of bone support on deflection and stresses generated in the teeth and their supporting structures. The loss of bone support increased the deflection and stresses generated in the constituent structures of the model. However, when the bridge was placed, a reduction of stress and deflection was observed in the supporting structures (H. Yang et al., 1999).

The development of the resin-bonded bridge technique has shown some advantages over conventional fixed partial dentures, such as the case of cantilever and fixed-fixed bridges, previously mentioned. One of the most used resin-bonded bridge is Maryland bridge, however fewer authors studied this type of dental bridge. Therefore, there is a lack of information regarding the resistance and longevity of adhesive bridges (Lopes et al., 2014).

As an alternative to the Maryland bridge appeared the direct fibre reinforced composite (FRC) bridge, technique that can improve the adhesion of the wing of the bridge to the abutment. In this way, the stresses applied at the interface between the bridge and the abutment tooth can be reduced (Li, Swain, Li, & Steven, 2005) (Vallittu & Sevelius, 2000). Many researchers study FRC bridges trying to develop an optimized design, which includes thickness, position and orientation of the fibres. Therefore, the fibres directions have to be aligned with those of the maximum principal stresses. Hence, it is necessary to discover the locations of higher stresses and directions of maximum principal stresses. Once high tensile stresses were found in the bottom of the pontic and in the connectors that link the pontic to the abutment teeth, it was concluded that fibres should be placed in the bottom of the pontic tooth extending to the connectors. Consequently, the optimized design is a U-shape substructure. The optimized design can improve fracture resistance of FPDs by reducing some of the failure-initiating stresses (Nakamura, Ohyama, Waki, & Kinuta, 2005) (Shi & Fok, 2009).

A study carried out a computer simulation of 96 cases of different adhesive bridges, to compare the impact of different bridge construction. Different materials were used in the study cases, concluding that, despite the stresses obtained when using FRCs are smaller, in none of the cases the applied stresses would be able to damage the construction of the bridge (Śmielak, Świniarski, Wołowiec-Korecka, & Klimek, 2016).

As it is perceptible, most of the articles focus on the study of the bridge itself, namely materials and design used. However, it is necessary to understand if the abutment teeth, as well as all the support structures, such as bone and periodontal ligament, can withstand the additionally applied loads. These studies, allow to understand the validity of using dental bridges as a dental reconstruction method.

2 MATERIAL AND METHODS

The present study aims to understand if the consequent distribution of loads produced by the use of adhesive bridges constitute or not a problem for the abutment teeth.

In this work, a 3D model was constructed from CT scans, Figure 1. Using anonymized CT scans, it was possible to obtain the geometric shape of the maxilla of the unknow patient. Then, a section of the maxilla was selected and a model consisting of the maxilla bone, the central incisor and a canine, was obtained. As it is possible to observe in Figure 2, this model simulates the lack of the lateral incisor. The structures considered were: dentin (Patch 3 and 4), cortical bone (Patch 1) and trabecular bone

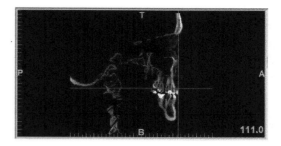

Figure 1. CT scans used to develop the three-dimensional model of the maxilla.

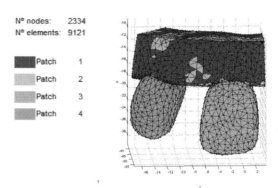

Figure 2. Maxilla three-dimensional representation, with respective materials identified, and element mesh discretizing the problem domain.

Table 1. Properties of each one of the materials consider in this article (Śmielak et al., 2016).

Part of the model	Material	Young's modulus (E) [MPa]	Poisson's ratio (υ)
Bone	Cortical bone	$1.1 \cdot 10^4$	0.30
	Trabecular bone	1370	0.30
Teeth	Dentin	$1.86 \cdot 10^4$	0.31

(Patch 2). To perform the numerical analysis of the problem, the biological structures were discretized into an element mesh, as demonstrated in Figure 2. The materials considered have an elastic, homogeneous and isotropic linear behaviour. The material properties of the biological structures presented in the model can be found in Table 1. It was investigated in the literature the ultimate tension stress for each of the materials, so it could then be compare to the maximum von Mises stress obtained with the present analyses. The ultimate tension stress of each of the materials is presented in Table 2.

For the case studied, the boundary conditions considered were applied on the top and on both sides of the bone, preventing either the rotation or the movement in any direction.

As mentioned previously, the loads applied to the pontic, because of chewing, are uniformly distributed to the abutment teeth. So, a bite force of 100 N, means that each abutment tooth will support 50 N. The abutment teeth, in addition to the support loads (which will be transmitted through the bridge), must also be able to withstand the loads directly applied to them. Thus, each tooth was subjected to a total of 150 N, applied in the direction of the Z axis (Li et al., 2005).

Table 2. Ultimate tension stress of each material (Śmielak et al., 2016) (Tavares & Jorge, 2012).

Part of the model	Material	Ultimate tension stress (MPa)
Bone	Cortical bone	300
	Trabecular bone	150
Teeth	Dentin	105.5

3 RESULTS AND DISCUSSION

The maximum stresses were found in the cervical region of each teeth and respective bone. These did not exceed 33 MPa.

To facilitate the interpretation of the results obtained, the analysis was performed for each teeth and surrounding bone separately. This means that it was examined a set of two variable fields: – the stresses obtained in the central incisor and the bone that surrounds this tooth (Figure 3); – the stresses obtained in the canine and the bone surrounding this tooth (Figure 4). The higher stresses were found on the bone surrounding the canine and in the central incisor. These areas of high stress are marked in Figure 3 and Figure 4.

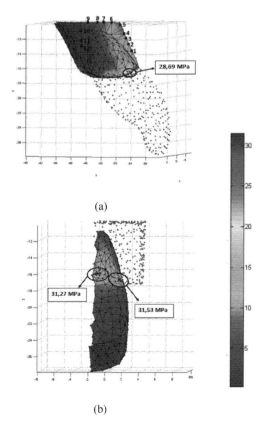

Figure 3. Stress map obtained to the: (a) bone surrounding the central incisor and (b) central incisor with maximum stresses selected [MPa].

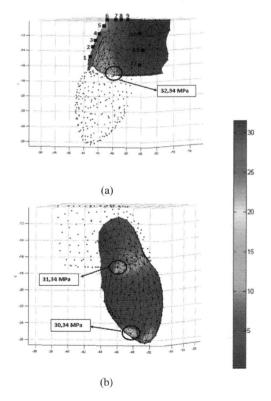

Figure 4. Stress map obtained to the: (a) bone surrounding the canine and (b) canine with maximum stresses selected [MPa].

The aim of this study was to understand if the use of dental bridges does not damage the abutment teeth. The loads applied to teeth corresponds to the masticatory forces applied to the crown of the bridge and to the abutment teeth. Comparing the stresses obtained throughout the model with the stresses listed in Table 2, it can be concluded that for the experimental conditions used, there is no risk to the maxilla or to the abutment teeth, since the stresses obtained are much lower than the ultimate stresses tension of each material.

4 CONCLUSIONS

The computer simulation of the abutment teeth submitted to an additional load (coming from the dental bridge) allowed to conclude that the abutment teeth are capable of supporting the additional loads applied. However, notice that this conclusion is only valid for the loading conditions studied in this work. Furthermore, the application of these loads does not appear capable of damage the abutment teeth. Consequently, the use of resin-bonded bridges can be a viable method for dental reconstruction.

ACKNOWLEDGEMENTS

The authors truly acknowledge the funding provided by Ministério da Ciência, Tecnologia e Ensino Superior—Fundação para a Ciência e a Tecnologia (Portugal) by project funding MIT-EXPL/ISF/0084/2017. Additionally, the authors gratefully acknowledge the funding of Project NORTE-01-0145-FEDER-000022—SciTech—Science and Technology for Competitive and Sustainable Industries, cofinanced by Programa Operacional Regional do Norte (NORTE2020), through Fundo Europeu de Desenvolvimento Regional (FEDER).

REFERENCES

Awadalla, H. A., Azarbal, M., Ismail, Y. H., & El-Ibiari, W. (1992). Three-dimensional finite element stress analysis of a cantilever fixed partial denture. *The Journal of Prosthetic Dentistry*, 68(2), 243–8.

Bushberg, J. T., Seibert, J. A., Leidholdt, E. M., Boone, J. M., & Goldschmidt, E. J. (2003). The Essential Physics of Medical Imaging. *Medical Physics*, 30(7), 1936. https://doi.org/10.1118/1.1585033.

Eraslan, O., Sevimay, M., Usumez, A., & Eskitascioglu, G. (2005). Effects of cantilever design and material on stress distribution in fixed partial dentures—a finite element analysis. *Journal of Oral Rehabilitation*, 32(4), 273–278.

Farah, J. W., Craig, R. G., & Sikarskie, D. L. (1973). Photoelastic and Finite Element Stress Analysis of a Restored Axisymmetric First Molar. *J. Biomechanics*, 6(5), 511–520.

Geng, J.-P., Tan, K. B. C., & Liu, G.-R. (2001). Application of finite element analysis in implant dentistry: A review of the literature. *J Prosthet Dent*, 85(6), 585–598. https://doi.org/10.1067/mpr.2001.115251.

Henyš, P., Ackermann, M., Čapek, L., Drahorád, T., Šimůnek, A., & Exnerová, M. (2017). Stress and fatigue analysis of cantilevered bridge during biting: a computer study. *Computer Methods in Biomechanics and Biomedical Engineering*, 20(sup1), 103–104. https://doi.org/10.1080/10255842.2017.1382882.

Li, W., Swain, M. V, Li, Q., & Steven, G. P. (2005). Towards automated 3D finite element modeling of direct fiber reinforced composite dental bridge. *Journal of Biomedical Materials Research Part B: Applied Biomaterials*, 74B(1), 520–528. https://doi.org/10.1002/jbm.b.30233.

Lin, C. L., Hsu, K. W., & Wu, C. H. (2005). Multi-factorial retainer design analysis of posterior resin-bonded fixed partial dentures: A finite element study. *Journal of Dentistry*, 33(9), 711–720. https://doi.org/10.1016/j.jdent.2005.01.009.

Lopes, I., Correia, A., Viana, P. C., Kovacs, Z., Viriato, N., Campos, J. C. R., & Vaz, M. A. (2014). All-ceramic CAD-CAM Maryland bridge—a numerical stress analysis. In *Biodental Engineering III—Proceedings of the 3rd International Conference on Biodental Engineering* (pp. 291–294). https://doi.org/10.1201/b17071.

Magne, P. (2007). Efficient 3D finite element analysis of dental restorative procedures using micro-CT data. *Dental Materials*, 23(5), 539–548. https://doi.org/10.1016/j.dental.2006.03.013.

Mokhtarikhoee, S., Jannesari, A., Behroozi, H., & Mokhtarikhoee, S. (2008). Effect of connector width on stress distribution in all ceramic fixed partial dentures (a 3D finite element study). In *Conference proceedings : 30th Annual International IEEE EMBS Conference* (pp. 1829–1832). Vancouver: IEEE. https://doi.org/10.1109/IEMBS.2008.4649535.

Nakamura, T., Ohyama, T., Waki, T., & Kinuta, S. (2005). Finite Element Analysis of Fiber-reinforced Fixed Partial Dentures. *Dental Materials Journal*, 24(2), 275–279.

Rappelli, G., Scalise, L., Procaccini, M., & Tomasini, E. P. (2005). Stress distribution in fiber-reinforced composite inlay fixed partial dentures. *The Journal of Prosthetic Dentistry*, 93(5), 425–432. https://doi.org/10.1016/j.prosdent.2005.02.022.

Reimann, Ł., Żmudzki, J., & Dobrzański, L. A. (2015). Strength analysis of a three-unit dental bridge framework with the Finite Element Method. *Acta of Bioengineering and Biomechanics*, 17(1), 51–59. https://doi.org/10.5277/ABB-00091-2014-02.

Shi, L., & Fok, A. S. L. (2009). Structural optimization of the fibre-reinforced composite substructure in a three-unit dental bridge. *Dental Materials*, 25(6), 791–801. https://doi.org/10.1016/j.dental.2009.01.001.

Śmielak, B., Świniarski, J., Wołowiec-Korecka, E., & Klimek, L. (2016). 2D-finite element analysis of inlay-, onlay bridges with using various materials. *International Scientific Journal*, 79(2), 71–78.

Tavares, J., & Jorge, N. (Eds.). (2012). Lectures Notes in Computational Vision and Biomechanics.

Thresher, R. W., & Saito, G. E. (1973). The stress analysis of human teeth. *Journal of Biomechanics*, *6*, 443–449. https://doi.org/10.1016/0021-9290(73)90003-1.

Trivedi, S. (2014). Finite element analysis: A boon to dentistry. *Journal of Oral Biology and Craniofacial Research*, *4*(3), 200–203. https://doi.org/10.1016/j.jobcr.2014.11.008.

Vallittu, P. K., & Sevelius, C. (2000). Resin-bonded, glass fiber-reinforced composite fixed partial dentures: a clinical study. *The Journal of Prosthetic Dentistry*, *84*(4), 413–418. https://doi.org/10.1067/mpr.2000.109782.

Walmsley, A. D., Walsh, T. F., Lumley, P., Burke, F. J. T., Shortall, A. C., Hayes-Hall, R., & Pretty, I. (2007). *Restorative Dentistry*. (Elsevier, Ed.) (Second Edi). Churchill Livingstone. Retrieved from https://www.sciencedirect.com/science/book/9780443102462.

Wang, C. H., Lee, H. E., Wang, C. C., & Chang, H. P. (1998). Methods to improve a periodontally involved terminal abutment of a cantilever fixed partial denture a finite element stress analysis. *Journal of Oral Rehabilitation*, *25*(4), 253–7. Retrieved from http://www.ncbi.nlm.nih.gov/pubmed/9610851.

Yang, H.-S., Chung, H.-J., & Park, Y.-J. (1996). Stress analysis of a cantilevered fixed partial denture with normal and reduced bone support. *The Journal of Prosthetic Dentistry*, *76*(4), 424–430. https://doi.org/10.1016/S0022-3913(96)90549-1.

Yang, H., Lang, L., & Felton, D. (1999). Finite element stress analysis on the effect of splinting in fixed partial dentures. *J Prosthet Dent*, *81*(6), 721–728.

Zhang, Z., Zhou, S., Li, E., Li, W., Swain, M. V., & Li, Q. (2015). Design for minimizing fracture risk of all-ceramic cantilever dental bridge. *Bio-Medical Materials and Engineering*, *26*, S19–S25. https://doi.org/10.3233/BME-151285.

Zienkiewicz, O. C., & Taylor, R. L. (1994). *The finite element method* (4th ed). London: McGraw-Hill.

Biodental Engineering V – Belinha et al. (Eds)
© 2019 Taylor & Francis Group, London, ISBN 978-0-367-21087-8

Predicting in-silico structural response of dental restorations using meshless methods

G.A.R. Caldas
Faculty of Engineering, University of Porto (FEUP), Porto, Portugal

J. Belinha
Department of Mechanical Engineering, School of Engineering, Polytechnic of Porto (ISEP), Porto, Portugal

R.M. Natal Jorge
Department of Mechanical Engineering, Faculty of Engineering, University of Porto (FEUP), Porto, Portugal

ABSTRACT: Failure of a dental restoration may cause even more problems for the patient than missing teeth. Therefore, there are a variety of options that should be considered and analysed. This work focuses on a specific type of dental restoration, the adhesive dental bridges. Adhesive dental bridges, also known as Maryland bridges, can be an alternative solution to conventional bridges or even implants, but it must guarantee the mechanical resistance of the bridge, to obtain a long and functional replacement. The main objective of this work was to study the effect of different resin-cements and the use of a two-retainer design or a single-retainer design on the mechanical resistance of an adhesive dental bridge. Three numerical methods were used: Finite Element Method (FEM), Radial Point Interpolation Method (RPIM) and Natural Neighbour Radial Point Interpolation Method (NNRPIM). The results showed that the connectors are the weakest areas because this is the area with highest stress concentration. The single-retainer design increases the risk of debonding. In addition, the results obtained using meshless methods are in agreement with the FEM.

1 STATE OF THE ART

1.1 Introduction

The loss of teeth has a negative impact on the individual's quality of life. Presently, in our society, aesthetics is very important, so the loss of a tooth can lead to low self-esteem, which can compromise individual's ability to socialize, adversely affecting performance at work and in daily activities. Thus, many patients have the desire to replace missing teeth, which can be done through a variety of treatment alternatives, like adhesive dental bridges.

Adhesive bridges are a type of fixed prosthesis in which the pontic tooth (replaced tooth) is attached to a structure that is cemented on the abutment teeth (patient's natural teeth) (Walmsley et al., 2007). With this type of restoration, the replaced teeth are sealed primarily to enamel, and therefore the fixed dental prosthesis is supported by natural teeth. Enamel has to be etched to provide mechanical retention for the resin cement (Lopes et al., 2014). This type of restoration distinguishes from the others because it is a conservative method and it is reversible, once it requires minimal tooth preparation and does not compromise the

abutment tooth (Walmsley et al., 2007) (Durey, Nixon, Robinson, & Chan, 2011).

However, there are still some concerns in using these bridges, which require a more complex geometry design and have a low retention rate. This low retention rate between the retainer wing and the abutment tooth leads to debonding, which is the main cause of failure of this type of dental restoration (Śmielak, Świniarski, Wołowiec-Korecka, & Klimek, 2016) (Vallittu & Sevelius, 2000).

1.2 Numerical simulation

Numerical simulation allows the development of virtual models, which permits the analysis of complex problems with a difficult analytical solution (Magne, 2007).

In the field of mechanical simulation, the use of modern medical imaging allows to obtain detailed three-dimensional (3D) architecture data, which then allows to simulate and study natural phenomena (Bushberg, Seibert, Leidholdt, Boone, & Goldschmidt, 2003). With the evolution of computer technology, it has become possible to develop increasingly robust and reliable models. Therefore, numerical simulation has become an essential tool in engineering and science, being indispensable in the diagnosis and treatment of diseases.

One of the most popular numerical tool used is the Finite Element Method (FEM) (Zienkiewicz & Taylor, 1994). FEM was initially developed in the 60's to solve aeronautic problems and it was first introduced in dental medicine in the early 1970s (Geng, Tan, & Liu, 2001) (Farah, Craig, & Sikarskie, 1973) (Thresher & Saito, 1973). The first works focused on the displacement field and the stress field in human tooth, aiming to study numerically the transferring of occlusal loads from the tooth into the surrounding structures (Thresher & Saito, 1973) (Farah et al., 1973). This method has several advantages. It allows to predict (and interpolate) the stress/strain state of virtually any point inside the geometric 3D model. (Moratal, 2016) (Li, Swain, Li, Ironside, & Steven, 2004) Additionally, FEM provides quick solutions and results can be obtained with a reasonable degree of accuracy. (Srirekha & Bashetty, 2010) However, FEM has limitations, mostly because it is a mesh-dependent discretization method. Therefore, the FEM solution is directly influenced by element mesh arrangement and so distorted or poor-quality meshes lead to high-errors (C. Tavares, Belinha, Dinis, & Jorge, 2015).

Thus, a family of meshfree advanced discretization techniques were developed to address some of the limitations of FEM (Jorge Belinha, 2014).

1.3 *Meshfree advanced discretization techniques*

The main difference between FEM and meshless methods is that in the latter, the domain of the problem is discretized in arbitrarily distributed nodes without any pre-established relation between them. Nodal connectivity is established by influence-domains, so field functions are approximated within an influence-domain, rather than an element. In meshless methods, influence-domains must overlap each other (Jorge Belinha, 2014).

Meshless methods can be divided into two categories: approximation meshless methods and interpolation meshless methods (Jorge Belinha, 2014).

The first meshless methods developed were approximation methods. These methods use approximation functions, as they allow to obtain smoother solutions. The influence-domains were obtained through fixed radial searches and the background integration mesh (used to integrate the integral-differential equations that govern the study of a physical phenomenon) was constructed through integration cells, independent on the nodal distribution. For this reason, these methods inherited the FEM integration scheme. (C. S. S. Tavares, Belinha, Dinis, & Natal Jorge, 2015)

As mentioned in the work of Belinha (Jorge Belinha, 2014), the first meshless approximation

method was the Smoothed-Particle Hydrodynamics (SPH), developed for astronomy. This was the origin of the Reproducing Kernel Particle Method (RKPM). One of the oldest methods is the Diffuse Element Method (DEM). This method uses the Moving Least Square approximants (MLS), proposed by Lancaster and Salkauskas, in the construction of the approximation function. Belytschko evolved DEM by developing one of the most popular meshless methods, the Element Free Galerkin Method (EFGM) (Dinis, Natal Jorge, & Belinha, 2007) (Jorge Belinha, 2014).

However, these approximation methods present a limitation in the imposition of essential and natural boundary conditions, due to the lack of the delta Kronecker property, for which the interpolation methods were developed. Several interpolation methods have been developed, such as the Point Interpolation Method (PIM), the Radial Point Interpolation Method (RPIM), the Natural Neighbour Finite Element Method (NNFEM) and the Natural Element Method (NEM), as mentioned in (Dinis et al., 2007) and (Jorge Belinha, 2014).

The RPIM had its origin in the PIM, through the addition of an extra functional base, an RBF (Radial Basis Function). The combination of NEM and RPIM originated the Natural Neighbour Radial Point Interpolation Method (NNRPIM) (Jorge Belinha, 2014).

An issue causing discussion among the numerical methods community is the dependency and the construction of a background mesh for integration purposes. Notice that some meshless methods do not promote a truly meshless discretization method since they require a secondary mesh: the background integration mesh. Some of these methods are the EFGM and the RPIM. Alternatively, other meshless method formulations are capable to construct the integration mesh and to impose the nodal connectivity using only the nodal distribution, being truly meshless methods. Some of these techniques are the NNRPIM and the NREM (C. Tavares et al., 2015) (Dinis et al., 2007).

The meshless methods used in this work, along with FEM, are the RPIM and the NNRPIM.

Meshless methods require the combination of three parts: nodal connectivity, numerical integration scheme, and shape functions (Jorge Belinha, 2014).

When using these advanced numerical methods, the first step should be the study of the geometry of the problem and the establishment of a solid domain, its boundaries and boundary conditions. Then, the solid must be numerically discretized by a nodal set, with regular or irregular distribution. The spatial location of each discrete node is the only information required. It is necessary to consider that the nodal discretization has a direct effect on the result of the numerical analysis, affecting the performance of the method. As such, a uniform nodal distribution leads to more accurate results. Then, it is necessary to impose nodal connectivity through influence-domains, in the case of RPIM, or influence-cells, in the case of NNRPIM. Next, a background integration mesh is created. For RPIM, a regular background lattice is built (disregarding completely the nodal spatial position) and then each integration cell is filled with integration points following the Gauss-Legendre quadrature scheme. For the NNRPIM, the Voronoï diagram is used to define the required integration cells, which are filled with integration points following the same procedure as the RPIM (Jorge Belinha, 2014). Notice that, since the NNRPIM procedure (only) depends on the Voronoï diagram, it (only) depends on the nodal spatial position. Thus, the NNRPIM constructs the integration mesh using the nodes spatial position. Therefore, the NNRPIM is a truly meshless method. Lastly, it is possible to obtain the field variables under study using approximation or interpolation functions, based on the combination of RBFs with polynomial basis functions.

1.4 *Meshless methods in biomechanics*

These advanced discrete methods have not yet been widely applied in dentistry. Therefore, most of the work done so far was to validate this approach.

The results obtained in different analysis—by using this advanced discretization computational technique—were compared with those obtained either experimentally or with other numeric methods. Meshless methods proved to be useful for: (1) the analysis of the biomechanical behaviour of dental prostheses (Andrade, Belinha, Dinis, & Natal Jorge, 2013); (2) predicting the loads that should be applied to dental implants to maximize bone density near the implant (by combining meshless methods with bone remodelling algorithms) (J. Belinha, Dinis, & Jorge, 2014) (J. Belinha, Dinis, & Natal Jorge, 2013); (3) predicting osseointegration around the contact area between bone and implant (J. Belinha, Dinis, & Jorge, 2015); (4) studying the interactions between bone tissue and an implant, which will allow to select the best clinical solution (by combining meshless methods with an elasto-plastic model) (C. S. S. Tavares et al., 2015); (5) predicting the biomechanical behaviour of restored teeth (C. Tavares et al., 2015) (C. S. Tavares, Belinha, Dinis, & Natal, 2016) (C. S. Tavares, Belinha, Dinis, & Natal Jorge, 2014); and (6) predicting the principal and secondary trabecular structures (by combining meshless methods with bone remodelling algorithms) (J. Belinha et al., 2015). Like in FEM, it is imperative to consider the presence of adjacent teeth, since these are important for the prevention of possible fractures (C. S. Tavares et al., 2016).

Meshless methods were also applied to study a cantilever bridge supported by two implants, by varying the bar material and subjecting the bridge to two different load cases. It was possible to verify that as the stiffness of the bar increases, the stresses in the bone tissue also increase and the stresses in the implants decrease (Duarte, Belinha, Dinis, & Natal Jorge, 2013).

2 MATERIAL AND METHODS

This work aims to simulate the effect of the resin-cement used on the mechanical resistance of a resin-bonded dental bridge.

A single-retainer design was introduced in the beginning of the 1980s, as a way to try avoiding the debonding of one of the retainer wings, that frequently occurred in the two-retainer design (Hopkins, 1981). Therefore, both designs were also simulated.

The materials' behaviour was considered as elastic, homogeneous and isotropic. The mechanical properties are given in Table 1.

A two-dimensional (2D) model was constructed based on an anonymized orthopantomography of an unknown patient. Using an image analysis software, with this medical imaging exam, it was possible to obtain the measurements and geometry of each teeth considered. The obtained model consists of mandibular central incision, lateral incisor and canine. In this model, the central incisor and the canine represent the abutment teeth, and the lateral incisor the pontic tooth. Moreover, wings with 0.4 mm of thickness were built on each side of the pontic tooth, thus simulating the presence of the adhesive, as represented in Figure 1.

To simulate the presence of only one wing, to the right-side wing was assigned the following properties: E = 0.0841 MPa and $\upsilon = 0.3$.

The domain of the problem was discretized in a mesh of triangular elements, represented in Figure 1.

Table 1. Mechanical properties (Cornacchia, Las Casas, Cimini, & Peixoto, 2010) (Moreira, Belinha, Dinis, & Jorge, 2014) (Della Bona, Donassollo, Demarco, Barrett, & Mecholsky, 2007) (Manicone, Rossi Iommetti, & Raffaelli, 2007).

Material		Young's Modulus (E) [GPa]	Poisson's Ratio (υ)
Enamel		84.1	0.33
Dentin		14.7	0.31
Pulp		0.02	0.45
Zirconia		245	0.26
Resin-cement	Admira Fusion VOCO (A)	3.6	0.3
	Brilliant Coltene (B)	2.3	0.3
	NC Coltene (NC)	2.3	0.3

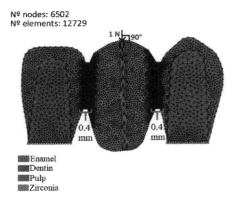

Figure 1. Representation of the global 2D geometric model, boundary and load conditions considered and element mesh.

In this study as a natural boundary condition it was assumed a 1 N load, with 90° of inclination with the longitudinal axis of the tooth. The bottom nodes of the central incisor and the canine were constrained in both Ox and Oy directions.

Three numerical methods were used: FEM, RPIM and NNRPIM. Thus, the results of all methods were compared, and their performance was evaluated.

3 RESULTS AND DISCUSSION

In Figure 2 are represented the colour dispersion maps of principal stress σ1, for the presence of both "one-wing" or "two-wings" solutions and for the resin-cement Admira, once all the adhesives seemed to present a similar behaviour. These results are shown for FEM.

As it can be verified in Figure 2, when using the single-retainer design, the maximum principal stress obtained is ten times higher than the one obtained when using the two-retainer design. In Figure 2(b), is possible to observe a peak of stress concentration in the left inferior area of the central incisor. However, this is due to element mesh distortion.

To better evaluate the stress distribution along the retainer wing and understand the effect of one or two wings, it was graphically represented the principal stress σ1 and maximum shear stress τ_{max}, obtained with Equation (1), along selected points of the left wing, marked by the red line in Figure 3. This distribution was obtained for the three methods (FEM, RPIM and NNRPIM), to better understand the differences between them.

$$\tau_{max} = |\sigma_{11} - \sigma_{22}|/2 \qquad (1)$$

As it can be seen in Figure 4, the three methods present similar results: the values of principal stress σ1 and maximum shear stress τ_{max}, along the left wing, are higher for the single-retainer design. However, RPIM presents a higher variation of values along the retainer wing.

It was also evaluated the total displacement in the node marked in Figure 3, for the three methods, and for the different adhesive materials. These data are presented in Figure 5.

It can be verified that the total displacement is higher for the single-retainer design and for the

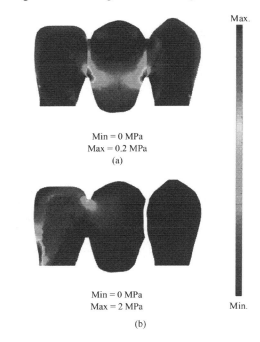

Figure 2. The principal stress σ1 map for: (a) two-retainer design and (b) single-retainer design. The colour maps are for Admira resin-cement and FEM analysis.

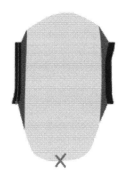

Figure 3. The red line indicates the nodes where the principal stresses σ1 and σ2 were analysed. The red cross indicates de node where the total displacement was analysed.

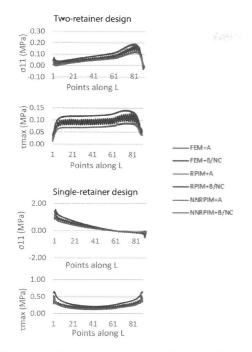

Figure 4. Graphic representation of principal stress σ1 and maximum shear stress τmax, in points along left retainer wing of the dental bridge.

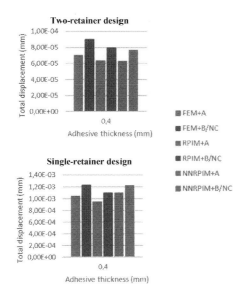

Figure 5. Histograms of total displacement for a node in the inferior portion of the pontic.

adhesive Brilliant and NC Coltene. The results for the three methods are very similar, being FEM and NNRPIM the closest.

4 CONCLUSIONS

In the two-retainer design, there is a high concentration of tensile stresses in the inferior part of the connector, while in the single-retainer design occurs the opposite, i.e. there is a high concentration of tensile stresses in the superior area of the connector (Figure 2 and Figure 4). As it can be seen in Figure 4, the values of principal stress σ1 and maximum shear stress τ_{max}, along the left wing, are higher for the single-retainer design. Also, for the total displacement of the pontic it was verified that this is higher for the single-retainer design (Figure 5).

Therefore, it can be concluded that the connectors are the weakest areas, once this is the area with highest stress concentration. Moreover, the single-retainer design increases the risk of debonding.

Regarding the resin-cement, all materials presented a similar behaviour, except for the total displacement, that was higher for Brilliant and NC Coltene adhesives.

In addition, the results obtained using meshless methods are in agreement with the FEM. RPIM presented more inconstant results, which was due to the lower thickness of the adhesive. Therefore, when the radial search is performed, the influence-domains of the point of interest include alternately nodes from the adhesive and the more resistant material, either enamel or zirconia, depending on the side. Thus, when analysing materials with lower thickness, FEM and NNRPIM, provide more reliable results.

ACKNOWLEDGEMENTS

The authors truly acknowledge the funding provided by Ministério da Ciência, Tecnologia e Ensino Superior—Fundação para a Ciência e a Tecnologia (Portugal) by project funding MIT-EXPL/ISF/0084/2017. Additionally, the authors gratefully acknowledge the funding of Project NORTE-01-0145-FEDER-000022—SciTech—Science and Technology for Competitive and Sustainable Industries, cofinanced by Programa Operacional Regional do Norte (NORTE2020), through Fundo Europeu de Desenvolvimento Regional (FEDER).

REFERENCES

Andrade, J.R., Belinha, J., Dinis, L.M.J.S., & Natal Jorge, R.M. (2013). Analysis of dental implant using a meshless method. In *Biodental Engineering II—Proceedings of the 2nd International Conference on Biodental Engineering* (pp. 145–150).

Belinha, J. (2014). Meshless Methods in Biomechanics: Bone Tissue Remodelling Analysis. In *Lecture Notes in Computational Vision and Biomechanics*. Springer. https://doi.org/https://doi.org/10.1007/978-3-319-06400-0

Belinha, J., Dinis, L.M.J.S., & Jorge, R.M.N. (2014). The bone tissue remodelling analysis in dentistry using a meshless method. In *Biodental Engineering III—Proceedings of the 3rd International Conference on Biodental Engineering* (pp. 213–220). https://doi.org/10.1201/b17071-40.

Belinha, J., Dinis, L.M.J.S., & Jorge, R.M.N. (2015). The Mandible Remodeling Induced By Dental Implants: a Meshless Approach. *Journal of Mechanics in Medicine and Biology*, *15*(4), 1550059-1-31. https://doi.org/10.1142/S0219519415500591.

Belinha, J., Dinis, L.M.J.S., & Natal Jorge, R.M. (2013). Mandible bone tissue remodelling analysis using a new numerical approach. In *Biodental Engineering II—Proceedings of the 2nd International Conference on Biodental Engineering* (pp. 151–157).

Bushberg, J.T., Seibert, J.A., Leidholdt, E.M., Boone, J.M., & Goldschmidt, E.J. (2003). The Essential Physics of Medical Imaging. *Medical Physics*, *30*(7), 1936. https://doi.org/10.1118/1.1585033.

Cornacchia, T.P.M., Las Casas, E.B., Cimini, C.A., & Peixoto, R.G. (2010). 3D finite element analysis on esthetic indirect dental restorations under thermal and mechanical loading. *Medical & Biological Engineering & Computing*, *48*(11), 1107–1113. https://doi.org/10.1007/s11517-010-0661-7.

Della Bona, A., Donassollo, T.A., Demarco, F.F., Barrett, A.A., & Mecholsky, J.J. (2007). Characterization and surface treatment effects on topography of a glass-infiltrated alumina/zirconia-reinforced ceramic. *Dental Materials*, *23*(6), 769–775. https://doi.org/10.1016/j.dental.2006.06.043.

Dinis, L.M.J.S., Natal Jorge, R.M., & Belinha, J. (2007). Analysis of 3D solids using the natural neighbour radial point interpolation method. *Computer Methods in Applied Mechanics and Engineering*, *196*, 2009–2028. https://doi.org/10.1016/j.cma.2006.11.002.

Duarte, H.M.S., Belinha, J., Dinis, L.M.J.S., & Natal Jorge, R.M. (2013). Analysis of a bar-implant using meshless method. In *Biodental Engineering II—Proceedings of the 2nd International Conference on Biodental Engineering* (pp. 139–144).

Durey, K.A., Nixon, P.J., Robinson, S., & Chan, M.F.W.Y. (2011). Resin bonded bridges: Techniques for success. *British Dental Journal*, *211*(3), 113–118. https://doi.org/10.1038/sj.bdj.2011.619.

Farah, J.W., Craig, R.G., & Sikarskie, D.L. (1973). Photoelastic and Finite Element Stress Analysis of a Restored Axisymmetric First Molar. *J. Biomechanics*, *6*(5), 511–520.

Geng, J.-P., Tan, K.B.C., & Liu, G.-R. (2001). Application of finite element analysis in implant dentistry: A review of the literature. *J Prosthet Dent*, *85*(6), 585–598. https://doi.org/10.1067/mpr.2001.115251.

Hopkins, C. (1981). An immediate cantilever Rochette bridge. *British Dental Journal*, *151*(9), 292–295. https://doi.org/10.1038/sj.bdj.4804691.

Li, W., Swain, M.V., Li, Q., Ironside, J., & Steven, G.P. (2004). Fibre reinforced composite dental bridge. Part II: Numerical investigation. *Biomaterials*, *25*(20), 4995–5001. https://doi.org/10.1016/j.biomaterials.2004.01.011.

Lopes, I., Correia, A., Viana, P.C., Kovacs, Z., Viriato, N., Campos, J.C.R., & Vaz, M.A. (2014). All-ceramic CAD-CAM Maryland bridge—a numerical stress analysis. In *Biodental Engineering III—Proceedings of the 3rd International Conference on Biodental Engineering* (pp. 291–294). https://doi.org/10.1201/b17071.

Magne, P. (2007). Efficient 3D finite element analysis of dental restorative procedures using micro-CT data. *Dental Materials*, *23*(5), 539–548. https://doi.org/10.1016/j.dental.2006.03.013.

Manicone, P.F., Rossi Iommetti, P., & Raffaelli, L. (2007). An overview of zirconia ceramics: Basic properties and clinical applications. *Journal of Dentistry*, *35*(11), 819–826. https://doi.org/10.1016/j.jdent.2007.07.008.

Moratal, D. (2016). *Finite Element Analysis: From Biomedical Applications to Industrial Developments*. (D. Moratal, Ed.) (Second Edi). InTech.

Moreira, S.F., Belinha, J., Dinis, L.M.J.S., & Jorge, R.M.N. (2014). A global numerical analysis of the "central incisor/local maxillary bone" system using a meshless method. *Molecular & Cellular Biomechanics: MCB*, *11*(3), 151–184. https://doi.org/10.3970/mcb.2014.011.151.

Srirekha, A., & Bashetty, K. (2010). Infinite to finite: An overview of finite element analysis. *Indian Journal of Dental Research*, *21*(3), 425. https://doi.org/10.4103/0970-9290.70813.

Tavares, C., Belinha, J., Dinis, L., & Jorge, R.N. (2015). The numerical analysis of a restored tooth using meshless methods. *Proceedings—2015 IEEE 4th Portuguese Meeting on Bioengineering, ENBENG 2015*. https://doi.org/10.1109/ENBENG.2015.7088872.

Tavares, C.S., Belinha, J., Dinis, L., & Natal, R. (2016). The biomechanical response of a restored tooth due to bruxism : a mesh- less approach. In *BioMedWomen: Proceedings of the International Conference on Clinical and Bioengineering for Women's Health* (pp. 49–56).

Tavares, C.S.S., Belinha, J., Dinis, L.M.J.S., & Natal Jorge, R.M. (2014). Numerical analysis of a teeth restoration: A meshless method approach. In *Biodental Engineering III—Proceedings of the 3rd International Conference on Biodental Engineering* (pp. 207–211).

Tavares, C.S.S., Belinha, J., Dinis, L.M.J.S., & Natal Jorge, R.M. (2015). The elasto-plastic response of the bone tissue due to the insertion of dental implants. *Procedia Engineering*, *110*, 37–44. https://doi.org/10.1016/j.proeng.2015.07.007.

Thresher, R.W., & Saito, G.E. (1973). The stress analysis of human teeth. *Journal of Biomechanics*, *6*, 443–449. https://doi.org/10.1016/0021-9290(73)90003-1.

Vallittu, P.K., & Sevelius, C. (2000). Resin-bonded, glass fiber-reinforced composite fixed partial dentures: a clinical study. *The Journal of Prosthetic Dentistry*, *84*(4), 413–418. https://doi.org/10.1067/mpr.2000.109782.

Walmsley, A.D., Walsh, T.F., Lumley, P., Burke, F.J.T., Shortall, A.C., Hayes-Hall, R., & Pretty, I. (2007). *Restorative Dentistry*. (Elsevier, Ed.) (Second Edi). Churchill Livingstone. Retrieved from https://www.sciencedirect.com/science/book/9780443102462.

Zienkiewicz, O.C., & Taylor, R.L. (1994). *The finite element method* (4th ed). London: McGraw-Hill.

Śmielak, B., Świniarski, J., Wołowiec-Korecka, E., & Klimek, L. (2016). 2D-finite element analysis of inlay-, onlay bridges with using various materials. *International Scientific Journal*, *79*(2), 71–78.

Biodental Engineering V – Belinha et al. (Eds)
© 2019 Taylor & Francis Group, London, ISBN 978-0-367-21087-8

Using meshless methods to analyse bone remodelling after the insertion of a femoral implant

A.T.A. Castro
Faculty of Engineering, University of Porto (FEUP), Porto, Portugal

M.M.A. Peyroteo
Institute of Mechanical Engineering (IDMEC), Unit of Design and Experimental Validation, Porto, Portugal

J. Belinha
Department of Mechanical Engineering, School of Engineering, Polytechnic of Porto (ISEP), Porto, Portugal

R.M. Natal Jorge
Department of Mechanical Engineering, Faculty of Engineering, University of Porto (FEUP), Porto, Portugal

ABSTRACT: Over the years, the number of hip arthroplasties has increased significantly, and the literature indicates that the number of new cases, in the coming decades around the world, will continue to grow. There are several factors that lead to failure of the implant, one of the most critical being the phenomenon of stress shielding. This phenomenon is responsible for triggering the process of bone resorption as a result of the change in the typical stress field to which the bone is subjected after insertion of an implant. The main objective of this work was to analyse the bone remodelling process in the surrounding bone tissue after the insertion of a femoral implant, combining a material law of bone tissue recently developed by Belinha, and three numerical discretization methods: Finite Element Method (FEM) and two meshless methods—the Radial Point Interpolation Method RPIM and Natural Neighbour Radial Point Interpolation Method (NNRPIM). The results obtained allow to conclude that the algorithm of bone remodelling used accurately predicts the main and secondary trabecular structure. Finally, comparing both numerical methods, it was possible to observe that the RPIM and NNRPIM meshless methods produce smoother stress fields when compared to FEM, which corroborates the literature. The results presented in this work, shows that meshless methods provide a viable and reliable alternative to the FEM, with respect to biomechanical problems.

1 INTRODUCTION

Every year, about one million total hip arthroplasties (THA) are performed worldwide. The aging of the population, the decrease in the average age of the patients who need this surgical intervention, as well as the limited lifespan of the prosthesis components are factors that inevitably will cause an increase in the number of people who need this surgery in the future (Holzwarth & Cotogno, 2012).

Orthopedic prostheses are considered one of the most innovative products in the field of biomedical engineering, being subjected to continuous research and development. Most THA prostheses are commonly composed of four distinct parts: two acetabular components, the femoral head and the neck/femoral stem assembly. There are several factors that lead to failure of the implant, one of the most critical being the

femoral bone loss observed after insertion of the implant into the intramedullary cavity, caused by the stress shielding phenomenon. This phenomenon is responsible for triggering the process of bone resorption as a result of the change in the stress field to which the bone is subjected after insertion of an implant.

Therefore, bone tissue presents itself as a dynamic material with the ability to adapt to different mechanical environments. Wolff was the first investigator to defend the idea that bone remodelling is induced by stress or strain. Wolff has found that the orientation of the trabecular bone tissue coincides with the direction of the stress lines, i.e. the bone adapts its internal structure according to the loads applied (Wolff, 1986).

In an attempt to better understand the dynamics of bone remodelling, a large number of researchers dedicated themselves to the development of empirical laws capable of mathematically describe this phenomenon.

Fyhrie and Carter (Fyhrie & Carter, 1986) developed a 'self-optimization' theory in order to predict the apparent bone density (or density fraction), as well as the trabecular orientation of the bone tissue. The numerical model proposed by Carter et al. allows to consider several mechanical cases and assumes that the mechanical stimulus is proportional to the equivalent stress field.

In the following years, several authors proposed numerous versions of the Carter algorithm. Beaupré et al., expanded Carter's idea by developing a time-dependent modelling/remodelling theory, based on the response to daily loading history. The theory basically argues that the bone needs a certain level of stimulation for its maintenance, and when superior stimulation is applied, additional bone will be deposited, otherwise the bone will be reabsorbed (Beaupré, Orr, & Carter, 1990a). Pettermann et al. (Pettermann, Reiter, & Rammerstorfer, 1997) proposed a new version of Carter's algorithm. These authors used the optimization criterion of Strain Energy Density (SED), combining the adaptation of the bone spatial distribution with the reorientation of the main axis of the material and the rigidity parameters.

The theory of adaptive elasticity was developed by Cowin et al., and argues that living tissues alter their shape to fit the mechanical loads (S. C. Cowin & Hegedus, 1976) (S. C. Cowin, Sadegh, & Luo, 1992) (Stephen C. Cowin, 1985). This theory is based on the theory of linear elasticity, complemented by equations that allow to express the changes in the density and external shape of the bone. At first, this theory was modelled to simulate the external remodelling, and this was later complemented to simulate the trabecular bone adaptation. Cowin et al. introduced the notion of fabric tensor with the ability to manifest the anisotropy of the trabecular bone. The fabric tensor is a second-order symmetric tensor that describes the arrangement of trabeculae and pores (Stephen C. Cowin, 1985). The equilibrium state of bone remodelling is reached when the stress (and strain) principal directions are in accordance with the fabric tensor principal axes, i.e. characterized by the condition that there is no realignment of the trabecular architecture, nor absorption or deposition of trabecular bone tissue.

Bone tissue is clearly an anisotropic heterogeneous material. However, the initial bone models were considered isotropic. Carter and Hayes were the first authors to correlate the apparent density of bone tissue with various mechanical properties such as elastic modulus and ultimate compressive stress (Carter & Hayes, 1977). Later several authors established new laws of anisotropic bone material, based on experimental studies, being Lotz the pioneer (Lotz, Gerhart, & Hayes, 1991).

This work uses the phenomenological law proposed by Belinha (Jorge Belinha, 2014). Following the work of Zioupus, Belinha proposed a mathematical relation correlating the elastic modulus in the axial and transverse direction, with the apparent density of the bone. Based on the results obtained by Lotz, Belinha also suggested the curves for the ultimate compressive stress in the axial and transverse directions.

These mathematical formulations are then incorporated into an algorithm and can be tested using the Finite Element Method (FEM) with the aim of predicting and simulating changes in bone structures. The FEM is the numerical discretization technique most frequently found in the literature. However, due to the increasingly rapid evolution of both science and engineering, computational challenges are increasingly complex (Gu, 2005). Faced with these new challenges, the FEM began to show several limitations, especially in the analysis of some complex problems. The origin of all problems is mainly due to the use of meshes (Gu, 2005). A detailed explanation of the FEM formulation, described by Zienklewicz, can be found in the literature (Zienklewicz & Taylor, 1977).

In the last decades several alternative methods, such as meshless methods, have started to appear (Belytshko, Krongauz, Organ, Fleming, & Krysl, 1996) (Nguyen, Rabczuk, Bordas, & Duflot, 2008). In meshless methods the solid domain is discretised into an unstructured nodal cloud. These methods have presented very precise and flexible results.

In this work, besides FEM, two meshless methods are used—the Radial Point Interpolation Method (RPIM) and the Natural Neighbour Radial Point Interpolation Method (NNRPIM). In the RPIM formulation, nodal connectivity is obtained by overlapping the influence-domain of each node, whereas in the NNRPIM, it is established by overlapping the Voronoï cells. Next, a numerical integration mesh is created adapted to the problem's physical domain. In the particular case of RPIM, the integration mesh is obtained with a background grid, in which the integration cells are filled with integration points respecting the Gauss-Legendre quadrature rule. In the case of NNRIPIM the influence-cells are obtained using geometric and mathematical constructs, such as the Voronoï diagrams and the Delaunay triangulation. Finally, the field variables under study are obtained using approximation or interpolation functions, based on the combination of the radial basis functions (RBF) with polynomial base functions (Jorge Belinha, 2014).

Gradually, meshless methods began to be applied to the analysis of bone structures. Liew et al. (Liew, Wu, & Ng, 2002), presented one of the first studies. Through a femoral bone model, these authors performed a simple stress analysis. However, some limitations were identified, namely the difficulty in manipulating nonconvex limits as well as discontinuities of the material in the bone structure. Later, the first works in bone remodelling began to appear. Doblaré et al. (Doblaré et al., 2005), implemented an anisotropic bone remodelling model using a meshless discretization method. Fernandez et al., presented a study for a better understanding of the mechanisms of remodelling of cortical bone tissue (Fernandez et al., 2013).

Belinha et al., developed a novel bone tissue remodelling algorithm in conjunction with the meshless method, NNRPIM (Jorge Belinha, 2014). This method presents great precision, not presenting the limitations observed in the first studies on the subject. Initially, the model of bone remodelling proposed by Belinha was applied to the microscale (J. Belinha, Natal Jorge, & Dinis, 2012) and was later extended to the macroscale of bone structures such as the calcaneus bone (Jorge Belinha, Jorge, & Dinis, 2013), the femoral bone (Jorge Belinha et al., 2013) (J. Belinha, Dinis, & Natal Jorge, 2016), the mandibula bone (J. Belinha, Dinis, & Jorge, 2015) and maxillary bone (Moreira, Belinha, Dinis, & Jorge, 2014). The results obtained demonstrate a distribution of local apparent bone density and anisotropic bone behaviour entirely in agreement with the structural architecture and the distribution of apparent bone density observed in x-ray images of both the natural bone (J. Belinha et al., 2012) (Jorge Belinha et al., 2013), and the bone with implant (J. Belinha et al., 2015) (J. Belinha et al., 2016). More recently, Peyroteo et al. completed the work developed by Belinha, combining the proposed bone remodelling algorithm with the meshless method, RPIM, and combining three numerical discretization techniques RPIM, NNRPIM and the FEM (Peyroteo, Belinha, Vinga, Dinis, & Natal Jorge, 2018). The remodelling algorithm was able to reproduce typical trabecular bone distributions and all numerical approaches were validated. However, meshless solutions produced smoother and more accurate results, closer to the radiograph images.

2 REMODELLING ALGORITHM

The bone remodelling algorithm adopted in this study was developed by Belinha and consists of an adaptation of the model proposed by Carter (Jorge Belinha, 2014). The process of bone remodelling is activated by a mechanical stimulus, the SED (Strain Energy Density). Figure 1 outlines the algorithm that was implemented in this work. This algorithm is a non-linear procedure that iteratively determines the apparent local bone density and the orientation of the material, and that assumes the phenomenological law proposed by Belinha (Jorge Belinha, 2014). This model of bone remodelling allows its combination with several numerical methods.

In a designated pre-processing phase, the problem domain is discretized in an unstructured nodal mesh, and the numerical integration mesh is then constructed taking into account the chosen numerical method (FEM, RPIM or NNRPIM). The initial properties of the material are then assigned in their domain areas. At this stage, the properties of the material are considered isotropic.

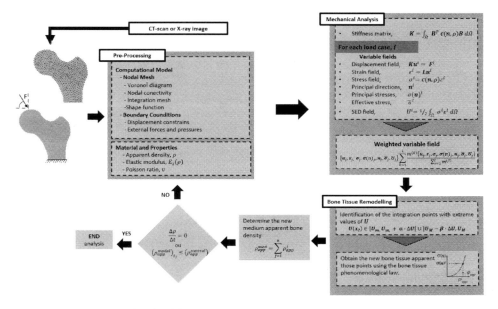

Figure 1. Bone tissue remodelling algorithm.

To obtain the principal directions of the stress field at each integration point, an elasto-static analysis, called a "zero" step, j = 0, is required.

Subsequently, the shape functions for each integration point, x_I, are constructed, $\varphi(x_I)$, and finally the essential and natural boundary conditions are imposed. Only now the iterative remodelling algorithm can be truly initiated. Throughout the iterative process, an analysis is always performed for each instant t_j. The local stiffness matrices, K_I, for each integration point are determined. At the end the local stiffness matrices, K_I, are assembled into global stiffness matrix, K_j. Then, the displacement field can be obtained, $u_j^k = K_j^{-1} f_j^k$, where u_j^k is the unknown displacement field, and f_j^k is the vector of applied forces. After defining the displacement field, u_j^k, it is possible to obtain the stress field, σ_j^k, and strain field, ε_j^k. The strain and stress fields obtained can be used to establish the SED field, U_j^k, the von Mises effective stress, $\bar{\sigma}_j^k$, and also the principal stresses, $\sigma(n)_j^k$ and directions, n_j^k, for each point of interest. Since the algorithm allows to consider numerous load cases, f_j^k, the variable fields obtained for each load case are weighted by the equation observed in the Figure 1.

Then, the algorithm selects the integration points with lower SED weighting values, which are submitted to the density remodelling process, unlike all other points of interest that maintain the previous density. Taking into account the weighted principal stress field, each one of the selected points of interest will update the apparent density using the chosen material law, which in this case is the phenomenological law proposed by Belinha (Jorge Belinha, 2014). Subsequently, after determining the new apparent density, the algorithm progresses to the next iteration step. Next, using the new apparent density field, at each point of interest, the material properties are updated.

The bone tissue remodelling process ends if two consecutive iteration steps present the same medium apparent density, or if the medium apparent density of the model, ρ_{app}^{model}, reaches a controlled value, $\rho_{app}^{control}$, which is a control value determined by the user based on clinical observations The complete description of the remodelling algorithm can be found in the literature (Jorge Belinha, 2014).

3 NUMERICAL ANALYSIS

3.1 Geometrical and numerical model

The present numerical study analyses the remodelling process of bone tissue surrounding the femoral implant, in order to compare the performance of the three methods of numerical discretization previously discussed—FEM, RPIM and NNRPIM.

The two-dimensional numerical model used in this study was based on medical radiographs. In Figure 2 it is presented a detailed description of the dimensions of the analysed numerical model. The femoral bone presents a constant natural cortical layer with 0.5 mm of thickness. The domain of the problem considered was discretized into a mesh of irregular triangular elements. The femur is a bone that is daily subjected to various loads. In this study as natural boundary conditions, the three load cases suggested by Beaupré et al. were considered. As for the essential boundary condition, it was considered the constraint of the lower base of the model, preventing its movement along the Ox and Oy directions (Beaupré et al., 1990a; Beaupré, Orr, & Carter, 1990b). Each case consists of a load distributed parabolically on the femoral head and another distributed parabolically on the greater trochanter. In this model the head of the femur was replaced by a femoral stem, therefore the first load of each case considered is applied to the head of the femoral stem following a uniform distribution. Table 1 shows the magnitude of each load, the corresponding direction and the number of cycles per day, for load case 1 (LC1), load case 2 (LC2) and load case 3 (LC3). The natural and essential boundary conditions are schematically represented in Figure 2.

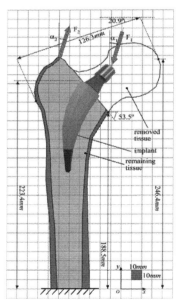

Figure 2. Representation of the global 2D geometric model and boundary and load conditions considered.

Table 1. Load cases.

Load cases	F_1	α_1	F_2	α_2	Load cycles
LC1	2317	24°	703	28°	6000
LC2	1158	−15°	351	−8°	2000
LC3	1548	56°	468	35°	2000

The analysed model assumes a uniform initial density distribution, $\rho_{app}^{max} = 2,1 \, g/cm^3$, and a constant Poisson ratio $v = 0.3$. Regarding the mechanical properties of the bone tissue, these depend on the current apparent density and are obtained through the phenomenological law described above. The femoral stem of Titanium has the following mechanical properties: $E = 110$ GPa and $v = 0.32$. In this study, a cemented interface between the stem and the bone tissue was not considered.

Next, the numerical analysis was performed with FEMAS-Finite Element and Meshless Analysis Software. This software is capable of analysing computationally diverse mechanical problems, using FEM and meshless methods (more details in cmech.webs.com).

3.2 Results

The numerical model presented previously was then analysed using the bone remodelling algorithm, assuming an apparent density control medium value $\rho_{app}^{control} = 1,2 \, g/cm^3$, and considering the three numerical approaches: FEM, RPIM, NNRPIM. The literature suggests that human long bones have apparent density between 0,9 e 1,2 g/cm^3 (Keyak, Kaneko, Tehranzadeh, & Skinner, 2005).

In Figure 3 and Figure 4 are presented the colour maps of the final von Mises effective stress distribution and the final trabecular architecture, respectively for FEM, RPIM and NNRPIM. The results regarding the evolution of the trabecular architecture are presented as isomaps of gray scale. In these isomaps the white colour represents the minimum apparent density of $\rho_{app}^{min} = 0,1 \, g/cm^3$, and the dark gray color represents the maximum apparent density $\rho_{app}^{max} = 2,1 \, g/cm^3$. All other shades of gray represent apparent transient densities.

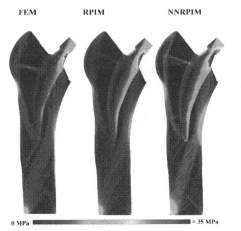

Figure 3. Final von Mises effective stress distribution using FEM, RPIM e NNRPIM and considering $\rho_{app}^{control} = 1,2 \, g/cm^3$.

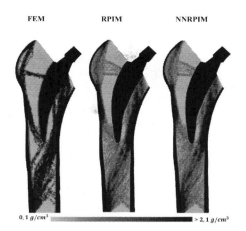

Figure 4. Final obtained bone tissue trabecular architecture, using FEM, RPIM e NNRPIM and considering $\rho_{app}^{control} = 1,2 \, g/cm^3$.

4 CONCLUSION

The aim of this study was to predict the remodelling of the femoral bone after insertion of a femoral implant, by combining three numerical discretization methods (FEM, RPIM and NNRPIM) with the bone remodelling algorithm considered. As described above, when the femoral head is removed and replaced by a femoral stem, the stress field on the bone will change, stress-shielding occurs. The results obtained allowed to conclude that the proposed methodology predicts the main and secondary trabecular structure. For the three numerical approaches used, it was possible to observe that in this type of stems the highest concentration of stresses is observed in the head of the implant and that the observed trabecular distribution is coherent with other results found in the literature (Gong, Kong, Zhang, Fang, & Zhao, 2013). Comparing both numerical methods, it was possible to observe that meshless methods produce smoother stress fields, when compared to the FEM, corroborating the literature that shows that meshless methods provide a viable and reliable alternative to FEM with respect to biomechanical problems. Finally, it is believed that the methodology presented here possesses a significant progression potential, namely in the prediction of bone remodelling after implant insertion.

ACKNOWLEDGEMENTS

The authors truly acknowledge the funding provided by Ministério da Ciência, Tecnologia e Ensino Superior—Fundação para a Ciência e a Tecnologia (Portugal), under grants: SFRH/

BD/133105/2017 and by project funding MIT-EXPL/ISF/0084/2017. Additionally, the authors gratefully acknowledge the funding of Project NORTE-01-0145-FEDER-000022—SciTech—Science and Technology for Competitive and Sustainable Industries, co-financed by Programa Operacional Regional do Norte (NORTE2020), through Fundo Europeu de Desenvolvimento Regional (FEDER).

REFERENCES

Beaupré, G., Orr, T.E., & Carter, D.R. (1990a). An Approach for Time-Dependent Bone Modeling and Remodeling—Theoretical Development. *Journal of Orthopaedic Research*, 8(3), 651–661.

Beaupré, G.S., Orr, T.E., & Carter, D.R. (1990b). An Approach for Time-Dependent Bone Modeling and Remodeling-Application: A Preliminary Remodeling Simulation. *Journal of Orthopaedic Research*, 8, 662–670.

Belinha, J. (2014). *Meshless Methods in Biomechanics: Bone Tissue Remodelling Analysis*. Springer Netherlands. https://doi.org/10.1007/978-94-007-4174-4.

Belinha, J., Dinis, L.M.J.S., & Jorge, R.M.N. (2015). The Mandible Remodeling Induced By Dental Implants: a Meshless Approach. *Journal of Mechanics in Medicine and Biology*, 15(4), 1–31. https://doi.org/10.1142/S0219519415500591.

Belinha, J., Dinis, L.M.J.S., & Natal Jorge, R.M. (2016). The analysis of the bone remodelling around femoral stems: A meshless approach. *Mathematics and Computers in Simulation*, 121, 64–94. https://doi.org/10.1016/j.matcom.2015.09.002.

Belinha, J., Jorge, R.M.N., & Dinis, L.M.J.S. (2013). A meshless microscale bone tissue trabecular remodelling analysis considering a new anisotropic bone tissue material law. *Computer Methods in Biomechanics and Biomedical Engineering*, 16(11), 1170–1184. https://doi.org/10.1080/10255842.2012.654783.

Belinha, J., Natal Jorge, R.M., & Dinis, L.M.J.S. (2012). Bone tissue remodelling analysis considering a radial point interpolator meshless method. *Engineering Analysis with Boundary Elements*, 36(11), 1660–1670. https://doi.org/10.1016/j.enganabound.2012.05.009.

Belytshko, T., Krongauz, Y., Organ, D., Fleming, M., & Krysl, P. (1996). Meshless methods: An overview and recent developments. *Computer Methods Appl. Mech. Engrg*, 139, 3–47. Retrieved from http://www.worldscientific.com/doi/abs/10.1142/S0219876205000673.

Carter, D.R., & Hayes, W.C. . (1977). The Compressive Behavior Porous of Bone Structure as a Two-Phase. *The Journal of Bone and Joint Surgery*, 59(7), 954–962. https://doi.org/10.1007/978-1-4471-5451-8_116.

Cowin, S.C. (1985). The relationship between the elasticity tensor and the fabric tensor. *Mechanics of Materials*, 4, 137–147.

Cowin, S.C., & Hegedus, D.H. (1976). Bone remodeling II: theory of adaptive elasticity. *Journal of Elasticity*, 6(3), 313–326. https://doi.org/10.1007/BF00041724.

Cowin, S.C., Sadegh, A.M., & Luo, G.M. (1992). An evolutionary Wolff's law for trabecular architecture. *Journal of Biomechanical Engineering*, 114(1), 129–136. https://doi.org/10.1115/1.2895436.

Doblaré, M., Cueto, E., Calvo, B., Martínez, M.A., Garcia, J.M., & Cegoñino, J. (2005). On the employ of meshless methods in biomechanics. *Computer Methods in Applied Mechanics and Engineering*, 194(6–8), 801–821. https://doi.org/10.1016/j.cma.2004.06.031.

Fernandez, J.W., Das, R., Cleary, P.W., Hunter, P.J., Thomas, C.D.L., & Clement, J.G. (2013). Using smooth particle hydrodynamics to investigate femoral cortical bone remodelling at the Haversian level. *International Journal for Numerical Methods in Biomedical Engineering*, 29(1), 129–43. https://doi.org/10.1002/cnm.

Fyhrie, D.P., & Carter, D.R. (1986). A unifying principle relating stress to trabecular bone morphology. *Journal of Orthopaedic Research*, 4(3), 304–317. https://doi.org/10.1002/jor.1100040307.

Gong, H., Kong, L., Zhang, R., Fang, J., & Zhao, M. (2013). A femur-implant model for the prediction of bone remodeling behavior induced by cementless stem. *Journal of Bionic Engineering*, 10(3), 350–358. https://doi.org/10.1016/S1672-6529(13)60230-9.

Gu, Y.T. (2005). Meshfree methods and their comparison. *International Journal of Computational Methods*, 2(4), 477–515. https://doi.org/10.1142/S0219876205000673.

Holzwarth, U., & Cotogno, G. (2012). *Total Hip Arthroplasty. Journal of Bone and joint surgery inc* (Vol. 85). https://doi.org/10.2788/31286.

Keyak, J.H., Kaneko, T.S., Tehranzadeh, J., & Skinner, H.B. (2005). Predicting proximal femoral strength using structural engineering models. *Clinical Orthopaedics and Related Research*, (437), 219–228. https://doi.org/10.1097/01.blo.0000164400.37905.22.

Liew, K.M., Wu, H.Y., & Ng, T.Y. (2002). Meshless method for modeling of human proximal femur: treatment of nonconvex boundaries and stress analysis. *Computational Mechanics*, 28(5), 390–400. https://doi.org/10.1007/s00466-002-0303-5.

Lotz, J.C., Gerhart, T.N., & Hayes, W.C. (1991). Mechanical properties of metaphyseal bone in the proximal femur. *Journal of Biomechanics*, 24(5), 317–329. https://doi.org/10.1016/0021-9290(91)90350-V.

Moreira, S.F., Belinha, J., Dinis, L.M.J.S., & Jorge, R.M.N. (2014). A Global Numerical analysis of the "central incisor/local maxillary bone" system using a meshless method. *Molecular & Cellular Biomechanics : MCB*, 11(3), 151–84. https://doi.org/10.3970/mcb.2014.011.151.

Nguyen, V.P., Rabczuk, T., Bordas, S., & Duflot, M. (2008). Meshless methods: A review and computer implementation aspects. *Mathematics and Computers in Simulation*, 79(3), 763–813. https://doi.org/10.1016/j.matcom.2008.01.003.

Pettermann, H.E., Reiter, T., & Rammerstorfer, F. .-. (1997). Computational Simulation of Internal Bone Remodeling, 4, 295–323.

Peyroteo, M.M.A., Belinha, J., Vinga, S., Dinis, L.M.J.S., & Natal Jorge, R.M. (2018). Mechanical bone remodelling: Comparative study of distinct numerical approaches. *Engineering Analysis with Boundary Elements*, 0(January), 1–15. https://doi.org/10.1016/j.enganabound.2018.01.011.

Wolff, J. (1986). *The law of bone remodelling*. (P. Maquet & R. Furlong, Eds.), *Journal of Biomechanics* (Vol. 22). Springer. https://doi.org/10.1016/0021-9290(89)90043-2.

Zienklewicz, O.C., & Taylor, R.L. (1977). *The Finite Element Method - Fifth edition - Volume 1: The Basis* (Fifth, Vol. 1). Butterworth.

Biodental Engineering V – Belinha et al. (Eds)
© 2019 Taylor & Francis Group, London, ISBN 978-0-367-21087-8

Using meshless methods to predict *in-silico* the stress distribution around bone sarcoma

A.T.A. Castro
Faculty of Engineering, University of Porto (FEUP), Porto, Portugal

J. Belinha & E.M.M. Fonseca
Department of Mechanical Engineering, School of Engineering, Polytechnic of Porto (ISEP), Porto, Portugal

R.M. Natal Jorge
Department of Mechanical Engineering, Faculty of Engineering, University of Porto (FEUP), Porto, Portugal

V.C.C. Oliveira & A.F. Oliveira
Institute of Biomedical Sciences Abel Salazar, University of Porto (ICBAS), Porto, Portugal

ABSTRACT: The main concern associated with the presence of bone sarcoma is the weakening of the host bone, which potentially leads to bone fractures. Such unexpected rupture frequently occurs in the proximal femur due to the high loads that this bone is submitted during the gait. Nowadays, the existent methods to predict the risk of bone failure are not sufficient. Therefore, it is necessary to explore new tools, such as computational simulation. The main objective of this work is to study the mechanical effect of the size of a bone sarcoma located in the femoral head, using numerical discretization techniques, such as the well-known Finite Element Method (FEM) and two meshless methods—the Radial Point Interpolation Method (RPIM) and the Natural Neighbour Radial Point Interpolation Method (NNRPIM). The obtained results show that with the progression of the disease, there is a significant increase in the stress field around the sarcoma. In addition, it was possible to verify that meshless methods can produce softer stress fields when compared to FEM. Such conclusions are in concordance with the clinical observation and the literature.

1 STATE OF THE ART

1.1 Introduction

Primary bone sarcoma is rare, however bone is one of the sites of the human body most affected by metastatic cancer (Roodman, 2004) (Coleman, 1997).The main complication associated with this pathology is bone fracture due to bone weakening. These fractures occur in 71% of the cases in the proximal and diaphysis areas of the femur due to significant mechanical stresses, resulting from flexion and torsion during walking (Tanck et al., 2009). Currently, the major problem encountered by orthopedic medicine is the identification of high and low risk cases based on medical imaging. There are no indicators that can accurately predict the imminent risk of a fracture (Miller & Whitehill, 1984) (Hipp, Springfield, & Hayes, 1995).

The finite element models (FE) have demonstrated to be a promising tool for evaluating the mechanical behaviour of bone under load, in order to predict the phenomenon of bone failure (Tanck

et al., 2009). In the literature there is a lack of information regarding the study of femoral bone failure (Spruijt et al., 2006) (Cheal, Spector, & Hayes, 1992).

1.2 Numerical methods

With the development of computer technology, numerical simulation has now become an essential tool in engineering and science. The finite element method (FEM) is the discretization numerical technique most frequently used in academic research and industrial applications. This numerical method was first presented to orthopedic biomechanics in 1972. Since then, several complex problems have been addressed, boosting the development of biomechanics (Brown, 2004).

Due to the rapid evolution of both science and engineering, computational challenges are increasingly complex (Gu, 2005). Faced with these new challenges, the FEM began to show several limitations. The origin of all problems is mainly due to the use of structured meshes (Gu, 2005). Therefore, in the last decades several alternative methods have started to appear, such as the meshless methods (Belytshko, Krongauz, Organ, Fleming, & Krysl, 1996), (Nguyen, Rabczuk, Bordas, & Duflot, 2008).

1.3 *Meshfree advanced discretization techniques*

The main advantage of meshless methods is the capability to discretize virtual models using only scattered nodes (following or not a structured distribution). Such advantage eliminates part of the limitations of the finite element method associated with the dependence of a mesh.

The meshfree methods are subdivided into two different classes: the strong form and the weak form. In a strong formulation, the partial differential equations that describe the problem are directly used to set the problem's equilibrium equations and the final solution is acquired. In a weak formulation the residual weight of each equation is minimized. This residue is given by an approximate or interpolated function that is influenced by a test function (Jorge Belinha, 2014).

The method of Smooth Particle Hydrodynamics (SPH) was one of the first meshless methods (Gingold & Monaghan, 1977). This method is based on a strong formulation. However, in the 1990s other methods were developed based on a weak formulation. This has shown great progress in the last years, being applied mainly in solid mechanics (Nguyen et al., 2008). One of the first meshless methods developed using the weak form was the Diffuse Element Method (DEM) (Nayroles, Touzot, & Villon, 1992). Later, other methods began to emerge, namely the Element Free Galerkin Method (EFGM), which is one of the most well-known methods developed by Belytschko et al. (T. Belytschko & Lu, 1994). Many other meshless methods have been developed, such as the Reproducing Kernel Particle Method (RKPM) (W. K. Liu, Jun, & Zhang, 1995), the Local Pretov-Galerkin Method (MLPG) (S.N. Atluri and T. Zhu, 1998), the Finite Point Method (FPM) (Onate, Idelsohn, & Zienkiewicz, 1996) and the Method of the Finite Spheres (MFS) (De & Bathe, 2000). Nevertheless, despite the success of these methods in computational mechanics, there are still some problems that have not been fully solved (Dinis, Natal Jorge, & Belinha, 2007). The limitations are mainly due to the lack of the Kronecker delta property in the shape functions. This property allows the direct imposition of the essential boundary conditions. The previously mentioned meshless methods use approximation functions instead of interpolation functions, which include this property.

To solve the problem, several interpolated meshless methods have been developed in recent years. Some of the most relevant methods are the Point Interpolation Method (PIM) (G. R. Liu & Gu, 2001), the Radial Point Interpolation Method (RPIM) (Wang & Liu, 2002), the Natural Neighbour Finite Element Method (NNFEM) (Sukumar, Moran, Semenov, & Belikov, 2001) and the Natural Element Method (NEM) (Sukumar, Moran, & Belytschko, 1998). All the methods mentioned use the interpolation functions of Sibson (Jorge Belinha, 2014). A combination of NEM and RPIM gave rise to the Natural Neighbour Radial Point Interpolation Method (NNRPIM) (Dinis et al., 2007). More recently, another method was developed, the Natural Radial Element Method (NREM), that showed to be an effective and truly meshfree method (J. Belinha, Dinis, & Natal Jorge, 2013).

In this study, two meshless methods along with the FEM were used, the RPIM and the NNRPIM. With these advanced discretization methods, the domain of the problem is discretized using a nodal set. Subsequently, it is necessary to establish nodal connectivity through influence-domains, in the case of RPIM, or influence-cells, in the case of NNRPIM. Regarding the numerical integration scheme, RPIM uses a stabilized nodal integration or Gauss integration schemes, while NNRPIM uses numerical integration based on Voronoï cells and Delaunay triangulation (Jorge Belinha, 2014).

1.4 *Meshless methods in biomechanics*

Recently, meshless methods were introduced in the field of biomechanics, proving their usefulness to analyse the behaviour of biological structures. The results obtained using meshless methods present much more accurate stress, strain and displacement fields, when compared with other numerical analysis methods (J Belinha, 2016).

In the biomechanics area, meshless methods present significant advantages when compared to the finite element method, mainly because it allows the simulation of soft materials, such as muscles or internal organs. In addition, it allows to accurately simulate body fluids. Due to the higher precision of this advanced discretization computational techniques in the calculation of stress and strain fields, it becomes pertinent to use meshless methods to predict the adaptive phenomenon of bone remodelling. Studies have shown that the combination of meshless methods with CT (Computed Tomography) and MRI (Magnetic Resonance Imaging) techniques present a higher efficiency than the FEM (Wong, Wang, Zhang, Liu, & Shi, 2010), (Chen et al., 2010).

Doweidar et al. simulated the human collateral ligament and the knee joint, using NEM. The results obtained showed advantages of using this advanced numerical technique, when compared to the finite element method (Doweidar, Calvo, Alfaro, Groenenboom, & Doblaré, 2010). The EFGM was used by Zhang et al. to simulate the brain tissue reaction, demonstrating its ability to manipulate nonlinear hyperelastic materials (Zhang, Wittek, Joldes, Jin, & Miller, 2014). Meshless methods are repeatedly used in hemodynamic studies. In this sense, some authors simulated the movement experienced by blood cells, such as a deformable red blood cell in the blood flow. Other authors have also presented a study on the effect of red blood cells on the primary formation of a blood clot (Mori et al., 2008).

Liew et al. (Liew, Wu, & Ng, 2002) presented one of the first studies on bone structures, using RKPM. Through a femoral bone model, these authors performed a simple stress analysis. However, some limitations were identified, namely the difficulty in manipulating nonconvex limits, as well as discontinuities of the material in the bone structure.

Over time, meshless methods began to be gradually applied in the study of bone remodelling. Doblaré et al. implemented a model of bone remodelling of anisotropic nature, previously developed, in order to prove the applicability of meshless methods (Doblaré et al., 2005). The model of bone remodelling applied is based on the principles of mechanics of continuous damage, correlating the damage with the local porosity of the bone tissue. Numerical studies demonstrated a good performance of the meshless method, NEM. Thus, NEM appears as an efficient alternative to be applied in problems that comprise large deformations.

Subsequently, Lee et al. and Taddei et al. used meshless methods for analysis of bone tissue. Lee et al. used CT images of trabecular bone tissue from the femoral neck to obtain a meshless geometric model (Lee, Chen, Zeng, Eskandarian, & Oskard, 2007). The phenomenon of trabecular bone fracture at the microscale level was modelled and simulated, thus predicting osteoporosis. Taddei et al. presented a study of prediction of deformations in long bones, particularly in femur (Taddei, Pani, Zovatto, Tonti, & Viceconti, 2008).

Fernandez et al. carried out a study in order to understand better the mechanisms of remodelling of cortical bone tissue (Fernandez et al., 2013). Thus, it was possible to better interpret the mechanisms that increase the vulnerability of bones, making them more susceptible to fracture. The numerical approach adopted was based on the meshless method SPH, capable of representing the characteristics of bone remodelling at the level of the Havers channels.

More recently, Belinha et al. developed a new bone tissue remodelling algorithm combined with the meshless method NNRPIM (J. Belinha, Natal Jorge, & Dinis, 2012), (Jorge Belinha, Jorge, & Dinis, 2013). This method presents high accuracy, eliminating the limitations observed in the first studies on the subject. However, the main disadvantage associated with this approach is the significant computational cost in a three-dimensional analysis. The developed works have demonstrated that the precision and flexibility of the NNRPIM technique may in the future improve the numerical analysis of the process of bone regeneration after fracture and the process of osseointegration. Belinha et al. extended the approach described previously, presenting a study analysing the remodelling of the femoral bone after insertion of an implant (J. Belinha, Dinis, & Natal Jorge, 2016). The main purpose of this work was to numerically analyse the remodelling of the bone tissue surrounding the implant to predict the necrosis of the femoral head and to understand what requests cause this pathology. The results obtained demonstrated a distribution of local apparent bone density and anisotropic bone behaviour entirely in agreement with the structural architecture and the distribution of apparent bone density observed in x-ray images of both the natural bone, (J. Belinha et al., 2012), (Jorge Belinha et al., 2013), and bone with implant (J. Belinha, Dinis, & Jorge, 2015), (J. Belinha et al., 2016).

2 NUMERICAL ANALYSIS

2.1 Geometrical and numerical models

This work aims to simulate the effect of size of a bone sarcoma located in the proximal femur and to compare the performance of the three numerical methods: FEM, RPIM and NNRPIM. To replicate this pathology, three numerical models were constructed. In these models, it was represented a bone sarcoma in the region of the femoral neck. The position of the sarcoma is always the same, schematically represented in Figure 1(a). However, its size varies for each model. The shape of the sarcoma respects an ellipse, as Figure 1(a) shows. In each model, the size of the ellipse (ruled by radius a and b) varies accordingly with the values presented in Table 1.

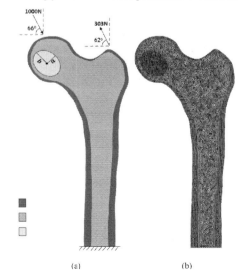

Figure 1. (a) Representation of the global 2D geometric model and boundary and load conditions considered. (b) Element mesh.

Table 1. Description of the three models used.

Models	Size of bone sarcoma a (mm)	b (mm)	Nodes	Elements
Model 1	6	10	6764	13081
Model 2	10	14	6795	13143
Model 3	14	18	6882	13317

Table 2. Mechanical properties.

Materials	Young's modulus (E) [GPa]	Poisson's ratio (υ)
Cortical bone	17	0.3
Trabecular bone	2.13	0.3
Sarcoma	2.5×10^{-6}	0.3

The domain of the three geometric models considered was discretized in a mesh of triangular elements, being the number of nodes and elements of each model listed in Table 1. The three numerical models presented in this work have a uniform nodal distribution as shown in Figure 1 (b).

The three bone models are composed of a layer of cortical bone (external), with minimum thickness of 0.5 mm and maximum thickness of 5 mm, trabecular bone and a bone sarcoma. The materials considered have an elastic, homogeneous and isotropic linear behaviour, and the mechanical properties are summarized in Table 2.

In this study as a natural boundary condition, a representative load was assumed for a patient weighing 100 kg, consisting of a parabolic load distributed on the femoral head and another parabolic load distributed in the greater trochanter. The essential boundary condition imposed was the restriction of the lower surface of the models, constraining their movement in all directions. In Figure 1(a), it is possible to observe the result of each applied load and the corresponding direction, adapted from the first load case suggested by Beaupré et al., as well as the essential boundary condition (Beaupré, Orr, & Carter, 1990).

Next, the numerical analysis was performed with FEMAS-Finite Element and Meshless Analysis Software. This software is capable of analysing computationally diverse mechanical problems, using FEM and meshless methods (more details in cmech.webs.com).

2.2 *Results*

The results obtained from the computational analysis of the three previously described models are presented, using the three numerical methods: FEM, RPIM and NNRPIM. The colour maps of the equivalent von Mises stress for the three models are presented in the Figure 2.

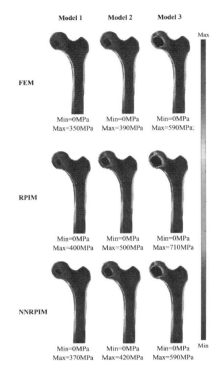

Figure 2. The von Mises stress map for Model 1, Model 2 and Model 3 for FEM, RPIM and NNRPIM analysis.

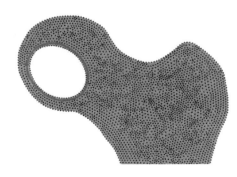

Figure 3. The red line indicates the nodes that surround the sarcoma, where the principal stress 1 was analysed.

To understand the effect of sarcoma size, the red nodes observed in the Figure 3 were selected (these nodes are in the boundary of the sarcoma). Then, the stress value on each of these nodes was obtained and documented. Thus, it was possible to construct a graph showing the variation of the stress along the sarcoma boundary, Figure 4. The results plotted in Figure 4 only correspond to the NNRPIM analyses (for the three studied models).

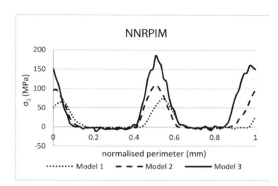

Figure 4. Graphic distribution of principal stress 1 along selected nodes that surround sarcoma, for model 1, 2 and 3.

3 CONCLUSION

In conclusion, observing the colour dispersion maps, it was verified that regardless of the methodology used, the maximum stress observed increases with the increase of sarcoma size, especially in the cortical bone, as would be expected. It is concluded that this case of bone sarcoma is critical, since the maximum stress observed is superior to the ultimate compressive stress of the bone, which will result in fracture of the femoral neck. Additionally, with the growth of the sarcoma, it was possible to observe in Figure 4 a consequent increase of principal stress in the nodes surrounding the sarcoma, which is in concordance with the equivalent von Mises stress colour maps. Regarding the different methodologies used, it was possible to conclude that meshless methods (RPIM and NNRPIM), allow to achieve smoother distribution stress maps, which is in agreement with the literature. In addition, the solution obtained using meshless methods is in agreement with the FEM, corroborating the literature that shows that meshless methods provide a viable and reliable alternative to the FEM for biomechanical analysis (Jorge Belinha, 2014). Finally, this study shows that the biomechanical effect of bone sarcoma is relevant and its size and position significantly influences the structural resistance of the femur bone.

ACKNOWLEDGEMENTS

The authors acknowledge the funding provided by Ministério da Ciência, Tecnologia e Ensino Superior—Fundação para a Ciência e a Tecnologia (Portugal) by project funding MIT-EXPL/ISF/0084/2017. The authors acknowledge the funding of Project NORTE-01-0145-FEDER-000022—SciTech—Science and Technology for Competitive and Sustainable Industries, cofinanced by Programa Operacional Regional do Norte (NORTE2020), through Fundo Europeu de Desenvolvimento Regional (FEDER).

REFERENCES

Atluri, S.N. and T. Zhu. (1998). A new Meshless Local Petrov-Galerkin (MLPG) approach in computational mechanics. *Computational Mechanics*, 22, 117–127.

Beaupré, G.S., Orr, T.E., & Carter, D.R. (1990). An Approach for Time-Dependent Bone Modeling and Remodeling-Application: A Preliminary Remodeling Simulation. *Journal of Orthopaedic Research*, 8, 662–670.

Belytschko, T., L.G., & Lu, Y.Y. (1994). Fracture and crack growth by element free Galerkin methods. *Model. Simul. Mater. Sci. Engrg.*, 2, 519–534.

Belinha, J. (2014). *Meshless Methods in Biomechanics: Bone Tissue Remodelling Analysis*. Springer Netherlands. https://doi.org/10.1007/978-94-007-4174-4.

Belinha, J. (2016). Meshless Methods: The Future of Computational Biomechanical Simulation. *Journal of Biometrics & Biostatistics*, 7(4). https://doi.org/10.4172/2155-6180.1000325.

Belinha, J., Dinis, L.M.J.S., & Jorge, R.M.N. (2015). The Mandible Remodeling Induced By Dental Implants: a Meshless Approach. *Journal of Mechanics in Medicine and Biology*, 15(4), 1–31. https://doi.org/10.1142/S0219519415500591.

Belinha, J., Dinis, L.M.J.S., & Natal Jorge, R.. (2013). The natural radial element method. *International Jornal For Numerical Methods in Engineering*, 93, 1286–1313. https://doi.org/10.1002/nme.

Belinha, J., Dinis, L.M.J.S., & Natal Jorge, R.M. (2016). The analysis of the bone remodelling around femoral stems: A meshless approach. *Mathematics and Computers in Simulation*, 121, 64–94. https://doi.org/10.1016/j.matcom.2015.09.002.

Belinha, J., Jorge, R.M.N., & Dinis, L.M.J.S. (2013). A meshless microscale bone tissue trabecular remodelling analysis considering a new anisotropic bone tissue material law. *Computer Methods in Biomechanics and Biomedical Engineering*, 16(11), 1170–1184. https://doi.org/10.1080/10255842.2012.654783.

Belinha, J., Natal Jorge, R.M., & Dinis, L.M.J.S. (2012). Bone tissue remodelling analysis considering a radial point interpolator meshless method. *Engineering Analysis with Boundary Elements*, 36(11), 1660–1670. https://doi.org/10.1016/j.enganabound.2012.05.009.

Belytschko, T., Krongauz, Y., Organ, D., Fleming, M., & Krysl, P. (1996). Meshless methods: An overview and recent developments. *Computer Methods Appl. Mech. Engrg*, 139, 3–47. Retrieved from http://www.worldscientific.com/doi/abs/10.1142/S0219876205000673.

Brown, T.D. (2004). Finite element modeling in musculoskeletal biomechanics. *Journal of Applied Biomechanics*, 20(4), 336–366. https://doi.org/10.1123/jab.20.4.336.

Cheal, E.J., Spector, M., & Hayes, W.C. (1992). Role of loads and prostheses material properties on the mechanics of the proximal femur after total hip arthroplasty. *J Orthop Res.*, 10, 405–422.

Chen, T., Kim, S., Goyal, S., Jabbour, S., Zhou, J., Rajagopal, G., … Yue, N. (2010). Object-constrained meshless deformable algorithm for high speed 3D nonrigid registration between CT and CBCT. *Medical Physics*, 37(1), 197–210. https://doi.org/10.1118/1.3271389.

Coleman, R.E. (1997). Skeletal complications of malignancy. *Cancer*, *80*(8 Suppl), 1588–94. https://doi.org/10.1002/(SICI)1097-0142(19971015)80:8+<1588::AID-CNCR9 > 3.0.CO;2-G.

De, S., & Bathe, K.J. (2000). The method of finite spheres. *Computational Mechanics*, *25*(4), 329–345. https://doi.org/10.1007/s004660050481.

Dinis, L.M.J.S., Natal Jorge, R.M., & Belinha, J. (2007). Analysis of 3D solids using the natural neighbour radial point interpolation method. *Computer Methods in Applied Mechanics and Engineering*, *196*(13–16), 2009–2028. https://doi.org/10.1016/j.cma.2006.11.002.

Doblaré, M., Cueto, E., Calvo, B., Martínez, M.A., Garcia, J.M., & Cegoñino, J. (2005). On the employ of meshless methods in biomechanics. *Computer Methods in Applied Mechanics and Engineering*, *194*(6–8), 801–821. https://doi.org/10.1016/j.cma.2004.06.031.

Doweidar, M.H., Calvo, B., Alfaro, I., Groenenboom, P., & Doblaré, M. (2010). A comparison of implicit and explicit natural element methods in large strains problems: Application to soft biological tissues modeling. *Computer Methods in Applied Mechanics and Engineering*, *199*(25–28), 1691–1700. https://doi.org/10.1016/j.cma.2010.01.022.

Fernandez, J.W., Das, R., Cleary, P.W., Hunter, P.J., Thomas, C.D.L., & Clement, J.G. (2013). Using smooth particle hydrodynamics to investigate femoral cortical bone remodelling at the Haversian level. *International Journal for Numerical Methods in Biomedical Engineering*, *29*(1), 129–43. https://doi.org/10.1002/cnm.

Gingold, R. ., & Monaghan, J.J. (1977). Smoothed particle hydrodynamics: theory and application to non-sherical stars. *Mon. Not. R. Astr. Soc*, *181*, 375–389.

Gu, Y.T. (2005). Meshfree methods and their comparison. *International Journal of Computational Methods*, *2*(4), 477–515. https://doi.org/10.1142/S0219876205000673.

Hipp, J.A., Springfield, D.S., & Hayes, W.C. (1995). Predicting pathologic fracture risk in the management of metastatic bone defects. *Clinical Orthopaedics and Related Research*, (312), 120–35. Retrieved from http://www.ncbi.nlm.nih.gov/pubmed/7634597.

Lee, J.D., Chen, Y., Zeng, X., Eskandarian, A., & Oskard, M. (2007). Modeling and simulation of osteoporosis and fracture of trabecular bone by meshless method. *International Journal of Engineering Science*, *45*(2–8), 329–338. https://doi.org/10.1016/j.ijengsci.2007.03.007.

Liew, K.M., Wu, H.Y., & Ng, T.Y. (2002). Meshless method for modeling of human proximal femur: treatment of nonconvex boundaries and stress analysis. *Computational Mechanics*, *28*(5), 390–400. https://doi.org/10.1007/s00466-002-0303-5.

Liu, G.R., & Gu, Y.T. (2001). A point interpolation method for two dimensional solids. *International Journal for Numerical Methods in Engineering*, *50*(4), 937–951. https://doi.org/10.1002/1097-0207(20010210)50.

Liu, W.K., Jun, S., & Zhang, Y. (1995). Reproducing kernel particle methods. *International Journal for Numerical Methods in Fluids*, *20*(8–9), 1081–1106. https://doi.org/10.1002/fld.1650200824.

Miller, F., & Whitehill, R. (1984). Carcinoma of the breast metastatic to the skeleton. *Clin Orthop Relat Res*.

Mori, D., Yano, K., Tsubota, K. ichi, Ishikawa, T., Wada, S., & Yamaguchi, T. (2008). Computational study on effect of red blood cells on primary thrombus formation.

Thrombosis Research, *123*(1), 114–121. https://doi.org/10.1016/j.thromres.2008.03.006.

Nayroles, B., Touzot, G., & Villon, P. (1992). Generalizing the finite element method: Diffuse approximation and diffuse\n elements. *Comput. Mech.*, *10*(5), 307–318. https://doi.org/10.1007/BF00364252.

Nguyen, V.P., Rabczuk, T., Bordas, S., & Duflot, M. (2008). Meshless methods: A review and computer implementation aspects. *Mathematics and Computers in Simulation*, *79*(3), 763–813. https://doi.org/10.1016/j.matcom.2008.01.003.

Onate, E., Idelsohn, S., & Zienkiewicz, O. (1996). A finite point method in computational mechanics. Applications to convective transport and fluid flow. *For Numerical Methods …*, *39*(December 1995), 3839–3866. Retrieved from http://onlinelibrary.wiley.com/doi/10.1002/(SICI)1097-0207(19961130)39:22%3C3839::AID-NME27%3E3.0.CO;2-R/full.

Roodman, G.D. (2004). Mechanisms of Bone Metastasis. *New England Journal of Medicine*, *350*(16), 1655–1664. https://doi.org/10.1056/NEJMra030831.

Spruijt, S., Van Der Linden, J., Sander Dijkstra, P., Wiggers, T., Oudkerk, M., Snijders, C., … Swierstra, B. (2006). Prediction of torsional failure in 22 cadaver femora with and without simulated subtrochanteric metastatic defects: A CT scan-based finite element analysis. *Acta Orthopaedica*, *77*(3), 474–481. https://doi.org/10.1080/17453670610046424.

Sukumar, N., Moran, B., & Belytschko, T. (1998). The natural element method in solid mechanics. *International Journal for Numerical Methods in Engineering*, *43*, 839–887.

Sukumar, N., Moran, B., Semenov, A.Y., & Belikov, V.V. (2001). Natural neighbour Galerkin methods. *International Journal for Numerical Methods in Engineering*, *50*(1), 1–27. https://doi.org/10.1002/1097-0207(20010110)50:1 < 1::AID-NME14 > 3.0.CO;2-P.

Taddei, F., Pani, M., Zovatto, L., Tonti, E., & Viceconti, M. (2008). A new meshless approach for subject-specific strain prediction in long bones: Evaluation of accuracy. *Clinical Biomechanics*, *23*(9), 1192–1199. https://doi.org/10.1016/j.clinbiomech.2008.06.009.

Tanck, E., van Aken, J.B., van der Linden, Y.M., Schreuder, H.W.B., Binkowski, M., Huizenga, H., & Verdonschot, N. (2009). Pathological fracture prediction in patients with metastatic lesions can be improved with quantitative computed tomography based computer models. *Bone*, *45*(4), 777–783. https://doi.org/10.1016/j.bone.2009.06.009.

Wang, J.G., & Liu, G.R. (2002). A point interpolation meshless method based on radial basis functions. *International Journal for Numerical Methods in Engineering*, *54*(11), 1623–1648. https://doi.org/10.1002/nme.489.

Wong, K.C.L., Wang, L., Zhang, H., Liu, H., & Shi, P. (2010). Meshfree implementation of individualized active cardiac dynamics. *Computerized Medical Imaging and Graphics*, *34*(1), 91–103. https://doi.org/10.1016/j.compmedimag.2009.05.002.

Zhang, G.Y., Wittek, A., Joldes, G.R., Jin, X., & Miller, K. (2014). A three-dimensional nonlinear meshfree algorithm for simulating mechanical responses of soft tissue. *Engineering Analysis with Boundary Elements*, *42*, 60–66. https://doi.org/10.1016/j.enganabound.2013.08.014.

Biodental Engineering V – Belinha et al. (Eds)
© 2019 Taylor & Francis Group, London, ISBN 978-0-367-21087-8

Using meshless methods to predict the biomechanical behaviour of red blood cells

S.D. Ferreira
Faculty of Engineering, University of Porto (FEUP), Porto, Portugal

J. Belinha
Department of Mechanical Engineering, School of Engineering, Polytechnic of Porto (ISEP), Porto, Portugal

R.M. Natal Jorge
Department of Mechanical Engineering, Faculty of Engineering, University of Porto (FEUP), Porto, Portugal

ABSTRACT: The Red Blood Cells (RBCs) occupy the highest percentage of the blood's volume. These cells have a very important biological function since they are responsible for the oxygenation of all the tissues of the body. In certain pathologies, the biomechanical properties of RBCs appear to be altered. The treatment of these pathologies is often expensive and not always effective. In this work, it was constructed a three-dimensional model of an RBC. Two different boundary conditions were applied to the virtual model of the cell and several output variables were analysed, such as the displacement, the Von Mises effective stress and the equivalent strain. Two numerical methods were used: The Finite Element Method (FEM) and the Radial Point Interpolation Method (RPIM)—a meshless method. Comparing the results of both techniques, it was possible to conclude that meshless methods are capable to provide smoother stress/strain fields.

1 STATE OF THE ART

1.1 Introduction

Structurally, the Red Blood Cells (RBCs) are relatively simple cells since they do not have organelles or nucleus. The membrane of these cells works as a complex structure, in which the components interact with each other to ensure the integrity of the cells, as well as their properties and biological functions. In RBCs constitution it is possible to find a protein (of red colour) denominated hemoglobin. This protein is responsible for transporting oxygen to all parts of the body, as well as for the elimination of carbon dioxide. To ensure its function, RBCs must navigate through the circulatory system, through blood vessels of small calibre, such as capillaries. Within these vessels, high shear stresses predominate. (Buys, Rooy, Soma, Papendorp, & Lipinski, 2013).

The RBCs in healthy mammals have the form of a biconcave disc with a volume of approximately 90 m³ and a surface area of 140 m². (Yawata, 2003). The high capacity of reversible deformation of these cells is due to the high ratio between the surface and the volume of these cells.

Important structural and functional characteristics of the RBC membrane have been maintained over the years. Nowadays, it is known that four layers constitute this cell: two lipid monolayers, a network of elastic proteins and integral proteins. The elastic protein network can slide freely under the two lipid monolayers (Elgsaeter & Mikkelsen, 1991).

Several factors affect the deformability of RBCs, such as: geometry, elasticity and internal and external viscosity (Tse & Lux, 1999).

For decades many researchers have dedicated their studies to comprehend the behaviour and composition of RBCs. To understand and explain this behaviour it was necessary to determine the biomechanical properties of these cells, presented in Table 1 (Tomaiuolo, 2014).

1.2 Discretization Techniques

In the year of 1870, Rayleigh made the first steps developing an approximation technique that years later would be in the origin of the Finite Element Method (FEM). Today, the FEM is a well-known discretization technique used in several scientific

Table 1. Mechanical and geometric properties of healthy RBCs. (Tomaiuolo 2014).

Property	Healthy RBC
Volume (μm^3)	89.4 ± 17.6
Surface area (μm^2)	113.8 ± 27.6
Cytoplasmatic viscosity (mPa/s)	6.07 ± 3.8
Surface viscosity (μN s/m)	0.7 ± 0.2
Shear elastic modulus (μN/m)	5.5 ± 3.3
Bending elastic modulus ($\times 10^{-9}$ Nm)	1.15 ± 0.9
Relaxation time constant (s)	0.17 ± 0.08
Area compressibility modulus (mN/m)	399 ± 110
Young's modulus (KPa)	26 ± 7

fields to solve differential equation ruling the most diverse physical phenomena. In the literature, it is possible to find several documents explaining with detail the methodology (Campilho, 2012). Quickly, the FEM has become a solution to many problems involving complex structures.

The FEM principle consists in the discretization of a complex structure into several smaller elements (Reddy, 2005). The elements can take different forms, such as triangles or quadrilaterals, for the two-dimensional case, and hexahedrons or tetrahedrons, for the three-dimensional case. All elements must be interconnected by common nodes and the field function must be interpolated to each of them via shape functions.

Nowadays, there are many areas that use this numerical method to solve specific problems. These areas include: metallurgy; the automotive industry and mechanical engineering; naval; civil; aeronautics; aerospace; of structures, among others.

However, this numerical method is still limited and is not ideal to solve problems with high deformations (Belytschko, Krongauz, Organ, Fleming, & Krysl, 1996).

In the year of 1980 appeared the meshless methods (MMs) (Belytschko et al., 1996) technique. With these advanced discretization methods, the problem domain is discretized with only a nodal distribution (Pierre et al., 2008). In this type of method, and contrary to what happens in FEM with its elements, the influence-domains can and should overlap one another. The solution obtained with these methods, although approximate, is more accurate than that obtained for FEM (Belinha, 2014).

The meshless methods require de combination of three basic parts: nodal connectivity, numerical integration scheme and shape functions. Initially, the geometry and contour of the structure are studied. In this way, it is possible to discretize the domain and the contour of the structure. The nodes resulting from the discretization process can be distributed arbitrarily, without having to follow

a structured mesh. To determine the field functions only the position of the nodes is necessary. Therefore, it is not necessary to know the relation between the different nodes.

The accuracy of the results obtained with the MMs depends on the spatial distribution and the number of nodes used. If more nodes are used, the higher the accuracy will be. However, if the node number increases, the computational cost also increases.

2 NUMERICAL ANALYSIS

In this paper two meshless methods will be presented, the Radial Point Interpolation Method (RPIM) and the Natural Neighbour Radial Point Interpolation Method (NNRPIM).

2.1 *RPIM*

After the discretization process is completed, it is necessary to determine the nodal connectivity.

In RPIM the weak formulation is applied, and the nodal connectivity is obtained by the overlap of influence-domains.

That is, around points of interest are defined areas and concentric volumes and all nodes contained in these areas and volumes belong to the influence-domain.

The shape and size of the influence-domains will affect the final solution(Belinha, 2014).

After this step, it is necessary to define the integration points, thus it is applied the Gauss-Legendre quadrature rule (Wriggers, 2006). Therefore, it becomes necessary to create a background integration mesh. In this mesh, the integration points are distributed. The weight and location of the integration points depends on the shape of the mesh elements.

2.2 *NNRPIM*

In NNRPIM, unlike RPIM, nodal connectivity is imposed not by influence-domains, but by influence-cells. To obtain the influence-cells, the Voronoï diagrams and the Delaunay triangulation method can be applied. After the discretization, for each node n_I is determined a Voronoï cell V_I defined by a polygon with P_{Ii} vertices. Each Voronoï cell, in the case of an irregular mesh, can be further divided into n smaller quadrilaterals S_{Ii}. The midpoint between node n_I and node n_i is designated M_{Ii}. In the case of a regular mesh, the midpoints M_{Ii} coincide with the midpoints of the edges giving rise to triangles instead of quadrilaterals.

This method is advantageous because for the elaboration of the background integration scheme it is only necessary to know the position in the space of the nodes belonging to the domain (Belinha, 2014).

Influence-cells can be divided into two types: first and second degree. The first degree contains the first natural neighbours only. The second-degree on the other hand also contain the natural neighbours of the first natural neighbours.

After the construction of the Voronoï diagram the Delaunay rule is applied, obtaining smaller areas inside the Voronoï cells. In the two-dimensional case, the size (A_{V_I}) of a Voronoï cell V_I is the sum of the size of all S_{I_i} sub-cells, as represented in Equation (1) (Belinha, 2014).

$$A_{VI} = \sum_{i=1}^{n} A_{S_{Ii}}, \quad \forall A_{S_{Ii}} \geq 0 \qquad (1)$$

For the two-dimensional and three-dimensional case A represents an area and a volume, respectively. It is assumed that in NNRPIM the weight assigned to any integration point is calculated by the sum of the areas S_{Ii}. The sub-cells alternate essentially between the form of squares and triangles. From these forms, it is possible to apply different methods of integration methods.

Finally, after the determination of the nodal connectivity and integration scheme, it is necessary to calculate the shape function $u(x_I)$. This function, calculated by the same way for RPIM and NNRPIM, consists of a radial basis function ($R_i(x_I)$) combined with a polynomial function ($p_j(x_I)$), as demonstrated in Equation (2) (Belinha, 2014; Dai & Liu, 2006).

$$\begin{aligned} u(x_I) &= \sum_{i=1}^{n} R_i(x_I) a_i(x_I) + \sum_{j=1}^{m} p_j(x_I) b_j(x_I) = \\ &= R^T(x_I) a + p^T(x_I) b \\ &= \{R^T(x_I), p^T(x_I)\} \begin{Bmatrix} a \\ b \end{Bmatrix} \end{aligned} \qquad (2)$$

The equation above can also be written as follows:

$$\begin{aligned} \begin{bmatrix} R & p \\ p^T & 0 \end{bmatrix} \begin{Bmatrix} a \\ b \end{Bmatrix} &= \begin{Bmatrix} u_s \\ 0 \end{Bmatrix} \Rightarrow \begin{Bmatrix} a \\ b \end{Bmatrix} \\ &= \begin{bmatrix} R & p \\ p^T & 0 \end{bmatrix}^{-1} \begin{Bmatrix} u_s \\ 0 \end{Bmatrix} \Rightarrow \begin{Bmatrix} a \\ b \end{Bmatrix} = G^{-1} \begin{Bmatrix} u_s \\ 0 \end{Bmatrix} \end{aligned} \qquad (3)$$

Finally, it is possible to represent the shape function in the following way:

$$\begin{aligned} u(x_I) &= \{R^T(x_I), p^T(x_I)\} G^{-1} \begin{Bmatrix} u_s \\ 0 \end{Bmatrix} \\ &= \varphi(x_I) \begin{Bmatrix} u_s \\ 0 \end{Bmatrix} \end{aligned} \qquad (4)$$

3 NUMERICAL ANALYSIS

3.1 *Geometrical and numerical models*

In this work, it was performed a static analysis of a RBC subject to a force of $1,2 \times 10^{-7}$ N (blood pressure). The methods used were FEM and RPIM.

A three-dimensional model of a RBC was developed in CAD software, and a regular mesh with 14750 triangles and 4013 nodes was generated (Figure 1).

The software used to perform the analyses was FEMAS—Finite Element and Meshless Analysis Software, which is an academic software capable to perform several kinds of computational mechanics analysis, using both the FEM and meshless methods (more details in cmech.webs.com). The mechanical properties of a healthy RBC were defined: Young's Modulus was 2.6×10^{-8} N/m² (Tomaiuolo, 2014) and Poisson's ratio was 0.45. Afterwards, two distinct essential boundary conditions were considered, allowing to study two different cases, as it is possible to visualize in Figure 2. Finally, a distributed pressure was applied along the Oy-axis ($1,6 \times 10^{-10}$ N/μm) on one face of the RBC (the pressure aims to simulate the surrounding fluid pressure due to the fluid motion).

After this step, using the available output files it was possible to compare the FEM and RPIM results, for the two distinct cases of boundary conditions.

Initially the displacement of the RBC membrane was studied to estimate the displacement of the cell subjected to a force with a certain intensity and direction. This situation can be compared to what happens to the RBC during its circulation

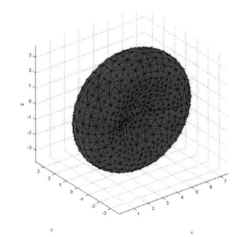

Figure 1. Model 3D of a RBC obtained after the creation of a mesh.

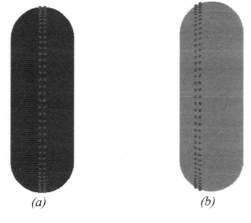

Figure 2. a) boundary condition 1 (b) boundary condition 2.

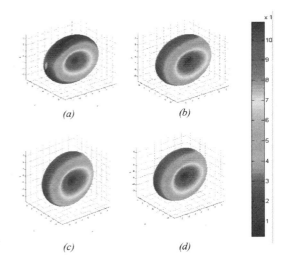

Figure 3. (a) Displacement field |u|, in microns, for FEM and boundary condition 1. (b) Displacement field |u|, in microns for FEM and boundary condition 2. (c) Displacement field |u|, in microns, for RPIM and boundary condition 1. (d) Displacement field |u|, in microns for RPIM and boundary condition 2.

through the bloodstream, where are restrictions on their movement. One example of these restrictions is when they move to a blood vessel of diameter smaller than their diameter (border condition).

In a second step, the von Mises effective stress was analysed in order to understand what happens in the walls of the RBC when these are submitted to the internal pressures of the blood vessels.

In the last stage of the work, the deformation obtained by a RBC was simulated.

In this way, it was possible to infer, to visualize and to calculate the displacement, the Von Mises effective stress and the equivalent strain for the conditions imposed (boundary conditions and forces) and for the two methods (FEM and RPIM).

3.2 Results

The displacement of the RBC was obtained, and it was possible to verify that when a RBC is submitted to the considered pressure, it undergoes a certain displacement, as it can be seen in Figure 3. It is also observed that the degree of displacement varies with the different boundary conditions imposed, since the shape acquired by the cells with the application of the force of $1,6 \times 10^{-10}$ N/μm differs in the two studied cases. The displacement values, |u|, are maximum for the central region (red/orange colour) and decrease as it moves away from the centre of the cell (region where the force is applied), assuming values close to zero.

As for the equivalent von Mises stresses it was possible to infer that this is maximum in the areas where a boundary condition was applied, for both FEM and RPIM, as it is possible to visualize in Figure 4.

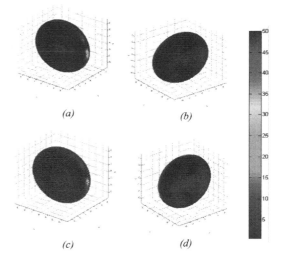

Figure 4. (a) von Mises effective stress in Pascal for FEM and boundary condition 1. (b) von Mises effective stress in Pascal for FEM and boundary condition 2. (c) von Mises effective stress in Pascal for RPIM and boundary condition 1. (b) von Mises effective stress in Pascal for RPIM and boundary condition 2.

With respect to strain, in Figure 5 it is possible to verify that the equivalent strain was maximum in the zone where the boundary conditions were applied, both for FEM and RPIM.

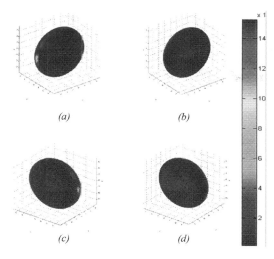

Figure 5. (a) Equivalent strains for FEM and boundary condition 1 (b) Equivalent strains for FEM and boundary condition 2. (c) Equivalent strains for RPIM and boundary condition 1 (b) Equivalent strains for RPIM and boundary condition 2.

4 CONCLUSIONS

As expected, it is possible to conclude that the displacement field is higher in the centre of the cell (for a force of equal intensity and direction). Additionally, the strain increases near the boundary conditions.

It is also possible to visualize that the von Mises effective stress is maximum in centre of the cell.

Moreover, the results of FEM and RPIM were similar. Therefore, this study shows that meshless methods are a robust alternative to the finite element method for biomechanical applications.

ACKNOWLEDGEMENTS

The authors truly acknowledge the funding provided by Ministério da Ciência, Tecnologia e Ensino Superior—Fundação para a Ciência e a Tecnologia (Portugal) by project funding MIT-EXPL/ISF/0084/2017. Additionally, the authors gratefully acknowledge the funding of Project NORTE-01-0145-FEDER-000022—SciTech—Science and Technology for Competitive and Sustainable Industries, cofinanced by Programa Operacional Regional do Norte (NORTE2020), through Fundo Europeu de Desenvolvimento Regional (FEDER).

REFERENCES

Belinha, J. (2014). *Meshless Methods in Biomechanics: Bone Tissue Remodelling Analysis.*

Belytschko, T., Krongauz, Y., Organ, D., Fleming, M., & Krysl, P. (1996). Meshless Methods: An Overview and Recent Developments.

Buys, A. V, Rooy, M. Van, Soma, P., Papendorp, D. Van, & Lipinski, B. (2013). Changes in red blood cell membrane structure in type 2 diabetes : a scanning electron and atomic force microscopy study Changes in red blood cell membrane structure in type 2 diabetes : a scanning electron and atomic force microscopy study.

Campilho, R. (2012). Método de elementos finitos.

Dai, K.Y., & Liu, G.R. (2006). Inelastic analysis of 2D solids using a weak-form RPIM based on deformation theory, *195*, 4179–4193. https://doi.org/10.1016/j.cma.2005.07.021.

Elgsaeter, A., & Mikkelsen, A. (1991). Shapes and shape changes invitro in normal red blood cells. *Bio, 1071*, 273–290.

Pierre, S., Bordas, A., Duflot, M., Ñóò, Æ.Ù.Ý.Ò.Î.Ò.È.Ù.Ì., Ëø, Ê.Þ.Ù., Ôö, Ð., ... Òøö, Ò. (2008). Meshless methods : A review and computer implementation aspects, (October 2017). https://doi.org/10.1016/j.matcom.2008.01.003.

Reddy, J.N. (2005). *An Introduction to The Finite Element Method.*

Tomaiuolo, G. (2014). Biomechanical properties of red blood cells in health and disease towards microfluidics. *Biomicrofluidics, 8*(5). https://doi.org/10.1063/1.4895755.

Tse, W.T., & Lux, S.E. (1999). Red blood cell membrane disorders. *British Journal of Haematology, 104*(2), 2–13.

Wriggers, P. (2006). *Computational Contact Mechanics.* Retrieved from https://link.springer.com.

Yawata, Y. (2003). *Cell Membrane.*

The computational mechanical simulation of healthy and pathological red blood cells with meshless methods

S.D. Ferreira
Faculty of Engineering, University of Porto (FEUP), Porto, Portugal

J. Belinha
Department of Mechanical Engineering, School of Engineering, Polytechnic of Porto (ISEP), Porto, Portugal

R.M. Natal Jorge
Department of Mechanical Engineering, Faculty of Engineering, University of Porto (FEUP), Porto, Portugal

ABSTRACT: Red Blood Cells (RBCs) have a high deformability capability that allows them to reach all parts of the body. In certain pathologies this capacity is affected. The high rates of new diagnoses of these diseases have attracted the interest of the scientific community, which has performed a significant amount of research in this area. In this article, a two-dimensional simulation was performed using healthy and pathological red cells (ovalocytosis and sickle cell anemia). The aim, of this article, is to understand the behaviour of healthy and pathological cells when subjected to a force and a boundary condition. In the simulation, it was applied the Finite Element Method (FEM) and two meshless methods: The Radial Point Interpolation Method (RPIM) and the Natural Neighbour Radial Point Interpolation Method (NNRPIM).

1 STATE OF THE ART

1.1 Introduction

In pathologies such as diabetes (Bommer et al., 2017; Buys, Rooy, Soma, Papendorp, & Lipinski, 2013; Pereira, Carreira, Lunet, & Azevedo, 2013; Sørensen, Arneberg, Line, & Berg, 2016; Sousa-uva et al., 2016; Tomaiuolo, 2014), sickle cell anemia (Li, Dao, Lykotra, & Em, 2017; Suresh, 2006), ovalocytosis (Paquette et al., 2015; Wong, 2004) or malaria (Biology, Tilley, Dixon, & Kirk, 2011; Castillo-riquelme, Mcintyre, & Barnes, 2008; Fedosov, Lei, Caswell, Suresh, & Karniadakis, 2011; Hanssen, Mcmillan, & Tilley, 2010; Hennessee et al., 2017; Hosseini & Feng, 2012; Shretta et al., 2017; Wu, Feng, Wu, & Feng, 2013; Ye, Phan-thien, Khoo, & Lim, 2013), the structure and certain properties of red blood cells (RBCs) appear to be altered (Kozlov & Markin, 1987). These shape alterations can function as biomarkers of these pathologies. Thus, a more in-depth knowledge of the functioning of these RBCs has a high patho-physiological importance.

All pathological RBCs have the following characteristics: reduction of surface area and capacity of deformation and alteration in cell morphology (Suresh, 2006).

In the healthy RBCs the maintenance of the biomechanical properties is achieved by the articulation of all the components present in these cells. There are two modes of interaction between the components within the RBCs: horizontal interactions and vertical interactions (Figure 1) (Elgsaeter & Mikkelsen, 1991).

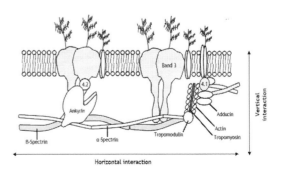

Figure 1. Diagram of the RBCs membrane.

The lipid bilayer interacts with the spectrin network through vertical interactions, whereas the constituents of the spectrin network interact through horizontal interactions.

During a blood circulation the RBCs have to cross capillaries of very small dimensions. For that reason, they must undergo a deformation. The reduced dimensions of the capillary will act as a boundary condition imposed to RBCs, whereas the blood pressure acts as a force applied to the cells.

It is known that when a RBC is subjected to a force, its components will articulate so that the cell deforms. After removal of the force, the cell must return to its initial shape (reversible deformation) (Chasis & Shohet, 1987).

Sickle cell anemia is originated from a mutation in the amino acid sequence encoding the hemoglobin protein. In this condition the RBCs change their shape to take the form of a sickle. Clinically, sickle cell anemia can range from mild to severe cases, in which patients suffer severe pain crises due to the creation of clots within small blood vessels. With sickle cell anemia, the Young's modulus of RBCs becomes higher, and therefore pathologic RBCs are stiffer than healthy RBCs (Suresh, 2006) (Li et al., 2017).

Another pathology that changes the shape and biomechanical properties of RBCs is ovalocytosis. This pathology occurs due to a mutation in the band 3 protein. As a consequence of this mutation, the RBCs increase their stiffness and become more oval. Some evidence seem to show that the carriers of this pathology are more resistant to several parasites that cause malaria (Paquette et al., 2015; Wong, 2004).

Pathologies, such as those previously mentioned, imply high monetary costs for the state and for the patients' families. Thus, a policy of prevention, together with a detailed knowledge of the RBCs, can lead to a reduction of costs and an improvement in the well-being of the population.

1.2 Discrete techniques

Currently, many numerical methods are known. In this paper, it will be discussed two of these methods: the Finite Element Method (FEM) and the Meshless Methods (MMS).

The Finite Element Method is widely used in several fields of activity, from mechanical engineering to the prosthesis industry, for example. This method is based on the idea that all systems are continuous systems that can be represented by smaller parts. Thus, this method divides a complex problem into smaller elements (Reddy, 2005). Starting from the domain of the problem, a mesh is created, containing the elements and their

respective nodes, and the boundary conditions are defined. This step is called discretization. In FEM the unknown field functions are interpolated within each element by shape functions or interpolation functions. However, in some problems, this numerical method has some limitations. In problems where there are large deformations, the mesh takes a very distorted form, leading to less accurate results (Belytschko, Krongauz, Organ, Fleming, & Krysl, 1996).

Due to the FEM limitations, there has been a growing interest in Meshless Methods (MMs) (Belytschko et al., 1996). In the MMs, a set of nodes is arbitrarily distributed along the domain of the problem, and the field functions are obtained for each domain of influence (Belinha, 2014; Pierre et al., 2008).

In this article, FEM will be applied, as well as two meshless methods: the Radial Point Interpolation Method (RPIM) and the Natural Neighbour Radial Point Interpolation Method (NNRPIM).

In RPIM, nodal connectivity is determined by overlapping the existing influence-domains of each node. To determine the influence-domain, a sufficient number of nodes are considered within an area or volume of influence, for a 2D or 3D case, respectively. This area or volume can assume different sizes and shapes, influencing the solution obtained by the method.

In NNRPIM, nodal connectivity is determined by overlapping influence-cells, obtained from Voronoï cells.

After determining nodal connectivity, it is necessary to establish the integration scheme. For RPIM are used Gauss integration schemes (Wriggers, 2006) and for NNRPIM are used the Voronoï and Delaunay triangulation methods (Belinha, 2014).

2 NUMERICAL MODEL

In an initial phase of this work, three models were constructed (two-dimensional models), representative of the cells: healthy, with ovalocytosis and with sickle cell anemia.

In the creation of these models was used CAD software, which allowed the generation of the meshes represented in Figure 2.

For the healthy cell, in order to study the convergence path of each discrete numerical method, five different meshes were created. The five meshes possess an increasing number of nodes.

After the generation of the different meshes, the models were submitted to a numerical analysis software (FEMAS). FEMAS—Finite Element and Meshless Analysis Software—is an academic software capable to perform several kinds of computational mechanics analysis, using both the FEM

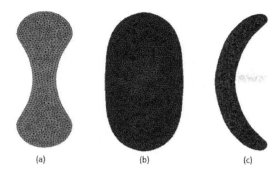

Figure 2. (a) Mesh of the model representative of a healthy cell (b) Mesh of the model representative of a cell with ovalocytosis (c) Mesh of the model representative of a cell with sickle cell anemia.

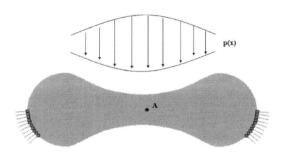

Figure 3. Two boundary conditions and a distributed force applied in a healthy cell.

and meshless methods (more details in cmech. webs.com).

In this work, the mechanical properties of the cells were defined as: E = 26000 kPa (Tomaiuolo, 2014) and υ = 0.45 (Young's modulus and Poisson's coefficient, respectively). These properties were the same for all models.

For the five meshes of the healthy cell model, after the mechanical properties were defined, two boundary conditions and a distributed force were applied as shown in Figure 3. The force applied had an intensity of 1.6×10^{-10} N/μm and is representative of the pressure applied to a RBC when passing on a blood vessel, where the blood pressure was 1.6×10^{-9} $N/\mu m$, to another vessel, where the blood pressure is 1.6×10^{-6} $N/\mu m$.

In an initial stage, the healthy RBC membrane displacement was studied for the five meshes constructed. Each of the meshes was analysed with the three numerical methods: FEM, RPIM and NNRPIM. The purpose of this preliminary study was to access the convergence path of the three methodologies (FEM, RPIM and NNRPIM).

In a second stage, simulations were performed assuming only one mesh (the mesh with the higher number of nodes) for RBCs: healthy, with ovalocytosis, and with sickle cell anemia. For each one of these cells, the membrane displacement, von Mises effective stress field and strain field were studied.

The properties of the cells were kept constant in order to determine the effect of the geometry change. For each of the models, the three numerical methods were also applied: FEM, RPIM, NNRPIM.

3 RESULTS

Regarding the convergence study, it was obtained the displacement on the centre of the cell for the five distinct meshes representing a healthy RBC. The results are shown in Figure 4.

The analysis of this figure allows to verify that the results obtained with the FEM, the RPIM and the NNRPIM tend to converge. That is, after a certain number of nodes the solution seems to maintain its value, towards a final converged solution.

The graphical interface in the FEMAS software allows to plot several variable fields. Thus, regarding the simulation of the healthy cell, the following variable fields were documented: displacement (Figure 5(a)), the von Mises effective stress (Figure 5(b)) and the strain (Figure 5(c)).

It is observed that the displacement is maximum in the central region of the cell (red colour) and decreases as the distance to the centre of the cell increases. The von Mises effective stress and the deformation also have their maximums in the central region of the cell.

When analysing the model representative of the cell with the ovalocytosis pathology, it was verified that the displacement is maximum in the central region of the cell (red colour) and decreases as the distance to the centre of the cell increases (Figure 6(a)). On the other hand, the von Mises effective stress (Figure 6(b)) and the equivalent strain (Figure 6(c)) have their maximum in

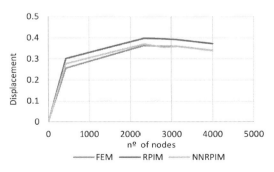

Figure 4. Displacement in function of the number of nodes that constitute the mesh.

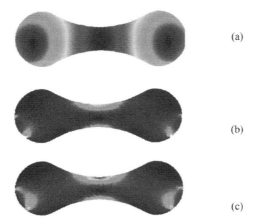

Figure 5. (a) The displacement predicted by the simulation for the healthy cell; (b) the von Mises effective stress predicted by the simulation for the healthy cell; and (c) the deformation predicted by the simulation for the healthy cell.

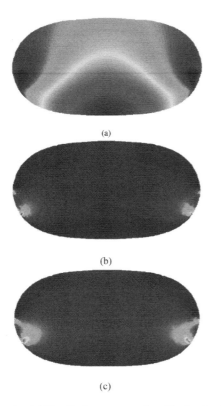

Figure 6. (a) The displacement predicted by the simulation for the cell with ovalocytosis; (b) the von Mises effective stress predicted by the simulation for the cell with ovalocytosis; and (c) the deformation predicted by the simulation for the cell with ovalocytosis.

the region where the boundary conditions were applied. This allows to verify that the geometry of the cell influences the obtained results.

Finally, when analysing the model representative of the cell with the pathology of sickle cell anemia, it was verified that the displacement is maximum in the central region of the cell (red colour) and decreases as the distance to the centre of the cell increases (Figure 7(a)). On the other hand, the von Mises effective stress (Figure 7(b)) and the deformation (Figure 7(c)) have higher values near the boundary condition.

From the obtained results, it was possible to obtain a graphic representation of the displacement (Figure 8), the von Mises effective stress (Figure 9)

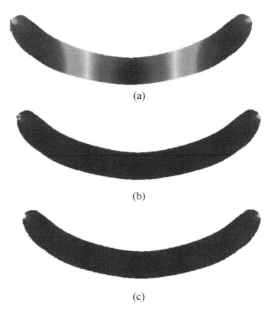

Figure 7. (a) The displacement predicted by the simulation for the cell with sickle cell anemia; (b) the von Mises effective stress predicted by the simulation for the cell with sickle cell anemia; and (c) the deformation predicted by the simulation for the cell with sickle cell anemia.

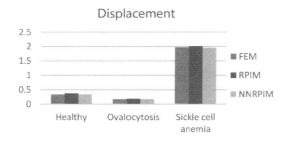

Figure 8. The displacement predicted by the simulation.

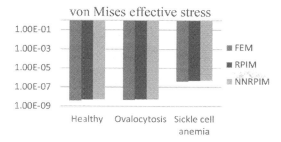

Figure 9. The effective stress of Von Mises predicted by the simulation.

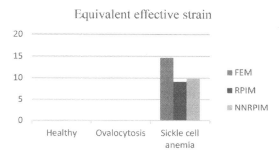

Figure 10. The effective strain predicted by the simulation.

and the equivalent strain (Figure 10). This graphics include the analysis of the three cell types.

By the analysis of the graphs it was verified that the values for the displacement, for the von Mises effective stress and for the effective deformation are maximum for the sickle-shaped cell.

4 CONCLUSIONS

With the simulations performed in this work, it was possible to conclude that all the methodologies converge very fast to the final converged solution. Additionally, it was verified that FEM and meshless provide very similar solutions.

In this paper, it was also possible to verify that the shape of the cell influences the obtained solution. It was observed that the sickle shape presents the highest displacement and equivalent strain. Thus, as expected, it is the most deformable shape.

ACKNOWLEDGEMENTS

The authors truly acknowledge the funding provided by Ministério da Ciência, Tecnologia e Ensino Superior—Fundação para a Ciência e a Tecnologia (Portugal) by project funding MIT-EXPL/ISF/0084/2017. Additionally, the authors gratefully acknowledge the funding of Project NORTE-01-0145-FEDER-000022—SciTech—Science and Technology for Competitive and Sustainable Industries, cofinanced by Programa Operacional Regional do Norte (NORTE2020), through Fundo Europeu de Desenvolvimento Regional (FEDER).

REFERENCES

Belinha, J. (2014). *Meshless Methods in Biomechanics: Bone Tissue Remodelling Analysis.*

Belytschko, T., Krongauz, Y., Organ, D., Fleming, M., & Krysl, P. (1996). Meshless Methods: An Overview and Recent Developments.

Biology, C., Tilley, L., Dixon, M.W.A., & Kirk, K. (2011). The Plasmodium falciparum-infected red blood cell Leann. *International Journal of Biochemistry and Cell Biology*, *43*(6), 839–842. https://doi.org/10.1016/j.biocel.2011.03.012.

Bommer, C., Heesemann, E., Sagalova, V., Manne-goehler, J., Atun, R., Bärnighausen, T., & Vollmer, S. (2017). The global economic burden of diabetes in adults aged 20–79 years: a cost-of-illness study. *Lancet Diabetes Endocrinol*, *8587*(17), 1–8. https://doi.org/10.1016/S2213-8587(17)30097-9.

Buys, A. V, Rooy, M. Van, Soma, P., Papendorp, D. Van, & Lipinski, B. (2013). Changes in red blood cell membrane structure in type 2 diabetes: a scanning electron and atomic force microscopy study Changes in red blood cell membrane structure in type 2 diabetes: a scanning electron and atomic force microscopy study.

Castillo-riquelme, M., Mcintyre, D., & Barnes, K. (2008). Household burden of malaria in South Africa and Mozambique: is there a catastrophic impact?, *13*(1), 108–122. https://doi.org/10.1111/j.1365-3156.2007.01979.x.

Chasis, J.A., & Shohet, S.B. (1987). Red cell biochemical anatomy and membrane properties.

Elgsaeter, A., & Mikkelsen, A. (1991). Shapes and shape changes invitro in normal red blood cells. *Bio*, *1071*, 273–290.

Fedosov, D.A., Lei, H., Caswell, B., Suresh, S., & Karniadakis, G.E. (2011). Multiscale Modeling of Red Blood Cell Mechanics and Blood Flow in Malaria, *7*(12). https://doi.org/10.1371/journal.pcbi.1002270.

Hanssen, E., Mcmillan, P.J., & Tilley, L. (2010). Cellular architecture of Plasmodium falciparum—infected erythrocytes. *International Journal for Parasitology*, *40*(10), 1127–1135. https://doi.org/10.1016/j.ijpara.2010.04.012.

Hennessee, I., Chinkhumba, J., Hagen, M.B., Bauleni, A., Shah, M.P., Chalira, A., … Mathanga, D.P. (2017). Household costs among patients hospitalized with malaria: evidence from a national survey in Malawi, 2012. *Malaria Journal*, 1–12. https://doi.org/10.1186/s12936-017-2038-y.

Hosseini, S.M., & Feng, J.J. (2012). How Malaria Parasites Reduce the Deformability of Infected Red Blood Cells. *Biophysj*, *103*(1), 1–10. https://doi.org/10.1016/j.bpj.2012.05.026.

Kozlov, M.M., & Markin, V.S. (1987). Model of Red Blood Cell Membrane Skeleton: Electrical and Mechanical Properties, 439–452.

Li, X., Dao, M., Lykotra, G., & Em, G. (2017). Biomechanics and biorheology of red blood cells in sickle cell anemia, *50*, 34–41. https://doi.org/10.1016/j.jbiomech.2016.11.022.

Paquette, A.M., Harahap, A., Laosombat, V., Patnode, J.M., Satyagraha, A., Sudoyo, H., … Wilder, J.A. (2015). Infection, Genetics and Evolution The evolutionary origins of Southeast Asian Ovalocytosis. *INFECTION, GENETICS AND EVOLUTION*, *34*, 153–159. https://doi.org/10.1016/j.meegid.2015.06.002.

Pereira, M., Carreira, H., Lunet, N., & Azevedo, A. (2013). Trends in prevalence of diabetes mellitus and mean fasting glucose in Portugal (1987 e 2009): a systematic review. *Public Health*, *128*(3), 214–221. https://doi.org/10.1016/j.puhe.2013.12.009.

Pierre, S., Bordas, A., Duflot, M., Ñóò, Æ.Ù.Ý.Ò.Î.Ò.È.Ù.Ì., Ëø, Ê.Þ.Ù., Ôö, Ð., … Òøö, Ò. (2008). Meshless methods: A review and computer implementation aspects, (October 2017). https://doi.org/10.1016/j.matcom.2008.01.003.

Reddy, J.N. (2005). *An Introduction to The Finite Element Method*.

Shretta, R., Zelman, B., Birger, M.L., Haakenstad, A., Singh, L., Liu, Y., & Dieleman, J. (2017). Tracking development assistance and government health expenditures for 35 malaria—eliminating countries: 1990–2017. *Malaria Journal*, 1–11. https://doi.org/10.1186/s12936-017-1890-0.

Sørensen, M., Arneberg, F., Line, T.M., & Berg, T.J. (2016). Cost of diabetes in Norway 2011, *2*, 0–8. https://doi.org/10.1016/j.diabres.2016.10.012.

Sousa-uva, M. De, Antunes, L., Nunes, B., Rodrigues, A.P., Simões, J.A., Ribeiro, R.T., & Boavida, J.M. (2016). Trends in diabetes incidence from 1992 to 2015 and projections for 2024: A Portuguese General Practitioner's Network study. *Primary Care Diabetes*, *10*(5), 329–333. https://doi.org/10.1016/j.pcd.2016.05.003.

Suresh, S. (2006). Mechanical response of human red blood cells in health and disease: Some structure-property-function relationships. https://doi.org/10.1557/JMR.2006.0260.

Tomaiuolo, G. (2014). Biomechanical properties of red blood cells in health and disease towards microfluidics. *Biomicrofluidics*, *8*(5). https://doi.org/10.1063/1.4895755.

Wong, P. (2004). A hypothesis of the erythrocyte rigidity in Southeast Asian ovalocytosis. *Medical Hypotheses*, *62*(6), 1024. https://doi.org/10.1016/j.mehy.2004.03.003.

Wriggers, P. (2006). *Computational Contact Mechanics*. Retrieved from https://link.springer.com.

Wu, T., Feng, J.J., Wu, T., & Feng, J.J. (2013). Simulation of malaria-infected red blood cells in microfluidic channels: Passage and blockage Simulation of malaria-infected red blood cells in microfluidic channels: Passage and blockage, *44115*. https://doi.org/10.1063/1.4817959.

Ye, T., Phan-thien, N., Khoo, B.C., & Lim, C.T. (2013). Stretching and Relaxation of Malaria-Infected Red Blood Cells. *Biophysj*, *105*(5), 1103–1109. https://doi.org/10.1016/j.bpj.2013.07.008.

Biodental Engineering V – Belinha et al. (Eds)
© 2019 Taylor & Francis Group, London, ISBN 978-0-367-21087-8

Predicting the stress distribution in the mandible bone due to the insertion of implants: A meshless method study

H.I.G. Gomes
Faculty of Engineering, University of Porto (FEUP), Porto, Portugal

J. Belinha
Department of Mechanical Engineering, School of Engineering, Polytechnic of Porto (ISEP), Porto, Portugal

R.M. Natal Jorge
Department of Mechanical Engineering, Faculty of Engineering, University of Porto (FEUP), Porto, Portugal

ABSTRACT: The number of dental implants has increased exponentially over the years, mainly because the number of partially edentulous patients is increasing as a consequence of the aging of the population. Thus, it is necessary to study the response of the bone when submitted to different loads, which may be either axial, horizontal, or a combination of these two. This work aims to simulate the mechanical behaviour of the mandible with distinct numerical methods, such as the Finite Element Method (FEM), and two meshless methods—the Radial Point Interpolation Method (RPIM) and the Natural Neighbour Radial Interpolation Method (NNRPIM). Additionally, this study aims to study the effect of the occlusal load orientation. Thus, a virtual model of the mandible was constructed and analysed with the distinct numerical techniques. The results obtained showed significant differences in the stress distribution when axial or horizontal loads are considered. Loads aligned with the horizontal direction produce stresses four times higher than loads applied in the axial direction.

1 STATE OF THE ART

1.1 Introduction

Dental implants are currently considered an efficient treatment, possessing a high success rate (Zupnik, Kim, Ravens, Karimbux, & Guze, 2011). Its use has increased exponentially in recent years, with more than 5 million implants per year in the United States, which is equivalent to about 800 billion euros.

This treatment consists of a biocompatible device, placed in the maxilla/mandible bone, providing support for a prosthetic reconstruction. After its insertion, dental implants are subjected to various loads during its life-span (occlusal loads), which are produced by the muscles involved in mastication.

When applying numerical methods for dental implant analysis, it is important to consider not only the axial and horizontal loads, but also the oblique loads. These represent more realistic bite directions and can produce larger forces, which consequently cause higher stresses and strains in the implant and in the bone (Watanabe, Hata, Komatsu, Ramos, & Fukuda, 2003). Therefore, in the case of oblique loads, it is important to specify the magnitude and angle to be used in the simulation.

Several FEM studies have demonstrated that an increase in force angle increases stress/strain concentrations in the neck region and, thus, such effect increases maximum stress/strain values in the bone (Barbier, Sloten, Krzesinski, Schepers, & Van Der Perre, 1998), (Watanabe et al., 2003), (Holmgren, Seckinger, Kilgren, & Mante, 1998), (Qian, Todo, Matsushita, & Koyano, 2009). The oblique load is considered the most severe loading condition, and it is suggested in the literature that such load should be avoided as much as possible (Barbier et al., 1998), (Watanabe et al., 2003), (Holmgren et al., 1998), (Qian et al., 2009).

1.2 Numerical methods

In recent years, computational mechanics has been widely used in the numerical simulation of biological structures, due to the need to predict their behaviour in the presence of mechanical stresses. The constant evolution of computers enabled the creation of increasingly robust and reliable models for biomechanical analysis. Therefore, nowadays, computational mechanics is considered a very useful tool in the diagnosis and treatment of diseases.

Currently, the most commonly used method is the Finite Element Method (FEM). This numerical method was introduced in the area of implantology by Weinsteim in 1976, who developed the first two-dimensional model of finite elements (Weinstein, Klawitter, Anand, & Richard, 2015). Later, the same author extended his study, developing a three-dimensional model (Cook, Weinstein, & Klawitter, 1982). In the FEM, it is necessary to create a discrete mesh geometrically identical to the object to be studied. Therefore, the problem domain has to be divided into multiple subdomains, called finite elements. Each element is constituted by nodes. Then, the mechanical properties of the materials building the model, and the essential and natural boundary conditions of the model have to be set. After solving the system of equations, it is possible to obtain the displacement of each node and consequently, it is possible to obtain the stress/strain fields, throughout the problem's domain.

The FEM analysis, in several problems, can have a high computational cost due to its dependence on the mesh (Duarte, 1995). Thus, to overcome this disadvantage, in recent years, a family of advanced discretization techniques—called meshless methods—has been under strong development. Today, meshless methods are being successfully applied to solve several distinct physical problems (Belinha, 2014). The main advantages of meshless methods, when compared to FEM, is their meshing/remeshing flexibility and their higher accuracy.

1.3 Meshless methods

Meshless methods are divided into two distinct categories, according to the formulation used: the strong formulation system, or the weak formulation, which is preferably used to obtain an approximate solution.

One of the first meshless methods developed, using the strong formulation, was the Smooth Particle Hydrodynamics Method (SPH) (Gingold & Monaghan, 1977). Since the 1990's, several methods have been developed, especially methods based on weak formulation. Examples of such methods include, the Diffuse Element Method (DEM) (Nayroles, Touzot, & Villon, 1992) and the Element Free Galerkin Method (EFGM) (Belytschko, Lu, & Gu, 1994). The EFGM was developed based on the DEM, which, in turn, was the first meshless method to use the Moving Least Square (MLS) approximations (Lancaster & Salkauskas, 1981) in the construction of the shape functions. One year later, the Reproducing Kernel Particle Method (RKPM) (W. K. A. M. Liu, Jun, & Zhang, 1995) was developed, based on two different methods, the

SPH and the Petrov-Galerkin Method (MLPG) (Atluri & Zhu, 1998).

Despite all the advantages of these meshless methods when compared to FEM, these methods also have limitations. The shape functions of these meshless methods do not satisfy the delta Kronecker property, which hinders the imposition of the essential and natural boundary conditions.

To solve this problem, several interpolating meshless methods have been developed in recent years. Some of these methods are the Point Interpolation Method (PIM) (G. R. Liu & Gu, 2001), Point Assembly Method (G. R. Liu, 2002), Meshless Finite Element Method (MFEM) (Calvo, Pin, Idelsohn, & Eugenio, 2003), Natural Neighbour Finite Element Method (NNFEM) (Traversoni, 1994) or the Natural Element Method (NEM) (Braun & Sambridge, 1995). Through evolution of the PIM, which used the original polynomial base function, it was possible to develop the RPIM (Wang & Liu, 2002). This method uses a Radial Basis Function (RBF) to construct the shape functions, combined with the polynomial base function. Recently, through the combination of NEM and RPIM, it was possible to develop the NNRPIM (Dinis, Jorge, & Belinha, 2007).

The generic procedure of the meshless methods requires the combination of three basic parts: nodal connectivity, numerical integration scheme and shape functions. First, it is necessary to consider the geometry of the problem, through the location of each node. Nodal connectivity in RPIM is obtained by overlapping the influence-domain of each node. Whereas, in NNRPIM it is established by the overlapping of influence-cells obtained through Voronoï cells. As for numerical integration, RPIM uses Gauss integration schemes, and NNRPIM uses an integration scheme based on Voronoï cells and Delaunay triangulation (Belinha, 2014).

In this work it was used, in addition to the FEM, the RPIM and NNRPIM.

1.4 Meshless methods in biomechanics

In recent years, meshless methods have been widely applied in numerical simulation. These methods have less dependence on the nodal distribution, which makes it a valid option to solve some problems found in the FEM. Additionally, some recent studies have demonstrated that meshless simulations, with models obtained through CT and MRI imaging, are more efficient when compared to FEM (Wong, Wang, Zhang, Liu, & Shi, 2010), (Chen et al., 2010).

Regarding applications in biomechanics, it is still not possible to find a significant number of papers in the literature.

Zhang et al. developed an algorithm based on meshless methods to simulate the response of biological soft tissues subject to large deformations (Zhang, Wittek, Joldes, Jin, & Miller, 2014). The results obtained confirmed the accuracy and predictability of the algorithm.

One of the oldest meshless methods is SPH. This method is usually used in biomechanics to simulate hemodynamic problems. Through this method, a two-dimensional simulation was performed to analyse the movement of a deformable red blood cell in the blood plasma (Tsubota, Wada, & Yamaguchi, 2006). It was also possible to study the mechanical effect that the red blood cells have in the formation of a primary thrombus (Mori et al., 2008). Both studies have demonstrated the ability of this method to express phenomena that occur in blood flow.

NEM has a clear advantage over FEM when applied to problems with large mesh distortions or complex geometry (Braun & Sambridge, 1995), (Sukumar, Belytschko, & Moran, 1998). These problems are usually encountered in simulations of biological structures involving soft tissues. Doblaré et al. consider NEM as the most suitable method for biomechanical applications (Doblaré et al., 2005). In this work, the authors simulated the internal remodelling of the bone, the behaviour of the meniscus subjected to normal loads, and the behaviour of the tendon, considering it as a hyperelastic and almost incompressible material. The obtained results were compared with FEM simulations, demonstrating that the two methods were in agreement. Later, a detailed model of the human knee was developed to simulate the behaviour of the ligament under knee flexion. The ligament surface geometries were reconstructed from a set of Magnetic Resonance Images (MRI), while the femur and the tibia were reconstructed through Computed Tomography (CT) images. In this work, it was verified that the NEM presents several advantages, when compared with the FEM (Doweidar, Calvo, Alfaro, Groenenboom, & Doblaré, 2010).

Liew et al. used a meshless method for mechanical simulation of the proximal femur (Liew, Wu, & Ng, 2002). Stress analyses were performed, showing very interesting biomechanical characteristics. Lee et al. converted CT images of the trabecular bone of the femur into a meshless model, which was used to simulate the osteoporosis process (Lee, Chen, Zeng, Eskandarian, & Oskard, 2007). This work was used to understand fracture related to osteoporosis. Taddei et al. used a meshless method to predict deformation in a femur from CT images (Taddei, Pani, Zovatto, Tonti, & Viceconti, 2008). More recently, Belinha and co-workers, presented a new bone tissue remodelling algorithm, based on a meshless method (NNRPIM) (Belinha, Jorge, & Dinis, 2013). The viability and efficiency of the method were successfully tested by applying the algorithm in several examples, namely, in the femur bone and the calcaneus bone. The NNRPIM method has been applied in implantology, namely to study the elasto-plastic behaviour of bone tissue in the presence of dental implants (Tavares, Belinha, Dinis, & Natal Jorge, 2015), and to predict the remodelling of the mandible bone tissue caused by the placement of dental implants (Belinha, Dinis, & Jorge, 2015).

2 NUMERICAL ANALYSIS

2.1 Geometrical and numerical models

This study aims to evaluate the behaviour of the mandibular bone when submitted to loads applied at different angles. For this purpose, the mandible was sectioned according to a plane of analysis Oxy, represented in Figure 1. Then, it was analysed considering a two-dimensional approach.

The model was based on the mandibular bone structure, being composed of trabecular bone and a thin layer of cortical bone (approximately 1 mm thick). The dimensions of the titanium implant were based on the study of (Kayabasi, Yuzbasıoglu, & Erzincanlı, 2006), presenting a diameter of 4.1 mm and 12 mm of length. All materials were considered linear elastic, isotropic and homogeneous, and their mechanical properties are summarized in Table 1.

The obtained model was discretized into a mesh of triangular elements, composed by 10834 elements and 5578 nodes, as represented in Figure 2(b). Then,

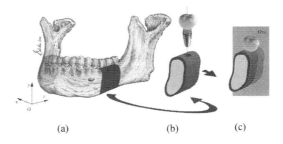

Figure 1. (a) Mandible. (b) Fragment of mandible with dental implant. (c) Model obtained through a cut according to the Oxy axis (BELINHA et al., 2015).

Table 1. Mechanical properties of all materials used in the analysis.

Material	Young's modulus (E) (MPa)	Poisson's ratio (v)
Titanium alloy	110000	0.32
Cortical bone	13700	0.3
Trabecular bone	1000	0.3

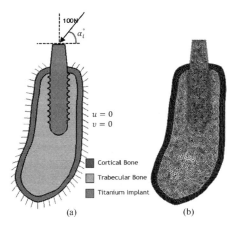

Figure 2. (a) Representation of the geometric model, with the essential and natural boundary conditions applied; (b) Element mesh.

the natural and essential boundary conditions were defined. Thus, an occlusal load distributed over the upper surface of the implant was applied with a magnitude of 100 N, as used in Chou's work (Chou, Jagodnik, & Muftu, 2008). The angle of application varied between $0° \geq \alpha \leq 180°$, with intervals of 15°. As for the application of the essential boundary conditions, the model was constrained along Ox and Oy directions, as seen in Figure 2(a).

The numerical model was analysed with FEMAS—Finite Element and Meshless Analysis Software, which is an academic software capable to perform several kinds of computational mechanics analysis, using both the FEM and meshless methods (more details in cmech.webs.com).

2.2 Results

After the analysis of the geometric model using the three discretization techniques, it was possible to obtain the colour distribution maps of the von Mises equivalent stresses and principal stress, for each method: FEM, RPIM and NNRPIM. Since the stress distribution of the three methodologies is very close, only the results obtained with the NNRPIM are shown, Figure 3. Thus, although several load cases were analysed, assuming several loading angles, in Figure 3 it is possible to observe only the stress maps for the angles: 0°, 45° and 90°.

Table 2 lists the total displacement values obtained at a point of interest located on the upper surface of the implant (Figure 4) for all analysed loading angles. To better interpret these data, a corresponding graph was constructed (Figure 5). This shows a decrease of the total displacement between 0° and 90°, and an increase between 90° and 180°.

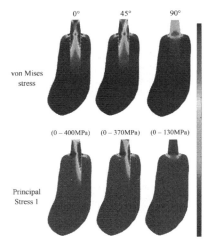

Figure 3. The von Mises and Principal stress 1 colour map, for NNRPIM analysis and the variation of the force angle.

Table 2. Total displacement obtained for all force angles.

Angle	Total displacement (mm)
0°	0.03574
15°	0.03451
30°	0.03102
45°	0.025546
60°	0.018572
75°	0.011028
90°	0.006529
105°	0.011359
120°	0.018914
135°	0.025834
150°	0.031226
165°	0.034617
180°	0.03574

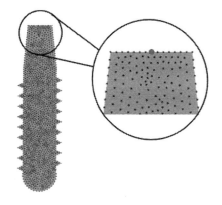

Figure 4. The red point indicates the node located in the implant where the total displacement was analysed.

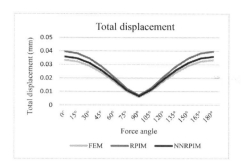

Figure 5. Graphical representation of the values obtained for the total displacement, considering the different angles of application of the load, and for the FEM, RPIM and NNRPIM methods.

3 CONCLUSIONS

With the colour maps of Figure 3, it is possible to observe that the maximum stresses in the implant were located in the region of the neck, near the superior edge of the cortical bone. When submitted to horizontal (0°) and oblique (45°) loads, the stress fields presented an asymmetric pattern, with maximum values located on the lingual side (in the direction of the force). In the case of axial loading (90°), as expected, the stress fields exhibited a symmetrical pattern. The same was observed in the distribution of stress in the bone. As for the distribution of the principal stress 1, maximum stress (compression and tensile stresses) were verified when the horizontal load (0°) and oblique (45°) were applied, being the compression stresses more pronounced in the crest of cortical bone, and tensile stresses on the opposite side.

This study allowed to compare the different numerical methods used, namely FEM, RPIM and NNRPIM, by analysing the total displacement at a chosen point on the upper surface of the implant (Figure 4). It was then possible to verify that there was an agreement between the different methods used. It was also observed a decrease of the displacement when the angle of application of the load varies between 0° and 90°, and an increase between 90° and 180° (Figure 5).

ACKNOWLEDGEMENTS

The authors truly acknowledge the funding provided by Ministério da Ciência, Tecnologia e Ensino Superior—Fundação para a Ciência e a Tecnologia (Portugal) by project funding MIT-EXPL/ISF/0084/2017. Additionally, the authors gratefully acknowledge the funding of Project NORTE-01-0145-FEDER-000022—SciTech—Science and Technology for Competitive and Sustainable Industries, cofinanced by Programa Operacional Regional do Norte (NORTE2020), through Fundo Europeu de Desenvolvimento Regional (FEDER).

REFERENCES

Atluri, S.N., & Zhu, T. (1998). A new Meshless Local Petrov-Galerkin (MLPG) approach in computational mechanics. *Computational Mechanics*, 22, 117–127.

Barbier, L., Sloten, J. Vander, Krzesinski, G., Schepers, E., & Van Der Perre, G. (1998). Finite element analysis of non-axial versus axial loading of oral implants in the mandible of the dog. *Journal of Oral Rehabilitation*, 25, 847–858.

Belinha, J. (2014). *Meshless Methods in Biomechanics: Bone Tissue Remodelling Analysis*. (Springer International Publishing, Ed.) (Vol. 16).

Belinha, J., Dinis, L.M.J.S., & Jorge, R.M.N. (2015). The Mandible Remodeling Induced By Dental Implants: a Meshless Approach. *Journal of Mechanics in Medicine and Biology*, 15(4), 1550059 (31 pages). https://doi.org/10.1142/S0219519415500591.

Belinha, J., Jorge, R.M.N., & Dinis, L.M.J.S. (2013). A meshless microscale bone tissue trabecular remodelling analysis considering a new anisotropic bone tissue material law. *Computer Methods in Biomechanics and Biomedical Engineering*, 16(11), 1170–1184. https://doi.org/10.1080/10255842.2012.654783.

Belytschko, T., Lu, Y.Y., & Gu, L. (1994). Element-free galerkin methods. *International Journal For Numerical Methods In Engineer*, 37, 229–256.

Braun, J., & Sambridge, M. (1995). A numerical method for solving partial differencial equantions on highly irregular evolving grids. *Nature*, 376(24), 655–660.

Calvo, N., Pin, F. Del, Idelsohn, S.R., & Eugenio, O. (2003). The meshless finite element method. *International Journal For Numerical Methods In Engineering*, 58, 893–912. https://doi.org/10.1002/nme.798.

Chen, T., Kim, S., Goyal, S., Jabbour, S., Zhou, J., Rajagopal, G., … Yue, N. (2010). Object-constrained meshless deformable algorithm for high speed 3D nonrigid registration between CT and CBCT. *Medical Physics*, 37(1), 197–210. https://doi.org/10.1118/1.3271389.

Chou, H.-Y., Jagodnik, J.J., & Muftu, S. (2008). Predictions of bone remodeling around dental implant systems. *Journal of Biomechanics*, 41, 1365–1373. https://doi.org/10.1016/j.jbiomech.2008.01.032.

Cook, S.D., Weinstein, A.M., & Klawitter, J.J. (1982). Materials Science: A Three-dimensional Finite Element Analysis of a Porous Rooted Co-Cr-Mo Alloy Dental Implant. *Journal of Dental Research*, 61(1), 25–29. https://doi.org/10.1177/00220345820610010501.

Dinis, L.M.J.S., Jorge, R.M.N., & Belinha, J. (2007). Analysis of 3D solids using the natural neighbour radial point interpolation method. *Computer Methods in Applied Mechanics and Engineering*, 196, 2009–2028. https://doi.org/10.1016/j.cma.2006.11.002.

Doblaré, M., Cueto, E., Calvo, B., Martínez, M.A., Garcia, J.M., & Cegoñino, J. (2005). On the employ of meshless methods in biomechanics. *Computer Methods in Applied Mechanics and Engineering*, 194(6–8), 801–821. https://doi.org/10.1016/j.cma.2004.06.031.

Doweidar, M.H., Calvo, B., Alfaro, I., Groenenboom, P., & Doblaré, M. (2010). A comparison of implicit and explicit natural element methods in large strains problems: Application to soft biological tissues modeling. *Computer Methods in Applied Mechanics and Engineering, 199*(25–28), 1691–1700. https://doi.org/10.1016/j.cma.2010.01.022.

Duarte, C.A. (1995). A Review of Some Meshless Methods to Solve Partial Differential Equations, (October). https://doi.org/10.13140/RG.2.2.21361.48489.

Gingold, R.A., & Monaghan, J.J. (1977). Smoothed particle hydrodynamics: theory and application to non-spherical stars. *Monthly Notices of the Royal Astronomical Society, 181*, 375–389.

Holmgren, E.P., Seckinger, R.J., Kilgren, L.M., & Mante, F. (1998). Evaluating Parameters Of Osseointegrated Dental Implants Using Finite Element Analysis—A Two-Dimensional Comparative Study Examining The Effects Of Implant Diameter, Implant Shape, And Load Direction. *The Journal of Oral Implantology, 24*(2), 80–88.

Kayabasi, O., Yuzbasıoglu, E., & Erzincanlı, F. (2006). Static, dynamic and fatigue behaviors of dental implant using finite element method. *Advances in Engineering Software, 37*, 649–658. https://doi.org/10.1016/j.advengsoft.2006.02.004.

Lancaster, B.P., & Salkauskas, K. (1981). Surfaces Generated by Moving Least Squares Methods. *Mathematics of Computation, 37*(155).

Lee, J.D., Chen, Y., Zeng, X., Eskandarian, A., & Oskard, M. (2007). Modeling and simulation of osteoporosis and fracture of trabecular bone by meshless method. *International Journal of Engineering Science, 45*(2–8), 329–338. https://doi.org/10.1016/j.ijengsci.2007.03.007.

Liew, K.M., Wu, H.Y., & Ng, T.Y. (2002). Meshless method for modeling of human proximal femur: Treatment of nonconvex boundaries and stress analysis. *Computational Mechanics, 28*(5), 390–400. https://doi.org/10.1007/s00466-002-030-5.

Liu, G.R. (2002). A point assembly method for stress analysis for two-dimensional solids. *International Journal of Solids and Structures, 39*(1), 261–276. https://doi.org/10.1016/S0020-7683(01)00172-X.

Liu, G.R., & Gu, Y.T. (2001). A point interpolation method for two-dimensional solids. *INTERNATIONAL JOURNAL FOR NUMERICAL METHODS IN ENGINEERING, 50*, 937–951.

Liu, W.K.A.M., Jun, S., & Zhang, Y.I.F.E.I. (1995). Reproducing kernel particle methods. *International Journal For Numerical Methods In Fluids, 20*, 1081–1106.

Mori, D., Yano, K., Tsubota, K. ichi, Ishikawa, T., Wada, S., & Yamaguchi, T. (2008). Computational study on effect of red blood cells on primary thrombus formation. *Thrombosis Research, 123*(1), 114–121. https://doi.org/10.1016/j.thromres.2008.03.006.

Nayroles, B., Touzot, G., & Villon, P. (1992). Computational Mechanics Generalizing the finite element method : Diffuse approximation and diffuse elements. *Computational Mechanics, 10*, 307–318.

Qian, L., Todo, M., Matsushita, Y., & Koyano, D.D.S.K. (2009). Effects of Implant Diameter, Insertion Depth, and Loading Angle on Stress/Strain Fields in Implant/Jawbone Systems: Finite Element Analysis. *The International Journal of Oral & Maxillofacial Implants, 24*, 877–886.

Sukumar, N., Belytschko, T., & Moran, B. (1998). The natural element method in solid mechanics. *International Journal for Numerical Methods in Engineering, 43*(5), 839–887. https://doi.org/10.1002/(SICI)10970207 (19981115)43:5 <839::AID-NME423>3.0.CO;2-R.

Taddei, F., Pani, M., Zovatto, L., Tonti, E., & Viceconti, M. (2008). A new meshless approach for subject-specific strain prediction in long bones: Evaluation of accuracy. *Clinical Biomechanics, 23*(9), 1192–1199. https://doi.org/10.1016/j.clinbiomech.2008.06.009.

Tavares, C.S.S., Belinha, J., Dinis, L.M.J.S., & Natal Jorge, R.M. (2015). The elasto-plastic response of the bone tissue due to the insertion of dental implants. *Procedia Engineering, 110*, 37–44. https://doi.org/10.1016/j.proeng.2015.07.007.

Traversoni, L. (1994). Natural neighbour finite elements. *Transactions on Ecology and the Environment, 8*.

Tsubota, K. ichi, Wada, S., & Yamaguchi, T. (2006). Particle method for computer simulation of red blood cell motion in blood flow. *Computer Methods and Programs in Biomedicine, 83*(2), 139–146. https://doi.org/10.1016/j.cmpb.2006.06.005.

Wang, J.G., & Liu, G.R. (2002). A point interpolation meshless method based on radial basis functions. *International Journal For Numerical Methods In Engineering, 54*, 1623–1648. https://doi.org/10.1002/nme.489.

Watanabe, F., Hata, Y., Komatsu, S., Ramos, T.C., & Fukuda, H. (2003). Finite element analysis of the influence of implant inclination, loading position, and load direction on stress distribution. *Odontology, 91*, 31–36. https://doi.org/10.1007/s10266-003-0029-7.

Weinstein, A.M., Klawitter, J.J., Anand, S.C., & Richard, S. (2015). Stress Analysis of Porous Rooted Dental Implants. *Journal of Dental Research, 55*(5), 772–777.

Wong, K.C.L., Wang, L., Zhang, H., Liu, H., & Shi, P. (2010). Meshfree implementation of individualized active cardiac dynamics. *Computerized Medical Imaging and Graphics, 34*(1), 91–103. https://doi.org/10.1016/j.compmedimag.2009.05.002.

Zhang, G.Y., Wittek, A., Joldes, G.R., Jin, X., & Miller, K. (2014). A three-dimensional nonlinear meshfree algorithm for simulating mechanical responses of soft tissue. *Engineering Analysis with Boundary Elements, 42*, 60–66. https://doi.org/10.1016/j.enganabound.2013.08.014.

Zupnik, J., Kim, S., Ravens, D., Karimbux, N., & Guze, K. (2011). Factors Associated With Dental Implant Survival: A 4-Year Retrospective Analysis. *Journal of Periodontology, 82*(10), 1390–1395. https://doi.org/10.1902/jop.2011.100685.

Biodental Engineering V – Belinha et al. (Eds)
© 2019 Taylor & Francis Group, London, ISBN 978-0-367-21087-8

Studying the mandible bone tissue remodelling in the vicinity of implants using a meshless method computational framework

H.I.G. Gomes
Faculty of Engineering, University of Porto (FEUP), Porto, Portugal

J. Belinha
Department of Mechanical Engineering, School of Engineering, Polytechnic of Porto (ISEP), Porto, Portugal

R.M. Natal Jorge
Department of Mechanical Engineering, Faculty of Engineering, University of Porto (FEUP), Porto, Portugal

ABSTRACT: The use of dental implants has increased exponentially over the years. Today, dental implant therapy is a reliable treatment with a high success rate. Thus, it is necessary to continually study the response of the surrounding bone tissue, since the implant changes the biomechanical environment of the mandible bone tissue, triggering the adaptation and remodelling of the bone tissue around the implant. Thus, the main objective of this work was to investigate the behaviour of remodelling of the mandibular bone structure, after the placement of a dental implant. In this way, computational simulation methods and techniques were used to simulate biological structures in a non-invasive and time efficient way. The numerical method used was a recently developed method: Natural Neighbour Radial Point Interpolation Method (NNRPIM). Moreover, to predict the remodelling of bone tissue, an algorithm was used, based on the assumption that bone reorganization depends mainly on mechanical stimuli. It was possible to observe that the algorithm predicts critical regions of high and low density, as found the ones found in clinical observations.

1 INTRODUCTION

The placement of dental implants is currently a valid treatment and with a high success rate (Zupnik, Kim, Ravens, Karimbux, & Guze, 2011). Nowadays, there are several types of implants, which can be classified according to their macro and microstructure. The characteristics of the implant aim to increase primary stability, a factor that is essential for osseointegration. Although there is no concrete definition for "primary stability", this is usually understood as the lack of mobility of the implant immediately after its placement (Neukam & Flemmig, 2006). Thus, for implant success to occur, bone tissue development must occur during osseointegration and bone remodelling. Osseointegration usually occurs in the peri-implant region within the first three to six months after surgery. Subsequently, the implant increases the stability through the deeper bone remodelling, that is, in the deeper cortical and trabecular bone. After a certain healing period, a state of equilibrium remodelling is achieved, where bone loss is minimal, and the implant failure rate is low.

Thus, it is possible to affirm that the bone tissue continually passes through processes of growth, reinforcement and resorption, collectively known as bone remodelling. Julius Wolff, in 1892, considered that the bone adapts its morphology in response to external loads (Wolff, 1986). Based on this assumption, several theories have been proposed to explain how the mechanical environment influences the growth, maintenance and degeneration of bone tissue. These theories can be formulated in terms of computational algorithms and are described below.

Fyhrie and Carter assumed that bone material tends to optimize its structural integrity. Thus, the trabeculae are aligned and the apparent density is adjusted in order to optimize some objective function, introducing the concept of self-optimization (Fyhrie & Carter, 1986). Later, Carter expanded the single-load approach, and described a theory that considers the daily loading history, which is characterized in terms of stress magnitude, cyclic strain energy density, and number of loading cycles (Carter, Fyhrie, & Whalen, 1987) (Carter, Orr, & Fyhrie, 1989). Several models based on these studies were developed. Beaupré modified and expanded these ideas in order to develop a theory of time-dependent remodelling (Beaupré, Orr, & Carter, 1990b) (Beaupré, Orr, & Carter, 1990a). Later, Petterman used the Strain Energy Density (SED) optimization criterion,

219

combining the adaptation of the bone spatial distribution with the reorientation of the main axes of the material and the stiffness parameters (Petterman, Rejter, & Rammerstorfer, 1997). Also based on the Carter model, a continuous damage repair algorithm was developed by Doblaré (Doblaré & García, 2002).

The theory of adaptive elasticity was proposed by Cowin and Hegedus (Cowin & Hegedus, 1976). These researchers have developed a model that is capable of predicting density changes and reorientation of the trabecular architecture, through the stress applied to the bone and certain bone parameters. The proposed model was based on an elastic constitutive relation for the trabecular bone that includes the second-order tensor, called a fabric tensor (as a measure of microstructure), as well as stress and strain tensors (Turner, Cowin, Rho, Ashman, & Rice, 1989), (Cowin, 1985). The state of bone equilibrium is reached when the principal directions of strain and stress are concordant with the main axes of the fabric tensor. In this state of equilibrium there is no realignment of the trabecular architecture, nor absorption or deposition of bone tissue.

Furthermore, several material laws have been proposed over time. Carter proposed an isotropic law of bone, which showed that the elastic modulus was proportional to the apparent density: $E = 3790 \, \varepsilon^{0.06} \rho^3$. This mathematical model was able to predict the mechanical properties of bone but does not consider the influence of bone microstructure and mechanical behaviour in different directions. Thus, new material laws have been proposed considering bone anisotropy ((Lotz, Gerhart, & Hayes, 1991), (Zioupos, Cook, & Hutchinson, 2008)). Based on these works, Belinha proposed a new unified orthotropic mathematical law for the cortical and trabecular bone, which will be used in the present work (Belinha, Jorge, & Dinis, 2013). This law allows to calculate the elastic modulus and ultimate compressive stress as a function of the apparent bone density.

These theories can be formulated in terms of computational algorithms and can be tested using the Finite Element Method (FEM). This method is the most used and has a fundamental role in biomechanical analysis, allowing to solve engineering problems for which it is difficult to obtain an exact analytical solution. However, due to the constant development of engineering and science, the problems of computational mechanics are increasingly complex and challenging. Faced with these new challenges, the FEM has some limitations, mainly since it is dependent on the mesh (Duarte, 1995). To overcome this problem, the meshless methods have appeared, in which it is possible to construct a geometric structure through a completely nodal approximation. In this work, the NNRPIM is used. This advanced numerical method uses mathematical concepts, such as the Voronoï diagrams and the Delaunay triangulation, for the construction of the influence-cells and the numerical integration mesh, completely dependent on the nodal mesh (Belinha, 2014).

Regarding applications in biomechanics, it is still not possible to find a significant number of papers in the literature. Doblaré et al. simulated the internal remodelling of the bone, the behaviour of the meniscus under normal loads, and the behaviour of the tendon, considering it as a hyperelastic and almost incompressible material (Doblaré et al., 2005). The obtained results were compared with finite element simulations, showing a good agreement with the NEM (Natural Element Method). Lee et al. converted CT images of the trabecular bone of the femur into a meshless model, which in turn was used to simulate the osteoporosis process (Lee, Chen, Zeng, Eskandarian, & Oskard, 2007). Belinha and his colleagues, presented a new bone tissue remodelling algorithm, based on the NNRPIM (Belinha et al., 2013). The viability and efficiency of the method were, in turn, successfully tested by applying the algorithm in several examples, namely the femur bone and the calcaneus bone. The NNRPIM method was also applied in the area of implantology, specifically to predict remodelling of the mandible caused by the placement of dental implants (Belinha, Dinis, & Jorge, 2015). More recently, Peyroteo et al. applied a mechanical bone remodelling algorithm, combined with three distinct discretization techniques, namely FEM, RPIM (Radial Point Interpolation Method) and NNRPIM (Peyroteo, Belinha, Vinga, Dinis, & Natal Jorge, 2018). Thus, a bone patch and a femur were analysed, and the trabecular bone architecture was accurately verified in both numerical methods used. However, it was found that the meshless methods produced smoother and more accurate results, closer to radiography images.

2 REMODELLING ALGORITHM PROCEDURE

This work, uses a non-linear bone remodelling algorithm, combined with a meshless method (the NNRPIM), which is presented in Figure 1 and described with detail in this section. First, it is possible to discretize the domain of the problem in an unstructured nodal mesh, by obtaining the Voronoï diagram, determining the nodal connectivity (influence-cells) and constructing the integration mesh. This phase is called pre-processing and ends with the definition of the natural and essential boundary conditions and the definition of material properties in the respective areas of the domain. Before starting the iterative remodelling process, a first linear analysis is performed to evaluate the problem. In

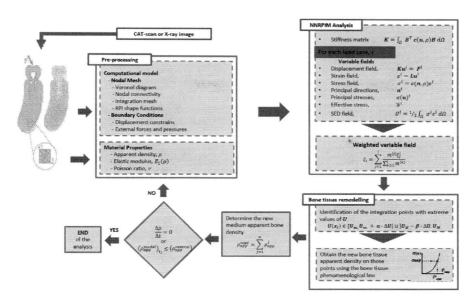

Figure 1. Algorithm of bone remodelling used in this work (Belinha, 2014).

this step, the principal directions of the stress field for each integration point are obtained and the material is oriented following that direction. Thus, in this first iteration no remodelling takes place.

The NNRPIM procedure requires the construction of a local stiffness matrix for each integration point, and then all these local stiffness matrices are assembled, forming a global stiffness matrix, K_i. The remodelling algorithm used in this work allows to consider simultaneously several load cases, f_i^j, and thus, it is possible to determine: (1) the displacement field for each load case, $u_i^j = K_i^{-1} f^j$; (2) the respective strain field, ε_i^j; (3) the stress field, σ_i^j; and (4) the SED field, U_i^j.

Finally, the variable fields obtained for each load case are weighted by the equation shown in Figure 1. Thus, the interest points presenting SED values belonging to the interval of the equation presented in Figure 1 are submitted to a remodelling process of the apparent density, according to the phenomenological law proposed by Belinha (Belinha et al., 2013). All other points maintain the previous density.

Then, considering the weighted principal stresses field at the points of interest selected, it is possible to estimate the new individual apparent density. Once the new density is established, the process proceeds to the next iteration step, and the material properties are updated at each point of interest. The bone tissue remodelling process ends when the medium apparent density of the model reaches a controlled value, or if two consecutive iteration steps present the same medium apparent density. The controlled value can be established by the user, based on clinical observations.

The complete description of the remodelling algorithm can be found in the literature (Belinha, 2014).

3 NUMERICAL ANALYSIS

3.1 Geometrical and Numerical Models

This work aims to numerically evaluate the remodelling of the bone tissue of the mandible surrounding a dental implant. For this purpose, the mandible was sectioned according to an Oyz analysis plane, represented in Figure 2, and then, it was analysed considering a two-dimensional approach.

The model under study is based on the mandibular bone structure, being composed of trabecular bone and a thin layer of cortical bone, approximately 1 mm thick. The dimensions of the titanium implant were based on the study of (Lian et al., 2010), presenting a diameter of 4.5 mm and 11 mm in length. Regarding its mechanical properties, it presents an elastic modulus E = 105 GPa and Poisson's ratio $\upsilon = 0.3$. In relation to bone tissue, its properties depend on the current apparent density and were obtained with the phenomenological law presented previously (Belinha et al., 2013).

After constructing the model and defining the materials, it was possible to discretize the domain of the problem with an irregular nodal mesh composed of 4700 nodes. Subsequently, the natural and essential boundary conditions were defined. Thus, an occlusal load with a magnitude of 100 N, oriented at 11° with respect to the longitudinal axis of the implant, and a pressure (P = 500 Pa) uniformly distributed on the external surface of the

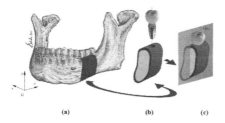

Figure 2. (a) Mandible. (b) Fragment of mandible with dental implant. (c) Model obtained through a cut according to the Oyz axis (Belinha et al., 2015).

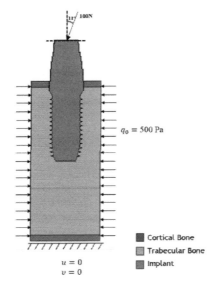

Figure 3. Representation of the geometric model, with the essential and natural boundary conditions applied.

cortical bone, were applied, to simulate the effect of flexion of the mandible. As for the application of the essential boundary conditions, the model is restricted at the base along the Ox and Oy directions, as seen in Figure 3.

Finally, the numerical model described was analysed using a bone remodelling algorithm and an academic software (FEMAS—Finite Element and Meshless Analysis Software) capable to perform several kinds of computational mechanics analysis, using both the FEM and meshless methods (more details in cmech.webs.com).

All materials considered in this analysis assume an initial uniform density distribution, $\rho_{app}^{max} = 2.1\,g/cm^3$, and a constant Poisson's ratio, $\upsilon = 0.3$. Three average densities of the bone were assumed, namely $\rho_{app} = 0.90\,g/cm^3$, $\rho_{app} = 0.65\,g/cm^3$ e $\rho_{app} = 0.40\,g/cm^3$. Notice that the bone remodelling process ends when the medium bone density reaches the controlled value.

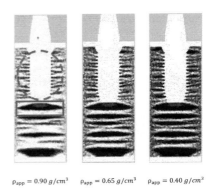

Figure 4. Trabecular architecture obtained for the respective control values considered: 0.90 g/cm³, 0.65 g/cm³ e 0.40 g/cm³. Label: A— B--.

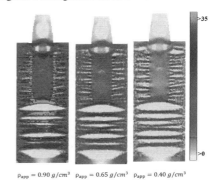

Figure 5. Distribution of the von Mises stress for the respective control values considered: 0.90 g/cm³, 0.65 g/cm³ e 0.40 g/cm³.

3.2 *Results*

The results obtained for the model under study and the changes in the trabecular architecture obtained for each of the controlled apparent densities, are presented in Figure 4. From the analysis, it was possible to obtain the respective von Mises stress distribution maps using the NNRPIM method (Figure 5).

4 CONCLUSION

Below the implant it is possible to observe that the algorithm predicts high density regions oriented horizontally, which connect the cortical sections. However, in the region just below the implant (apical region), large resorption zones are observed. Thus, it is possible to observe in Figure 4 that the distributions of general density in the three images are similar in the following aspects: the trabecular pattern around the implant, as observed by region A; and the area of lower density (bone resorption) just below the implant, as highlighted by region B. The results presented, obtained with the remodelling algorithm, combined with the numerical method NNRPIM, are in agreement with other studies found in the literature, but using FEM (Chou, Jagodnik, & Muftu, 2008) (Lian et al., 2010).

ACKNOWLEDGEMENTS

The authors acknowledge the funding provided by Ministério da Ciência, Tecnologia e Ensino Superior—Fundação para a Ciência e a Tecnologia (Portugal) by project funding MIT-EXPL/ISF/0084/2017. The authors acknowledge the funding of Project NORTE-01-0145-FEDER-000022—SciTech—Science and Technology for Competitive and Sustainable Industries, cofinanced by Programa Operacional Regional do Norte (NORTE2020), through Fundo Europeu de Desenvolvimento Regional (FEDER).

REFERENCES

Beaupré, G.S., Orr, T.E., & Carter, D.R. (1990a). An Approach for Time-Dependent Bone Modeling and Remodeling-Application: A Preliminary Remodeling Simulation. *Journal of Orthopaedic Research*, *8*, 662–670.

Beaupré, G.S., Orr, T.E., & Carter, D.R. (1990b). An Approach for Time-Dependent Bone Modeling and Remodeling-Theoretical Development. *Journal of Orthopaedic Research*, *8*, 651–661.

Belinha, J. (2014). *Meshless Methods in Biomechanics: Bone Tissue Remodelling Analysis.* (Springer International Publishing, Ed.) (Vol. 16).

BELINHA, J., DINIS, L.M.J.S., & JORGE, R.M.N. (2015). The Mandible Remodeling Induced By Dental Implants: a Meshless Approach. *Journal of Mechanics in Medicine and Biology*, *15*(4), 1550059 (31 pages). https://doi.org/10.1142/S0219519415500591.

Belinha, J., Jorge, R.M.N., & Dinis, L.M.J.S. (2013). A meshless microscale bone tissue trabecular remodelling analysis considering a new anisotropic bone tissue material law. *Computer Methods in Biomechanics and Biomedical Engineering*, *16*(11), 1170–1184. https://doi.org/10.1080/10255842.2012.654783.

Carter, D.R., Fyhrie, D.P., & Whalen, R.T. (1987). Trabecular Bone Density And Loading History: Regulation Of Connective Tissue Biology By Mechanical Energy. *Journal of Biomechanics*, *20*(8), 785–794.

Carter, D.R., Orr, T.E., & Fyhrie, D.P. (1989). Relationships Between Femoral Loading History and Femoral Cancellous Bone Architecture. *Journal of Biomechanics*, *22*(3), 231–244. https://doi.org/10.1016/0021-9290(89)90091-2.

Chou, H.-Y., Jagodnik, J.J., & Muftu, S. (2008). Predictions of bone remodeling around dental implant systems. *Journal of Biomechanics*, *41*, 1365–1373. https://doi.org/10.1016/j.jbiomech.2008.01.032.

Cowin, S.C. (1985). The Relationship Between the Elasticity Tensor and the Frabic Tensor. *Mechanics of Materials*, *4*, 137–147.

Cowin, S.C., & Hegedus, D.H. (1976). Bone remodeling I : theory of adaptive elasticity. *Journal of Elasticity*, *6*(3), 313–326.

Doblaré, M., Cueto, E., Calvo, B., Martínez, M.A., Garcia, J.M., & Cegoñino, J. (2005). On the employ of meshless methods in biomechanics. *Computer Methods in Applied Mechanics and Engineering*, *194*(6–8), 801–821. https://doi.org/10.1016/j.cma.2004.06.031.

Doblaré, M., & García, J.M. (2002). Anisotropic bone remodelling model based on a continuum damage-repair theory. *Journal of Biomechanics*, *35*(1), 1–17. https://doi.org/10.1016/S0021-9290(01)00178-6.

Duarte, C.A. (1995). A Review of Some Meshless Methods to Solve Partial Differential Equations, (October). https://doi.org/10.13140/RG.2.2.21361.48489.

Fyhrie, D.P., & Carter, D.R. (1986). A Unifying Principle Relating Stress to Trabecular Bone Morphology. *Journal of Orthopaedic Research*, *4*, 304–317.

Lee, J.D., Chen, Y., Zeng, X., Eskandarian, A., & Oskard, M. (2007). Modeling and simulation of osteoporosis and fracture of trabecular bone by meshless method. *International Journal of Engineering Science*, *45*(2–8), 329–338. https://doi.org/10.1016/j.ijengsci.2007.03.007.

Lian, Z., Guan, H., Ivanovski, S., Loo, Y., Johnson, N.W., & Effect, H.Z. (2010). Effect of bone to implant contact percentage on bone remodelling surrounding a dental implant. *The International Journal of Oral and Maxillofacial Surgery*, *39*, 690–698. https://doi.org/10.1016/j.ijom.2010.03.020.

Lotz, J.C., Gerhart, T.N., & Hayes, W.C. (1991). Mechanical Properties Of Metaphyseal Bone In The Proximal rpimur. *Journal of Biomechanics*, *24*(5), 317–329.

Neukam, F.W., & Flemmig, T.F. (2006). Local and systemic conditions potentially compromising osseointegration. *Clinical of Oral Implantology and Research*, *17*, 160–162.

Petterman, H.E.P., Rejter, T.J., & Rammerstorfer, F.G. (1997). Computational Simulation of Internal Bone Remodeling. *Archives of Computational Methods in Engineering*, *4*(4), 295–323.

Peyroteo, M.M.A., Belinha, J., Vinga, S., Dinis, L.M.J.S., & Natal Jorge, R.M. (2018). Mechanical bone remodelling: Comparative study of distinct numerical approaches. *Engineering Analysis with Boundary Elements*, *0*(July 2017), 1–15. https://doi.org/10.1016/j.enganabound.2018.01.011.

Turner, C.H., Cowin, S.C., Rho, Y., Ashman, R.B., & Rice, J.C. (1989). The Fabric Dependence Of The Orthotropic Elastic Constants Of Cancellous Bone. *Journal of Biomechanics*, *23*(6), 549–561.

Wolff, J. (1986). *The law of bone remodeling (Das Gesetzder Transformationder Knochen, Hirschwald, 1892).* Berlin Heidelberg New York: Springer.

Zioupos, P., Cook, R.B., & Hutchinson, J.R. (2008). Some basic relationships between density values in cancellous and cortical bone. *Journal of Biomechanics*, *41*, 1961–1968. https://doi.org/10.1016/j.jbiomech.2008.03.025.

Zupnik, J., Kim, S., Ravens, D., Karimbux, N., & Guze, K. (2011). Factors Associated With Dental Implant Survival: A 4-Year Retrospective Analysis. *Journal of Periodontology*, *82*(10), 1390–1395. https://doi.org/10.1902/jop.2011.100685.

Biodental Engineering V – Belinha et al. (Eds)
© 2019 Taylor & Francis Group, London, ISBN 978-0-367-21087-8

Computational structural analysis of dental implants using radial point interpolation meshless methods

C.C.C. Coelho
Faculty of Engineering, University of Porto (FEUP), Porto, Portugal

J. Belinha
Department of Mechanical Engineering, School of Engineering, Polytechnic of Porto (ISEP), Porto, Portugal

R.M. Natal Jorge
Department of Mechanical Engineering, Faculty of Engineering, University of Porto (FEUP), Porto, Portugal

ABSTRACT: Over the years, several studies have shown that dental implants are the best solution to restore the natural dental dynamics. With the increasing demand for oral care, favourable times for its continuous evolution are approaching. Currently, numerical methods are essential computational techniques to respond effectively to problems encountered in the dental practice. The objective of this study was to understand the biomechanical behaviour of the implants and investigate how the nodal discretization of the model and the constituent material of the medical device influence the displacement and stress distribution. Therefore, this work used the Finite Element Method (FEM) and radial point interpolation meshless methods, namely the Radial Point Interpolation Method (RPIM) and the Natural Neural Radial Point Interpolation Method (NNRPIM), to accomplish these objectives. The solutions obtained with the three methodologies were compared. In the end, it was verified that the meshless methods have smoother and more precise variable fields.

1 STATE OF THE ART

1.1 Introduction

With the incessant search for "perfection", the smile becomes one of the most important factors for the human being. Thus, its care and treatment became an indispensable factor. Over the years, it is inevitable to escape tooth decay. Unbalanced diet, lack of oral hygiene care and smoking are some of the causes that aggravate this procedure and may contribute to the appearance of pathologies such as dental caries and periodontal diseases.

Currently, dental implants are the best solution for dental absence (Bicudo, Reis, Deus, Reis, & Vaz, 2016), providing to the patient a regain of function, comfort and aesthetics (Van Staden, Guan, Johnson, Loo, & Meredith, 2008).

From the biomechanical point of view, the key factor for the success of a dental implant depends on how stress and strain are transmitted to the surrounding tissues. These distributions of stress and strain are affected by a number of variables, such as geometry, dimensions and material properties, load conditions, nature of the bone-implant interface and bone density (Bicudo et al., 2016), (Van Staden et al., 2008), (Eskitascioglu, Usumez, Sevimay, Soykan, & Unsal, 2004), (Ichim, Hu, Bazen, & Yi, 2016). Relating all these variables to find an ideal solution becomes a challenging task.

1.2 Numerical methods

There has always been a need to understand and explain the physical phenomena of nature, such as heat conduction, electromagnetic fields, fluid mechanics, or stress in mechanical structures. These phenomena can be described by mathematical formulations and predicted through partial differential equations. However, these equations are extremely complex to be solved analytically because they involve a variety of intervening factors such as multidimensional domains, nonlinear systems, complex structures, load systems, and boundary conditions. Therefore, approximation numerical methods are a powerful computational tool to obtain fields of precise and immediate solutions to such problems (Heckbert, 1993). Due to the development of high-speed digital computers, the cost-effectiveness of numerical procedures was significantly improved and these methods became very efficient and reliable (Chao & Chow, 2002). Computational mechanics thus became a fundamental ally, without which many issues would remain unresolved.

1.2.1 *Finite elements method*

The FEM consists in dividing the domain of the problem into a finite number of small parts called finite elements. These elements represent the continuous domain of the problem, being interpolated by base functions, the shape functions (Heckbert, 1993). The discretization of the domain into finite elements, that are interconnected with each other by points denominated nodes, construct a mesh. It is then possible to reduce a problem of extreme complexity, into a simpler problem, which enables to solve it more effectively. These elements can have different shapes, depending on the type and size of the problem, and can have different properties that allow the discretization of structures with different materials (Chao & Chow, 2002), (Liu & Quek, 2013). The solution to the overall system is obtained by pooling the results for each element. The precision of the results obtained by the Finite Element Method depends on the number of nodes and elements and the size of the mesh. That is, the higher the number of nodes and elements of the discretization, the higher the precision will be (Nguyen, Rabczuk, Bordas, & Duflot, 2008).

The FEM is a well-known numerical method and it is used in large scale in several areas of engineering. However, this method has limitations. Because interpolation is dependent on the mesh generated, distorted or poor-quality meshes lead to high errors. Moreover, it is not suitable for treating problems with discontinuities that do not align with the ends of the elements (Nguyen et al., 2008). Therefore, a family of widely developed methods, meshless methods, emerged as an attractive alternative for a growing variety of problems (Doblaré et al., 2005).

1.2.2 *Meshless methods*

In meshless methods, the physical domain of the problem is discretized with an unstructured nodal distribution, since the field functions are approximated within a domain of influence rather than an element (Belinha, 2014), (Tavares, Belinha, Dinis, & Natal Jorge, 2015). As opposed to the non-overlap rule between elements of the finite element method, in meshless methods, influence-domains can and should overlap one another. It is possible to define and classify a numerical method by three fundamental phases: the construction of shape functions, formulation and integration (Belinha, 2014).

Depending on the formulation used, meshless methods can be classified into two categories.

The first is the strong formulation, that directly uses the partial differential equations that govern the physical phenomenon studied to obtain the solution (Belinha, 2014). Smooth Particle Hydrodynamics (SPH) was the first meshless method to be proposed in this category, as mentioned in (Tavares et al., 2015), being responsible for the origin of the Reproducing Kernel Particle Method (RKPM). A parallel pathway on the development of meshless methods began in the 1990s. This alternative pathway used weak formulation. The weak formulation uses a variable principle to minimize the residual weight of the differential equations that govern the phenomenon. This residue is obtained by replacing the exact solution with an approximate function affected by a test function (Belinha, 2014). The first mature meshless method to be used with this formulation in computational mechanics was the Diffuse Element Method (DEM) (Belinha, 2014), (Tavares et al., 2015) based on the approximation method, the least squares moving (Lancaster & Salkauskas, 1981).

As mentioned in (Belinha, 2014), with the development of these formulations many new methods have been developed and proposed, such as the Element Free Galerkin Method (EFGM), being this one of the most well-known meshless method. Meshless Local Petrov-Galerkin Method (MLPG), another important meshless method, that was initially developed to solve problems of linear and nonlinear potential. Later, Oñate and co-workers developed a new meshless method, the Finite Point Method (FPM), which uses a stabilization technique to perform numerical integration. Another method of approximation also proposed was the Radial Basis Function Method (RBFM), as cited in (Belinha, 2014). Although approximate meshless methods have been applied successfully in computational mechanics, several problems have not been completely solved, because many differential equations governing real-world phenomena do not admit sufficiently soft solutions (Belinha, 2014). The most important and unresolved problem is the lack of the delta Kronecker property in the approximation functions, which makes it difficult to impose essential and natural conditions that have to be imposed by computationally expensive numerical techniques such as Lagrange multipliers (Belinha, 2014), (Tavares et al., 2015), (Dinis, Natal Jorge, & Belinha, 2007). As mentioned in (Belinha, 2014), to overcome this problem, several meshless interpolation methods have been developed, such as the Point Interpolation Method (PIM), the Radial Point Interpolation Method (RPIM), the Natural Neighbour Finite Element Method (NNFEM), and the Natural Element Method (NEM). More recently, the Natural Radial Element Method (NREM) was developed. NREM is an effective and accurate, truly meshless method that has low order nodal connectivity. The combination between the NEM and the RPIM originated the Natural Neighbour Radial Point Interpolation Method (NNRPIM) (Belinha, 2014).

1.2.2.1 *RPIM e NNRPIM*

Meshless methods require the presence and the combination of three basic parts: nodal connectivity, numerical integration, and shape functions. These three concepts will be briefly described for the meshless methods used in this study.

In RPIM, nodal connectivity is obtained by overlapping the influence-domain of each node. These influence-domains are found through a search of a specific number of nodes, within a given area, for a 2D problem (as demonstrated in Figure 1) (Belinha, 2014), (Wang & Liu, 2002), (Liu & Gu, 2001), or a determined volume, for a 3D problem, (Nguyen et al., 2008), (Doblaré et al., 2005), (Wang & Liu, 2002), and may present several forms with fixed or variable size that affect the performance of this method (Belinha, 2014).

To impose the nodal connectivity in the NNRPIM, the influence-domain is replaced by the concept of influence-cell that depends on geometric and mathematical concepts, such as the Voronoï diagrams (Belinha, 2014). Influence-cells may be first-order influence-cells or second-order influence-cells, as shown in Figure 2.

Since RPIM and NNRPIM use the weak Galerkin formulation, a background integration mesh is required. For the RPIM, numerical integration is established using the Gaussian integration scheme. In the NNRPIM, the integration mesh is based on the nodal distribution, that is, on the Voronoï diagram and the Delaunay triangulation (Belinha, 2014).

The interpolation functions for both methods are determined using the RPI technique, which

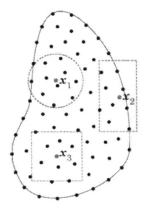

Figure 1. Influence-domains with different sizes and shapes.

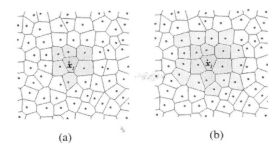

Figure 2. (a) First-degree influence cells, (b) second degree influence cells. The x_I represents the selected interesse node.

requires the combination of a polynomial basis with a radial basis function (RBF) (Wang & Liu, 2002).

1.3 *Meshless methods and dental implants*

In the literature, it is possible to find some studies that use the meshless methods in the field of biomechanics (Doblaré et al., 2005), (Tsubota, Wada, & Yamaguchi, 2006), (Belinha, Dinis, & Natal Jorge, 2015), however, Duarte et al. were the first to use a meshless method, the NNRPIM, for the 2D numerical analysis of dental implants (Duarte, Andrade, Dinis, Jorge, & Belinha, 2015). In this study, numerical models for a single implant system and a bar implant system were built. In the analysis of the single implant system, the maximum stresses obtained with the NNRPIM were very similar to the FEM. However, comparing the stress field obtained with the NNRPIM with the strain field obtained in FEM, it is noticeable that the NNRPIM solution is softer than the solution obtained with the formulation of the finite element method. The authors found that bone tissues (which present a higher rigidity) induce higher levels of stress in the implant structure and lower stress levels in the bone tissues, which may lead to a lower remodelling in the surrounding bone tissue. In the numerical analysis of the bar-implant system, it was verified that the increase of rigidity of the bar material leads to higher levels of stress in the bone tissue and lower levels of stress in the implant, which potentially can increase the remodelling of the mandibular bone tissue. The results obtained allowed to conclude that the NNRPIM is a valid and alternative method in the linear elastostatic biomechanical analysis of dental implant systems (Duarte et al., 2015).

Tavares et al. performed an elastoplastic analysis of bone tissue due to the insertion of dental implants through NNRPIM and 2D modelling. In this work only the trabecular bone was assumed as a non-linear material. It was verified that the trabecular bone begins to enter the plastic region for an occlusal load with a magnitude of 113N and 10° from the implant's longitudinal line. When the load value reaches 223N, most of the trabecular bone surrounding the implant is already in the plastic region (Tavares et al., 2015).

2 NUMERICAL ANALYSIS

2.1 Geometrical and numerical models

The geometric model was obtained from the literature (Tian et al., 2012), which allowed to adapt a 2D model from a 3D model.

As shown in Figure 3(a), the implant has 4 mm of diameter and 14.8 mm of height. It was inserted into the bone in an axial position. The abutment was aligned with the mandibular bone at an angle of 90° with the horizontal plane. The bone tissue is composed of two dissimilar layers: trabecular bone (internal layer) and cortical bone (outer layer). Both bone layers were considered. In addition, a portion of the gum was also assumed inserted into the lateral parts of the implant, as represented in Figure 3(b).

Subsequently, the nodal mesh was constructed. For the convergence study, five different meshes were created and are listed in Table 1.

The number of nodes that each patch should have was obtained from the length of the curves that outlined it, in order to reach a more uniform mesh. The abutment and the implant were considered to be a single body of Ti-6Al-4V alloy.

Selecting the model discretized with 5281 nodes, the most uniform mesh, it was possible to study the biomechanical behaviour of the two-dimensional model by varying the material of the dental implant.

Table 1. Nodal meshes used in the convergence study.

	Nodes	Elements
Mesh 1	1627	3083
Mesh 2	2408	4617
Mesh 3	3232	6241
Mesh 4	4337	8421
Mesh 5	5281	10284

Table 2. Mechanical properties of materials used in numerical analysis.

		Young's modulus (E) [MPa]	Poisson's ratio (υ)
Implant	Ti-6Al-4V	110000	0.30
	3Y-TZP	210000	0.30
	Ti-15Zr	112000	0.30
	CFR-PEEK	150000	0.35
Bone	Cortical	13700	0.30
	Trabecular	1370	0.30
Gum		19.6	0.30

The following materials were assumed (tested) for the implant: Titanium (Ti-6Al-4V), Zirconia (3Y-TZP), Titanium-Zirconium (Ti-15Zr) (Saini, Singh, Arora, Arora, & Jain, 2015), and Polyetheretherketone with carbon fibres (CFR-PEEK).

In Table 2 are shown the mechanical properties of the materials used in this study. These mechanical properties are described in the literature (Tian et al., 2012), (Madfa, Al-Sanabani, Al-Qudami, Al-Sanabani, & Amran, 2014), (Schwitalla, Abou-Emara, Spintig, Lackmann, & Müller, 2015), (Kayabaşi, Yüzbasioğlu, & Erzincanli, 2006). All materials were considered homogeneous, linear elastic and isotropic.

For both the convergence study and the study of stress distribution, the same boundary conditions and the same loads were defined.

As represented in Figure 4, the peripheral parts of the bone were fully constrained.

Simulating the initial periods of bruxism, the occlusal force exerted will shift in its direction due to the manifested friction force. Thus, it was considered a force with a magnitude of 1N and an angulation of 84.29° (Zheng, Zhou, Zhang, Li, & Yu, 2003). This force is applied into the upper part of the abutment, as shown in Figure 4.

2.2 Results

In the convergence study the vertical displacement was evaluated for the six different nodal meshes

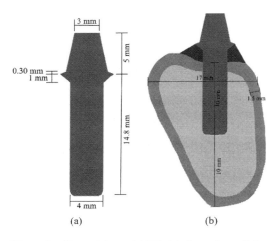

Figure 3. Geometric model 2D; (a) dimensions of the dental implant, (b) dimensions of the bone tissue.

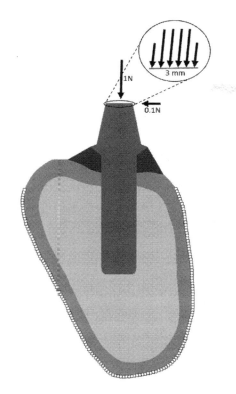

Figure 4. Load case and boundary conditions applied in the two-dimensional model.

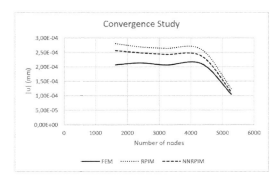

Figure 5. Total displacement obtained for the different nodal discretization and for the different numerical methods.

and for the three numerical methods. The point of interest selected for this study was the highest and intermediate point located at the top of the abutment.

It can be seen from the results in Figure 5 that the values obtained with FEM are lower when compared with values obtained with the two meshless methods. In addition, it should be noted that

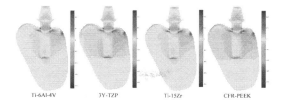

Figure 6. Main stress maps, $\sigma 11$, for analysis performed in FEMAS software by NNRPIM.

the results obtained are already very close to the final converged value (all lines are almost flat).

The distributions of the principal stress, for the model with 5281 nodes, as a function of implant material were obtained for the three numerical methods. It was found that all the three solutions presented very similar values. Therefore, only the results obtained with the NNRPIM are shown in Figure 6.

3 CONCLUSIONS

Through the convergence study it can be concluded that the nodal mesh influences the biomechanical behaviour of the model. As the number of nodes increases, the obtained displacement fields are more accurate for the three numerical discretization methods. It was verified that the values from the meshless methods are more accurate and smooth when compared to the FEM.

It was verified that the minimum stresses were verified in the implant neck and the maximum stresses in the apical zone of the implant and in the interface with cortical bone, for the four materials analysed. Metal alloys have a better stress distribution when compared to ceramic and composite materials.

With these studies is possible to conclude that the meshless methods are a good alternative to the finite element method for biomechanical applications.

In future works, it is recommended that other variable fields, in addition to displacement and stress, are evaluated for the different implant materials in more complex models, such as three-dimensional analyses, to find more viable therapeutic solutions for the dental reality. Elastoplastic behaviour and anisotropic materials are other important factors to consider.

ACKNOWLEDGEMENTS

The authors truly acknowledge the funding provided by Ministério da Ciência, Tecnologia e

Ensino Superior—Fundação para a Ciência e a Tecnologia (Portugal) by project funding MIT-EXPL/ISF/0084/2017. Additionally, the authors gratefully acknowledge the funding of Project NORTE-01-0145-FEDER-000022—SciTech—Science and Technology for Competitive and Sustainable Industries, cofinanced by Programa Operacional Regional do Norte (NORTE2020), through Fundo Europeu de Desenvolvimento Regional (FEDER).

REFERENCES

Belinha, J. (2014). *Meshless Methods in Biomechanics—Bone Tissue Remodelling Analysis*. (J.M.R.S. Tavares & R.M. Natal Jorge, Eds.) (Vol. 16). Springer Netherlands. https://doi.org/10.1007/978-94-007-4174-4.

Belinha, J., Dinis, L.M.J.S., & Natal Jorge, R.M. (2015). The meshless methods in the bone tissue remodelling analysis. *Procedia Engineering, 110*, 51–58. https://doi.org/10.1016/j.proeng.2015.07.009.

Bicudo, P., Reis, J., Deus, A.M., Reis, L., & Vaz, M.F. (2016). Performance evaluation of dental implants: An experimental and numerical simulation study. *Theoretical and Applied Fracture Mechanics, 85*, 74–83. https://doi.org/10.1016/j.tafmec.2016.08.014.

Chao, T.Y., & Chow, W. (2002). A review on the applications of finite element method to heat transfer and fluid flow. *International Journal on Architectural Science, 3*(1), 1–19.

Dinis, L.M.J.S., Natal Jorge, R.M., & Belinha, J. (2007). Analysis of 3D solids using the natural neighbour radial point interpolation method. *Computer Methods in Applied Mechanics and Engineering, 196*(13), 2009–2028. https://doi.org/10.1016/j.cma.2006.11.002.

Doblaré, M., Cueto, E., Calvo, B., Martínez, M.A., Garcia, J.M., & Cegoñino, J. (2005). On the employ of meshless methods in biomechanics. *Computer Methods in Applied Mechanics and Engineering, 194*(6–8), 801–821. https://doi.org/10.1016/j.cma.2004.06.031.

Duarte, H.M.S., Andrade, J.R., Dinis, L.M.J.S., Jorge, R.M.N., & Belinha, J. (2015). Numerical analysis of dental implants using a new advanced discretization technique. *Mechanics of Advanced Materials and Structures, 23*(4), 467–479. https://doi.org/10.1080/15376494.2014.987410.

Eskitascioglu, G., Usumez, A., Sevimay, M., Soykan, E., & Unsal, E. (2004). The influence of occlusal loading on stresses transferred to implant-supported prostheses and supporting bone: A three dimensional finite element study. *Journal Prosthetic Dentistry, 91*(2), 144–150. Retrieved from njcmindia.org/uploads/5-1_81-84.pdf.

Heckbert, P.S. (1993). Introduction to finite element methods, 1–10.

Ichim, P.I., Hu, X., Bazen, J.J., & Yi, W. (2016). Design optimization of a radial functionally graded dental implant. *Journal of Biomedical Materials Research—Part B Applied Biomaterials, 104*(1), 58–66. https://doi.org/10.1002/jbm.b.33345.

Kayabaşı, O., Yüzbasioğlu, E., & Erzincanli, F. (2006). Static, dynamic and fatigue behaviors of dental implant using finite element method. *Advances in Engineering Software, 37*(10), 649–658. https://doi.org/10.1016/j.advengsoft.2006.02.004.

Lancaster, P., & Salkauskas, K. (1981). Surface generated by moving least square methods. *Mathematics of Computation, 37*(155), 141–158. https://doi.org/10.1090/S0025-5718-1981-0616367-1.

Liu, G.R., & Gu, Y.T. (2001). A point interpolation method for two dimensional solids. *International Journal for Numerical Methods in Engineering, 50*(4), 937–951. https://doi.org/10.1002/1097-0207(20010210)50.

Liu, G.R., & Quek, S.S. (2013). *The finite element method: a practical course* (2th ed.). Elsevier Butterworth Heinemann.

Madfa, A.A., Al-Sanabani, F.A., Al-Qudami, N.H., Al-Sanabani, J.S., & Amran, A.G. (2014). Use of zirconia in dentistry: An overview. *Biomaterials, 5*(1), 1–7. https://doi.org/10.2174/1876502501405010001.

Nguyen, V.P., Rabczuk, T., Bordas, S., & Duflot, M. (2008). Meshless methods: A review and computer implementation aspects. *Mathematics and Computers in Simulation, 79*(3), 763–813. https://doi.org/10.1016/j.matcom.2008.01.003.

Saini, M., Singh, Y., Arora, P., Arora, V., & Jain, K. (2015). Implant biomaterials: A comprehensive review. *World Journal of Clinical Cases, 3*(1), 52–57. https://doi.org/10.12998/wjcc.v3.i1.52.

Schwitalla, A.D., Abou-Emara, M., Spintig, T., Lackmann, J., & Müller, W.D. (2015). Finite element analysis of the biomechanical effects of PEEK dental implants on the peri-implant bone. *Journal of Biomechanics, 48*(1), 1–7. https://doi.org/10.1016/j.jbiomech.2014.11.017.

Tavares, C.S.S., Belinha, J., Dinis, L.M.J.S., & Natal Jorge, R.M. (2015). The elasto-plastic response of the bone tissue due to the insertion of dental implants. *Procedia Engineering, 110*, 37–44. https://doi.org/10.1016/j.proeng.2015.07.007.

Tian, K., Chen, J., Han, L., Yang, J., Huang, W., & Wu, D. (2012). Angled abutments result in increased or decreased stress on surrounding bone of single-unit dental implants: A finite element analysis. *Medical Engineering and Physics, 34*(10), 1526–1531. https://doi.org/10.1016/j.medengphy.2012.10.003.

Tsubota, K. ichi, Wada, S., & Yamaguchi, T. (2006). Particle method for computer simulation of red blood cell motion in blood flow. *Computer Methods and Programs in Biomedicine, 83*(2), 139–146. https://doi.org/10.1016/j.cmpb.2006.06.005.

Van Staden, R.C., Guan, H., Johnson, N.W., Loo, Y., & Meredith, N. (2008). Step-wise analysis of the dental implant insertion process using the finite element technique. *Clinical Oral Implants Research, 19*(3), 303–13. https://doi.org/10.1111/j.1600-0501.2007.01427.x.

Wang, J.G., & Liu, G.R. (2002). A point interpolation meshless method based on radial basis functions. *International Journal for Numerical Methods in Engineering, 54*(11), 1623–1648. https://doi.org/10.1002/nme.489.

Zheng, J., Zhou, Z.R., Zhang, J., Li, H., & Yu, H.Y. (2003). On the friction and wear behaviour of human tooth enamel and dentin. *Wear, 255*(7–12), 967–974. https://doi.org/10.1016/S0043-1648(03)00079-6.

Biodental Engineering V – Belinha et al. (Eds)
© 2019 Taylor & Francis Group, London, ISBN 978-0-367-21087-8

The biomechanical simulation of a zygomatic bar implant using meshless methods

C.C.C. Coelho
Faculty of Engineering, University of Porto (FEUP), Porto, Portugal

J. Belinha
Department of Mechanical Engineering, School of Engineering, Polytechnic of Porto (ISEP), Porto, Portugal

R.M. Natal Jorge
Department of Mechanical Engineering, Faculty of Engineering, University of Porto (FEUP), Porto, Portugal

ABSTRACT: The combination of several implants presents itself as a safe and efficient (with a high success rate) therapeutic option for edentulism and bone atrophy. In this study, the stress fields of the 3D geometric model of a bar implant with one zygomatic implant and three conventional implants were numerically analysed, using FEM, RPIM and NNRPIM. Based on the results obtained, it is possible to affirm that meshless methods allow to obtain more precise and smoother solutions when compared with the most popular technique – the finite element method. Thus, meshless methods have the potential to be the future of computational biomechanics.

1 STATE OF THE ART

1.1 Introduction

The prevalence of the elderly population, as well as the increase in average life expectancy in recent decades, gradually increases the number of people who use dental prostheses (De Vico et al., 2011). Implanted prostheses became commonplace in the late 1960s because of their long-term success. Although the same investigators had hypothesized to use one implant for each missing tooth, this procedure is not possible in all situations, especially where bone height is insufficient (Ozdemir Doğan, Polat, Polat, Seker, & Gul, 2014).

The edentulous condition, and consequently the bone reabsorption, restricts the use of dental implants and often the use of cantilever prostheses or bone graft procedures (Brånemark, Brånemark, Rydevik, & Myers, 2001). In the presence of a cantilever, excessive implant tension can be observed, with an increase in biomechanical complications and consequently implant failure (de Souza Batista et al., 2017). Bone graft surgery has some limitations, including multiple surgical procedures, increased risk of complications, longer treatment period, higher costs and low patient acceptance (Maló, de Araujo Nobre, & Lopes, 2008), (Bhering et al., 2016).

Thus, combinations of several dental implants have led to the development of solutions to solve these problems, ensuring less invasive and shorter treatment intervals, lower cost, lower patient morbidity and better quality of life (Bhering et al., 2016), (Peixoto et al., 2017), (Gümrükçü, Korkmaz, & Korkmaz, 2017).

1.2 Numerical methods

The use of numerical methods has revolutionized current science, leaving behind experimental studies which, in addition of being very dependent on assumptions (due to the impossibility of obtaining experimental models in humans), require very high costs and observation periods. The most popular discretization technique is the Finite Element Method (FEM) (Zienkiewicz, Taylor, & Zhu, 2005). This method allows to discretize the domain of the problem into a set of not overlapping elements that can present a variety of forms depending on the type and dimension of the problem. These elements are connected by nodes, forming the finite element mesh. The solution fields are obtained by interpolating shape functions in each one of the elements that make up the mesh. The FEM performance depends on the mesh quality, that influences the accuracy of the results (Zienkiewicz et al., 2005).

However, FEM generally exhibits some numerical perturbations in the stress fields, particularly in areas of discontinuities and areas of material change. Therefore, to overcome these limitations, the scientific community dedicated themselves to the development of other methods of discretization, the meshless methods (Belinha, 2014). These methods have the potential to contribute with more precise and smooth analyses, providing better solutions and improving clinical performances.

1.3 *Meshless advanced discretization techniques*

It was from the mid-twentieth century that meshless methods began to be used to solve partial differential equations (Gingold & Monaghan, 1977), (Atluri & Zhu, 1998). Since then, new methods have been developed (Wang & Liu, 2002), (Dinis, Natal Jorge, & Belinha, 2007) and applied to computational biomechanics (Belinha, 2014), (Belinha, 2016).

The main difference of the meshless methods in relation to the method traditionally used is in the discretization of the problem. The domain of the problem is discretized in arbitrarily distributed nodes, rather than elements (Belinha, 2014), (Tavares, Belinha, Dinis, & Natal Jorge, 2015). In biomechanics, this flexibility of discretization is very advantageous because it allows the domain of the problem to be discretized directly from medical imaging techniques, such as computer tomography or magnetic resonance imaging (Belinha, 2016).

In this study, two meshless methods were used, namely the Radial Point Interpolation Method (RPIM) and Natural Neighbour Radial Point Interpolation Method (NNRPIM). After discretization, nodal connectivity can be imposed using influence-domains for the RPIM, or influence-cells for the NNRPIM. The influence-domains are found by searching a specific number of nodes within a given area (for a 2D problem), or a given volume (for a 3D problem), and can present variable size and shape (Belinha, 2014). To obtain the influence-cells, the NNRPIM depends on geometric and mathematical constructs, such as the Delaunay triangulation and Voronoï diagrams (Belinha, 2014).

For numerical integration it is necessary to build a background mesh. As in FEM, it is common to use background Gaussian integration meshes fitted to the problem domain. For the meshless methods, there are other approaches, such as the use of nodal integration, that directly use the nodal distribution to obtain the integration weight at each node. The meshless methods using this integration scheme are called "truly meshless methods" (Belinha, 2014).

The system of equations is obtained with the weak formulation of Galerkin. To write such system of equations, it is necessary to obtain shape functions. In both meshless methods, the shape functions are constructed using the radial point interpolator technique (Wang & Liu, 2002), which requires the combination of a polynomial base with a Radial Basis Function (RBF). The interpolation functions possess the delta Kronecker property, which means that the function obtained passes through all points scattered in an influence-domain. This property is very important, since it allows the use of the same simple techniques used in the FEM to establish the essential boundary conditions, thus reducing the computational cost (Belinha, Dinis, & Natal Jorge, 2013), (Belinha, 2014).

1.4 *Meshless methods in biomechanics*

Meshless methods are used in a wide variety of fields, but their attention is focused on the biomechanical field due to their important discretization flexibility feature, which allows the discretization of the problem domain through medical imaging. Then, it is possible to directly analyse the biomechanical behaviour of biological structures (Belinha, 2016).

Recently, several studies have applied the meshless methods to the biomechanical field. Today, NNRPIM is a popular meshless discretization technique because NNRPIM is more accurate than other meshless methods and the Finite Element Method, producing smoother stress and strain fields (Belinha, Natal Jorge, & Dinis, 2012).

Belinha and his collaborators (Belinha et al., 2012) presented a new algorithm to predict bone remodelling. Through the NNRPIM and radiography medical images, it was possible to evaluate the remodelling in the femoral bone (Belinha et al., 2012), (Belinha, Dinis, & Natal Jorge, 2015b), calcaneus bone (Belinha et al., 2012) and with the insertion of a femoral implant (Belinha, Dinis, & Natal Jorge, 2016). The remodelling model was also applied to the molar region of the mandible, analysing the presence of a dental implant (Belinha, Dinis, & Natal Jorge, 2015a). The biomechanical behaviour of simple and bar dental implants (Duarte, Andrade, Dinis, Jorge, & Belinha, 2015) and natural teeth (Moreira, Belinha, Dinis, & Jorge, 2014) were also analysed by the advanced discretization technique, the NNRPIM. Geometric models were developed to predict non-linear behaviour of bone structures in the presence of a dental implants (Tavares et al., 2015). Recently, the meshless methods were also used to analysed the vestibular system (Santos et al., 2017).

2 NUMERICAL ANALYSIS

2.1 Geometrical and numerical models

The geometric model of a right maxillary prosthesis was obtained from the literature (Miyamoto, Ujigawa, Kizu, Tonogi, & Yamane, 2010).

The prosthesis consists of three conventional implants: Brånemark System® standard implants (Norbel Biocare AB, Goteborg, Sweden), with 3.75 mm in diameter and 13 mm in length. But also, a zygomatic implant. The abutment has a height of 3 mm. The implants and their respective abutments were connected in one body. The three commercial implants had an inclination of 90° in relation to the vertical plane, and the zygomatic implant an inclination of 90° with respect to the resection plane. The bar, 8 mm long and 10 mm high, supported all implants. The construction and simulation of the three-dimensional model was developed in FEMAS—Finite Element and Meshless Analysis Software, which is an academic software capable to perform several kinds of computational mechanics analysis, using both the FEM and meshless methods (more details in cmech.webs.com).

The numerical analysis was performed by the most popular technique, the FEM and by recently developed techniques and of enormous interest in the biomechanics, the meshless methods, namely RPIM and NNRPIM. A three-dimensional mesh with 8221 nodes and 38112 elements was generated for the three numerical methods.

The properties of the materials used in this study are listed in Table 1 and were obtained from reference values described in the literature (Geng, Tan, & Liu, 2001). All materials were considered homogeneous and isotropic, with linear elastic behaviour.

The application of a vertical force with a magnitude of 150 N was assumed normal to the Oxy plane of the zygomatic implant (Ujigawa, Kato, Kizu, Tonogi, & Yamane, 2007), as show in Figure 2. The interface zones between the implants and the bar were defined as restriction of the prosthesis, assuming osseointegrated implants, in such a way that no movement occurs in these regions.

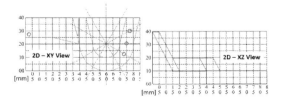

Figure 1. Bar implant design with 1 zygomatic implant and three conventional implants.

Table 1. Mechanical properties of the materials considered.

	Young's modulus (E) [MPa]	Poisson ratio (ν)
Implants		
Ti-6 Al-4V	110000	0.33
Bar		
Type 3 gold alloy	100000	0.30

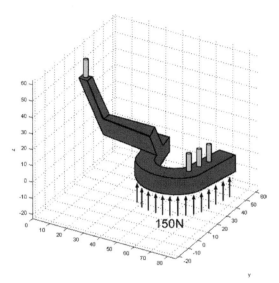

Figure 2. Boundary conditions and applied load.

All these conditions were assumed for the three numerical methods under study.

2.2 Results

In Figure 3 is observed the von Mises stress distribution for the three numerical methods. The regions of higher stress were recorded near the zygomatic implant, in the conventional implant placed in the position of the superior premolar and posteriorly in the interconnection of the upper part with the lower part of the bar. It is also possible to observe that the results obtained for the three numerical methods are very similar.

Then von Mises stress was studied individually for each one of the implants that constitute the dental prosthesis.

In Figure 4 is displayed the stresses recorded for each one of the implants as a function of the numerical methods.

It is notorious that meshless methods present stress fields more precise and smooth than the

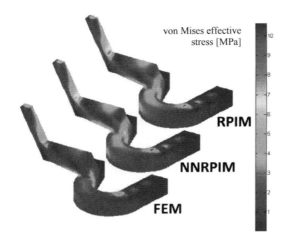

Figure 3. Effective stress maps for the three numerical methods.

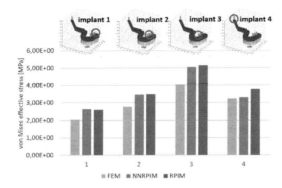

Figure 4. von Mises stress for each implant of the dental prosthesis and for the three numerical methods.

ones obtained with the FEM. The implant located at the position of the upper premolar presents the highest stress. Therefore, this implant is more susceptible to fracture. One solution to combat the areas of greatest stress would be to increase the number of implants to have a better distribution of stress and thus obtain a more stable model

3 CONCLUSIONS

Since all methodologies were programmed following the same layout, the computational framework permits a more pragmatic comparison regarding the performance and the accuracy of each numeric approach. Thus, the experience acquired with the developed work permits to assert the following conclusions: (1) meshless methods are capable to produce variable fields very similar to FEM, however those fields are smoother, and accordingly to the literature, the variable fields (stresses/strains/displacements) are more accurate than FEM for the same discretization (number of nodes); (2) the number and the location of the implants significantly change the maximum stress obtained; (3) meshless methods present a much higher computational cost, comparing with FEM.

The developed work and the obtained results permit to conclude that meshless methods, being accurate and flexible numerical method, have the potential to progress on the immediate future in several biomechanics fields.

ACKNOWLEDGEMENTS

The authors truly acknowledge the funding provided by Ministério da Ciência, Tecnologia e Ensino Superior—Fundação para a Ciência e a Tecnologia (Portugal) by project funding MIT-EXPL/ISF/0084/2017. Additionally, the authors gratefully acknowledge the funding of Project NORTE-01-0145-FEDER-000022—SciTech—Science and Technology for Competitive and Sustainable Industries, cofinanced by Programa Operacional Regional do Norte (NORTE2020), through Fundo Europeu de Desenvolvimento Regional (FEDER).

REFERENCES

Atluri, S.N., & Zhu, T. (1998). A new Meshless Local Petrov-Galerkin (MLPG) approach in computational mechanics. *Computational Mechanics*, 22(2), 117–127. https://doi.org/10.1007/s004660050346.

Belinha, J. (2014). *Meshless Methods in Biomechanics – Bone Tissue Remodelling Analysis*. (J.M.R.S. Tavares & R.M. Natal Jorge, Eds.) (Vol. 16). Springer Netherlands. https://doi.org/10.1007/978-94-007-4174-4.

Belinha, J. (2016). Meshless Methods: The Future of Computational Biomechanical Simulation. *Journal of Biometrics & Biostatistics*, 7(4), 1–3. https://doi.org/10.4172/2155-6180.1000325.

Belinha, J., Dinis, L.M.J.S., & Natal Jorge, R.M. (2013). The natural radial element method. *International Journal for Numerical Methods in Engineering*, 93(12), 1286–1313. https://doi.org/10.1002/nme.4427.

Belinha, J., Dinis, L.M.J.S., & Natal Jorge, R.M. (2015a). The Mandible Remodeling Induced by Dental Implant: a Meshless Approach. *Journal of Mechanics in Medicine and Biology*, 15(4), 31. https://doi.org/10.1142/S0219519415500591.

Belinha, J., Dinis, L.M.J.S., & Natal Jorge, R.M. (2015b). The meshless methods in the bone tissue remodelling analysis. *Procedia Engineering*, 110, 51–58. https://doi.org/10.1016/j.proeng.2015.07.009.

Belinha, J., Dinis, L.M.J.S., & Natal Jorge, R.M. (2016). The analysis of the bone remodelling around femoral stems: A meshless approach. *Mathematics and Computers in Simulation, 121,* 64–94. https://doi.org/10.1016/j.MATCOM.2015.09.002.

Belinha, J., Natal Jorge, R.M., & Dinis, L.M.J.S. (2012). Bone tissue remodelling analysis considering a radial point interpolator meshless method. *Engineering Analysis with Boundary Elements, 36*(11), 1660–1670. https://doi.org/10.1016/j.enganabound.2012.05.009.

Bhering, C.L.B., Mesquita, M.F., Kemmoku, D.T., Noritomi, P.Y., Consani, R.L.X., & Barão, V.A.R. (2016). Comparison between all-on-four and all-on-six treatment concepts and framework material on stress distribution in atrophic maxilla: A prototyping guided 3D-FEA study. *Materials Science and Engineering C, 69,* 715–725. https://doi.org/10.1016/j.msec.2016.07.059.

Brånemark, R., Brånemark, P.-I., Rydevik, B., & Myers, R.R. (2001). Osseointegration in skeletal reconstruction and rehabilitation. *J Rehabil Res Dev, 38*(2), 1–4.

de Souza Batista, V.E., Verri, F.R., Almeida, D.A. de F., Santiago Junior, J.F., Lemos, C.A.A., & Pellizzer, E.P. (2017). Finite element analysis of implant-supported prosthesis with pontic and cantilever in the posterior maxilla. *Computer Methods in Biomechanics and Biomedical Engineering, 20*(6), 663–670. https://doi.org/10.1080/10255842.2017.1287905.

De Vico, G., Bonino, M., Spinelli, D., Schiavetti, R., Sannino, G. Pozzi, A., & Ottria, L. (2011). Rationale for tilted implants: FEA considerations and clinical reports. *ORAL & Implantology, 4*(3–4), 23–33. Retrieved from http://www.pubmedcentral.nih.gov/articlerender.fcgi?artid=3530969&tool=pmcentrez&rendertype=abstract.

Dinis, L.M.J.S., Natal Jorge, R.M., & Belinha, J. (2007). Analysis of 3D solids using the natural neighbour radial point interpolation method. *Computer Methods in Applied Mechanics and Engineering, 196*(13), 2009–2028. https://doi.org/10.1016/j.cma.2006.11.002.

Duarte, H.M.S., Andrade, J.R., Dinis, L.M.J.S., Jorge, R.M.N., & Belinha, J. (2015). Numerical analysis of dental implants using a new advanced discretization technique. *Mechanics of Advanced Materials and Structures, 23*(4), 467–479. https://doi.org/10.1080/15376494.2014.987410.

Geng, J.P., Tan, K.B., & Liu, G.R. (2001). Application of finite element analysis in implant dentistry: A review of the literature. *The Journal of Prosthetic Dentistry, 85*(6), 585–598. https://doi.org/10.1067/mpr.2001.115251.

Gingold, R.A., & Monaghan, J.J. (1977). Smoothed particle hydrodynamics: theory and application to non-spherical stars. *Monthly Notices of the Royal Astronomical Society, 181,* 375–389.

Gümrükçü, Z., Korkmaz, Y.T., & Korkmaz, F.M. (2017). Biomechanical evaluation of implant-supported prosthesis with various tilting implant angles and bone types in atrophic maxilla: A finite element study.

Computers in Biology and Medicine, 86, 47–54. https://doi.org/10.1016/j.compbiomed.2017.04.015.

Maló, P., de Araujo Nobre, M., & Lopes, I. (2008). A new approach to rehabilitate the severely atrophic maxilla using extramaxillary anchored implants in immediate function: A pilot study. *Journal of Prosthetic Dentistry, 100*(5), 354–366. https://doi.org/10.1016/S0022-3913(08)60237-1.

Miyamoto, S., Ujigawa, K., Kizu, Y., Tonogi, M., & Yamane, G.Y. (2010). Biomechanical three-dimensional finite-element analysis of maxillary prostheses with implants. Design of number and position of implants for maxillary prostheses after hemimaxillectomy. *International Journal of Oral and Maxillofacial Surgery, 39*(11), 1120–1126. https://doi.org/10.1016/j.ijom.2010.06.011.

Moreira, S.F., Belinha, J., Dinis, L.M.J.S., & Jorge, R.M.N. (2014). A Global Numerical analysis of the "central incisor/local maxillary bone" system using a meshless method. *Molecular & Cellular Biomechanics: MCB, 11*(3), 151–84. https://doi.org/10.3970/mcb.2014.011.151.

Ozdemir Doğan, D., Polat, N.T., Polat, S., Seker, E., & Gul, E.B. (2014). Evaluation of "All-on-Four" concept and alternative designs with 3D finite element analysis method. *Clinical Implant Dentistry and Related Research, 16*(4), 501–510. https://doi.org/10.1111/cid.12024.

Peixoto, H.E., Camati, P.R., Faot, F., Sotto-Maior, B.S., Martinez, E.F., & Peruzzo, D.C. (2017). Rehabilitation of the atrophic mandible with short implants in different positions: A finite elements study. *Materials Science and Engineering C, 80,* 122–128. https://doi.org/10.1016/j.msec.2017.03.310.

Santos, C.F., Belinha, J., Gentil, F., Parente, M., Jorge, R.N., & Roberto Frias, R. (2017). An alternative 3D numerical method to study the biomechanical behaviour of the human inner ear semicircular canal, *19*(1), 3–15. https://doi.org/10.5277/ABB-00498-2015-03.

Tavares, C.S.S., Belinha, J., Dinis, L.M.J.S., & Natal Jorge, R.M. (2015). The elasto-plastic response of the bone tissue due to the insertion of dental implants. *Procedia Engineering, 110,* 37–44. https://doi.org/10.1016/j.proeng.2015.07.007.

Ujigawa, K., Kato, Y., Kizu, Y., Tonogi, M., & Yamane, G.-Y. (2007). Three-dimensional finite elemental analysis of zygomatic implants in craniofacial structures. *International Journal of Oral and Maxillofacial Surgery, 36*(7), 620–625. https://doi.org/10.1016/J.IJOM.2007.03.007.

Wang, J.G., & Liu, G.R. (2002). A point interpolation meshless method based on radial basis functions. *International Journal for Numerical Methods in Engineering, 54*(11), 1623–1648. https://doi.org/10.1002/nme.489.

Zienkiewicz, O.C., Taylor, R.L., & Zhu, J.Z. (2005). *Method: Its Basis and Fundamentals* (6th ed.). London: Elsevier Butterworth-Heinemann.

Biodental Engineering V – Belinha et al. (Eds)
© 2019 Taylor & Francis Group, London, ISBN 978-0-367-21087-8

Wound healing angiogenesis: An overview on mathematical models

A.C. Guerra
Institute of Science and Innovation in Mechanical and Industrial Engineering (INEGI), Porto, Portugal

J. Belinha
Department of Mechanical Engineering, School of Engineering, Polytechnic of Porto (ISEP), Porto, Portugal

R.M. Natal Jorge
Department of Mechanical Engineering, Faculty of Engineering, University of Porto (FEUP), Porto, Portugal

ABSTRACT: Angiogenesis, the formation of new blood vessels from pre-existent ones, is a fundamental process in wound healing since it allows the reestablishment of the normal blood flow and the sufficient exchange of oxygen and nutrients, essential for cell proliferation and viability. In the last three decades, computational mathematical modelling have been under focus due to its possibility to mimic biological processes and to test new therapies using non-invasive procedures. With this paper, we provided a global view of the current approaches to model wound healing angiogenesis, pointing out the advantages and disadvantages of using different mathematical models in order to identify possible improvements. The development of wound healing angiogenesis models with higher dimension and that incorporate multiscale analysis remains a challenge.

1 INTRODUCTION

Wounds in several tissues, such as skin, are very frequent during human life and may have a negative impact in health (Posnett & Franks 2008, Sen et al. 2009). After the tissue is damaged wound healing takes place in order to restore the tissue's homeostasis. Accordingly, understand the wound healing process in order to improve its treatment is demanded.

The effectiveness of the wound healing process is dependent on sufficient oxygen and nutrient supply, functional vascular network and accurate diffusion of growth factors. Therefore, angiogenesis consisting in the formation of new blood vessels from pre-existing ones is an indispensable process during wound healing (Carmeliet & Jain 2011). Several *in vitro* (Herman & Leung 2009, Staton et al. 2009) and *in vivo* (Wong et al. 2011, Chen et al. 2013) studies have already been developed in order to fully describe angiogenesis. However, this biological process is very complex and comprises several mediators and regulatory factors. Accordingly, it is difficult to establish a relationship between changing one biological parameter and its influence in angiogenesis. Consequently, mathematical models capable of reproducing biological systems are

powerful tools that can be used to understand the complexity of biological systems and their regulatory processes (Morel et al. 2001, Galle et al. 2005).

The aim of this paper is to perform an overview through the continuum, discrete and hybrid models of wound healing angiogenesis described in the literature. Moreover, the relevance of using meshless methods, as an advanced discretization technique able to simulate angiogenesis, will also be addressed. In order to understand the importance of wound healing angiogenesis, a briefly description of the angiogenic process will be performed.

2 WOUND HEALING ANGIOGENESIS

Angiogenesis is essential during wound healing since it provides the reestablishment of the normal blood flow and consequently the sufficient exchange of oxygen and nutrients and the removal of metabolic wastes (Carmeliet & Jain 2011).

In healthy tissues, mature vessels are in a quiescent state. These blood vessels are composed by a monolayer of endothelial cells surrounded by a basement membrane and coated with smooth muscle cells and pericytes, promoting endothelial cell survival and allowing vessel stability (Carmeliet 2003). However,

237

during wound healing, quiescent vessels are exposed to proangiogenic factors and the angiogenic process is initiated. Therefore, in the region where the new blood vessel will be formed, a previously quiescent endothelial cell is converted into a tip cell. This tip cell forms filopodia, cytoplasmic elongations sensible to the growth factors gradients in the environment, which allows cell migration. The adjacent endothelial cells become stalk cells that start to proliferate and to migrate in the direction of the tip cell, resulting in vessel's sprouting elongation. Afterwards, blood vessel density increases and the vascular sprout will fuse with another neighbouring vessel. This process is called anastomosis and allows the blood flow's reestablishment. The unperfused vessels regress by apoptotic processes. Finally, the vasculature returns to a quiescent state, the basement membrane is restored and the new blood vessel is coated by smooth muscle cells and pericytes that stabilize it (Carmeliet, & Jain 2011). If the tissue wound healing was correctly performed, the number of vessels normalizes and returns to a level close to the one observed in uninjured tissue (Yamashita et al. 2014).

Angiogenesis is modulated by several chemical factors capable of activate cellular related pathways. However, the main regulator of angiogenesis is the vascular endothelial growth factor (VEGF-A or simple VEGF). This soluble factor bind specifically to the tyrosine kinases receptor (VEGFR1 and VEGFR2) on the cell surface and to non-tyrosine kinase receptors of the neuropilin (NRP-1 and NRP-2), which function as co-receptor for VEGFRs. The specific binding of VEGF to its receptor allows the activation of cellular pathways downstream, which stimulates endothelial cells to proliferate, to migrate, to differentiate and to survive, allowing new blood vessel formation. Indeed, the binding of VEGF to VEGFR2 is the principal pathway known for stimulating endothelial cells proliferation and migration and for increasing the vascular permeability (Koch & Claesson-Welsh 2012). Moreover, cutaneous wounds present high levels of VEGF that is produced in response to injury by multiple cells types, such as keratinocytes, macrophages and fibroblasts (Brown et al. 1992, Willenborg et al. 2012).

Besides VEGF, angiogenesis is stimulated by other growth factors, such as basic fibroblast growth factor, interleukin-8, platelet derived growth factor (PDGF), transforming growth factor β, hypoxia-inducible factor and placental growth factor (Bao et al. 2009, Penn et al. 2012).

As already mentioned, angiogenesis is a complex process. In recent years, *in silico* models have been under focus since they allow to model angiogenesis with more economic and less time-consuming approaches, comparatively to laboratory methodologies.

3 MATHEMATICAL MODELS OF WOUND HEALING ANGIOGENESIS

Mathematical models are powerful tools to virtually simulate interactions between biochemical and biomechanical effects and to better understand the role of these factors in the wound healing as a whole (Kitano 2002).

The first step when simulating a biological process is to create a mathematical model suitable to address the biological feature that we want to study. Since the mathematical model is not analytically tractable, it is necessary to convert them into a computational model, composed by the algorithmic solution of these equations. This methodology, nominated as discretization, allows to simulate the biological phenomena in various degrees of complexity. In the context of wound healing there are two mathematical approaches available: continuum models and discrete models.

Continuum models are often used to modulate chemical mediators' concentrations and mechanical factors, such as forces and deformation. In these models the evolution of different fields is governed through partial differential equations (PDEs) that need to be discretize both in time and space. Time is frequently discretize into small intervals using the finite difference method. Space may be discretized by several ways, being one of them by using advanced discretization techniques (finite element method or meshless methods). Discrete models are frequently used to modulate cell populations, allowing to study the behaviour of individual cells. These models are typically represented through ordinary differential equations (ODEs), which are solved locally to predict the evolution of each individual entity in time. Discrete models are conceptually simpler than continuum models but, because each entity needs to be represented through its own equation, they are computational more expensive (Buganza-Tepole & Kuhl 2013). Since biological processes are very complex, some authors have developed hybrid models. These models allow to describe explicitly the behaviour of cells at the microscale and, simultaneously, to predict the variation of the chemical species' concentration due to reaction and diffusion at the macroscale. Nevertheless, it is the scale of interest that will determine which modelling approach is more appropriate. Components at molecular or cellular level can be modulated using discrete models. At tissue, organ or system levels the continuum models are a better approach

In the last 30 years, several modelling strategies for wound healing angiogenesis have been developed. The most relevant approaches in this area are presented below.

3.1 Continuum models

In angiogenesis' computational research, continuum models are extensively used to describe the behaviour of cell populations and chemical concentration.

Balding & McElwain (1985) developed the first model of angiogenesis to study the tumour angiogenic factor concentration's effect in blood vessel and capillary tip density. Although this model has been used to study tumour-induced angiogenesis, it attended the subsequent mathematical models of wound healing angiogenesis. Sherratt & Murray (1990) developed the first mathematical model that introduced several aspects about cell migration, proliferation and death that the upcoming models have adopted.

Pettet et al. (1996) developed the first two truly models of wound healing angiogenesis. These models include a system of PDEs to describe the evolution of dependent variables in space and time: capillary-tip density, chemo-attractant concentration and blood vessel density. The model assumes that tip cell production is proportional to the product of the attractant concentration and the vessel density. Natural death was modelled by a linear decay of tips and the tip-to-tip anastomosis was modelled using a term proportional to the square of the tip density. With this approach the authors successfully modelled the propagation of wound healing angiogenesis and several other authors used this model as a base for the upcoming studies.

Several other authors used PDEs and the same parameters analysed by Pettet et al. (1996) to model angiogenesis with different levels of complexity (Byrne et al. 2000, Maggelakis 2003, Schugart et al. 2008, Flegg et al. 2010). Byrne et al. (2000) included in the model the effect of vascular remodelling. Maggelakis (2003) studied the effect of the oxygen concentration through the wound space and the production, depletion and absorption of macrophage derived growth factors (MDGFs). Schugart et al. (2008) studied for the first time the effect of tissue oxygen tension on cutaneous wound healing. This model also incorporated more variables, such as capillary sprouts, inflammatory cells (macrophages and neutrophils), fibroblasts and extracellular matrix (ECM) density. Flegg et al. (2010) studied for the first time the role of hyperbaric oxygen therapy in the healing process. The model described the interactions in space and time of oxygen and chemo-attractant concentrations, and the densities of capillary tip, blood vessel, fibroblast and ECM.

Contrary to the models previously mentioned, Olsen et al (1997) and Gaffney et al. (2002) described wound healing angiogenesis without considering chemical factors regulation. Olsen et al. (1997) addressed for the first time the interactions between endothelial cells and ECM involved in wound angiogenesis. The model was composed by two coupled of PDEs, for endothelial cells and for ECM densities. The results showed that angiogenesis occurs because the endothelial cells and ECM moving inside from both the wound margins and the wound base. Gaffney et al. (2002) established a model focused only on endothelial cells and capillary tips, allowing to understand the capillary tip migration.

Xue et al. (2009) developed the first model that incorporates ECM mechanical properties in the study of ischemic dermal wounds. The authors described the ECM by its density and velocity using a growth and decay term due to collagen secretion by fibroblasts and degradation by matrix metalloproteinase. Similarly with other models, this model combined biological and chemical factors: concentration of oxygen, VEGF and PDGF, densities of macrophages, fibroblasts, capillary tips and capillary sprouts.

Javierre et al. (2008), Vermolen & Javierre (2011) and Valero et al. (2013) established different models to study the wound closure process. Javierre et al. (2008) studied the effect of oxygen concentration on the rate of wound closure. Moreover, this model incorporated the epidermal growth factor (EGF) concentration that regulates cell mitosis and motility allowing wound closure. An adaptive mesh algorithm was implemented because of the discontinuous production of EGF. Vermolen & Javierre (2011) coupled for the first time wound contraction, angiogenesis and wound closure in the same model. The temporal evolution of fibroblasts, ECM, VEGF, capillary profiles, oxygen, EGF and epidermal cell density were modelled in a dermal wound gap. Valero et al. (2013) incorporated the effect of fibroblasts contraction in their model, coupling angiogenesis and wound contraction. The model included biological (capillaries and fibroblasts), chemical (oxygen and MDGF concentrations) and mechanical factors (cell traction forces and ECM deformation) that regulate the skin wound healing. It was also considered the stress of one fibroblast cell per unit of ECM that corresponds to the mechanical stimulus that regulates the forces exerted by the cells. The model included two types of wound of the same size and different shapes (circular and elliptical). The numerical simulation demonstrated that elongated wounds had faster vascularization. However, the contraction experienced by both wounds was similar.

As presented above, continuum models are very useful to describe angiogenesis during wound healing. However, the prediction of the vascular network structure of these models is limited.

3.2 Discrete models

Discrete models are a better approach to determine the effect of nutrients, oxygen and growth factors in capillary's morphology. These cell-based models include cellular automata and cellular Potts models. Cellular automata models consist in particles that occupy some or all sites of a regular lattice (Deutsch & Dormann 2005). Each particle is characterized by one or more state variables, by a set of rules describing the evolution of their state and position and by their neighbouring. The change of state and the movement of the particles depend on their current state and of their neighbouring particles. At each time step, each cell will move to a neighbouring site according to its corresponding instantaneous velocity. Accordingly, cells are treated as point-like objects but its shape during migration is not accounted. However, eukaryotic cells normally move by remodelling of their cytoskeleton and consequently change their shapes. Thus, shape change can influence the cell migration pattern and this characteristic needs to be taken into account in modelling. Consequently, cellular Potts models that describe cell volume and shape more realistic aroused the interest of researchers. Cellular Potts models describe the individual cell behaviour and the interaction with the ECM, allowing to modulate cell growth, proliferation, motility, adhesion, apoptosis, differentiation and polarity (Merks & Glazier 2005).

The first discrete model to describe angiogenesis was developed by Stokes & Lauffenburger (1991). The model was based in cell speed and chemotactic responsiveness that allows endothelial cells migration and vessel branching. The obtained results showed that microvessel endothelial cells motility and chemotaxis affect the vascular network structure, being essential in angiogenesis.

More recently, other authors developed cell based models to study angiogenesis (Peirce et al. 2004, Bentley et al. 2008, Matsuya et al. 2016). Matsuya et al. (2016) verified that the deterministic interaction between endothelial cells could lead to cell-mixing behaviour, elongation and bifurcation. Peirce et al. (2004) developed a cellular automata model to predict microvascular network patterning. The model allowed to study the living multicellular systems growth, the cell behaviour adaptation and the epigenetic engineering of vascular tissues. Moreover, the results for the maturation response reported by in vivo rodent models were statistically similar to those predicted by the cellular automata simulation. Bentley et al. (2008) investigated how notch signalling due to different concentrations of VEGF and filopodia dynamics modulate tip cell angiogenic sprouting. The numerical simulation demonstrated that VEGF gradients and filopodia extension are determine in the robustness of tip/stalk morphology.

Some authors combined cellular Potts model with PDEs. Merks et al. (2004) implemented a preferential motion for the endothelial cells along gradients of the chemo-attractant. The results obtained with the simulations allowed to study intercellular adhesion and cell morphology and showed that endothelial cell adhesion is essential for stable vessels' formation. Scianna et al. (2015) established a model that included reaction–diffusion equations to describe VEGF diffusion, decay, uptake and production and oxygen diffusion and consumption. In the model, the endothelial cells, upon VEGF stimulation turn from a quiescent phenotype to a stalk or a tip one. The numerical simulation results showed that the model could reproduce the formation of a functional network by sprouting angiogenesis. van Oers et al. (2014) developed a cellular Potts model to study endothelial cells' motility, and combined them with the finite element method to study cells' deformation. This approach allowed to study the interaction between endothelial cells and ECM components and also the cell behaviour that permits the formation of vessels network and sprouting.

3.3 Hybrid models

The accurate simulation of angiogenesis requires several distinct interdependent variables and entities. Accordingly, some authors developed hybrid models to simultaneously predict the cell behaviour and the evolution of species' concentration along distinct time and space scales.

Sun et al. (2005) developed a nonlinearly system of equations to study the effect of chemotactic growth factors distributions in capillary network. In the model, the traditional endothelial cell density was replaced by the capillary indicator function, allowing to model the capillary network precisely at fine scales. The computational simulations created capillary networks with a very realistic structure and morphology, comparatively to data described in vitro studies. Machado et al. (2011) simulated cells' migration through chemotaxis, in response to VEGF gradients, and through haptotaxis, in response to gradients in the ECM. In the model, the endothelial cells produce matrix-degrading enzymes, allowing the haptotaxis response. The results obtained in the computational simulation for wound areas, vessel densities and vessel junction densities were in excellent agreement, in both time and space response, with the results obtained in vivo. Bookholt et al. (2016) studied the effect of local chemical conditions in endothelial cells' differentiation into tip and stalk cells. The model combined cell motility with diffusion-reaction equations in order to study the proteases' effect in the substrate degradation. Moreover, it was also performed an *in vitro* assay, using dermal endothelial cells, to analyse the effect of several VEGF concentrations in the angiogenic sprouting. The results obtained for the sprout's morphology were similar in both methodologies. Pillay et al. (2017) analysed the spatiotemporal evolution of tip cells and endothelial cell densities, using PDEs. The simulation results showed that the vessel formation due to tip cells movement can be modelled as a source term of tip cells on the macroscale. Moreover, it was demonstrated that anastomosis imposes cell occupancy and density restrictions on the discrete and continuum models, respectively.

Several approaches can be used to model wound healing angiogenesis. The numerical approaches described above present relevant differences between them, such as the model's dimension, the assumed angiogenic factors and the biological scale-level of interest (molecular, cellular or tissue). Moreover, the numerical method used to perform the simulation is determinant for its success. Accordingly, in the last years meshless methods arouse the interest of scientific community due to their usefulness to simulate biologic systems (Belinha et al. 2016, Santos et al. 2017). In the next section, the applicability of using meshless methods to simulate angiogenesis will be discussed.

4 USING MESHLESS METHODS TO STUDY ANGIOGENESIS

Meshless methods present some advantages when compared with the finite element method, such as the re-meshing efficiency. This property allows to deal with the large distortions of soft materials, such as the skin. Therefore, meshless methods are successfully used to numerically solved differential equations (Belinha 2014).

One of the most relevant meshless methods is the Radial Point Interpolation Method (RPIM). This method possess the Kronecker delta property, which facilitates the imposition of the essential and natural boundary conditions. Given its relevance, the applicability of using RPIM to model wound healing angiogenesis will be discussed in this section.

RPIM combines three basic concepts: the nodal connectivity, the numerical integration and the shape functions. Since there is no predefined nodal interdependency in this numerical method, the nodal connectivity has to be enforced after the nodal discretization. Consequently, the influence-domain of each node, obtained by searching enough nodes inside of a fixed area or volume, has to be determined. Then, the integration mesh, using the Gauss-Legendre quadrature scheme, is constructed. Afterwards, the discrete equations system is established, using the approximation or interpolations shape functions. In RPIM, the interpolation shape function combines a radial basis function with a polynomial basis function (Belinha 2014).

In the field of wound healing angiogenesis, RPIM can be used to analyse individual endothelial cells' migration accordingly to the VEGF diffusion gradient. As already mentioned, VEGF is a powerful proangiogenic factor. This biological factor is produced by several cell types that participate in wound healing: endothelial cells, fibroblasts, smooth muscle cells, keratinocytes, macrophages, neutrophils and platelets (Bao et al. 2009).

The chemical diffusion can be numerically simulated as a field problem (Liu & Quek 2003) using the following general form of the Helmholtz, presented in the equation:

$$D_x \frac{\partial^2 \phi}{\partial x^2} + D_y \frac{\partial^2 \phi}{\partial y^2} - g\phi + Q = 0 \qquad (1)$$

where ϕ is the field variable, D_x corresponds to VEGF diffusion coefficient along dimension x, D_y represents the VEGF diffusion coefficient along dimension y, g is the chemical infusibility matrix that will be neglected ($g = 0$) and Q is the VEGF concentration. The chemical diffusion gradients and the VEGF concentration were obtained from the available literature (Karayiannakis et al. 2003, Sun et al. 2005). Using the weighted residual approach, it is possible to formulate the meshless system equations:

$$\left[\boldsymbol{K}_D + \boldsymbol{K}_g \right] \boldsymbol{\Phi} - q = 0 \qquad (2)$$

Solving the above equation, it is possible to obtain the final VEGF concentration in each node, $\boldsymbol{\Phi}$. Accordingly, Figure 1 represents the

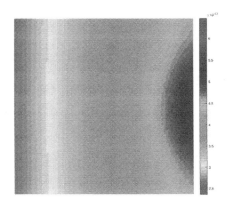

Figure 1. VEGF gradient concentration. The basal concentration of VEGF used was 2.35×10^{-13} g m^{-3} and the VEGF flux was 6.43×10^{-13} g mm^{-3}.

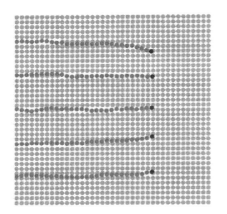

Figure 2. Simulation results for endothelial cells migration pattern obtained with the RPIM software.

VEGF diffusion gradient obtained with the RPIM methodology.

After obtaining the VEGF gradient concentration, the position of the new tip cell is determined. By repetition of this process, the capillary pattern network is obtained, as presented in Figure 2.

5 FINAL REMARKS

Mathematical models became a focus of interest since they allow to study biological processes with a non-invasive procedure. For the development of a mathematical model for wound healing angiogenesis some simplifications, assumptions and decisions have to be considered. The spatial dimensional is an important aspect to deliberate. Frequently, it is considered that wounds are much longer than wide or deep, and in these situations 1D models are a proper approach. In fact, several studies modelled angiogenesis in a 1D framework (Byrne et al. 2000, Flegg et al. 2010, Gaffney et al. 2002, Maggelakis 2003, Olsen et al. 1997, Schugart et al. 2008, Xue et al. 2009). These models are conceptually simpler, numerical tractable and present less computational costs. However, if it is intended to study more realistic geometries, similar to those visualized in real wounds, it is necessary to add more complexity to the model and extend them to two dimensions, as some authors have showed (Javierre et al. 2008, Machado et al. 2011, Matsuya et al. 2016, Peirce et al. 2004, Sun et al. 2005, Valero et al. 2013, Vermolen & Javierre 2011). The 3D models (Bentley et al. 2008, Bookholt et al. 2016) simulate skin structure and cell-ECM interactions more closely to reality and allow an accurate representation of the involved phenomena. Nevertheless, these models are analytically more complex and represent a high computational cost. For these reasons, there is still a lack in the literature of 3D models for the simulation of wound healing angiogenesis.

Another crucial aspect is to decide how many interacting species the model will include. Olsen et al. (1997) and Gaffney et al. (2002) modelled angiogenesis considering only endothelial cells and blood vessels. Several other authors (Bookholt et al. 2016, Peirce et al. 2004, Schugart et al. 2008, Xue et al. 2009) developed more complex models, which included several chemical species (oxygen, VEGF, MDGFs, EGF, PDGF and TGF-β), different cell types (capillary tip, capillary sprout, fibroblasts, inflammatory cells and smooth muscle cells) and also ECM. The number of variants can be changed substantially depending on the scope of the model. In general, most of the studies were focussed in the endothelial cells and do not consider the inflammatory cells (required for the establishment of chemical gradients) that allow to attract different cell populations. Moreover, smooth muscle cells and pericytes, required to stabilize the formed new blood vessels, are frequently not included. Vessel maturation is an important step in angiogenesis that allows the stability of vascular network and, for this reason, should be included in the upcoming mathematical models. Nevertheless, a model with a larger number of variants may be difficult to implement.

The tissues' mechanical properties is also an important subject to deliberate. *In vivo* and *in vitro* studies have shown that modelling the skin as a hyperelastic material is a better option. Indeed, hyperelastic models provides a more accurate approximation of the mechanical state of the tissue and allow the incorporation of fibre remodelling (Valero et al. 2013). Frequently, skin is considered as an isotropic matrix (Machado et al. 2011, Scianna et al. 2015, Valero et al. 2013, van Oers et al. 2014). However, anisotropic skin behaviour is clearly observed in experimental studies. The use of skin anisotropy on the mechanical model improve the accuracy of healing kinetics in the simulation. Accordingly, the mechanical behaviour of human tissues is as important parameter to include in the upcoming models.

The current models allow to model angiogenesis and help to understand this complex biological process. However, some specific steps of angiogenesis are less explored. Therefore, vessel maturation, reperfusion with another vessel, vascular network remodelling and the involvement of ECM components are parameters that the upcoming models should include.

Meshless methods are suitable numerical tools to simulate biomechanical problems (Belinha et al. 2016, Gomes et al. 2017, Peyroteo et al. 2018) due to theirs flexibility to represent complex geometries and large deformations and also their robustness and accuracy. However, presently, the use of these numerical methods to model angiogenesis is less explored. Since meshless methods allow to analyse any phenomenon that is governed by differential equation, their application in the field of angiogenesis should be explored.

In silico models need the proper feedback from experimental *in vitro* and *in vivo* studies. These experimental works help to validate the computational models and also to determine how close the wound healing model is to the reality. Nevertheless, computational models are usually focused in human wounds and the experimental studies are developed in animal models, typically rodent. Thus, it is only possible to obtain a tendency of wound healing and the parameters analysed should be adjusted to be used in human models.

Accordingly, the development of wound healing angiogenesis models with higher dimension and incorporating multiscale analysis at molecular, cellular and tissue level, remain a challenge. Thus, there is still room for further research and improvement.

ACKNOWLEDGEMENTS

The authors truly acknowledge the funding provided by Ministério da Ciência, Tecnologia e Ensino Superior—Fundação para a Ciência e a Tecnologia (Portugal), under grants: SFRH/BD/133894/2017 and by project funding MIT-EXPL/ISF/0084/2017. Additionally, the authors gratefully acknowledge the funding of Project NORTE-01-0145-FEDER-000022—SciTech—Science and Technology for Competitive and Sustainable Industries, cofinanced by Programa Operacional Regional do Norte (NORTE2020), through Fundo Europeu de Desenvolvimento Regional (FEDER).

REFERENCES

Arnold, J.S. & Adam, J.A. 1999. A simplified model of wound healing II: The Critical Size Defect in two dimensions. Mathematical and Computer Modelling 30(11): 47–60.

Balding, D. & McElwain, D.L. 1985. A mathematical model of tumour-induced capillary growth. Journal of Theoretical Biology 114(1): 53–73.

Bao, P., Kodra, A., Tomic-Canic, M., Golinko, M.S., Ehrlich, H.P. & Brem, H. 2009. The Role of Vascular Endothelial Growth Factor in Wound Healing. The Journal of Surgical Research 153(2): 347–358.

Belinha, J. 2014. Meshless Methods in Biomechanics—Bone Tissue Remodelling Analysis (Vol.16). Lecture Notes in Computational Vision and Biomechanics. Netherlands: Springer.

Belinha, J., Dinis, L.M.J.S. & Jorge, R.M.N. 2016. The analysis of the bone remodelling around femoral stems. Mathematics and Computers in Simulation 121(C): 64–94.

Bentley, K., Gerhardt, H. & Bates, P.A. 2008. Agent-based simulation of notch-mediated tip cell selection in angiogenic sprout initialisation. Journal of Theoretical Biology 250(1): 25–36.

Bookholt, F.D., Monsuur, H.N., Gibbs, S. & Vermolen, F.J. 2016. Mathematical modelling of angiogenesis using continuous cell-based models. Biomechanics and Modeling in Mechanobiology 15(6): 1577–1600.

Brown, L.F., Yeo, K.T., Berse, B., Yeo, T.K., Senger, D.R., Dvorak, H.F. & van de Water, L. 1992. Expression of vascular permeability factor (vascular endothelial growth factor) by epidermal keratinocytes during wound healing. The Journal of Experimental Medicine 176(5): 1375–1379.

Buganza-Tepole, A. & Kuhl, E. 2013. Systems-based approaches toward wound healing. Pediatric Research 73(4–2): 553–563.

Byrne, H.M., Chaplain, M.A.J., Evans, D.L. & Hopkinson, I. 2000. Mathematical Modelling of Angiogenesis in Wound Healing: Comparison of Theory and Experiment. Journal of Theoretical Medicine 2(3): 175–197.

Carmeliet, P. 2003. Angiogenesis in health and disease. Nature Medicine 9(6): 653–660.

Carmeliet, P. & Jain, R.K. 2011. Molecular mechanisms and clinical applications of angiogenesis. Nature 473(7347): 298–307.

Chen, J.S., Longaker, M.T. & Gurtner, G.C. 2013. Murine models of human wound healing. Methods in Molecular Biology (Clifton, N.J.) 1037: 265–274.

Deutsch, A. & Dormann, S. 2005. Cellular Automaton Modeling of Biological Pattern Formation. Boston, Mass, USA: Birkhauser.

Flegg, J.A., Byrne, H.M. & McElwain, D.L. 2010. Mathematical model of hyperbaric oxygen therapy applied to chronic diabetic wounds. Bulletin of Mathematical Biology 72(7): 1867–1891.

Gaffney, E.A., Pugh, K., Maini, P.K. & Arnold F. 2002. Investigating a simple model of cutaneous wound healing angiogenesis. Journal of Mathematical Biology 45(4): 337–374.

Galle, J., Loeffler, M. & Drasdo, D. 2005. Modeling the effect of deregulated proliferation and apoptosis on the growth dynamics of epithelial cell populations in vitro. Biophysical Journal 88(1): 62–75.

Gomes, J., Belinha, J., Dinis, L.M.J.S. & Jorge, R.M.N. 2017. The structural analysis of chitosan tubes using meshless methods. 2017 IEEE 5th Portuguese Meeting on Bioengineering (ENBENG).

Herman, I.M. & Leung, A. 2009. Creation of human skin equivalents for the in vitro study of angiogenesis in wound healing. Methods in Molecular Biology (Clifton, N.J.) 467: 241–248.

Javierre, E., Vermolen, F.J., Vuik, C. & van der Zwaag, S. 2008. Numerical Modelling of Epidermal Wound Healing. Numerical Mathematics and Advanced Applications: Proceedings of ENUMATH 2007, the 7th European Conference on Numerical Mathematics and Advanced Applications.

Karayiannakis, A.J., Zbar, A., Polychronidis, A. & Simopoulos, C. 2003. Serum and drainage fluid vascular endothelial growth factor levels in early surgical wounds. European Surgical Research 35(6): 492–496.

Kitano, H. 2002. Computational systems biology. Nature 420(6912): 206–210.

Koch, S. & Claesson-Welsh, L. 2012. Signal transduction by vascular endothelial growth factor receptors.

Cold Spring Harbor Perspectives in Medicine 2(7): a006502.

Liu, G.R. & Quek, S.S. 2003. The finite element method: a practical course, Elsevier Science—Butterworth-Heinemann.

Machado, M.J., Watson, M.G., Devlin, A.H., Chaplain, M.A., McDougall, S.R. & Mitchell, C.A. 2011. Dynamics of angiogenesis during wound healing: a coupled in vivo and in silico study. Microcirculation (New York, N.Y.: 1994) 18(3): 183–197.

Maggelakis, S.A. 2003. A mathematical model of tissue replacement during epidermal wound healing. Applied Mathematical Modelling 27(3): 189–196.

Matsuya, K., Yura, F., Mada, J., Kurihara, H. & Tokihiro, T. 2016. A Discrete Mathematical Model for Angiogenesis. SIAM Journal on Applied Mathematics 76(6): 2243–2259.

Merks, R.M.H. & Glazier, J.A. 2005. A cell-centered approach to developmental biology. Physica A: Statistical Mechanics and its Applications 352(1): 113–130.

Merks, R.M.H., Newman, S.A. & Glazier, J.A. 2004. Cell-Oriented Modeling of In Vitro Capillary Development. Cellular Automata: 6th International Conference on Cellular Automata for Research and Industry, ACRI 2004.

Morel, D., Marcelpoil, R. & Brugal, G. 2001. A proliferation control network model: the simulation of two-dimensional epithelial homeostasis. Acta Biotheoretica 49(4): 219–234.

Olsen, L., Sherratt, J.A., Maini, P.K. & Arnold, F. 1997. A mathematical model for the capillary endothelial cell-extracellular matrix interactions in wound-healing angiogenesis. IMA Journal of Mathematics Applied in Medicine and Biology 14(4): 261–281.

Peirce, S.M., Van Gieson, E.J. & Skalak, T.C. 2004. Multicellular simulation predicts microvascular patterning and in silico tissue assembly. FASEB journal 18(6): 731–733.

Penn, J.W., Grobbelaar, A.O. & Rolfe, K.J. 2012. The role of the TGF-beta family in wound healing, burns and scarring: a review. International Journal of Burns and Trauma 2(1): 18–28.

Pettet, G., Chaplain, M.A.J., Mcelwain, D.L.S. & Byrne, H.M. 1996. On the role of angiogenesis in wound healing. Proceedings of the Royal Society of London. Series B: Biological Sciences 263(1376): 1487–1493.

Pettet, G.J., Byrne, H.M., McElwain, D.L. & Norbury, J. 1996. A model of wound-healing angiogenesis in soft tissue. Mathematical Biosciences 136(1): 35–63.

Peyroteo, M.M.A., Belinha, J., Vinga, S., Dinis, L.M.J.S. & Jorge, R.M.N. 2018. Mechanical bone remodelling: Comparative study of distinct numerical approaches. Engineering Analysis with Boundary Elements. in press.

Pillay, S., Byrne, H.M. & Maini, P.K. 2017. Modeling angiogenesis: A discrete to continuum description. Physical Review E 95(1): 012410.

Posnett, J. & Franks, P.J. 2008. The burden of chronic wounds in the UK. Nursing Times 104(3): 44–45.

Santos, C.F., Belinha, J., Gentil, F., Parente, M., Areias, B. & Jorge, R.N. 2017. Biomechanical study of the vestibular system of the inner ear using a numerical method. Procedia IUTAM 24: 30–37.

Schugart, R.C., Friedman, A., Zhao, R. & Sen, C.K. 2008. Wound angiogenesis as a function of tissue oxygen tension: A mathematical model. Proceedings of the National Academy of Sciences 105(7): 2628–2633.

Scianna, M., Bassino, E. & Munaron, L. 2015. A cellular Potts model analyzing differentiated cell behavior during in vivo vascularization of a hypoxic tissue. Computers in Biology and Medicine 63: 143–156.

Sen, C.K., Gordillo, G.M., Roy, S., Kirsner, R., Lambert, L., Hunt, T.K., Gottrup, F., Gurtner, G.C. & Longaker, M.T. 2009. Human skin wounds: a major and snowballing threat to public health and the economy. Wound Repair and Regeneration 17(6): 763–771.

Sherratt, J.A. & Murray, J.D. 1990. Models of epidermal wound healing. Proceedings. Biological sciences 241(1300): 29–36.

Staton, C.A., Reed, M.W.R. & Brown, N.J. 2009. A critical analysis of current in vitro and in vivo angiogenesis assays. International Journal of Experimental Pathology 90(3): 195–221.

Stokes, C.L. and Lauffenburger, D.A. 1991. Analysis of the roles of microvessel endothelial cell random motility and chemotaxis in angiogenesis. Journal of Theoretical Biology 152(3): 377–403.

Sun, S., Wheeler, M.F., Obeyesekere, M. & Patrick, C.W., Jr. 2005. A deterministic model of growth factor-induced angiogenesis. Bulletin of Mathematical Biology 67(2): 313–337.

Sun, S., Wheeler, M.F., Obeyesekere, M. & Patrick, C., Jr. 2005. Nonlinear behaviors of capillary formation in a deterministic angiogenesis model. Nonlinear Analysis: Theory, Methods & Applications 63(5–7): e2237–e2246.

Valero, C., Javierre, E., Garcia-Aznar, J.M. & Gomez-Benito, M.J. 2013. Numerical modelling of the angiogenesis process in wound contraction. Biomech Model Mechanobiol 12(2): 349–360.

van Oers, R.F.M., Rens, E.G., LaValley, D.J., Reinhart-King, C.A. & Merks, R.M.H. 2014. Mechanical cell-matrix feedback explains pairwise and collective endothelial cell behavior in vitro. PLOS Computational Biology 10(8): e1003774.

Vermolen, F.J. & Javierre E. 2011. A finite-element model for healing of cutaneous wounds combining contraction, angiogenesis and closure. Journal of Mathematical Biology 65(5): 967–996.

Willenborg, S., Lucas, T., van Loo, G., Knipper, J.A., Krieg, T., Haase, I., Brachvogel, B., Hammerschmidt, M., Nagy, A., Ferrara, N., Pasparakis, M. & Eming, S.A. 2012. CCR2 recruits an inflammatory macrophage subpopulation critical for angiogenesis in tissue repair. Blood 120(3): 613–625.

Wong, V.W., Sorkin, M., Glotzbach, J.P., Longaker, M.T. & Gurtner, G.C. 2011. Surgical approaches to create murine models of human wound healing. Journal of Biomedicine & Biotechnology 2011: 969618.

Xue, C., Friedman, A. & Sen, C.K. 2009. A mathematical model of ischemic cutaneous wounds. Proceedings of the National Academy of Sciences 106(39): 16782–16787.

Yamashita, K., Yotsuyanagi, T., Yamauchi, M. & Young, D.M. 2014. Klotho mice: a novel wound model of aged skin. Plastic and Reconstructive Surgery Global Open 2(1): e101.

Biodental Engineering V – Belinha et al. (Eds)
© 2019 Taylor & Francis Group, London, ISBN 978-0-367-21087-8

The influence of a blood clot in hemodynamics: A meshless method study

M.I.A. Barbosa
Faculty of Engineering, University of Porto (FEUP), Porto, Portugal

J. Belinha
Department of Mechanical Engineering, School of Engineering, Polytechnic of Porto (ISEP), Porto, Portugal

R.M. Natal Jorge
Department of Mechanical Engineering, Faculty of Engineering, University of Porto (FEUP), Porto, Portugal

ABSTRACT: Cardiovascular diseases are one of the leading causes of death in the world, with about 15 million deaths per year. Therefore, it is important to develop strategies to allow the study of this type of diseases, in order to understand how to oppose these numbers. To this end, biomechanical simulation using discrete numerical techniques, such as Finite Element Method (FEM) and Radial Point Interpolation Method (RPIM), emerge as unique techniques to study haemodynamics. The aim of the present work is to compare the velocity profile of a discretized model of a tubular straight artery, using two methods, FEM and RPIM, in order to compare the results obtained with each one. FEMAS software was used and allowed to conclude that RPIM is preferable to FEM since, the first, presents a more uniform velocity profile of the blood flow when compared to the results obtained with FEM, being more suitable for this type of analysis. However, the RPIM parameters need to be calibrated since the clot presented a larger size than what should be expected when using this model.

1 INTRODUCTION

According to the World Health Organization, cardiovascular diseases kill 15 million people per year and represent 49% of deaths in Europe and 30% of global deaths in 2010, being the most common cause of death and disability in the world [1, 2]. Cardiovascular diseases are a major issue in modern society and occur in specific vascular parts of the body associated with low wall shear stress, such as vascular stenosis, regions of curvature, bifurcated area, vessel branches and junctions. It can also be associated with quick changes in flow or when the flow is unstable [1, 3, 4].

The vascular system refers to the heart and blood vessels. The main role of arteries is to carry blood to the organs. However, while doing so, they play another extremely important role, arteries adapt to local changes and maintain overall homeostasis of the circulatory system [5]. In normal conditions, they can adapt to changes in blood flow and blood pressure [5]. However, sometimes the adaptive and healing processes fail and arteries are unable to respond to the imposed forces, leading to its inability to provide blood to important organs [5].

An injury of a blood vessel promotes loss of blood. Therefore, an intervention of the hemostatic system is required, in order to repair the wound as fast as possible [6]. Platelets are instantly activated and become capable of strong adhesion to the wall and to each other [6]. The formation of a blood clot normally starts with the exposure of tissue factor and collagen, in the subendothelium, to blood components after a vascular injury [6, 7]. A clot is an aggregation of blood components that becomes pasted up and acts as a barrier to prevent blood loss and reestablishes hemostasis [6, 7]. However, in this process, the small diameter, extended length, degree of curvature, flow characteristics, vessel geometry, flow waveform shape and shape of the inlet velocity profile can influence hemodynamics [8, 9]. Additionally, some pathological phenomena, such as rupture of atherothrombotic plaque or hypercoagulable states, can promote clot formation inside intact vessels, preventing the passage of blood flow (i.e., thrombosis) [7, 10].

Cardiovascular diseases lead to abnormal blood flows, some of which are linked to hemolysis and thrombus formation [11]. Thrombus stagnation is a dangerous event that leads to its growth, which in turn affects the normal flow of the region. Besides that, it may embolize, propagate down to other arteries, and become lodged to then [4].

Thrombosis can generate vessel occlusion and this may lead to myocardial infarction or stroke [10]. Stroke is a condition that affects a large number of individuals per year and, consequently, it is the number one cause of long-term illness and the third leading cause of death in the United States with more than 700000 persons affected each year [4, 12]. Annually, in the United States alone, this condition costs about $15 billion to $30 billion and 15% to 45% of all strokes are caused by emboli [12], either due to the occlusion of arteries or the downstream propagation of the thrombus in them [4, 13].

Central aortic shunts, for example, have a thrombosis incidence of 16–53%, with clotting being the major cause of shunt failure [8].

Since arterial thrombosis is the source of a wide variety of cardiovascular diseases, it becomes necessary to develop models to understand and study the influence of a clot or the blood flow in an artery [14]. To understand the normal and pathologic behavior of the vascular system, it is required to have detailed knowledge of blood flow and the response of blood vessels [5]. However, the complexity of the vascular system hinders the analysis and prediction of its behavior. Thus, to obtain this kind of information, numerical studies are essential [3].

In recent years, non-intrusive and virtual computational techniques have been used to understand vascular hemodynamics and numerous two dimensional artery analyses were performed [5]. Today, the use of computational fluid dynamics to monitor/predict the blood flow characteristics is common. Furthermore, such techniques are currently capable of providing detailed and accurate information on the haemodynamics associated with malformations [15].

Numerical methods have been used for almost 30 years to understand the biomechanics and biofluidity of the body, by assuming/constructing simplified models of the human body and its haemodynamics [15]. For example, Rindt *et al.* in 1987 studied the stationary flow in a 2D model of the carotid artery bifurcation [16].

Nowadays, the advances in computer technology have enabled the application of numerical methods to simulate physical phenomena more realistically and this allowed to increase the intense research of the blood flow in the cardiovascular system [17].

The Finite Element Method (FEM) is a popular method to represent and analyze complex 3D geometries efficiently. Thus, the FEM is capable to successfully perform biomechanical analyses, by modeling and simulating the cardiovascular system with accuracy and robustness [18].

This numerical technique is a continuous parametric methodology with high modeling precision that can simulate complex geometry structures and adjust the parameters of different shape [1]. The calculation process is complex and the computation time is very high. However, optimizing the model and the solution algorithm, the computational efficiency can be improved, allowing the FEM to be more widely applicable [1].

Therefore, some studies were performed over the years. Chesnutt JK, *et al.*, based on computational simulations, verified that thrombosis was caused by increased fluid shear stress with the alteration of the fluid flow due to bending of the venules [10].

A study of LN He *et al.,* using the FEM, analyzed an arterial model with different shapes and its influence in the vascular flow, taking into account several parameters, such as the blood velocity and the wall pressure. The objective of their work was to provide the theoretical bases of haemodynamics for a real vessel. They verified that blood flow is significantly influenced by the vessel geometry and that abnormal changes of geometry could result in aneurysm. This type of study proved that computational fluid dynamics is helpful to analyze and predict the development of aneurysms [19].

Sotelo J. *et al.* used computational methods to estimate the in-plane velocity gradients in 2D sections in the aorta of healthy volunteers using finite-element methodology [18].

On the other hand, meshless methods have been developed as an alternative to FEM, and achieved notable progress in recent years. RPIM, is one example of this type of methods, and the numerical techniques used in FEM can be applied with minimal modifications. Besides that, this method presents higher accuracy and stable results however, it is more expensive, when compared to FEM [20].

The aim of this work is to analyze an artery with a clot, in order to understand their influence in the results obtained with FEM and RPIM. Furthermore, this study aims to determine which method is more suitable to use in fluid flow analysis.

2 METHODS

2.1 *Finite Element Method (FEM)*

The FEM emerged in the 1950's decade, in order to facilitate the resolution of a large number of complex equations. However, it only started to be more commonly used with the development of computer technologies [21, 22], reaching high popularity around 1980 [23].

This method promotes an easy analysis of a body with an irregular surface, it has a large range of application fields, a capacity to deal with bodies with different materials, the ability to analyze different boundary conditions and it is easy to use and of low cost [24].

Briefly, the FEM consists in a mathematical approximation method that discretizes a continuous medium in finite elements, connected by nodes, in order to obtain an approximate solution, maintaining the same properties of the original medium [25, 26].

Afterwards, in each element, linear functions are defined in order to obtain the approximate distribution of the variable under study, establishing the equations that represent the global system, which allows the calculation of the variables [27].

2.2 *Radial Point Interpolation Method (RPIM)*

The RPIM is a meshless method used in several fields, as an alternative to FEM [28], besides that, it has been successfully applied to 2D solid mechanics problems [29].

In RPIM, the approximated solution is constructed from a set of nodes without an interrelationship between them [30]. Then, the background integration mesh is constructed using the Gauss-Legendre quadrature rule. Afterwards, the influence domains of each integration point are established and the nodal connectivity is obtained overlapping the influence domains. Thus, for each integration point the shape functions are constructed using the radial point interpolator technique [28]. In the end, the integro-differential equations governing the fluid flow phenomenon are considered and numerically integrated, allowing to achieve the global system of equations.

3 NUMERICAL ANALYSIS

3.1 *Geometric and numerical model*

The aim of this work is to analyze a tubular straight artery with a clot. Thus, the first step (model construction and discretization) of this work was performed using FEMAP commercial software directly (student version). Therefore, using FEMAP, it was possible to create a 2D model representing a tubular straight artery. Based on other articles of human arteries and blood flow, the artery models were defined with 1.6 cm of diameter, a reference value for the aorta [31], and 10.0 cm of length.

The clot has a circular geometry (spherical in 3D), and, in order to study its influence on the velocity of blood flow, different sizes for the clot were plotted in the same model.

With FEMAP, it was possible to design the model and to obtain the input files (INP file), used in FEMAS academic software (cmech.webs.com). The biomechanical fluid analyses of these models were studied using FEMAS software, since it allows the analysis of fluids with lows velocities, performing a static fluid flow analysis of blood using the original Zienkiewicz's formulation for FEM [32].

The mesh of the tubular straight model (Fig. 1) was made of triangular elements and composed of 1793 nodes and 3352 elements.

For this model four patches were defined. Patch one was defined as blood and the first two were defined as clot (the inner patch and the middle).

3.2 *Materials*

The fluid flow formulation encoded in FEMAS requires two parameters to define viscous fluids: the density and the viscosity. Accordingly to the literature, the value for the blood's density is 1050 kg/m3 and the viscosity 3.5×10^{-9} Pa.s [31]. These were the values used for this work and assumed as constants. Besides that, it was assumed that the blood was isotropic.

Blood is rheologically complex, however in this work it was considered a homogeneous flow. In large diameter arteries, blood can be considered as an incompressible viscous Newtonian fluid [17], a good approximation for blood flow in this type of arteries, where shear rates are high [8].

The blood clot is considered as a homogenous viscous fluid, with the same density of blood, but with upper viscosity. The viscosity was assumed as 3.5 Pa.s.

3.3 *Boundary conditions*

The hemodynamics in the arteries are strongly dependent on the geometry and the essential boundary conditions [19].

It was imposed that the artery's wall is fixed over its length, in Ox and Oy directions, preventing its movement/slipping (Fig. 2). This condition leads to a velocity of 0 along the wall.

The initial velocity affects the blood flow distribution along the artery [19]. Assuming a laminar flow, a parabolic velocity profile was used for

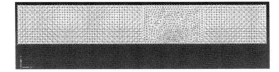

Figure 1. Regular and irregular mesh of the tubular model with a clot, obtain in FEMAP program.

the inlet (Fig. 3), with a maximum velocity at the center point of the parabola.

The general equation of a parabola is given by:

$v(y) = a_0 + a_1 x + a_2 x^2$

Taking into account the previous assumptions (velocity in the walls is 0 and in the center of the artery is maximum) and knowing that x varies from 0 to 16 mm, it is possible to obtain the parameters a_0, a_1 and a_2, for a given velocity.

In this work, an initial velocity of 0.18 mm/s was selected and imposed to the model, as observed in Figure 4.

Besides that, it was assumed that the artery's wall is rigid since the duration of the simulation is short.

3.4 Results

Before running the fluid flow analysis in FEMAS, the following results were obtained.

The velocity maps, which can be observed, present a color gradient that varies from blue to red, being the blue color the lower velocity and the red the highest velocity.

The next figures represent the velocity maps of the models, taking into account the selected velocity and using the FEM and RPIM.

The aim of the present work was to analyze the velocity profile of a model of an artery, with a clot.

It was expected that the model would present a parabolic constant velocity profile, as mentioned previously, along its length, when there would be no obstacle. For example, in the work of M. W. Siebert et al., a tubular model was presented with a parabolic profile, similar to those obtained in this work [34]. Taking into account the results presented, it is possible to verify that all the results tend to have this characteristic, at the beginning and at the end of the model.

The clot was defined as a highly viscous body, in order to ensure that it would act as a barrier to the blood flow. In the clot area, the velocity is zero since the blood flow could not pass under the clot. In the area where blood could flow, the velocity increased, and this can be explained according to the equation of flow rate. This can be translated by $m = v \cdot \rho \cdot A \cdot \cos \theta$, being m the flow rate, v the velocity, ρ the density of the fluid, A the area where blood flows and θ the angle between the unit normal and the velocity of mass elements. Thereby, if the section area decreases, to maintain the flow rate, the velocity needs to increase. Therefore, the results are coherent with what was to be expected. The model showed a maximum velocity of around 0.30 mm/s, with FEM, and 0.55 mm/s, with RPIM, which confirms what was previously mentioned.

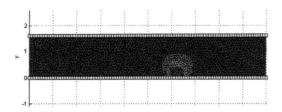

Figure 2. Representation of the boundary conditions in the artery's wall of the tubular model, in FEMAS.

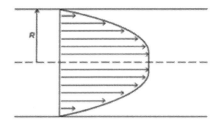

Figure 3. Schematic representation of the parabolic velocity profile on the artery, adapted from [33].

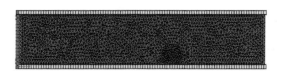

Figure 4. Representation of the imposed initial velocity in the artery, in FEMAS, following a parabolic shape.

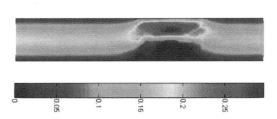

Figure 5. Color map of the velocity profile of the mixed mesh with the medium clot, using FEM.

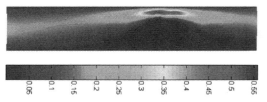

Figure 6. Color map of the velocity profile of the mixed mesh with the medium clot, using RPIM.

Using the RPIM method, it is noticeable that the change in the flow is smoother and more uniform when compared with FEM. However, the clot is more pronounced than expected, which influences the velocity profile along the model. Therefore, it is possible to conclude that the two methods are suitable for this type of analysis although, the parameters used in RPIM need to be improved/calibrated in order to achieve better results.

Besides, it is important to note that, the model presents some mesh irregularity, which influences the velocity profile. The introduction of a clot required further research and improvement, in order to obtain more realistic results.

4 CONCLUSIONS

As previously stated, cardiovascular diseases are a serious problem of current society, being one of the leading causes of mortality all around the world. Computational methods emerged as an innovation that allow the study of haemodynamics, which is vital for the prevention and treatment of this type of disease.

The present work analyzed the velocity profile of artery models with different meshes and shapes. For such purpose, four models were constructed and applied to the FEMAS software, using the FEM. Essential boundary conditions were applied along the artery wall as well as an initial velocity of 0.18 mm/s in all models. After this, the obtained results were analyzed and it was possible to conclude that RPIM presents better results. Comparing the results, the one using RPIM presents a softer and more uniform flow, when comparing to the other one using FEM. However, the parameters used in RPIM need to be calibrated in order to achieve even better results and closer to what should be expected. Thus, it is possible to conclude that, though the two methods work, RPIM is more suitable for this analysis. Despite this, the results were in accordance with the expectation in all cases.

However, it is important to improve on some aspects, namely, in the study of the presence of a clot, in which the mesh needs to be refined so that the results are less dependent on the type of mesh.

Besides, the use of DICOM files to build realistic 3D models, rather than 2D models, could be an important step to achieve more realistic results and will be further studied. The increase of the number of nodes and elements can provide more accurate results. Moreover, the walls were considered rigid and pulsate flow was for now neglected. However, these aspects, in a physiological environment, influence the blood flow. Future works will have to account these variables.

ACKNOWLEDGEMENTS

The authors truly acknowledge the funding provided by Ministério da Educação e Ciência–Fundação para a Ciência e a Tecnologia (Portugal), under project funding MIT-EXPL/ISF/0084/2017 (funding provided by the inter-institutional projects FCT/MIT-Portugal).

Additionally, the authors gratefully acknowledge the funding of Project NORTE-01-0145-FEDER-000022—SciTech—Science and Technology for Competitive and Sustainable Industries, cofinanced by Programa Operacional Regional do Norte (NORTE2020), through Fundo Europeu de Desenvolvimento Regional (FEDER).

REFERENCES

[1] Guo, S., et al. *Analysis of the elastic stress for the bifurcated region of blood vessel. in Mechatronics and Automation (ICMA), 2017 IEEE International Conference on.* 2017. IEEE.

[2] Sun, C.-K., et al., *High Sensitivity of T-Ray for Thrombus Sensing.* Scientific reports, 2018. **8**(1): p. 3948.

[3] Axner, L., et al., *Simulations of time harmonic blood flow in the Mesenteric artery: comparing finite element and lattice Boltzmann methods.* Biomedical engineering online, 2009. **8**(1): p. 23.

[4] Gay, M. and L.T. Zhang, *Numerical studies of blood flow in healthy, stenosed, and stented carotid arteries.* International journal for numerical methods in fluids, 2009. **61**(4): p. 453–472.

[5] Taylor, C.A., T.J. Hughes, and C.K. Zarins, *Finite element modeling of blood flow in arteries.* Computer methods in applied mechanics and engineering, 1998. **158**(1–2): p. 155–196.

[6] Tokarev, A., et al., *Continuous mathematical model of platelet thrombus formation in blood flow.* Russian Journal of Numerical Analysis and Mathematical Modelling, 2012. **27**(2): p. 191–212.

[7] Govindarajan, V., et al., *Impact of Tissue Factor Localization on Blood Clot Structure and Resistance under Venous Shear.* Biophysical journal, 2018. **114**(4): p. 978–991.

[8] Celestin, C., et al., *Computational fluid dynamics characterization of blood flow in central aorta to pulmonary artery connections: importance of shunt angulation as a determinant of shear stress-induced thrombosis.* Pediatric cardiology, 2015. **36**(3): p. 600–615.

[9] Myers, J., et al., *Factors influencing blood flow patterns in the human right coronary artery.* Annals of biomedical engineering, 2001. **29**(2): p. 109–120.

[10] Chesnutt, J.K. and H.-C. Han, *Tortuosity triggers platelet activation and thrombus formation in microvessels.* Journal of biomechanical engineering, 2011. **133**(12): p. 121004.

[11] Gülan, U., et al., *An in vitro investigation of the influence of stenosis severity on the flow in the ascending aorta.* Medical Engineering and Physics, 2014. **36**(9): p. 1147–1155.

[12] McNamara, R.L., et al., *Echocardiographic identification of cardiovascular sources of emboli to guide clinical management of stroke: a cost-effectiveness analysis.* Annals of internal medicine, 1997. **127**(9): p. 775–787.

[13] Abolfazli, E., N. Fatouraee, and B. Vahidi, *Dynamics of motion of a clot through an arterial bifurcation: a finite element analysis.* Fluid Dynamics Research, 2014. **46**(5): p. 055505.

[14] Jourdan, A., et al., *Experimental thrombosis model induced by free radicals. Application to aspirin and other different substances.* Thrombosis research, 1995. **79**(1): p. 109–123.

[15] Butty, V., et al., *Residence times and basins of attraction for a realistic right internal carotid artery with two aneurysms.* Biorheology, 2002. **39**(3, 4): p. 387–393.

[16] Baaijens, J., A. Van Steenhoven, and J. Janssen, *Numerical analysis of steady generalized Newtonian blood flow in a 2D model of the carotid artery bifurcation.* BIORHEOLOGY-OXFORD-, 1993. **30**: p. 63–63.

[17] Chakraborty, D. and J.R. Prakash, *Viscoelastic fluid flow in a 2D channel bounded above by a deformable finite-thickness elastic wall.* Journal of Non-Newtonian Fluid Mechanics, 2015. **218**: p. 83–98.

[18] Sotelo, J., et al., *3D quantification of wall shear stress and oscillatory shear index using a finite-element method in 3D CINE PC-MRI data of the thoracic aorta.* IEEE transactions on medical imaging, 2016. **35**(6): p. 1475–1487.

[19] He, L. and J. Pan. *Hemodynamics simulation of the intracranial bifurcation vessel with different shape. in Biomedical Engineering and Informatics (BMEI), 2010 3rd International Conference on.* 2010. IEEE.

[20] Liu, G., et al., *A nodal integration technique for meshfree radial point interpolation method (NI-RPIM).* International Journal of Solids and Structures, 2007. **44**(11–12): p. 3840–3860.

[21] Belinha, J., et al., *The analysis of laminated plates using distinct advanced discretization meshless techniques.* Composite Structures, 2016. **143**: p. 165–179.

[22] Belinha, J., et al., *The natural neighbor radial point interpolation method extended to the crack growth simulation.* International Journal of Applied Mechanics, 2016. **8**(01): p. 1650006.

[23] Fish, J. and T. Belytschko, *A first course in finite elements.* 2007.

[24] Lopes, A.M.R., *Vertebrae Bone Tissue Remodelling analysis using a meshless method.* 2013.

[25] Belinha, J., *Meshless Methods: The Future of Computational Biomechanical Simulation.* Journal of Biometrics & Biostatistics, 2016. **7**.

[26] Martin, R.B. *A genealogy of biomechanics. in 23rd Annual Conference of the American Society of Biomechanics.* 1999.

[27] Liu, G. and S. Quek, *The finite element method: a practical course. 2003.* Butterworth Heinemann, Oxford.

[28] Peyroteo, M., et al., *Mechanical bone remodelling: Comparative study of distinct numerical approaches.* Engineering Analysis with Boundary Elements, 2018.

[29] Liu, G.-R., et al., *A meshfree radial point interpolation method (RPIM) for three-dimensional solids.* Computational Mechanics, 2005. **36**(6): p. 421–430.

[30] Praveen Kumar, R. and G. Dodagoudar, *Two-dimensional modelling of contaminant transport through saturated porous media using the radial point interpolation method (RPIM).* Hydrogeology journal, 2008. **16**(8): p. 1497–1505.

[31] Khanafer, K.M., et al., *Modeling pulsatile flow in aortic aneurysms: effect of non-Newtonian properties of blood.* Biorheology, 2006. **43**(5): p. 661–679.

[32] Zienkiewicz, O.C., et al., *The Finite Element Method for Fluid Dynamics.* 2014: Butterworth-Heinemann.

[33] Rubenstein, D., W. Yin, and M.D. Frame, *Biofluid mechanics: an introduction to fluid mechanics, macrocirculation, and microcirculation.* 2015: Academic Press.

[34] Siebert, M.W. and P.S. Fodor. *Newtonian and non-newtonian blood flow over a backward-facing step–a case study. in Proceedings of the COMSOL Conference, Boston.* 2009.

Miscellaneous

Biodental Engineering V – Belinha et al. (Eds)
© 2019 Taylor & Francis Group, London, ISBN 978-0-367-21087-8

Masticatory muscles assessment with infrared imaging in oral rehabilitation—a case report

A. Moreira & R. Batista
Faculty of Dental Medicine, University of Porto (FMDUP), Porto, Portugal

J. Mendes
Faculty of Engineering, University of Porto (FEUP), Porto, Portugal

S. Oliveira, J.C. Reis Campos & M.H. Figueiral
FMDUP, Porto, Portugal

ABSTRACT: The association between removable prosthesis rehabilitation and the development of Temporomandibular Disorders (TMD) has been the focus of intense research efforts, as well as multiple controversies. Although an increased susceptibility to TMD in individuals wearing removable dentures is not completely clarified, a strong correlation between edentulous patients using unfitted or defective prosthesis and a higher incidence/intensity of TMD-related signs and symptoms has been suggested elsewhere. In the field of TMD, thermography has emerged as a valuable non-invasive and non-ionizing complementary diagnostic exam. In this context, a case report of a 60-year-old Caucasian female concerned with her unaesthetic smile and poor masticatory performance is described in this paper. A thermal imaging infrared camera was used to capture the patient before the oral rehabilitation, two weeks after the treatment and then, two months later. Despite preliminary, the results herein presented highlight the clinical potential of infrared medical imaging in the prosthodontic field.

1 INTRODUCTION

The past two centuries have witnessed a substantial increase in life expectancy, bringing new issues and challenges to the limelight. In the past, complete denture wearers were younger, therefore having less adaptation-related problems. Currently, with people experiencing tooth loss later in life, the development of neuromuscular capacities necessary for successful denture wearing is more difficult (Porwal *et al.* 2013). When an individual loses two molars in one quadrant his masticatory function on one side will be compromised (Malheiros *et al.* 2016). The absence of posterior teeth increases the overload force and may exceed the physiological resistance of intraarticular soft tissues. An imbalanced occlusion with unpaired masticatory forces decreases tissue homeostasis, thus raising the possibility of developing temporomandibular disorders (TMD; Ribeiro *et al.* 2014). TMD, whose diagnosis is sometimes difficult to ascertain, can be defined as a multifactorial pathology, characterized by an alteration of masticatory muscles, limitation of jaw movement, muscular and/or articular pain, joint noises and other signals and symptoms. In addition, the incorrect Vertical Dimension of Occlusion (VDO) has been historically associated with TMD (Bevilaqua-Grossi *et al.* 2007; Desmons *et al.* 2007;

Klasser *et al.* 2009; Stuginski-Barbosa *et al.* 2010). Edentulous patients presenting parafunctional habits, unstable prostheses and impaired masticatory function tend to have limited masticatory range of motion and muscle tenderness (Carlsson *et al.* 1999). Furthermore, subjects wearing unstable or poorly retentive dentures are more likely to clench their teeth in an attempt to improve denture retention during normal function. Supporting this concept, a cross-sectional study of Sipila *et al.* showed that wearing complete dentures or poor prostheses increases the prevalence of muscle pain on palpation (Sipila *et al.* 2013). Nevertheless, the association of denture wearers with TMD is tenuous and little solid evidence linking edentulism to TMD has been provided as well (Silva *et al.* 2015). It should be underlined, however, that occlusal and mechanical aspects appear to play a minor role in TMD development. The complex and multifactorial etiology of TMD make hard to prove that a patient with edentulism, unstable/unfitted denture or incorrect VDO will be more susceptible to TMD than an individual with ideal occlusal conditions (Maixner *et al.* 2011).

The Research Diagnostic Criteria for TMDs (RDC/TMD) is the only available TMD diagnostic system. It uses operationally defined measurement criteria to generate computer-derived diagnostic algorithms for the most common TMD forms and provides specifications for conducting a standardized clinical physical examination (Dworkin et al. 1992). Numerous complementary diagnostic methods have been proposed for TMDs. In this context, thermography has emerged as a valuable tool. The infrared thermography can be used to measure the skin surface temperature of masticatory muscles and temporomandibular joint (Dibai-Filho et al. 2015). In the presence of TMD the temperature of the assessed structures is altered due to the decrease in blood flow caused by the muscular hyperactivity (Barao et al. 2011; Desmons et al. 2007). Skin temperature over the TMJ is also increased in individuals with joint pain (Rodrigues-Bigaton et al. 2013).

The present case report brings together the thermographic analysis of the masticatory system with the process of an oral rehabilitation.

2 CASE DESCRIPTION

The patient was a 60-year-old Caucasian female seeking solutions to enhance her smile and improve the masticatory performance. From the clinical examination along with the panoramic (Figure 1) and periapical (Figure 2) radiographs, a reserved prognostic for both upper central incisors, upper left lateral incisor and the remaining mandibular teeth was established. The patient wore a misfit mandibular removable partial prosthesis, but no denture was used in the maxilla (Figure 3). Moreover, the VDO was lost and there was advanced mandibular alveolar ridge atrophy. After discussing the treatment plan with the patient, it was decided to extract the non-viable teeth and to place immediate upper and lower removable dentures to restore her smile and correct the VDO.

The prosthetic rehabilitation followed the conventional protocol for removable partial denture fabrication, whose starting point was a preliminary or diagnostic impression with alginate. At the second appointment the final or secondary impressions were obtained using an individual tray with alginate and functional movements, with the facebow records being performed as well. At the third appointment, the maxillomandibular relationships were recorded. In the fourth visit a try-in was made with little aesthetic adjustments and correction of some centric and eccentric occlusion contacts. At the denture insertion appointment teeth were extracted according to the pre-established plan, with the exception of the right lower second premolar which was maintained to increase the stability and retention of the mandibular denture (Figure 4). One month later two Klockner® implants were placed in the anterior region of the mandible. The second surgical phase will be conducted after implant osseointegration.

The thermal imaging infrared camera FLIR ONE® was used to photograph the patient. The following precautions were considered:

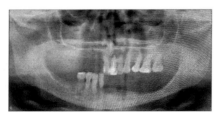

Figure 1. Panoramic radiograph at the beginning of the treatment.

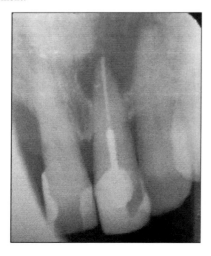

Figure 2. Periapical radiograph of tooth 21 (upper left central incisor).

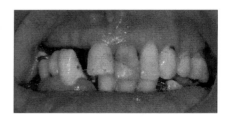

Figure 3. Initial intra-oral picture, frontal view.

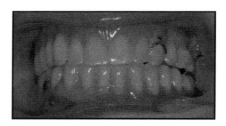

Figure 4. Immediate placement of upper and lower denture, frontal view.

a. Patient-related: ingestion of coffee, alcohol, tobacco or drugs was not allowed; no make-up, moisturizing cream or jewellery could be used; no bath was taken at least one hour before the exam; no physical exercise was made at least four hours before the exam; the patient rested for 15 minutes in a room without natural light.
b. Regarding the recording place: the same acclimatized room without natural light was used in the three recording moments.

For a precise evaluation of the landmarks of interest, the thermographs were interpreted using a dedicated software program, Flir Tools® version 6.3. In this particular clinical study, it was decided to assess the thermal behavior of the left and right temporomandibular joints, along with the temporal and masseter muscles. Flir Tools® allows to obtain the mean absolute temperature (T) averaged according to the selected Regions of Interest (ROIs). The thermographic characterization of the masticatory muscles during the three phases, before the oral rehabilitation, one week after the placement of the dentures and two months later is depicted in Figure 5.

Table 1 shows the mean absolute temperature obtained for the different landmarks at each recording time.

3 DISCUSSION

The primary goal of an oral rehabilitation is a long-lasting, comfortable dental restoration that provides a reasonable smile (Christensen et al. 2004). Although not meeting all the ideal aesthetic standards, the upper and lower removable partial dentures were able to make the patient pleased with her appearance in the clinical case here described. These days, with the increasingly prominent aesthetics concerns, dental professionals may lose their focus on one of the main objectives of prosthetic rehabilitation that is to improve the masticatory performance. A thorough analysis of the patients' initial condition revealed that only minimal occlusal contacts between natural dentition were present, besides the misfit lower denture whose function was likely lost a long-time ago.

As mentioned before, the impact of tooth loss, denture wear and denture status on TMDs is controversial. The study of Katyayan et al. reports that the majority of patients with most severe signs and symptoms of TMDs were individuals with zero teeth. A statistically significant number of cases presenting severe impairment of TMJ function was found in patients with 10–19 teeth. Finally, dentate patients with no removable dentures exhibited the least severe signs and symptoms (Katyayan et al. 2016).

Previous studies have presented thermography as a helpful complementary exam in identifying patients with TMD, with excellent intra- and inter-examiner reliability, as well as an efficient method to find miofascial trigger points in muscles like trapezium (Costa et al. 2013; Dibai-Filho et al. 2015; Woźniak et al. 2015). The thermographic analysis performed during the oral rehabilitation here described provided interesting results in terms of temperature differential (ΔT) at the three recording times (Table 1 and Figure 6). Apart from the masseter muscle, all the other ROIs increased ΔT from the first recording to the second, coinciding with denture placement. Furthermore, all ROIs decreased the ΔT from the second recording to the third, two months after the placement of the dentures.

To determine the presence of pathology, the clinician or researcher relies on the temperature differential of the left and right masticatory structures

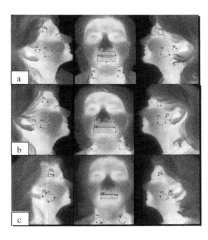

Figure 5. Right lateral, frontal and left lateral thermograms. a) before the oral rehabilitation, b) one week after the placement of the dentures, c) two months after the placement of the dentures.

Table 1. Temperature values of the studied landmarks at the three recording times. Temperature differential (ΔT) represents the difference between the values obtained for the left and right sides; in the case of lips, ΔT refers to the difference between the upper and lower lip.

	Left Side			Right Side			ΔT		
	Before	One week	Two months	Before	One week	Two months	Before	One week	Two months
Anterior triangle of the neck	37.9	35.4	34.1	37.2	36.3	33.6	0.7	0.9	0.5
Masseter	36.0	34.0	34.9	34.8	34.4	34.7	1.2	0.4	0.2
Temporal	37.4	36.1	36.6	37.7	37.1	36.3	0.3	1.0	0.3
TMJ	37.2	35.2	36.0	37.1	36.2	35.7	0.1	1.0	0.1
	Upper Lip			Lower Lip			ΔT		
	35.3	33.2	32.4	36.3	35.0	33.6	1.0	1.8	1.2

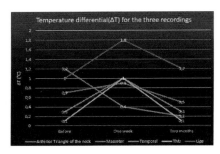

Figure 6. Evolution of the differential temperature for the three recordings moments (before intervention, one week after and two months after) on the five defined ROIs.

(contralateral). In the literature, reports of Fischer and Chang can be found describing miofascial trigger points with temperature differential ranging from 0.5°C to 1°C, while all other authors agree with variations between 0.3°C and 0.5°C (Haddad et al. 2012). In line with these results, Wozniak et al. showed that a cut-off point of 0.4°C of asymmetry is valid and efficient to predict the presence of a TMD in the assessed area of the stomatognathic system. Therefore, when comparing two bilateral structures, values over 0.4°C suggest a pathological stage, whereas values below 0.4°C suggest a healthy condition (Woźniak et al. 2015). Analyzing our results in light of Wozniak et al. findings, and assuming 0.4°C as cut-off value, it may be suggested that before the rehabilitation treatment the lip area, anterior triangle of the neck and masseter muscle had a settled inflammatory process. In particular, the highest initial asymmetry was observed in masseter muscles (1.2°C), which might be a consequence of the denture instability, reduced VDO and incorrect jaw position. Acting together, such conditions could lead to muscular changes and joint noises, with the masseter being particularly affected (Goiato, dos Santos et al. 2010). One week after the immediate placement of the dentures all structures assessed displayed values of asymmetry equal or greater than 0.4°C. Finally, after two months of denture wearing, the asymmetry recorded was overall reduced, with the exception being the lips and the anterior triangle of the neck, that still present pathological values. By reestablishing the correct VDO, increasing the occlusal stability of the mandible through a greater number of contact points and enhancing the denture retention, the oral condition of the patient was substantially improved, although the existence of an adaptation period should not be ignored. In fact, multiple studies report a significant increase in the masticatory force only after two months of adaptation (Lindquist et al. 1986; Muller et al. 2001; Wostmann et al. 2008). The last statement may, therefore, support the increased differential temperatures observed in the second recording, likely coinciding with the adaptation period of the patient, during which muscle growth and development are ongoing (Goldspink et al. 1998). Other significant aspect is that eight days after the immediate placement of the dentures, five alveolar sockets were still healing, a process that involves cytokines and inflammatory mediators. Human studies on post-extractional healing have demonstrated that mineralization begins at the end of the first week (Atwood et al. 1963). Hence, the healing process may have influenced the higher temperatures measured in the right structures in comparison to the left ROIs. Regarding the increased asymmetry registered in the lips on the third recording, it this conceivable that it tends to decrease or even disappear after concluding the mandibular rehabilitation with the implant-supported overdenture. Two locators will improve the prosthesis retention (Elsyad et al. 2016) and consequently a smaller muscular activity of the lower lip is expected.

Finally, and just as important, there are some limitations in the current paper. As a clinical case report, the presented results are from one single individual and cannot be generalized to all oral rehabilitations. A larger sample is therefore needed to strengthen the representativeness of the study. A more accurate and reliable thermal camera should be used in further studies to better validate the results obtained. The data collection process should also include a TMD diagnostic questionnaire, which would be useful to correlate the thermographic findings with the clinical examination and diagnosis. Considering the paucity of the literature available, however, these preliminary results encourage the use of thermography in other oral rehabilitation cases.

4 CONCLUSIONS

So far, the debate of our findings is mainly speculative. A thermal analysis of the masticatory system in oral rehabilitations may be a promising field in dental medicine, working side by side with the other medical imaging techniques. The thermographic study of the masticatory muscles throughout an oral rehabilitation may represent a helpful approach to all dental doctors to better understand the evolution of the stomatognathic system during the treatment. Future methodologies similar to the one herein presented may corroborate our evidence that replacement of a misfit denture, along with the reestablishment of VDO and rehabilitation of missing posterior teeth will balance the new occlusion, with repercussions in the thermal symmetry between the masticatory muscles.

REFERENCES

Atwood, D.A. 1963. Postextraction changes in the adult mandible as illustrated by microradiographs of midsagittal sections and serial cephalometric roentgenograms. *The Journal of Prosthetic Dentstry* 13(5): 810–824.

Barao, V.A. Gallo, A.K., Zuim, P.R., Garcia, A.R., Assunção, W.G. 2011. Effect of occlusal splint treatment on the temperature of different muscles in patients with TMD. *Journal of Prosthodontic Research* 55(1): 19–23.

Bevilaqua-Grossi, D., Chaves, T.C., de Oliveira, A.S. 2007. Cervical spine signs and symptoms: perpetuating rather than predisposing factors for temporomandibular disorders in women. *Journal of Applied Oral Science* 15(4): 259–264.

Carlsson, G.E. 1999. Epidemiology and treatment need for temporomandibular disorders. *Journal Orofacial Pain* 13(4): 232–237.

Christensen, G.J. 2004. Defining oral rehabilitation. *The Journal of the American Dental Association* 135(2): 215–217.

Costa, J.M., Grant, O.M., Chaves, M.M. 2013. Thermography to explore plant-environment interactions. *Journal of Experimental Botany* 64(13): 3937–3949.

Desmons, S., Graux, F., Atassi, M., Libersa, P., Dupas, P.H. 2007. The lateral pterygoid muscle, a heterogeneous unit implicated in temporomandibular disorder: a literature review. *Cranio* 25(4): 283–291.

Dibai-Filho, A V., Costa, A.S., Packer, A.C., de Castro, E.M., Rodrigues-Bigaton, D. 2015. Women with more severe degrees of temporomandibular disorder exhibit an increase in temperature over the temporomandibular joint. *The Scudi Dental Journal* 27(1): 44–49.

Dibai-Filho, A.V., Guirro, R.R. 2015. Evaluation of myofascial trigger points using infrared thermography: a critical review of the literature. *Journal of Manipulative and Physiological Therapeutics* 38(1): 86–92.

Dworkin, S.F., LeResche, L. 1992. Research diagnostic criteria for temporomandibular disorders: review, criteria, examinations and specifications, critique. *Journal of Craniomandibular Disorders* 6(4): 301–355.

Elsyad, M.A., Agha, N.N., Habib, A.A. 2016. Retention and Stability of Implant-Retained Mandibular Overdentures Using Different Types of Resilient Attachments: An In Vitro Study. *International Journal of Oral Maxillofacial Implants* 31(5): 1040–1048.

Goiato, M.C., dos Santos, D.M., Monteiro, D.R. 2010. Joint sounds in complete denture wearers. Literature review. The *New York State Dental Journal* 76(1): 46–49.

Goldspink, G. 1998. Cellular and molecular aspects of muscle growth, adaptation and ageing. *Gerodontology* 15(1): 35–43.

Haddad, D.S., Brioschi, M.L., Arita, E.S. 2012. Thermographic and clinical correlation of myofascial trigger points in the masticatory muscles. *Dentomaxillofacial Radiology* 41(8): 621–629.

Katyayan, P.A., Katyayan, M.K., Patel, G.C. 2016. Association of edentulousness and removable prosthesis rehabilitation with severity of signs and symptoms of temporomandibular disorders. *Indian Journal of Dental Research* 27(2): 127–136.

Klasser, G.D., Greene, C.S. 2009. Oral appliances in the management of temporomandibular disorders. *Oral*

Surgery Oral Medicine Oral Pathology Oral Radiology and Endodontics 107(2): 212–223.

Lindquist, L.W., Carlsson, G.E., Hedegard, B. 1986. Changes in bite force and chewing efficiency after denture treatment in edentulous patients with denture adaptation difficulties. *Journal of Oral Rehabilitation* 13(1): 21–29.

Maixner, W., Diatchenko, L., Dubner, R., Filingim, R.B., Greenspan, J.D., Knott, C., Ohrbach, R., Weir, B., Slade, G.D. 2011. Orofacial pain prospective evaluation and risk assessment study—the OPPERA study. *Journal of Pain.* 12(Suppl 11): T4–11.e11–12.

Malheiros, A.S., Carvalhal, S.T., Pereira, T.L., Filho, E.M., Tonetto, M.R., Gonçalves, L.M., Bandeca, M.C., de Jesus, R.R. 2016. Association between Tooth Loss and Degree of Temporomandibular Disorders: A Comparative Study. *The Journal of Contemporary Dental Practice* 17(3): 235–239.

Muller, F. Helath, M.R., Ott, R. 2001. Maximum bite force after the replacement of complete dentures. *Gerodontology* 18(1): 58–62.

Porwal, A., Sasaki, K. 2013. Current status of the neutral zone: a literature review. *Journal of Prosthetic Dentistry* 109(2): 129–134.

Ribeiro, J.A., de Resende, C.M., Lopes, A.L., Farias-Neto, A., Carreiro Ada, F. 2014. Association between prosthetic factors and temporomandibular disorders in complete denture wearers. *Gerodontology* 31(4): 308–313.

Rodrigues-Bigaton, D., Dibai Filho, A.V., Costa, A.C., Packer, A.C., de Castro, E.M. 2013. Accuracy and reliability of infrared thermography in the diagnosis of arthralgia in women with temporomandibular disorder. *Journal of Manipulative and Physiological Therapeutics* 36(4): 253–258.

Silva, J.V., Machado, F., Ferreira, M. 2015. Social Inequalities and the Oral health in Brazilian Capitals. *Ciência & Saúde Coletiva* 20(8): 2539–2548.

Sipila, K., Napankangas, R., Kononen, M., Alanen, P., Suominen, A.L. 2013. The role of dental loss and denture status on clinical signs of temporomandibular disorders. *Journal of Oral Rehabilitation* 40(1): 15–23.

Stuginski-Barbosa, J., Macedo, H.R., Bigal, M.E., Speciali, J.G. 2010. Signs of temporomandibular disorders in migraine patients: a prospective, controlled study. *The Clinical Journal of Pain* 26(5): 418–421.

Tallents, R.H., Macher, D.J., Kyrkanides, S., Katzberg, R.W., Moss, M.E. 2002. Prevalence of missing posterior teeth and intraarticular temporomandibular disorders. *The Journal of Prosthetic Dentistry* 87(1): 45–50.

Wostmann, B., Balbeknhol, M., Ferger, P., Rehmann, P. 2008. Changes in occlusal force at denture dislodgement after refabrication or optimization of complete dentures. *International Journal of Prosthodontics* 21(4): 305–306.

Woźniak, K., Szyszka-Sommerfeld, L, Trybek, G., Piatkowska, D. 2015. Assessment of the Sensitivity, Specificity, and Accuracy of Thermography in Identifying Patients with TMD. *Medical Science Monitor: International Medical Journal of Experimental and Clinical Research* 21: 1485–1493.

Biodental Engineering V – Belinha et al. (Eds)
© 2019 Taylor & Francis Group, London, ISBN 978-0-367-21087-8

Tips on implant screws tightening – an overview

A. Moreira & R. Batista
Faculty of Dental Medicine, University of Porto (FMDUP), Porto, Portugal

S. Oliveira, P. Ferrás, F. Góis & J.C. Reis Campos
FMDUP, Porto, Portugal

ABSTRACT: In the field of mechanical engineering, dental implant screws have improved their bio-mechanical behavior in the past decades. Once implant osseointegration has occurred, abutment screw loosening appears to be the most common problem. Several factors have been implicated in the aetiology of such technical failure, including occlusal overload, fatigue, improper screw engagement, superstructure non-passive fit, manufacture deficiencies and use of non-genuine implant components. Since the literature on this subject is vast and dispersed, the aim of this work was to perform an overview about dental implant screws, as an attempt to provide a list of clinical tips for practitioners, based on scientific evidence. The increasing use of dental implants has raised new concerns, particularly related to late failure, with screw retention representing a persistent clinical issue. Management of implant problems due to screw retention can be challenging, thus emphasizing the need for preventive efforts that preclude loss of the restoration.

1 INTRODUCTION

Since the beginning of implant-supported reha-bilitation, screws have been extensively studied to match the different implant connection systems and prosthetic requirements. A screw joint is estab-lished when the implant and abutment are con-nected by means of a screw. The torque applied to a screw inside a joint develops a force within the screw called preload (McGlumphy *et al.* 1998). Screw-tightening also causes its elongation, thus producing tension inside the joint with an associ-ated elastic recovery. The combination of forces acting at the joint generates a clamping force at the abutment-implant interface that maintains the parts together (Haack *et al.* 1995). Opposing the clamping force is a joint-separating force attempt-ing to uncouple the joint components. When this force overcomes the clamping force, loosening will be observed. If excessive separating forces are applied, a slippage of the screw threads may occur, resulting in the preload loss.

Despite these advances and according to some authors, once implant osseointegration has occurred, abutment screw loosening appears to be the most common problem associated with dental implants (Assenza *et al.* 2005; Cranin *et al.* 1990; Krishnan *et al.* 2014). Several factors have been linked to the aetiology of such technical failure, including occlusal overload, fatigue, improper screw engagement, superstructure's non-passive fit,

manufacture deficiencies and use of non-genuine implant components (Krishnan *et al.* 2014). The type of implant restoration is still a controversial issue, since cement-retained restorations are seen as non-retrieval despite their optimal occlusion and aesthetics, ease of fabrication and higher potential for passivity. Moreover, many techniques have been developed in order to improve the retrievability of such cement-retained restorations.

Given the insufficient number of randomised controlled trials available, conducting a complete systematic review on implant screws is challenging. Accordingly, the purpose of this work was to over-view the significant literature on implant screws topic, as an attempt to find clinical recommenda-tions that help reducing the likelihood of screw loosening in medical daily practice.

2 MATERIAL AND METHODS

The protocol for this review involved a database search on Pubmed® using the keywords "implant screw loosening", "dental implant screw", "screw-retained" and "abutment screw". Searches were restricted to full-text articles written in English and published before March 2018. The inclusion crite-ria considered for this review were research stud-ies, meta-analyses and reviews on screw-retained implant restorations or only on implant screw testing. Titles and abstracts were screened and the corresponding full-texts of potentially relevant publications were obtained and evaluated.

3 RESULTS AND DISCUSSION

From the 548 articles obtained in the initial search only 16 papers were selected according the overall relevance to the topic of interest. Posteriorly, the 16 articles allowed us to find other authors' research which was also included.

One of the most prominent factors affecting the longevity of an implant-supported prosthesis is retention (Michalakis *et al.* 2003). The choice of cement-retained or screw-retained implant rehabilitations has a major impact on the final occlusal design, directly affecting the transmission of forces to the components and to the bone-implant interface. The attachment mechanisms of cement retention and screw retention are dramatically different (Hebel 1997). Implant-supported prosthesis cemented using provisional cements are retrievable, being the cement used the essential factor controlling retention (Breeding *et al.* 1992). Some authors believe that this retention system represents a superior option in terms of occlusion, aesthetics, passivity and loading characteristics. In fact, cement retention has been used in fixed prosthodontics for decades and is very well documented (Hebel 1997).

Screw-retained implant restorations were validated by Branemark studies several years ago (Adell *et al.* 1990). Screws are used to connect abutments to implants and/or to prosthesis. At the edge of the abutment-implant connection fulcrum points are created. In the presence of an accurate fit, a continuity at the circumference joint is obtained, with vertical occlusal forces over the head of the implant being vertically transmitted to the screw with minimal stress, thus preventing the screw loosening phenomenon (Hebel 1997). By contrast, poorly fitting implant-abutment interfaces show gaps in the circumference, leading to casting compression followed by screw loosening. When offset loading is of greater magnitude than the clamping force, the screw can be stretched, loosened or broken due to rocking. Such separating force can be divided into vertical and horizontal components, whose sum of the moments [(Fv x L2) and (Fh x L1)] must be lower than the resisting moment of the screw to maintain equilibrium (Hurson 1995).

Guzaitis *et al.* showed that more than 10 screw insertion cycles should be avoided to guarantee maximum reverse torque values and maintain the preload conditions. In this study, four groups of 10 primary screws paired with OsseoSpeedTM system, Astra Tech implants were established. Each group received a number of screw insertion cycles as follows: 9, 19, 29 and 39 cycles. The authors

reported that increasing the number of screw insertion cycles resulted in decreased reverse torque values, suggesting that after 10 cycles a new prosthetic screw should be placed (Guzaitis *et al.* 2011).

In a single-unit implant-supported prosthesis the ideal occlusion can be settled with a cement-retained restoration, since there is no occlusal screw-access hole interfering with protrusive and lateral excursive movements that compromise the anterior guidance (Hebel *et al.* 1997). On the contrary, in screw-retained prosthesis it is difficult to achieve stable occlusal contacts due to wear of the material used to close the occlusal access hole. This restoration occupies nearly 50% of intercuspal occlusal table, affecting the direction of occlusal loads that will be distributed as lateral forces to the implant instead of being axially directed (Misch 2014). Nowadays and with new developments, this restoration occupies less occlusal surface which reduces but not eliminate its effect.

The assessment of passivity and fitness in multiple abutments has a remarkable literature (Hebel *et al.* 1997). When adaptability of the abutment is not achieved, microgaps are created that may lead to compression of the casting and shaking of the framework when exposed to vertical loading, being more significant in offset loading (Hebel *et al.* 1997). With this mentioned it is easy to understand that cemented prostheses over properly fitted abutments are more stable and passive than multiple screw retained ones (Hurson 1995). There are multiple studies concluding that screw loosening is a major problem in screw retained prostheses (Jemt *et al.* 1993; Kallus *et al.* 1994; Laney *et al.* 1994; Carlson *et al.* 1994; Misch 1993; Jemt *et al.* 1991; Jemt 1993; Kallus *et al.* 1994; Laney WR *et al.* 1994).

Misch *et al.* reported that apart from predictable retrievability and limited abutment height, arguments supporting the use of screw-retained prosthesis can hardly be found. As above-mentioned, cemented suprastructures provide a passive stable environment by being cemented on well-adapted machined abutments, with the possible discrepancies being mitigated by cement grouting (Misch 1993). In addition, the absence of screw holes enhances the physical properties of acrylic and ceramic materials in cemented prostheses.

There are many types of screws with diverse designs, materials and sizes, each one with a different purpose and mechanical properties. It was reported that screws made of gold can be tightened more effectively than the titanium ones (Andersson *et al.* 1992). Screw heads with internal hexagon remain tighter than those with slots (Kallus *et al.* 1994). Regarding the screw design, it is also worth mentioning that flat head screws 1:1 head/ shaft load ratio are preferred over tapered-head implants, since the latter have a 4:1 ratio that leads to strained interfaces, therefore increasing the possibility of screw loosening (Patterson *et al.* 1992). Multiple strategies have been developed to enhance the implant design. Accordingly, increasing the screw diameter has been used to improve the preload, while increasing the hex height and the implant platform diameter enhances stability and resistance to screw loosening (Boggan *et al.* 1999; Binon *et al.* 2000).

To achieve the optimal clamping force, screws should be tightened to implants with 50% to 75% of their yield strength, respecting the manufacturer's specifications and the appropriate mechanical wrench. Screw settling or embedment relaxation, that occurs shortly after screw tightening, is the result of compressing the microrough areas of the screw threads and opposing flanges during initial screw tightening (Haack *et al.* 1995). To limit this phenomenon and maintain preload values, retightening the screw 5 minutes after initial torquing and again a few weeks later is recommended (Binon *et al.* 2000). However, the amount of torque given to the screw is operator dependent (Jaarda *et al.* 1993), and is responsible for the preload in their threads (Jaarda *et al.* 1995). This preload also varies according to the presence and type of lubricant, the physical properties of the materials in contact, and the settling of the screw after initial torqueing (Burguete *et al.* 1995). Surface imperfections induce greater friction, therefore decreasing the preload. On the other hand, the use of lubricants, as well as removal or retorquing the screw, increases the preload by reducing imperfections (Haack *et al.* 1995). This is the rationale for not using cements and silicon as sealers, neither torque controllers, to avoid fracture of the screw (Scarano *et al.* 2004). By using high torque levels, screw loosening and fracture are both facilitated (Scarano *et al.* 2004).

After implant osseointegration, abutment screw loosening represents the major problem associated with dental implants. A one year multicentre prospective study showed that 26% of 107 implants were retightened during the observation period, while fistula formation coexisted with 10% of loose abutment screws (Jemt *et al.* 1991).

In a study performed by Scarano *et al.* involving patients with loosened suprastructures, a total of 58 screws were analysed by SEM and fractography to characterize the microstructure and fatigue crack initiation at thread level of the screws. A number of alterations and deformations in the concavities and convexities of threads were reported. Deformations were observed in convexities, while long fracture cracks were registered in concavities, generally throughout the long axis of the screws (Scarano *et al.* 2011). Fractography analysis of the external parts of the specimens revealed the presence of shear cracks and their propagation through the fine grain structures, which was accompanied by the formation of flake particles. The authors suggested that crack growth might be related to the coalescence of multiple crack events (Scarano *et al.* 2011). The early recognition of crack initiation, coupled to a thorough understanding of its growth pattern, is crucial in determining the fatigue life of implant screws (Scarano *et al.* 2011). The appearance of small cracks in titanium alloy under fatigue is mainly due to grain size and orientation (Scarano *et al.* 2011). The presence of cracks or other flaws increase the possibility of sudden fracture that depends on the size of the flaws, the stress placed on the component and the properties of the materials. An alternative mechanism of screw loosening occurs due to presence of microgaps between the implant and screw as previously discussed (Scarano *et al.* 2011; Hebel *et al.* 1997). Such microgaps, whose size is hard to control in clinical practice, allow the migration of bacteria to the internal portion of the implant (Scarano *et al.* 2005), where corrosion-related events may take place (Kawalec *et al.* 1995).

4 CONCLUSIONS

Prosthetic complications can be very expensive and very time consuming in its resolution. As such, companies and clinicians have tried to minimize these complications over time. Management of implant failure due to screw loosening can be very challenging, although essential for the success of the oral rehabilitation. Preventive efforts should begin on treatment study and planning from the surgery to the final prosthesis. Firstly, the implant should be placed where the occlusal forces are transmitted to the long axis of the implant. Secondly, cantilevers should be kept to a minimum. Thirdly, occlusal contacts are important, and establishing them in cusp-to-fossa relationships instead of cusp tip-to-cusp tip is preferable. It is essential that clinicians understand the rehabilitation process from the biological principles to the mechanical behaviour of screws. Through evidence-based knowledge and an accurate management of the factors herein discussed, increased success rates of screw-retained implant prosthesis can be envisaged, along with reduced number of screw loosening events.

REFERENCES

Adell, R., Eriksson, B., Lekholm, U., Branemark, P.I., Jemt, T. 1990. Long-term follow-up study of osseointegrated implants in the treatment of totally edentulous jaws. *The International Journal of Oral & Maxillofac Implants* 5(4): 347–359.

Andersson, B., Odmna, P., Carlsson, L., Branemark, P.I. 1992. A new Branemark single tooth abutment: handling and early clinical experiences. *The International Journal of Oral & Maxillofac Implants* 7(1): 105–110.

Assenza, B., Scarano, A., Leghissa, G., Carusi, G., Thams, U., Roman, F.S., Piattelli, A. 2005. Screw- vs cement-implant-retained restorations: an experimental study in the Beagle. Part 1. Screw and abutment loosening. *Journal of Oral Implantology* 31(5): 242–246.

Binon, PP. 2000. The external hexagonal interface and screw joint stability: a primer on threaded fasteners in implant dentistry. *Quintessence Dent Technol,* 91.

Boggan, R.S., Strong, J.T., Misch, C.E., Bidez, M.W. 1999. Influence of hex geometry and prosthetic table width on static and fatigue strength of dental implants. *Journal of Prosthetic Dentistry* 82(4): 436–440.

Breeding, L.C., Dixon, D.L., Bogacki, M.T., Tietge, J.D. 1992. Use of luting agents with an implant system: Part I. *Journal of Prosthetic Dentistry* 68(5): 737–741.

Burguete R.L., Johns, R.B., King, T., Patterson, E.A. 1994. Tightening characteristics for screwed joints in osseointegrated dental implants. *Journal of Prosthetic Dentistry* 71(6): 592–599.

Carlson, B., Carlsson, G.E. Prosthodontic complications in osseointegrated dental implant treatment. *The International Journal of Oral & Maxillofacial Implants* 9(1): 90–94.

Cranin, A.N., Dibling, J.B., Simons, A., Klein, M., Sirakian, A. Report of the incidence of implant insert fracture and repair of Core-Vent dental implants. *Journal of Oral Implantology* 16(3): 184–188.

Guzaitis, K.L., Knoernschild, K.L., Viana, M.A. 2011. Effect of repeated screw joint closing and opening cycles on implant prosthetic screw reverse torque and implant and screw thread morphology. *Journal of Prosthetic Dentistry* 106(3): 159–169.

Haack, J.E., Sakaguchi, R.L., Sun, T., Coffey, J.P. 1995. Elongation and preload stress in dental implant abutment screws. *The International Journal of Oral & Maxillofac Implants* 10(5): 529–536.

Hebel, K.S., Gajjar, R.C. 1997. Cement-retained versus screw-retained implant restorations: Achieving optimal occlusion and esthetics in implant dentistry. *Journal of Prosthetic Dentistry* 77(1): 28–35.

Hurson, S. 1995. Practical clinical guidelines to prevent screw loosening. *International Journal of Dentistry* 3(1): 22–25.

Jaarda, M.J., Razzog, M.E., Gratton, D.G.1993. Providing optimum torque to implant prostheses: a pilot study. *Implant Dentistry* 2: 20–52.

Jemt, T., Carlsson, L., Boss, A., Jorneus, L. 1991. In vivo load measurements on osseointegrated implants supporting fixed or removable prostheses: a comparative pilot study. *The International Journal of Oral & Maxillofac Implants* 6(4): 413–417.

Jemt, T., Pettersson, P. 1993. A 3-year follow-up study on single implant treatment. *Journal of Dentistry* 21(4): 203–208.

Jemt. T., Laney, W.R., Harris, D., Henry, P.J., Krogh, P.H., Polizzi, G., Zarb, G.A., Hermann, I. 1991. Osseointegrated implants for single tooth replacement: a 1-year report from a multicenter prospective study. *The International Journal of Oral & Maxillofacial Implants* 6(1): 29–36.

Kallus, T., Bessing, C. Loose gold screws frequently occur in full-arch fixed prostheses supported by osseointegrated implants after 5 years. *The International Journal of Oral & Maxillofac Implants* 9(2): 169–178.

Kawalec, J.S., Brown, S.A., Payer, J.H., Merritt, K. 1995. Mixed-metal fretting corrosion of Ti6 Al4V and wrought cobalt alloy. *Journal of Biomedical Materials Research* 29(7):867–873.

Krishnan, V., Thomas, C.T., Sabu, I. 2014. Management of abutment screw loosening: review of literature and report of a case. *Journal of Indian Prosthodontic Society* 14(3), 208–214.

Laney, W.R., Jemt, T., Harris, D., Henry, P.J., Krogh, P.H., Polizzi, G., Zarb, G.A., Hermann, I. 1994. Osseointegrated implants for single tooth replacement: progress report from a multicenter prospective study after 3 years. *The International Journal of Oral & Maxillofac Implants* 9(1): 49–54.

McGlumphy, E.A., Mendel, D.A., Holloway, J.A., Implant screw mechanics. *Dental Clinics of North America* 42(1): 71–89.

Michalakis, K.X., Hirayama, H., Garefis, P.D. 2003. Cement-retained versus screw-retained implant restorations: a critical review. *The International Journal of Oral & Maxillofac Implants* 18(5): 719–728.

Misch, C. (2014). Dental Implant Prosthetics (Vol. 2nd Edition): Mosby.

Misch 1993. Contemporary implant dentistry. St Louis: Mosby-Year Book Inc.

Patterson, E.A., Johns, R.B., 1992. Theoretical analysis of the fatigue life of fixture screws on osseointegrated dental implants. *The International Journal of Oral & Maxillofac Implants* 7(1):26–33.

Scarano, A., Assenza, B., Piatteli, M., Iezzi, G., Leghissa, G.C., Quaranta, A., Tortora,P., Piatelli, A. 2005. A 16-year study of the microgap between 272 human titanium implants and their abutments. *Journal of Oral Implantology* 31(6): 269–275.

Scarano, A., Murmura, G., Sinjari, B., Sollazzo, V., Spinelli, G., Carinci, F. 2011. Analysis and structural examination of screw loosening in oral implants. *International Journal of Immunopathology and Pharmacology* 24(2): 77–81.

Scarano A. 2004. Complicaciones mecànicas en implantes dentales con munòn atornillado o cementado: observaciones xperimentales *Gaceta Dental* 148: 20.

Zarb, G.A., Schmitt, A. 1990. The longitudinal clinical effectiveness of osseointegrated dental implants: the Toronto study. Part III: Problems and complications encountered. *Journal of Prosthetic Dentistry* 64(2): 185–194.

Biodental Engineering V – Belinha et al. (Eds)
© 2019 Taylor & Francis Group, London, ISBN 978-0-367-21087-8

Immediate loading in every dental implant protocol – is it safe?

D. Soares & João S. Marques
Faculty of Dental Medicine, University of Porto (FMDUP), Porto, Portugal

J.C. Reis Campos, M. Sampaio-Fernandes, C. Silva & J.C. Sampaio-Fernandes
FMDUP, Porto, Portugal

ABSTRACT: Immediate loading is a protocol in which the prosthesis is placed as soon as the implant is inserted. It is a controversial option and there still remain doubts for the clinicians on the immediate loading protocol decision. This review aims to clarify the possible factors influencing the success of immediate loading dental implants. A search in the PubMed® and Scielo® databases was performed, restricted to systematic reviews and meta-analyses published within a period time limit of the past 6 years. 18 out of 86 articles were selected to discussion, according to the relevance of the subject addressed. Although overall analysis tends to attribute similar results to immediate loading protocol as compared to non-immediate loading procedures, this differentiated technique demands specific clinical requirements, in which the surgeon experience should not be neglected, but rather a key success factor. More well-designed randomized, controlled clinical trials and long-term follow-up studies are emergent.

1 INTRODUCTION

Patient's growing demand for less invasive and faster procedures that optimize their highly aesthetic requirements, has turn immediate loading the preferable option for patients (Moraschini et al. 2016). The literature describes 3 types of dental implant loading protocols: conventional loading, with a 3 to 6 months healing period between implant placement and restoration; early loading, where healing period is less than 3 months; and immediate loading, in which the prosthesis is placed as soon as the implant is inserted (Koirala et al. 2016). Thereafter, during the Consensus Conference of the European Association for Osseointegration (EAO) in 2006, immediate loading was defined as loading within 72 h after implant installation (Engelhardt et al. 2015).

The main criterion for performing immediate loading of single implants is primary stability (Moraschini et al. 2016). Primary stability can be measured by parameters like insertion torque, measured in Newton-centimeters (N/cm), and implant stability quotient (ISQ), measured by Resonance Frequency Analysis (RFA) (Moraschini et al. 2016). Previous studies have shown that primary stability is a critical factor for immediate loading and that low initial stability is a significant risk factor in early failure of single implants (Moraschini et al. 2016).

In 2018, Pigozzo et al. recommended the use of a minimum insertion torque of 32 N/cm for immediate loading in order to allow osseointegration simultaneously with mechanical loading. There are three biological factors that can influence osseointegration with immediate loading: factors affecting osteogenesis; factors affecting peri-implant osteolysis; and effects of micromotion on peri-implant osteogenesis (Al-Sawaii et al. 2016). With that in mind, it seems that immediate mechanical loading and its biological factors could contribute to the development of well-organized bone and increased BIC (bone to implant contact), resulting in enhanced osseointegration (Al-Sawaii et al. 2016).

Two types of immediate loading have been described in the literature. One is the immediate functional loading (IFL), which refers to the placement of a prosthesis in occlusal contact with the opposing arch within the first 72 h after surgery; and the alternative approach – immediate non-functional loading (INFL) that consists in modifying the restoration avoiding occlusal contacts in centric and lateral excursions, in order to reduce the early risks of mechanical overload caused by functional or parafunctional forces. In this way, the modified restoration would still be involved in the masticatory process, but the mechanical loading stress is reduced (Chrcanovic et al. 2014).

Also, the impact of implant location (maxilla vs. mandible; anterior vs. posterior region), implant number and inclination, geometry and surface of implants, type of prosthesis (fixed vs. removable), the different anchorage systems, type of bone and surgical techniques need to be evaluated concerning their importance on immediate loading (Al-Sawaii et al. 2016, Menini et al. 2012, Schwarz et al. 2016).

The question of whether implants could be immediately loaded after their insertion has relevant clinical implications since the treatment period could be drastically reduced for the patient's benefit (Esposito et al. 2013).

Accordingly, this paper aims to clarify the influence of possible factors in the success of immediate loading in every dental implant protocol.

2 MATERIAL AND METHODS

In order to shed light on immediate implant loading checkpoints, a search in the PubMed® and Scielo® databases was performed using the keywords "immediate loading"; "esthetic zone"; and "provisional restoration". For this purpose, the boolean markers "AND" and "OR" were also used. The search was restricted to systematic reviews and meta-analyses published within a period time limit of the past 6 years.

3 RESULTS AND DISCUSSION

The highest level of scientific evidence needed to answer a clinical question comes from systematic reviews and meta-analyses that analyze results from RCTs (Koirala et al. 2016). According to that, from the original literature search, 86 articles were obtained, being selected 16 papers to discussion, according to the relevance of the subject addressed.

In this way, the systematic review and meta-analyze published in 2018 by Pigozzo et al. reveals that for single implant-supported crowns, similar success and implant survival rates as well as similar marginal bone loss rates at 1 and 3 years have been reported for early and immediate loading protocols, especially when implants are placed with insertion torques greater than 32 N/cm (Pigozzo et al. 2018).

This absence of difference between these protocols could be explained by the fact that implants were loaded according to a randomized allocation and to achieve high insertion torque, implant sites were under prepared to various degrees according to bone quality (Pigozzo et al. 2018). In addition, the fact that not all the studies define immediate loading the same way can led to false conclusions. For clinical purpose, it seems that to give a fixed implant restoration in the same day of surgery or until 72 h after surgery, there is a need, in most cases, to under prepare the bone in order to have enough primary stability for immediate loading. The question is, if there is any adverse effect of allowing the implant to be placed tightened.

In 2015, Chrcanovic et al. published a meta-analysis showing that immediate loaded implants are 1.78 times more likely to fail than submerged implants, being the relative risk reduction using the submerged and conventional approach of 78% (Crhcanovic et al. 2015). This is a surprising result comparing to other studies that show similar results between these approaches, being important to investigate if these results are a real finding or due to lack of statistical power.

The reason for these results could be in the observation of Pilliar et al. that assumes that a micro movement of 150 mm may be the critical level above which healing will undergo fibrous repair rather than the desired osseous regeneration. This micromotion of implant surface relative to the bone can be the result of immediate loading that can also disturb the early remodeling phase. Although this explanation, it is important to remember that implants placed in the submerged way also fail to osseointegrate (Crhcanovic et al. 2015).

Relative to marginal bone loss, Chrcanovic et al. showed no statistical differences between immediate and conventional loading, but there is a higher implant failure rate (78%) associated with immediate loading (Crhcanovic et al. 2015).

In opposition, Zhang et al. in a meta-analysis published in 2017 compared the 3 loading protocols in terms of marginal bone loss (MBL) and implant survival rate, which revealed no inferiority in immediate loading comparing to non-immediate loading protocols, but as said before several factors as implant location, number of implants, type of prostheses and follow up time period could affect these results (Zhang et al. 2017). For example, it was reported that titanium oxide thickness in implants surface was associated with a high degree of BIC and bone formation which may enhance the clinical efficacy of immediate loading (Schwarz et al. 2016 & Zhang et al. 2017). Therefore, in situations of doubt about bone density, clinicians can fall back on the utilization of implants with a modified surface to compensate situation of patients with spongy bone. Moreover, increasing implant length could further facilitate immediate loading by enhancing primary stability in borderline cases (Zhang et al. 2017). These results are in accordance with the ones from Engelhardt et al. systematic review and meta-analysis published in 2014 (Engelhardt et al. 2015).

With that in mind, it seems that several factors can influence the predictability of immediate loading. With respect to tilted implants, in 2012, a systematic review published by Menini et al. evaluated the outcome of immediate loading between tilted and upright implants in the rehabilitation of edentulous maxilla and discover that both lead to an excellent prognosis, at least in the short term, with a peri-implant bone resorption of 0.77 mm and 0.73 mm, respectively, at 1 year of function (Menini et al. 2012). Despite these results, the inclination required to be considered a tilted implant is not completely defined.

The geometry of implant is a main characteristic normally associated to primary stability. In 2018, a systematic review and meta-analyze published by Atieh et al. showed that although there are not significant differences between tapered and parallel-walled implants, the tapered ones demonstrated a tendency for improved implant stability both at time of implant placement as well as 8 weeks postoperatively (Atieh et al. 2018). In this way, it seems that the selection of implant design should depend not only on bone quality and quantity but also on the loading protocol.

It is important to reline that there are two types of immediate loading protocols described in the literature. The 2014 systematic review and meta-analysis by Chrcanovic et al. revealed that implant failures are 1.13 times more likely to happen applying IFL compared to implants loaded under the INFL protocol with a relative risk reduction of 13% for INFL. However, these results did not reach statistical differences in respect to implant failure (p = 0.70) (Chrcanovic et al. 2014). In this way, it seems that is not the absence of loading per se that is critical for osseointegration, but rather the absence of excessive micromotion at the interface, which in fact suggest that splinting implants could be a protective solution (Chrcanovic et al. 2014).

In order to determine if immediate loading can achieve comparable clinical outcomes against conventional loading protocols with respect to technical and biological complications, success rates and clinical outcome variables, a 2016 consensus was published (Schwarz et al. 2016). The Camlog Foundation consensus realized that immediate loading is indicated in the following situations: edentulous maxilla (fixed splinted reconstructions) and edentulous mandible (removable and fixed splinted reconstructions); single tooth rehabilitation in the esthetic zone including premolars and fixed partial dentures limited to short spans (Schwarz et al. 2016).

It is also said that the survival rates are high for both groups, but immediate loading may impose a greater risk for implant failure when compared to conventional loading (Schwarz et al. 2016). On the other hand, it is suggested that there is less marginal bone loss around immediately loaded implants compared to conventionally loaded implants and with regard to peri-implant soft tissue, there are no significant differences between these 2 procedures (Schwarz et al. 2016). This suggestion is opposite to Chrcanovic findings that revealed similar results for marginal bone loss for both types of loading protocol (Schwarz et al. 2016 & Crhcanovic et al. 2015).

It is important to remember that these articles are written, in most cases, by experienced and highly trained clinicians, and an inexperienced surgical clinician may feel more comfortable and consequently have better results with delayed and conventional protocols. In addition, once primary stability is an essential condition for immediate loading and it requires, in most cases, an under preparation of the socket, it demands a precise technique that an inexperienced clinician can struggle to achieve.

Once primary stability seems to be the key factor for performing immediate loading, the Camlog Foundation consensus defined 30 N/cm as a minimum value of primary stability for performing immediate loading plus avoiding patients with clenching and bruxism (Schwarz et al. 2016).

These statements must be interpreted with caution because there are a lot of confounding factors. One of the most important is probably the splinting of implants making them work as a group and thereby compensating the lateral forces. This protective effect with an optimal distribution of implants and a correct occlusal scheme may inhibit the critical micromotion at the bone-to-implant interface. Moreover, it is not referred what is the type of attachment or their importance on the predictability of immediate loading with respect to mandibular removable splinted reconstructions (Schwarz et al. 2016). With respect to overdentures, the systematic review and meta-analysis by Helmi et al. revealed similar results regarding marginal bone loss and implant survival rates, however there is no information about the influence of the localization of the implants (Helmi et al. 2018).

The incidence of high masticatory forces in posterior areas discourages many clinicians performing immediate loading in these areas. Although it is known that primary stability is the key factor for performing immediate loading, clinicians are concerned about the predictability of immediate loading on posterior areas. Moreover, the meta-analysis by Moraschini et al. published in 2016 revealed that there are no significant differences between immediate and conventional loading regarding survival of implants as well as marginal bone loss in single implant rehabilitation in the posterior mandible (Moraschini et al. 2016). Once, posterior areas do not demand such esthetic concerns, normally clinicians prefer to wait and do a more conservative approach, with conventional loading.

Another question about immediate loading is if this is a predictable procedure in the esthetic zone. Weigl et al. in 2016 published a paper that revealed excellent results for immediately placed and restored single implants in the anterior maxilla with an 98.25% survival rate after a mean follow-up period of 31.2 months (Weigl et al. 2016). It is also important to reline that the mean crestal bone and interproximal mucosa level changes were less than 1 mm compared to baseline levels, with no significant differences related to the thickness of the mucosa (Weigl et al. 2016). Del Fabro et al. corroborated the results of Weigl et al., once it was discovered an overall implant survival rate of immediately restored implants of 97.6%, even though knowing that the achievement of aesthetic success may depend on several factors such as proper three-dimensional implant positioning, maintenance of the crestal anatomy at the buccal side and the tissue bio-type (Del Fabro et al. 2015). In addition, Kinaia et al. in their 2017 systematic review and meta-analysis, revealed that there are no statistical differences between immediate and conventional loading related to mid-facial recession and papillae height loss (Kinaia et al. 2017). In opposition to Weigl et al., Kinaia et al. found that mid-facial recession was less in thick biotypes (Kinaia et al. 2017). This maintenance of soft tissues with immediate restorative protocols may be related to the decrease in tissue trauma from a second-stage surgical operation.

4 CONCLUSIONS

Regarding all these considerations, definitive conclusions concerning the predictability of immediate loading in every dental implant protocol could not be done. Even though, the consensus included in this paper assumed that there is a slight higher risk in implant failure by performing immediate loading comparing to conventional loading, it seems that the risk of implant failure could be substantially minimized by proper patient selection and when executed by an experienced clinician (Schwarz et al. 2016).

The absence of enough primary stability seems to be the key factor to avoid immediate loading, being advisable to wait for a conventional healing period (Schwarz et al. 2016). In addition to lower implant primary stability, the presence of other factors that can influence the early stability of implants can increase the risk of early failures (Chrcanovic et al. 2014). So, conventional loading still seems to be the gold standard protocol, although immediate loading in specific condition could be used successfully (Del Fabro et al. 2015). For future research, it is advisable to further understand the bone biology in immediate loading, as well as define a standard primary stability quotient needed to perform immediate loading to be used in every paper. To strengthen the conclusions, more well-designed randomized, controlled clinical trials and long-term follow-up studies are needed.

REFERENCES

Al-Sawai, A.-A., & Labib, H. 2016. Success of immediate loading implants compared to conventionally-loaded implants: a literature review. *Journal of Investigative and Clinical Dentistry* 7(3): 217–24.

Atieh, M.A., Alsabeeha, N., Duncan, W.J. 2018. Stability of tapered and parallel-walled dental implants: A systematic review and meta-analysis. *Clinical Implant Dentistry and Related Research* 20(4): 634–45.

Chrcanovic, B.R., Albrektsson, T., & Wennerberg, A. 2014. Immediate nonfunctional versus immediate functional loading and dental implant failure rates: A systematic review and meta-analysis. *Journal of Dentistry* 42(9): 1052–9.

Chrcanovic, B.R., Albrektsson, T., Wennerberg, A. 2015. Immediately loaded non-submerged versus delayed loaded submerged dental implants: A meta-analysis. *International Journal of Oral Maxillofacial Surgery* 44(4): 493–506.

Del Fabro, M., Ceresoli, V., Taschieri, S., Ceci, C., Testori, T. 2015. Immediate Loading of Postextraction Implants in the Esthetic Area: Systematic Review of the literature. *Clinical Implant Dentistry and Related Research* 17(1): 52–70.

Engelhardt, S., Papacosta, P., Rathe, F., Özen, J., Jansen, J.A., Junker, R. 2015. Annual failure rates and marginal bone-level changes of immediate compared to conventional loading of dental implants. A systematic review of the literature and meta-analysis. *Clinical Oral Implants Research* 26(6): 671–87.

Esposito, M., Grusovin, M.G., Maghaireh, H., Worthington H.V. 2013. Interventions for replacing missing teeth: different times for loading dental implants. *Cochrane Database of Systematic Reviews* (3): CD003878.

Helmy, M.H.E.-D., Alqutaibi, Y., El-Ella, A., Shawky, F. 2018. Effect of implant loading protocols on failure and marginal bone loss with unsplinted two-implant-supported mandibular overdentures: systematic review and meta-analysis. *International Journal of Oral Maxillofacial Surgery* 47(5): 642–50.

Kinaia, B.M., Ambrosio, F., Lamble, M., Hope, K., Shah, M., Neely, A.L. 2017. Soft Tissue Changes Around Immediately Placed Implants: A Systematic Review and Meta-Analyses With at Least 12 Months of Follow-Up After Functional Loading. *Journal of Periodontology* 88(9): 876–86.

Koirala, D.P., Singh, S.V., Chand, P., Siddharth, R., Jurel, S.K., Aggarwal, H., Tripathi S., Ranabhatt R.,Mehrotra, D. 2016. Early loading of delayed versus immediately placed implants in the anterior mandible: A pilot comparative clinical study. *The Journal of Prosthetic Dentistry* 116(3): 340–45.

Menini, M., Signori, A., Tealdo, T., Bevilacqua, M., Pera, F., Ravera, G., Pera, P. 2012. Tilted Implants in the immediate loading rehabilitation of the maxilla: A systematic review. *Journal of Dental Research* 91(9): 821–7.

Moraschini, V. & Porto Barboza, E. 2016. Immediate versus conventional loaded single implants in the posterior mandible: a meta-analysis of randomized controlled trials. *International Journal of Oral and Maxillofacial Surgery* 45(1): 85–92.

Pigozzo, M.N., da Costa T.R., Sesma, N., Laganá, D.C. 2018. Immediate versus early loading of single dental implants: A systematic review and meta-analysis. *The Journal of Prosthetic Dentistry* 120(1): 25–34.

Schwarz, F., Sanz-Martín, I., Kern, J-S., Taylor, T., Schaer, A., Wolfart, S., Sanz, M. 2016. Loading protocols and implant supported restorations proposed for the rehabilitation of partially and fully edentulous jaws. Camlog Foundation Consensus Report. *Clinical Oral Implants Research* 27(8): 988–92.

Weigl, P., Strangio, A. 2016. The impact of immediately placed and restored single-tooth implants on hard and soft tissues in the anterior maxilla. *European Journal of Oral Implantology* 9(Suppl1): S89–S106.

Zhang, S., Wang, S., Song, Y. 2017. Immediate loading for implant restoration compared with early or conventional loading: A meta-analysis. *Journal of Cranio-Maxillo-Facial Surgery* 45: 793–803.

Immediate loading of dental implants – planning and provisional restauration: A case report

João S. Marques & Diogo Soares
Faculty of Dental Medicine, University of Porto (FMDUP), Porto, Portugal

J.M. Rocha, P.J. Almeida, J.C. Sampaio-Fernandes & M.H. Figueiral
FMDUP, Porto, Portugal

ABSTRACT: Tooth loss in the esthetic area is a traumatic experience for the patient, however, the advances in dental implantology provide excellent solutions for restoring almost all functions of missing teeth. The treatment of partially edentulous patient can be challenging, including careful planning of dental implants, placement, and restoration. The present article reports a clinical case using the provisional restoration as the guide for the surgery, while 2 implants with immediate loading were installed immediately after the extraction of 4 teeth in the mandible. Despite all the progress achieved so far, the success of oral rehabilitation still depends on a careful case selection, appropriate treatment planning, precise surgical and prosthetic protocols and an adequate follow-up, as described in the present case.

1 INTRODUCTION

Tooth loss in the esthetic area is often a traumatic experience for the patient (Singh, Kumar, Anwar, & Chand, 2015). In the majority of cases, dental implant rehabilitation offers an optimal solution for tooth replacement with high survival rates, along with providing well-being and comfort to patients (Craddock, 2009). Patient's growing demand for less invasive and faster procedures as well as highly aesthetic requirements have turned the immediate loading as preferable option for the patients (Moraschini & Porto Barboza, 2016). The advantages of this procedure include fewer surgical interventions, reduction in overall treatment time, reduced soft and hard tissue loss and psychological satisfaction of patient (Singh et al., 2015).

This paper reports a case of an immediate loading of dental implant rehabilitation of the mandibular anterior region. The procedure included tooth extraction followed by immediate implant placement and fixed provisional prosthesis. Furthermore, the literature search was carried out using PubMed database, restricted to papers in English language, with no limit on publication date. The keywords used were: "dental implant immediate load" and "immediate implant placement".

2 CASE DESCRIPTION

A Caucasian 51-years-old female patient attended the Oral Rehabilitation Specialization at FMDUP Dental Clinic to resolve the tooth sensitivity and mobility in the mandible. Clinical examination revealed absence of almost all posterior teeth, gingival recession in the remaining teeth and rigid splinting between the 33 and 43 dental pieces (Figure 1).

In addition, patient had a medical history of tobacco consumption (heavy smoker). Radiographic examination corroborated the diagnosis of advanced periodontal disease, with a prognosis of tooth loss (as can be seen in Figures 2 and 3).

Treatment planning included the extraction of teeth 31, 32, 41, 42, immediate implant loading in 32 and 42 positions, followed by fixed provisional prosthesis performed with CAD-CAM guidance. This provisional prosthesis was also used as a "surgical guide", indicating the ideal implant position. As a complement, two distal fins were made to stabilize the prosthetic device during the surgery and to be able to use as Maryland if needed (Figure 4).

After atraumatic tooth extraction, sockets were thoroughly debrided and inspected with a periodontal probe.

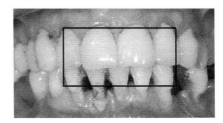

Figure 1. Initial aspect (detail of the square showing the bone loss in the area to be treated).

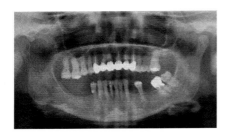

Figure 2. Initial orthopantomography (detail of the square showing the bone loss in the area to be treated).

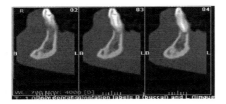

Figure 3. Sagital aspect of the computed tomography scan corresponding to the tooth 41.

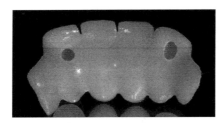

Figure 4. Temporary prosthesis CAD-CAM assisted Acrylate polymer material VITA CAD-Temp® (VITA Zahnfabrik, Germany).

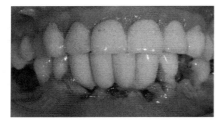

Figure 5. Final aspect and detail of the restoration in inocclusion after surgery.

Two implants Vega®NV Ø3,5 mm × 10 mm (Klockner® Implant System SA, Barcelona, Spain) were placed with 42 NCm torque insertion and adequate primary stability was confirmed by resonance frequency analysis (RFA) with the PenguinRFA® (Integration Diagnostics Sweden AB®, Sweden). The latter recorded an implant stability quotient (ISQ) of 78 for both implants, enough to perform immediate load, as will be further discussed.

3 DISCUSSION

In order to overcome the limitations related to the conventional implant placement, new strategies have significantly reduced the time of treatment, being now more predictable and successful than ever before (Del Fabbro, Testori, Francetti, Taschieri, & Weinstein, 2006; Singh et al., 2015). One of the strategies includes the immediate implant placement after the tooth extraction and provisional fixed prosthesis (as described in the present case report).

Anatomical limitations can make difficult to determine the implant location (Marchack, 2007), especially after tooth extraction. In order to overcome these limitations, surgery assisted by a guide and guided surgery may be considered.

The surgery assisted by a guide, involves a diagnostic tooth arrangement through one of the following ways: a diagnostic waxing, a trial denture teeth arrangement, or the duplication of a preexisting dentition/restoration (Garber, 1996). Guides can be classified as nonlimiting design, partially limiting design and completely limiting design (Stumpel, 2008). Nonlimiting designs only provide an indication to the surgeon where the proposed prosthesis is in relation to the selected implant site. This design indicates the ideal location of the implants without any emphasis on the angulation of the drill, thus allowing too much flexibility in the final positioning of the implant. In the partially limiting design, the first drill used for the osteotomy is directed using the surgical guide, but the remaining osteotomy and the implant placement is finished as desire of the surgeon. Finally, the completely limiting design restricts all of the instruments used for the osteotomy in a buccolingual and mesiodistal plane. Moreover, the addition of drill stops, limits the depth of the preparation, and thus the positioning of the prosthetic table of the implant. As the surgical guides become more restrictive, less of the decision-making and subsequent surgical execution is done intraoperatively.

Guided surgery uses data from computerized tomography scan (CT) and Computer-Aided Design/Computer-Aided Manufacturing (CAD/CAM) technology to plan implant rehabilitation (Marchack, 2007). In a simple way, the CT images are converted into data that are recognized by a CT imaging and planning software. This software then transfers this presurgical plan to the surgery site using stereolithographic drill guides (Nikzad & Azari, 2008). This type of surgery requires a proper system of drills. Accuracy of CAD/CAM technology in dental implant planning and predictable transfer of the presurgical plan to the surgical site has been documented previously by several authors (Arısan, Karabuda, & Özdemir, 2010; Jabero & Sarment, 2006; Schneider, Marquardt, Zwahlen, & Jung, 2009; Valente, Schiroli, & Sbrenna, 2009). However, complications including intrinsic errors during scanning, software planning, the rapid prototyping of the guide stent, and the transfer of information for the prosthetics have been related as well (Block & Chandler, 2009).

In the present clinical case, the combination of the CT scans along with the scanning of the patient study models were used, allowing the preparation of the temporary restoration prior to surgery. In the same surgical time, the position of the implants was captured using temporary abutments and self-curing acrylic in the mouth, while the acrylization was finished in the laboratory.

Regarding the placement of implants, the literature describes three types of dental implant loading protocols including conventional loading (with a 3 to 6 months healing period between implant placement and restoration); early loading (where healing period is less than 3 months); and immediate loading (prosthesis is placed as soon as the implant is inserted) (Koirala et al., 2016). In the present case we considered the last option due to functional, aesthetic and phonetic imperatives.

Two types of immediate loadings have been described in the literature, including the immediate functional loading (IFL) referring to the placement of a prosthesis in occlusal contact with the opposing arch within the first 72 h after surgery, and the alternative approach – immediate nonfunctional loading (INFL) that consists of modifying the restoration by avoiding occlusal contacts in centric and lateral excursions, in order to reduce the early risks of mechanical overload caused by functional or parafunctional forces (Al-Sawai & Labib, 2016). In this way, the modified restoration is still being involved in the masticatory process while mechanical loading stress is reduced (Chrcanovic, Albrektsson, & Wennerberg, 2014). This was also applied to this particular case (Figure 5).

The main criterion for performing the immediate loading of single implants is a primary stability. Primary stability can be measured by several parameters such as insertion torque – measured in Newton-centimeters (N/cm) and implant stability quotient (ISQ) – measured by Resonance Frequency Analysis (RFA). Previous studies have shown that primary stability is a critical factor for the immediate loading, and low initial stability is a significant risk factor of early failure of single implants with immediate loading (Moraschini & Porto Barboza, 2016). In this particular case, both the torque and ISQ indicated safe immediate implant loading.

4 CONCLUSIONS

Despite all the progress achieved so far, the success of oral rehabilitation still depends on a careful case selection, appropriate treatment planning, precise surgical and prosthetic protocols and adequate follow-up.

REFERENCES

Al-Sawai, A.-A. & Labib, H. 2016. Success of immediate loading implants compared to conventionally-loaded implants: a literature review. *Journal of Investigative and Clinical Dentistry* 7(3): 217–224.

Arısan, V., Karabuda, Z.C. & Özdemir, T. 2010. Accuracy of Two Stereolithographic Guide Systems for Computer-Aided Implant Placement: A Computed Tomography-Based Clinical Comparative Study. *Journal of Periodontology* 81(1): 43–51.

Block, M.S. & Chandler, C. 2009. Computed Tomography–Guided Surgery: Complications Associated With Scanning, Processing, Surgery, and Prosthetics. *Journal of Oral and Maxillofacial Surgery* 67(11): 13–22.

Chrcanovic, B.R., Albrektsson, T. & Wennerberg, A. 2014. Immediate nonfunctional versus immediate functional loading and dental implant failure rates: A systematic review and meta-analysis. *Journal of Dentistry* 42(9): 1052–1059.

Craddock, H.L. 2009. Consequences of Tooth Loss: 1. The Patient Perspective – Aesthetic and Functional Implications. *Dent Update* 36: 616–619.

Del Fabbro, M., Testori, T., Francetti, L., Taschieri, S. & Weinstein, R. 2006). Systematic review of survival rates for immediately loaded dental implants. *The International Journal of Periodontics & Restorative Dentistry* 26(3): 249–263.

Garber, D.A. 1996. The esthetic dental implant: letting restoration be the guide. *The Journal of Oral Implantology* 22(1), 45–50.

Jabero, M. & Sarment, D.P. 2006. Advanced surgical guidance technology: A review. *Implant Dentistry* 15(2): 135–42.

Koirala, D.P., Singh, S.V., Chand, P., Siddharth, R., Jurel, S.K., Aggarwal, H., *et al.* 2016. Early loading of delayed versus immediately placed implants in the anterior mandible: A pilot comparative clinical study. *The Journal of Prosthetic Dentistry* 116(3): 340–345.

Marchack, C.B. 2007. CAD/CAM-guided implant surgery and fabrication of an immediately loaded prosthesis for a partially edentulous patient. *The Journal of Prosthetic Dentistry* 97(6): 389–394.

Moraschini, V. & Porto Barboza, E. 2016. Immediate versus conventional loaded single implants in the posterior mandible: a meta-analysis of randomized controlled trials. *International Journal of Oral and Maxillofacial Surgery* 45(1): 85–92.

Nikzad, S. & Azari, A. 2008. A Novel Stereolithographic Surgical Guide Template for Planning Treatment Involving a Mandibular Dental Implant. *Journal of Oral and Maxillofacial Surgery* 66(7): 1446–1454.

Schneider, D., Marquardt, P., Zwahlen, M. & Jung, R.E. 2009. A systematic review on the accuracy and the clinical outcome of computer-guided template-based implant dentistry. *Clinical Oral Implants Research* 20(Suppl 4): 73–86.

Singh, M., Kumar, L., Anwar, M. & Chand, P. 2015. Immediate dental implant placement with immediate loading following extraction of natural teeth. *National Journal of Maxillofacial Surgery* 6(2): 252–255.

Stumpel, L.J. 2008. Cast-based guided implant placement: A novel technique. *Journal of Prosthetic Dentistry* 100(1): 61–69.

Valente, F., Schiroli, G. & Sbrenna, A. 2009. Accuracy of computer-aided oral implant surgery: a clinical and radiographic study. *The International Journal of Oral & Maxillofacial Implants* 24(2): 234–242.

Biodental Engineering V – Belinha et al. (Eds)
© 2019 Taylor & Francis Group, London, ISBN 978-0-367-21087-8

Local anesthetic administration—a rare necrotic ulcer on the palate: A case report

João S. Marques & Diogo Soares
Faculty of Dental Medicine, University of Porto (FMDUP), Porto, Portugal

J.M. Rocha, P. Ferrás, J.C. Reis Campos & M.H. Figueiral
FMDUP, Porto, Portugal

ABSTRACT: Local anesthesia is routinely used during dental procedures. Like any invasive procedure, local anesthesia can also lead to complications, which are fortunately rare. The present article reports a clinical case of necrosis of the palatal mucosa developed after the anesthetic infiltration. Furthermore, other complications of local anesthesia are discussed. The clinical prognosis in this type of case is influenced by the ability to make a differential diagnosis excluding the necrotizing sialometaplasia, aphthous ulcer and herpes ulcer as well as by the use of a suitable treatment protocol. Even though the anesthetic necrotic ulcers normally heal spontaneously, the patient's discomfort and possible complications could be avoided in some cases by the use of mepivacaine (reduced vasodilation effect). Particularly, the use of mepivacaine should be considered in patients with the history of necrotic ulcers or when palatal administration of anesthesia is required.

1 INTRODUCTION

The regular dental practice involves variety of dental procedures with the need for the application of local anesthetics (Khalil, 2014). Local anesthetics are the most commonly used drugs with great efficacy and safety to control pain (Pattni, 2013). Their mode of action is mediated by the selective blockage of pain transmission through the nerves (Ayoub & Coleman 1992). Every anesthesia comprises the vasoconstrictor property in order to maintain the effect as well as reduce bleeding (Haas, 2002). Local infiltration or nerve blockage are the most common forms of application (Baart & Brand, 2009).

Palatal infiltration, a common method of anesthesia, is deposition of solution close to the apex of the involved tooth. This infiltration method is usually free of complications, but sporadic problems have been documented, including local and systemic complications. Systemic complications are usual-ly multifactorial in origin and related to toxic drug overdose, rapid absorption, intravascular injection, cardiovascular, central nervous system, psychogenic or idiosyncratic reactions (Meechan, 2009; Sambrook et al. 2011). Local complications includes: needle breakage, prolonged pain, paresthesia and nerve damage (Smith & Lung, 2006), ocular troubles (Ravi et al. 2015) bruise, infection, edema, tissue necrosis and post

anesthetic intraoral ulcer lesions. The latter occurs commonly in the palatal region, as the mucosa is in close proximity to the underlying bone, leading to pressurized deposition of the local anesthetic solution and traumatic needle penetration (Ghanem & Suliman, 1983).

Additionally, a less common postoperative complication, referred to as anesthetic necrotic ulcer, may appear. This painful lesion usually develops several days after the procedure, therefore generating an uncomfortable situation for both the clinician and patient.

2 CASE DESCRIPTION

A 56-year-old female Caucasian patient came to our Dental Faculty Clinic, complaining of a 4 days painful lesion on the left palatal region. The patient had performed a dentistry procedure be-tween tooth 26 and 27 (first left molar and second left molar, respectively) one week before, under local anesthesia (LA) with articaine 4% and epinephrine 1:100000. The injection was performed using a 30 G, 12 mm needle.

During the clinical examination, a well-defined ulcer was evident on the hard palate in relation to the tooth 26. The lesion had an approximate size of 10 mm, circular shape, well-defined punched out margins and 2 mm of depth (Figure 1).

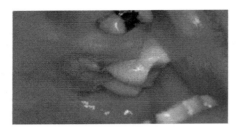

Figure 1. Ulcerated initial palatal lesion.

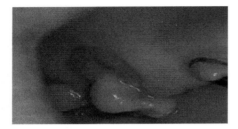

Figure 2. Appearance on 14th day control.

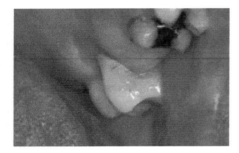

Figure 3. Appearance on 30th day control.

The central lesion area was covered by pseudomembranous slough that revealed a bleeding surface underneath (on palpation).

The medical history revealed absence of hyperthermia, no evident suppuration, increased metallic taste and local pain, exacerbated by the use of maxillary partial removable prosthesis of cobalt-chromium. The patient was medicated with systemic ibuprofen 600 mg (every 12 h, during 5 days), topical chlorhexidine antiseptic gel (3 times a day) and instructed to hygienize the affected area with a soft brush as well as to discontinue denture wearing for one week.

After 2 weeks, the patient reported an improvement of the clinical condition, along with the pain relief (Figure 2). The clinical examination showed partially healed ulcer.

After additional 4 weeks, the ulcerated lesion was completely healed with epithelialization of the mucosal surface (Figure 3).

3 DISCUSSION

Allergic reaction in some patients may be triggered by any drug, but the prediction of such response before the administration is challenging. Local anesthetics are some of the rarest drug allergens (Tomoyasu et al. 2011), thus we did not consider an articaine sensitivity test as it had been previously used in patient without the hypersensitivity reaction.

Ischemia resulting from the rapid pressurized administration of local anesthetic solution containing a vasoconstrictor may manifest as tissue necrosis, although its exact cause is unknown and may vary from case to case (Gracelin Ranjitha et al. 2015).

Regarding the differential diagnosis of post-anesthetic palatal ulcer, necrotizing sialometaplasia (NS), aphthous ulcer, and herpes ulcer need to be discarded (Garcia et al. 2012).

NS is a self-limiting, benign, inflammatory disease of the minor salivary glands. The majority of reported cases of NS affect the hard palate, while the other locations are along the upper respiratory tract, including major salivary glands, oral mucosa, and tonsils (Garcia et al. 2012). The lesion (1–3 cm) is normally painful with rapidly progressive swelling that becomes centrally ulcerated, frequently associated with erythema at the periphery of the lesion. The clinical presentation resembles a malignant salivary gland tumor of the palate, like mucoepidermoid carcinoma or adenoid cystic carcinoma, the history and rapid progression of NS helps in their diagnosis (Krishna & Bk 2011).

Herpes simplex, although most commonly observed extra orally, can also develop intraorally on tissues attached to the underlying bone; e.g. hard palate (Pattni 2013). In the present case, the ulcer was single, painless, persistent, and deep, not resembling the features of herpes ulcer.

In order to minimize the incidence of palatal lesions following lidocaine or articaine administration, certain precautions need to be taken including:

a. Deposition of the anesthetic solution should be applied with low pressure (Gracelin Ranjitha et al. 2015).
b. The anesthetic solutions containing relatively high concentrations of epinephrine (i.e., 1:50.000) should be used with caution (Haas 2002).
c. Anesthetic solutions without the vasoconstrictor such as 3% mepivacaine may be considered. (mepivacaine has less vasodilating activity than lidocaine that can be used reliably for procedures with short duration).

4 CONCLUSIONS

Anesthetic necrosis is generally self-limiting with no treatment required unless the ulceration fails to heal and the painful condition remains. In patients with the history of anesthetic necrotic ulcer or as a strategy for its prevention in palatal region, mepivacaine may be considered as an alternative local anesthetic (reduced vasodilation effect), depending on required duration of anesthesia and the location of injection.

REFERENCES

Ayoub, S.T. & Coleman, A.E. 1992. A review of local anesthetics. *General Dentistry* 40(4): 285–290.

Baart, J.A., Jacobus, A. & Brand, H.S. 2009. Local anaesthesia in dentistry. Wiley-Blackwell.

Garcia, N.G., Oliveira, D.T., Faustino, S.E.S. & Azevedo, A.L.R. 2012. Necrotizing Sialometaplasia of Palate: A Case Report. *Case Reports in Pathology* 2012: 679325.

Ghanem, H. & Suliman, A.M. 1983. Palatal ulceration: a complication of regional anesthesia of the oral cavity—a case report. *Anesthesia Progress* 30(4): 118–119.

Gracelin Ranjitha, E., Ramasamy, S. 2011. Austin, R.D., & Ramya, K. 2015. Necrotic Ulcer on the Palate: As Sequelae of Local Anesthetic Administration: A Rare Case Report. *International Journal of Advanced Health Sciences* 41(1): 35–38.

Haas, D.A. 2002. An Update on Local Anesthetics in Dentistry. *Journal Canadian Dental Association* 68(9): 546–551.

Khalil, H. 2014. Local anesthetics dosage still a problem for most dentists: A survey of current knowledge and awareness. *The Saudi Journal for Dental Research* 5(1): 49–53.

Krishna, S. & Romnarayan, Bk. 2011. Necrotizing sialometaplasia of palate: a case report. *Imaging Science in Dentistry* 41(1): 35–38.

Meechan, J.G. 2009. Local Anaesthesia: Risks and Controversies. *Dental Update* 36(5): 278–283.

Pattni, N. 2013. Superficial skin necrosis and neurological complications following administration of local anaesthetic: A case report. *Australian Dental Journal* 58(4): 522–525.

Ravi, P., Gopi, G., Shanmugasundaram, Raja, K.K. 2015. Ocular complications with dental local anaesthesia—a systematic review of literature and case report: clinical review. *South African Dental Journal* 70(8): 354–357.

Sambrook, P., Smith, W., Elijah, J. & Goss, A. 2011. Severe adverse reactions to dental local anaesthetics: systemic reactions. *Australian Dental Journal* 56(2): 148–153.

Smith, M.H. & Lung, K.E. 2006. Nerve injuries after dental injection: a review of the literature. *Journal Canadian Dental Association* 72(6): 559–564.

Tomoyasu, Y., Mukae, K., Suda, M., Hayashi, T., Ishii, M., Sakaguchi, M., *et al.* 2011. Allergic reactions to local anesthetics in dental patients: analysis of intracutaneous and challenge tests. *The Open Dentistry Journal* 5: 146–149.

Biodental Engineering V – Belinha et al. (Eds)
© 2019 Taylor & Francis Group, London, ISBN 978-0-367-21087-8

Retention of metal clips in overdentures

M.J. Roxo
Faculty of Dental Medicine, University of Porto (FMDUP), Porto, Portugal

M. Sampaio-Fernandes, P. Vaz, F. Góis, J.C. Reis Campos & M.H. Figueiral
FMDUP, Porto, Portugal

ABSTRACT: The success of implant supported overdentures depends on the retention capacity of their retainers to maintain their long term function. The aim of this study is to evaluate the retentive force of metal clips and to compare the strength of the fixed clips with two types of resins. A metal clip (MP-Clip®, Ackermann Bar®) was fixed in fourteen PMMA blocks with MegaCryl N and Quick-Up®. Another block presents a metal bar screwed to two parallel implants. Using a testing universal machine, a fatigue test up to 1080 cycles and a pull test were performed. The mean retentive force registered for the clip retained with MegaCryl-N is 33.85 N, which is lower than the one registered with Quick Up® (49.33 N). In the traction test, a mean force of 240.72 N is necessary to pull the metal clip from the MegaCryl N resin, while in the Quick-Up® resin it is 154.02 N. No fracture of the attachments occurred, but there was fracture of the Quick-Up® samples. It can be concluded that a metal clip fixed with Quick-Up® has more retentive force than a clip fixed with MegaCryl N. Most likely due to the composition differences between the two materials, the force required for pulling a clip is much lower with Quick-Up®.

1 INTRODUCTION

Conventional acrylic total dentures have been the traditional standard of care for edentulous patients for more than a century (Karabuda et al. 2008, Feine et al. 2002), although they are not fully competent in restoring masticatory function or in a satisfactory improvement of the quality of life of most patients (Fromentin et al. 2010, Carvalho et al. 2014, Savabi et al. 2013). These considerations are even more significant in the edentulous mandible, where bone resorption and muscle dynamics work with greater intensity (Fromentin et al. 2010).

The main problems in the treatment of total edentulous patients are residual ridge resorption subsequent to tooth loss (Andreiotelli et al. 2010), altered salivary flow and muscle tone reduction, that will lead to a decrease in the retention and stability of dentures, changing their biomechanical behavior (Carvalho et al. 2014, Savabi et al. 2013).

Because of the good prognosis of dental implants, these patients can be successfully treated with implant-supported overdentures (Andreiotelli et al. 2010). Success of this kind of dentures depends on two important factors: retention and stress distribution to its support elements (Shastry et al. 2016), being the retentive capacity of its attachment elements a determining factor to patient satisfaction (Carvalho et al. 2014, Savabi et al. 2013, Shastry et al. 2016).

Taking this in consideration, in 2002, the McGill Consensus established 2-implant overdenture as the first choice of treatment for the edentulous mandible (Feine et al. 2002), providing reliable and predictable treatment outcomes (Shastry et al. 2016, Kobayashi et al. 2014).

Implant-supported overdentures rely on the use of different retention systems, which can be categorized according to whether they will splint the implants or keep them independent (Kobayashi et al. 2014). The splinted attachment systems are generically denominated as bar and it can present diverse configurations, while the unsplinted systems comprise spherical/ball types, magnets, Locator® and telescopic crowns (Kobayashi et al. 2014).

Bar attachments have shown superior retention and stability when compared to unsplinted systems (Andreiotelli et al. 2010, Shastry et al. 2016, Kobayashi et al. 2014, Naert et al. 1999) allowing the union of the implants and correcting their inclinations and angulations (Sadig et al. 2003). Additionally they have the ability to mask excessive residual alveolar ridge atrophy (Sadig et al. 2003) and have fewer prosthetic complications (Naert et al. 1999).

They also present some disadvantages such as: higher initial cost, difficulty in repairing and a more complicated maintenance of oral hygiene, especially in case of patients with less manual dexterity (Shastry et al. 2016, Naert et al. 1999).

In addition, the screws that attach the bar to the implants will need to be retightened over time and, in the case of metal clips, they will need to be reactivated or even replaced so that the overdenture remains retentive (Kobayashi et al. 2014).

Therefore, the aim of this study is to assess the retentive force and fracture resistance of metal clips during insertion and deinsertion cycles and to compare the strength of fixed clips with two types of self-curing resins.

2 MATERIAL AND METHODS

This experimental work was carried out in collaboration with the Laboratory of Optics and Experimental Mechanics (LOME), which is a unit of the Institute of Science and Innovation in Mechanical and Industrial Engineering (INEGI), and the Faculty of Engineering of the University of Porto (FEUP).

For this study the attachment chosen was a metal clip: MP-Clip® from Ackermann-Bar® (Cendres + Métaux SA, Biel Switzerland). The two fixation materials tested were a self-curing composite resin used in-office—Quick-Up® (VOCO GmbH, Germany), and a self-curing acrylic resin used in laboratory—MegaCryl N 00 clear (megadental GmbH, Germany).

A block of polymethylmethacrylate (PMMA) was designed and manufactured in a CAD/CAM system, where two parallel Straumann SLA active® implants were placed. Subsequently, a metal bar (chromium-cobalt alloy) with circular section was cast, and then screwed into the implants (Figure 1).

To evaluate the metal clips 14 blocks were designed and milled with the same type of acrylic (PMMA). A cavity measuring 6.5 mm × 4.6 mm × 3 mm was designed for the placement of the materials used to fix the attachments (MegaCryl N and Quick-Up®). Inside the cavity a stop with the same height of the cavity was designed, always determining the same positioning of the attachment. The two materials were handled according to the manufacturer's instructions and placed in the PMMA blocks by the same operator, and one clip was fixed in each block (Figure 2).

Testing was carried out with a universal testing machine Instron Eletropuls E1000 (Figure 3).

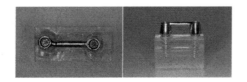

Figure 1. PMMA block with cast metal bar screwed to the implants.

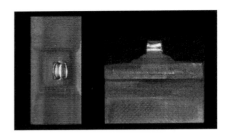

Figure 2. PMMA block milled in CAD/CAM after metal clip was fixed.

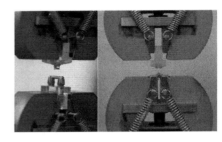

Figure 3. Universal testing machine with PMMA blocks during fatigue test and traction test.

Dislodging tensile forces were applied in a vertical direction at a speed of 50,8 mm/min.

A fatigue test was performed in two samples, one with the metal clip fixed with MegaCryl N and the other fixed with Quick-Up®. Considering that a complete cycle corresponds to the deinsertion and the respective insertion of the clip into the bar, the number of cycles per time periods was calculated considering that the patient removes the overdenture on average three times a day. The retentive force was evaluated from 0 cycles (initial force) to 1080 cycles (1 year).

Six samples of each material were used for the traction test. The PMMA block with the clip was placed and fixed manually at the top grip of the testing machine. In the active part of each clip was placed a portion of the cast bar that was cut after the fatigue tests were performed, so that no deformation or fracture of the active part of the attachment occurred during its removal from the acrylic block. The lower grip was secured to the active part of the clip. The grips were fixed and aligned manually to ensure equal distribution of forces by the attachment and its deinsertion on a vertical axis. The maximum force required for removing each clip from the PMMA blocks was recorded.

As a deterministic study, only descriptive statistical analysis was performed for both tests. Thus, maximum, minimum, mean and standard deviation values of each group of the samples were calculated.

3 RESULTS

3.1 *Fatigue test*

A total of 1080 cycles of deinsertion/insertion, corresponding to one year of use, were performed on two blocks, each with a different type of fixing material.

During the test, there was an initial increase of the retentive force in the two samples, remaining practically constant until the end of the test, when the force began to decrease.

Table 1 shows the maximum and minimum forces recorded on the deinsertion of the attachment during the 1080 cycles for the two materials. Table 2 shows the maximum and minimum forces on the insertion of the clip in the bar.

The values found are always lower in the MegaCryl samples, both on the deinsertion and the insertion of the clip. The mean values for both materials are always higher during deinsertion.

3.2 *Traction test*

In Table 3 the values of maximum force required for the removal of the metal clip of the acrylic

Table 1. Maximum, minimum and mean forces (N) on deinsertion of metal clips during fatigue test.

	Maximum force (N)	Minimum force (N)	Mean (N)
MegaCryl N	34.91	31.80	33.85
Quick-Up®	53.25	45.40	49.33

Table 2. Maximum, minimum and mean forces (N) on insertion of metal clips during fatigue test.

	Maximum force (N)	Minimum force (N)	Mean (N)
MegaCryl N	30.50	28.60	29.55
Quick-Up®	51.50	43.00	47.25

Table 3. Maximum, minimum and mean forces (N) for the removal of the metal clip of the acrylic block.

	MegaCryl N	Quick-Up®
Sample 1	164.60	73.06
Sample 2	244.18	124.38
Sample 3	240.72	149.79
Sample 4	252.63	165.23
Sample 5	207.58	154.02
Sample 6	239.61	189.20
Mean	240.72	154.02
Standard deviation	± 17.19	± 23.60

block were recorded. The values of samples 1 of MegaCryl N and Quick-Up® were considered outliers. Thus, the mean and standard deviation were calculated without the two atypical values.

In the traction test, a mean force of 240.72 N is necessary to pull the metal clip from the MegaCryl N resin, while in the Quick-Up® resin the mean force registered is 154.02 N. In the five samples considered, a higher force was required for pulling the clip fixed with MegaCryl, compared to Quick-Up®. In all the samples of MegaCryl, the resin tested was always kept in the PMMA block. Only the attachment was removed with no fracture of any parts of it.

In sample 2 of Quick-Up®, part of the resin tested was removed with the clip and the other part was kept in the PMMA block. In the other samples occurred total separation of Quick-Up® from the PMMA block during the pull of the clip.

4 DISCUSSION

Since there are no previous studies evaluating the retention of metal clips fixed with different materials, this work intends to be a preliminary study, testing the viability of the experiment performed so that subsequent research can be designed with greater understanding and precision using a larger and more meaningful sample.

There is no consensus in the literature regarding the matching of a number of cycles in vitro to a time of in vivo use (Carvalho et al. 2014, Kobayashi et al. 2014, Besimo et al. 2003). In this study, 1080 cycles were performed to simulate the in vivo function corresponding to 1 year, considering that on average a patient removes the overdenture three times a day, and considering that the manufacturer of the tested clips recommends its exchange at the end of 1 year, as a preventive measure.

In this work, only one clip was tested, guaranteeing its insertion and deinsertion on a vertical axis (unidirectional forces), thus reducing possible variables that may induce some confusion in the interpretation of the results.

It was verified that the maximum and minimum forces, both for insertion and for deinsertion, were always lower for MegaCryl N. The most relevant values are related to the force of deinsertion because it is related to the retentive force of the clip.

The results of the present study show an increase in retentive force in the initial cycles of the fatigue test in both MegaCryl N and Quick-Up®. A probable justification for this may be the lubrication of the retentive system components through their handling prior to testing. As the cycles were performed, the friction force increases and therefore raises the force required for insertion and deinsertion of the attachments on the bar. After this initial increase of force, it remains constant during the remaining cycles and practically until the end of the test, when it begins to decrease. For both materials, more cycles would be needed to better describe and infer the medium and long-term behavior of the clips.

In the traction test, a force of 240.72 N was required to remove the metal clip from MegaCryl N, while in Quick-Up® the average force recorded was 154.02 N.

No fracture of any part of the attachments occurred, but there was fracture of the Quick-Up® samples. The complete separation of the Quick-Up® from the PMMA blocks in samples 3, 4, 5 and 6 may be related to the fact that the composition of this material is very similar to a composite resin. Its main component is UDMA (urethane-dimethacrylate), an organic element that constitutes the chemically active part of the composite resins, being the main one responsible for giving resistance to the material.

Because it has a composition less similar to the PMMA blocks where it was placed, unlike MegaCryl, which is an acrylic polymer based on methylmethacrylate, its bonding may not be ideal, leading to the detachment of the Quick-Up® from the block. The mean retentive strength values obtained in the fatigue test for the two materials (33.85 N for MegaCryl N, 49.33 N for Quick-Up®) may also be related to their chemical composition, since the attachment used was always the same type. Quick-Up® may have a larger modulus of elasticity than MegaCryl N and consequently a higher stiffness, requiring greater force for the active part of the clip to exit the bar. It may also be for this reason that in the traction test the clip has been removed with Quick-Up®. However, the materials used should be tested to confirm this reading of the results.

5 CONCLUSIONS

Within the limits of this study, it can be concluded that a metal clip fixed with Quick-Up® has more retentive force than a clip fixed with MegaCryl N, and this force is, in both cases, constant over approximately one year. Most likely due to the differences between the two materials concerning their characteristics, the force required for pulling a clip is much lower with Quick-Up®.

In order to be representative for the dentist's practice, further research is needed, including other possible variables, to better understand the evaluation of retentive force of metal clips when fixed with different types of resins.

REFERENCES

Andreiotelli, M., Att, W., Strubb, J.R. 2010. Prosthodontic complications with implants overdentures: a systematic literature review. *The International Journal of Prosthodontics* 23(3): 195–203.

Besimo, C.E., Guarneri, A. 2003. In vitro retention force changes of prefabricated attachments for overdentures. *Journal of Oral Rehabilitation* 30(7): 671–8.

Carvalho, E.R., Figueiral, M.H., Fonseca, P., Vaz, M.A., Branco, F.M. 2014. In vitro study of the insertion and disinsertion effect on retention of two attachment systems of an overdenture on two implants. *Revista Odonto Ciência* 29(1): 1–5.

Feine, J.S., Carlsson, G.E., Awad, M.A., *et al.* 2002. The McGill consensus statement on overdentures. *The International Journal of Prosthodontics* 15(4): 413–4.

Fromentin, O., Lassauzay, C., Abi Nader, S., Feine, J., de Albuquerque Junior, R.F. 2010. Testing the retention of attachments for implant overdentures—validation of an original force measurement system. *Journal of Oral Rehabilitation* 37(1): 54–62.

Karabuda, C., Yaltirik, M., Bayraktar, M. 2008. A clinical comparison of prosthetic complications of implant-supported overdentures with different attachment systems. *Implant Dentistry* 17(1): 74–7.

Kobayashi, M., Srinivasan, M., Ammann, P., Perriard, J., Ohkubo, C., Müller, F., Belser, U.C., Schimmel, M. 2014. Effects of in vitro cyclic dislodging on retentive force and removal torque of three overdenture attachment systems. *Clinical Oral Implants Research* 25(4): 426–34.

Naert, I., Gizani, S., Vuylsteke, M., van Steenberghe, D. 1999. A 5-year prospective randomized clinical trial on the influence of splinted and unsplinted oral implants retaining a mandibular overdenture: prosthetic aspects and patient satisfaction. *Journal of Oral Rehabilitation* 26(3): 195–202.

Sadig, W.M. 2003. Special technique for attachment incorporation with an implant overdenture. *The Journal of Prosthetic Dentistry* 89(1): 93–6.

Savabi, O., Nejatidanesh, F., Yordshahian, F. 2013. Retention of implant-supported overdenture with bar/clip and stud attachment designs. *Journal of Oral Implantology* 39(2): 140–7.

Shastry, T., Anupama, N.M., Shetty, S., Nalinakshamma, M. 2016. An in vitro comparative study to evaluate the retention of different attachment systems used in implant-retained overdentures. *The Journal of Indian Prosthodontic Society* 16(2): 159–66.

Implant-tooth fixed supported prosthesis: A review

R. Batista & A. Moreira
Faculty of Dental Medicine, University of Porto (FMDUP), Porto, Portugal

M. Sampaio-Fernandes, P. Vaz, J.C. Sampaio-Fernandes & M.H. Figueiral
FMDUP, Porto, Portugal

ABSTRACT: The mismatch distribution of forces between a mobile element and a rigid element may induce a mechanical deficiency, eventually leading to the failure of the weakest link. The purpose of this paper is to review recent findings in the field of implantology and prosthodontics regarding the implant-tooth support. A PubMed® and Scopus® search were performed. From 1479 articles were included 19 in the review. Precise guidelines must be followed, along with a thorough understanding of the corresponding risks and complications. Choosing tooth-implant support allows the maintenance of proprioception and bone volume, also eliminating free-end saddles and/or cantilevers. However, the controversy regarding the success rate remains, with some studies reporting similar outcomes to implant support, whereas increased annual failure rates of implant-tooth support have been suggested by others. The paucity of longitudinal studies found in the literature reflects the need for further research in this field of prosthodontics and should inspire future work.

1 INTRODUCTION

For decades, dental implants have been recommended to improve the retention of removable dental prostheses (RDPs) placed in edentulous mandible (Rammelsberg et al. 2013). Moreover, prosthodontic options include fixed dental prosthesis (FDPs) on either, abutment teeth or abutment implants, a combination of abutment teeth and implants, implant-supported single crowns and resin-bonded prosthesis.

The mismatch distribution of forces between an implant that is ankylosed and a tooth that present function mobility due to the periodontal ligament may induce a mechanical deficiency, eventually leading to the failure of the weakest link. In oral implantology, therefore, the support created by a rigid connection between an implant and a natural tooth may represent an important cause of anxiety among clinicians (Lin et al. 2010; Lindh et al. 2001).

The purpose of this paper is to review recent findings in the field of implantology and prosthodontics regarding the tooth-implant supported prosthesis (TISP) (Figure 1). Particular attention will be given to the type of connection (rigid or non-rigid), the number of implants, average time of expectancy of the rehabilitations, as well as the dimension of the abutment (implants and teeth). Additionally, the clinical criteria to achieve good success rates in this type of rehabilitation will be also presented and discussed.

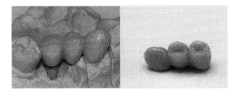

Figure 1. Three element tooth-implant supported prosthesis (TISP): Vestibular and lingual view.

2 MATERIAL AND METHODS

A PubMed® and Scopus® search were performed using the following keywords: "implant tooth support", "implant tooth bridge" and "connection tooth implant. The inclusion criteria were: 1) papers published from 1986 to March 2018; 2) documents written in English or Portuguese. The inclusion criteria were research or review studies on tooth-implant support done in-vitro, in animals or in humans. The exclusion criteria were all articles with only implant-implant or tooth-tooth support, case studies and short communications.

3 RESULTS AND DISCUSSION

From 773 PubMed's articles and 706 Scopus's articles, 24 articles were selected by the title. After reading the full-paper it was decided to include 19.

Posteriorly, these 19 articles allowed us to find other papers which were included in our review.

For a better comprehension on the subject this review was organized with an initial part of the discussion where multiple researches are going to be explored and posteriorly it will be bring to light important aspects that it should be in count during the process of the oral rehabilitation with tooth-to-implant support.

In the past few decades the discussion of extracting teeth to be substituted by implants to avoid the connection of teeth to implants has been one of the most controversial issues in field of prosthodontics. In 2001, the Committee of osteointegration and their authors did not found any risk by joining teeth and implants, although, they express concern that this kind of support could have higher level of complications or fractures (Weber *et al.* 2007). In 2004, a review of Lang and colleagues, about survival of implants in TISP was found to be 90.1%, and the prosthesis survival was found to be 94.1% (Lang *et al.* 2004). The corresponding figures for the 10-year survival were 82.1% for the implants and 77.8% for the prostheses. About the survival of prosthesis the studies included few cases in comparison to teeth or implant alone. (Lang *et al.* 2004). Later, Lindh and colleagues suggested that teeth should not be extracted in favour of placing dental implants without a specific indication and that a TISP should be considered as a viable prosthetic option (Lindh 2008). The number TISP's studies till 2008 are around 60, which are low when we compare to tooth support prosthesis (TSPs). In addition to the fact that long-term studies are few and do not have the same design.

In 2010, Weber and Zimering published a meta-analysis that included 555 patients with 538 TISP. The authors concluded that the TISP showed a lower survival rate for implants and FPDs (Weber *et al.* 2010), compared to similar meta-analysis of implant-only-supported fixed dental prosthesis (FDP).

The Gunne *et al.* study is a randomized-control clinical trial in which was used 23 patients that had a Kennedy Class I in the mandible and were rehabilitated. The comparison was intra individual with a split mouth design where randomization between three elements TISP versus three elements with implant support was left or right side of the patient, respectively. The dropout of this study was 13%. No difference in terms of implant survival or loss of marginal bone was found depending on the type support (Gunne *et al.* 1999). Bragger study is defined as a prospective long term case cohort. The initial aim was to observe peri-implant and periodontal conditions after one year of implant placement (Bragger *et al.* 1997). This cohort study was done retrospectively in patients treated at the university clinic. From this initial study a report of

4 to 5 years follow up was published (Bragger *et al.* 2001). After ten years, three studies were published by Karoussis *et al.*: one concerned the prognosis for implants in patients with and without a history of periodontitis (Karoussis *et al.* 2004); the second study about the association between periodontal and peri-implant conditions; and the third one about the effects of implant design on survival of the implant. In all of these studies the design of TISP was heterogeneous being difficult to compare with other studies.

Furthermore, when studied 19 cases of complete-arch fixed prostheses with combined tooth-implant-support, Cordaro *et al.* 2005 after a follow up of 94 months obtained a survival rate of 99% with only one implant lost in 90 implants, three implants had 2mm crestal bone loss and intrusion of teeth with intact periodontal was present when nonrigid connectors were used (Cordaro *et al.* 2005).

3.1 *Marginal bone loss*

Marginal loss is one of the characteristics which allows to determine the stability of TIPS. In a study of two year follow up with x-ray, it was found that in three elements FDP with premolars and molars, the implant support more load (Akca *et al.* 2006). At the end of 2 years there was a slight apposition of bone statistically more significant in the mesial side of the implant (Akca *et al.* 2006). Similar findings were observed in other studies (Lindh *et al.* 2001; Gunne *et al.* 1999; Hosny *et al.* 2000) however a study with follow up from 1.5 to 15 years founds a statistically significant loss of bone between free standing implant prosthesis and also in TISP (Naert *et al.* 2002).

3.2 *Technical complications*

Technical problems such as fracture of tooth or implant occurs in a low percentage and they are as common as with full implant supported prosthesis being below 2% at five years (Pjetursson *et al.* 2007). In the same study the cumulative rates are below 10% for most of complications were such as loosening of implant screws or abutments, and ceramic chipping. The most common complication is veneer fracture. In a 10 year follow up from the same group (Bragger *et al.* 2005), four out of 22 natural abutments developed carious lesions, leading to 19% failure. In other research with a similar follow up, the complication rate was 4% (Gunne *et al.* 1999). A reasonable conclusion is that even though the risk of complications of implant support prosthesis is low, we have to add the complications of teeth such as carious lesions and periodontal disease (Lindh 2008).

3.3 Type of connection

This is one of the most debated points in the issue of TIPS. Rigid connections consist in rigid screw retained abutment, coping with permanent cement (Figure 2) and soldered connectors (Greenstein et al. 2009, Nishimura et al. 1999). This type of connection for some authors is not rationale due to the adverse effects on the survival of the implants (Chee et al. 2006). In other in vivo and in vitro studies, it was shown that bending in implant components is sufficient to compensate the difference in mobility between tooth and implant (Gunne et al. 1997, Rangert et al. 1991, Rangert et al. 1995). In a later study, under clinical conditions the functional load is uniformly distributed to both abutments. In studies that evaluate bone loss around implants in TIPS with long periods of follow up indicate more loss in rigid connectors (Naert et al. 2001). However the difference between TIPS with rigid connection and control subjects (0.4 mm) is 0.3 mm in 15 year period of time and not affects the success of the prosthesis. Long term studies suggest that tooth and bone components of the implants go through certain deformation to compensate differences in resiliency under functional load (Naert et al. 1992, Nishimura et al. 1999, van Steenberghe 1989). The non-rigid connection consist in inter mobile elements that provide flexibility to compensate tooth mobility, and attachments. Some researchers concluded that using rigid connections has similar results has solely implant supported prosthesis (Nickenig et al. 2006). Most of recent studies show that rigid connections are superior to nonrigid. (Tsaousoglou et al. 2016, Mamalis et al. 2012; Hoffmann et al. 2012).

3.4 Tooth abutment displacement

Intrusion of the tooth is a common and unfavourable consequence that is well described in literature. This type of displacement is usually seen when non-rigid connectors or coping and telescopes with provisional cement or with no cement are used (Naert et al. 2001, Lindh et al. 2001, Garcia et al. 1998, Singer 1993). To avoid this phenomenon it has been observed that a rigid connection is more favourable than a connection with a disposer (or non-rigid) because it is able to attenuate the intrusion of the natural tooth. Furthermore, a pontic design short and straight as possible will prevent lateral displacement of the natural abutment (Naert IE. 2001). In cases where tooth-implant connection are required, it is necessary to follow-up the intrusion of the tooth abutment, since implants exhibit different displacement characteristics in response to loading when compared with natural teeth (Koyano et al. 2015). A study by Pesun and colleagues where TISP were placed in 30 mixed-breed dogs concluded that the vasculature and morphology of the histologic samples indicated stability and lack of inflammatory reaction from the periodontal ligament of the abutment tooth, but also lack of intrusion when using a rigid connector (Pesun et al. 1999).

3.5 Occlusal considerations

Overloading results from improper occlusion and once the implant lacks a supportive periodontal ligament the shock-absorbing function will be mostly cared by the tooth abutment (Alkharrat et al. 2017). Showed a lower fracture resistance in combined tooth-implant supported FDPs comparing to implant-supported regarding occlusal forces (Alkharrat et al. 2017). Due to the "inflexibility" of the implant system the implant will provide most of the support under light loading, but when loading exceeds 10 N the tooth begins sharing the load and contributes to support of the prosthesis (Rangert et al. 1995). Thus, it has been suggested placing minimal loading on teeth, and directing most of the load to implants in order to optimize the stress distribution. (Lin et al. 2010; Zhiyong et al. 2004; Ozçelik et al. 2007) Moreover, the occlusal force on the pontic should be minimized in centric position and lateral movements to maximize stress distribution (Lin et al. 2010).

3.6 Treatment considerations

The unbalance distribution of forces increases the risk of dislodging the prosthesis. Block and colleagues reported endodontically treated teeth being fractured at the interface of the post within the tooth (Block et al. 2002). Additionally, the quality of bone will influence the success of the rehabilitation, more failures of this treatment modality are associated with maxillary bone. So, short implants should be avoided to improve treatment success rate (Al-Omiri et al. 2017). A correct clinical examination and collection of the patient history is mandatory in all kind of treatments with no exception. Relatively to parafunctional habits, bruxism may be an unfavourable factor to a tooth-implant support rehabilitation. Menicucci and his colleagues, in 2002, tested a TISP prototype on finite element analyses and their results suggested that the load

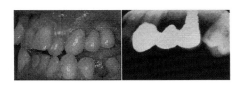

Figure 2. Cemented three element fixed prosthesis denture connecting tooth 23 to the implant 25 (rigid connection).

duration appeared to have a greater influence than load intensity on the stress distribution in the bone around an implant and a rigidly connected tooth (Menicucci *et al.* 2002). Static load showed to be potentially more harmful than a transitional load. Therefore, when present with a patient with centric bruxism (clenching) other treatment modalities should be considered or this parafunctional habit should be 'extinguished' before starting the oral rehabilitation. (Menicucci *et al.* 2002) Naert, in 2001, after evaluating over than 140 TISP and 329 freestanding (Branemark® system) implants, concluded that freestanding prostheses are more favourable when treating partial edentulism. The reason of Naert's preference is the clear tendency of more implant failures (mobility or fractures) and tooth complications in the tooth-implant connected prostheses (Naert *et al.* 2001).

3.7 Number of abutments

Lin *et al.* investigated the biomechanical interactions in TISP with variations in the periodontal support and number of splinted teeth using the non-linear finite element approach. Their results propose that when using two implants the stress on the bone is increased, from the opposite position the stress on the prosthesis decreased when compared when using one-piece implant. Interestingly, their model proposed that when splinting an implant to a compromised periodontal tooth the augment of stress increased was minimal compared to that of the splint system with a normal periodontal support. Moreover, when using two teeth as abutments the impact stress was not significant for the TISP (Lin *et al.* 2010).

4 CONCLUSIONS

Based on the literature reviewed, using implant-tooth support can be a reliable treatment option. If an attentive analysis at the risks-benefits is made to the patient requirements, this method may justify its application. From the present review we can conclude that:

– The success rate of TISP is admirable, although smaller when compared to the implant-implant support;
– A rigid connection is preferred;
– Greater bone loss may be expected around implant, although not clinically considerable;
– Both ends should be connected to the abutments equally, therefore cementing is preferred to screwing;
– Axial occlusal loading is preferred on the implant, oblique occlusal loading on the tooth

and minimum contact should be left on the pontic element;
– Complications such as caries lesions, intrusion, prostheses fracture, endodontic infections, loss of osteointegration, prostheses decementation are associated;
– Avoiding short implants, poor bone quality and compromised tooth abutment is recommended before opting the TISP.

There are still missing many aspects of this treatment paradigm, such as, the ideal number of abutments and units. More studies RCT with bigger samples are required.

REFERENCES

Akca, K., Uysal, S., Cehreli, M.C. 2006. Implant–tooth–supported fixed partial prostheses: correlations between in vivo occlusal bite forces and marginal bone reactions. *Clinical Oral Implants Research* 17(3): 331–336.

Al-Omiri, M., Maher. A., Mohannad, A., Lynch, E. 2017. Combined implant and tooth support: an up-to-date comprehensive overview. *International Journal of Dentistry* 2017: 6024565.

Alkharrat, A.R., Chmitter, M., Rues, S., Ramelsberg, P. 2017. Fracture behavior of all-ceramic, implant-supported, and tooth-implant-supported fixed dental prostheses. *Clinical Oral Investigations* (22): 1663–1673.

Block, M.S., Lirette, D., Gardiner D., Li, L., Finger, I.M., Hochstedler, L., Evans, G., Kent, J.N., Misiek, D.J., Mendez, A.J., Guerra, L., Larsen, H., Wood, W., Worthington, P. 2002. Prospective evaluation of implants connected t teeth. *The International Journal of Oral & Maxillofacial Implants* 17(4): 473–487.

Bragger, U., Aeschlimann, S., Burgin, W., Hammerle, C.H., Lang, N.P. 2001. Biological and technical complications and failures with fixed partial dentures (FPD) on implants and teeth after four to five years of function. *Clinical Oral Implants Research* 12(1): 26–34.

Bragger, U., Burgin, W.B., Hammerle, C.H., Lang, N.P. 1997. Associations between clinical parameters assessed around implants and teeth. *Clinical Oral Implants Research* 8(5): 412–421.

Bragger, U., Karoussis, I., Persson, R., Pjetursson, B., Salvi, G., Lang, N. 2005. Technical and biological complications/failures with single crowns and fixed partial dentures on implants: a 10-year prospective cohort study. *Clinical Oral Implants Research* 16(3): 326–334.

Chee, W., Jivraj, S. 2006. Connecting implants to teeth. *British Dental Journal.* 201(10): 629–632.

Cordaro, L., Erocli, C., Rossini, C., Torsello, F., Feng, C. 2005. Retrospective evaluation of complete-arch fixed partial dentures connecting teeth and implant abutments in patients with normal and reduced periodontal. *Journal of Prosthetic Dentistry* 94(4): 313–20.

Garcia, L.T., Oesterle, L.J. 1998. Natural tooth intrusion phenomenon. A survey. *The International Journal of Oral & Maxillofacial Implants* 13(2): 227–31.

Greenstein, G., Cavallaro, J., Smith, R., Tarnow, D. 2009. Connecting teeth to implants: A critical review of the literature and presentation of practical guidelines.

Compendium of continuing education in dentistry 30 (7):440–453.

Gunne, J., Astrand, P., Lindh, T., Borg, K., Olsson, M. 1999. Tooth—implant and implant supported fixed partial dentures: a 10- year report. *The International Journal of Prosthodontics* 12(3): 216–221.

Gunne, J., Rangert, B., Glantz, P.O., Svensson, A. 1997. Functional loads on freestanding and connected implants in three-unit mandibular prostheses opposing complete dentures: an in vivo study. *The International Journal of Oral & Maxillofacial Implants* 12(3): 335–341.

Hoffmann, O., Zafiropoulos, G.G. 2012. Tooth-implant connection: a review. *Journal of Oral Implantology* 38(2): 194–200.

Hosny, M.M., Duyck, J., van Stenberghe, D., Naert, I. 2000. Within—subject comparison between connected and nonconnected 375. tooth-to-implant fixed partial prostheses: up to 14-year follow-up study. *The International Journal of Prosthodontic* 13(4): 340–346.

Karoussis, I.K., Muller, S., Salvi, G.E., Heitz-Mayfield, L.J., Bragger, U., Lang, N.P. 2004. Association between periodontal and peri—implant conditions: a 10-year prospective study. *Clinical Oral Implants Research* 15(1): 1–7.

Koyano, K. Esaki, D. 2015. Occlusion on oral implants: current clinical guidelines. *Journal of Oral Rehabilitation* 42(2): 153–161.

Lang, N.P., Pjetursson, B.E., Tan, K., Bragger, U., Egger, M., Zwahlen, M. 2004. A systematic review of the survival and complication rates. II. Combined tooth–implant-supported FPDs. *Clinical Oral Implants Research* 15(6): 643–653.

Lin, C.L., Wang, J.C., Chang, S.H., Chen, S.T. 2010. Evaluation of stress induced by implant type, number of splinted teeth, and variations in periodontal support in tooth-implant-supported fixed partial dentures: a nonlinear finite element analysis. *Journal of Periodontology* 81(1): 121–130.

Lindh, T. 2008. Should we extract teeth to avoid tooth–implant combinations. *Journal of Oral Rehabilitation* 1: 44–54.

Lindh, T., Dahlgren, S., Gunnarsson, K., Josefsson, T., Nilson, H., Wilhelmsson, P., Gunne, J. 2001. Tooth–implant supported fixed prostheses: a retrospective multicenter study. *The International Journal of Prosthodontics* 14(4): 321–328.

Mamalis, A., Markopoulo, K., Kaloumenos, K., Analitis, A. 2012. Splinting osseointegrated implants and natural teeth in partially edentulous patients: a systematic review of the literature. *Journal of Oral Implantology* 38(4): 424–434.

Menicucci, G., Mossolov, A., Mozzati, M., Lorenzetti, M., Preti, G. 2002. Tooth-implant connection: some biomechanical aspects based on finite element analyses. *Clinical Oral Implants Research* 13(3): 334–41.

Naert, I., Koutsikakis, G., Quirynen, M., Duyck, J., van Steenberghe, D., Jacobs, R. 2002. Biologic outcome of implant-supported restorations in the treatment of partial edentulism. Part 2: a longitudinal radiographic study. *Clinical Oral Implants Research* 13(4): 390–395.

Naert, I.E., Duyck, J.A., Hosny, M.M., van Steenberghe, D. 2001. Freestanding and tooth implant connected prostheses in the treatment of partially edentulous patients. Part I: An up to 15 year clinical evaluation. *Clinical Oral Implants Research* 12(3): 237–244.

Naert I, Quirynen, M., van Steenberghe, D., Darius, P. 1992. A six-year prosthodontic study of 509 consecutively inserted implants for the treatment of partial edentulism. *Journal of Prosthetic Dentistry* 67(2): 236–245.

Nickenig, H.J., Schafer, C., Spiekermann, H. 2006. Survival and complication rates of combined tooth-implant-supported fixed partial dentures. *Clinical Oral Implants Research* 17(5): 506–511.

Nishimura, R.D., Ochiai, K.T., Caputo, A.A., Jeong, C.M. 1999. Photoelastic stress analysis of load transfer to implants and natural teeth comparing rigid and semirigid connectors. *Journal of Prosthetic Dentistry* 81(6): 696–703.

Ozçelik, T., Ahmet, E.E. 2007. An investigation of tooth-implant-supported fixed prosthesis designs with two-different stress analysis methods: an in vitro study. *Journal of Prosthodontics* 16(2): 107–116.

Pesun, I.J., Steflik, D.E., Parr, G.R., Haner, P.J. 1999. Histologic evaluation of the periodontium of abutment teeth in combination implant/tooth fixed partial denture. *The International Journal of Oral & Maxillofacial Implants* 14(3): 342–50.

Pjetursson, B.E., Bragger, U., Lang, N.P., Zwahlen, M. 2007. Comparison of survival and complication rates of tooth–supported fixed dental prostheses (FPDs) and implant-supported FPDs and single crowns (SCs). *Clinical Oral Implants Research* 18(3): 97–113.

Rammelsberg, P., Bernhart, G., Lorenzo Bermejo, J., Schmitter, M., Schwarz, S. 2013. Prognosis of implants and abutment teeth under combined tooth-implant-supported and solely implant-supported double-crown-retained removable dental prostheses. *Clinical Oral Implants Research* 25(7): 813–818.

Rangert, B., Gunne, J., Glantz, P.O., Svensson, A. 1995. Vertical load distribution on a three-unit prosthesis supported by a natural tooth and a single Branemark implant. An in vivo study. *Clinical Oral Implants Research* 6(1): 40–46.

Rangert, B., Gunne, J., Sullivan, D.Y. 1991. Mechanical aspects of a Branemark implant connected to a natural tooth: an in vitro study. *The International Journal of Oral & Maxillofacial Implants* 6(2): 177–186.

Singer, A. 1993. Apparent intrusion of natural teeth under an implant. *Journal of Prosthetic Dentistry* 70(1): 100.

Tsaousoglou, P., Michalakis, K., Kang, K., Weber, H.P., Sculean, A. 2016. The effect of rigid and non-rigid connections between implants and teeth on biological and technical complications: asystematic review and a meta-analysis. *Clinical Oral Implants Research* 28(7): 849–863.

van Steenberghe, D. 1989. A retrospective multicenter evaluation of the survival rate of osseointegrated fixtures supporting fixed partial prostheses in the treatment of partial edentulism. *Journal of Prosthetic Dentistry* 61(2): 217–223.

Weber, H.P., Sukotjo, C. 2007. Does the type of implant prosthesis. *International Journal of Oral and Maxillofacial Surgery* 22: 140–172.

Weber, H.P., Zimering, Y. 2010. Survival and complication rates of fixed partial dentures supported by a combination of teeth and implants. *Journal of Evidence-Based Dental Practice* 10(1): 58–60.

Biodental Engineering V – Belinha et al. (Eds)
© 2019 Taylor & Francis Group, London, ISBN 978-0-367-21087-8

Biomechanical behavior of dental implants—photoelastic analysis

V.N. Gomes & D. Tripak
Faculty of Dental Medicine, University of Porto (FMDUP), Porto, Portugal

S. Oliveira, J.C. Reis Campos & M.H. Figueiral
FMDUP, Porto, Portugal

ABSTRACT: Although oral rehabilitation with dental implants is worldwide accepted as an useful treatment option, failures still occur, particularly those related to implant stress distribution. The latter topic has benefited from the photoelastic analysis to gain further insights on the location of stress transmission areas. Additionally, such technique allows the identification of critical mechanical areas among implant components. This study aims to overview the contribution of the photoelastic analysis in the field of oral rehabilitation with dental implants.

1 INTRODUCTION

The biomechanical performance of implants in the mandible and its relationship with the stomatognathic system have been the focus of a number of studies. It is, therefore, elementary to comprehend the quantity and the quality of the forces produced and spread to the surrounding structures, such as the bone, from a biomechanical perspective (Pesqueira et al. 2014). For that reason, considering the mechanical properties of implant-prosthesis and the biomechanical aspects of the stomatognathic system is essential for a careful restorative treatment planning and design (Assunção et al. 2009).

The biomechanics of stress distribution around natural teeth and dental implants has fueled extensive research as well (Turcio et al. 2009). It has been described that under load, a dental implant displays considerably more restricted movements (10 μm) when compared to natural teeth (100 μm). In addition, the implant-bone interface is considered crucial for longterm implant success. Along with this, both stress and load distribution can lead to mechanical problems and bone loss (Pesqueira et al. 2014).

To assess the distribution of stress in implant-supported prosthesis, photoelastic analysis of tension and deformations has been widely used. The method of photoelastic analysis consists on evaluating the color change when colorless plastic materials are subjected to stress or deformation, as a result of refractive index changes. This analysis allows a qualitative assessment of stress, being commonly used to appraise the distribution of tension and deformations in implant-supported prosthesis (Pesqueira et al. 2014). It also enables the detection of critical points more susceptible to fracture, which occurs when the demanded forces are higher than the material resistance (Turcio et al. 2009). For that reason, and particularly in extensive oral rehabilitations, the evaluation of such critical points is crucial in order to use better materials that improve mechanical properties (Turcio et al. 2009).

Three major and classical techniques are available for photoelastic analysis: 2-dimensional, 3-dimensional and quasi 3-dimensional. In the last modality, the sample is assessed in 3D, whereas the fringes are analyzed in 2D. Another method, the reflective photoelasticity described by Pesqueira et al., allows an effective application in vivo, also enabling a quantitative evaluation (Pesqueira et al. 2014). In this review, the photoelasticity analysis will be discussed from a classical perspective, without distinguishing the different methods available.

The advantages of photoelastic analysis are multiple, being the possibility of directly assessing stress concentration, its location and the magnitude of stress forces one of the most prominent. Besides, the results can be measured and photographed without conversion into numerical data, and the method is applicable to irregular geometry (Pesqueira et al. 2014) (Assunção et al. 2009). This approach presents some drawbacks, however, since the method is limited in terms of the strength and force applied to the photoelastic material (Pesqueira et al. 2014). Accordingly, differentiating medullary from cortical bone is not possible, considering its non homogeneous and anisotropic characteristics. As an indirect technique, photoelastic analysis requires validation in a clinical context using identical conditions, but there are still limited quantitative data available (Pesqueira et al. 2014) (Assunção et al. 2009).

When compared to strain gauge systems and finite element methods, photoelastic analysis offers benefits to evaluate stress distribution, tissue response and physical properties of dental implants or prostheses (Assunção et al. 2009). Considering the multitude and diversity of studies relying on photoelastic analysis, the purpose of this work is to perform a literature review on this topic in the field of dental medicine, as a validated method for evaluating the behavior of dental implants and prostheses.

2 MATERIAL AND METHODS

For this study, a systematic review of the literature was conducted using Pubmed (Fig. 1). Articles dated between 2003 to 2018 were selected using the MESH terms. Firstly, the search aimed at finding descriptive information about the principal methods used to test stress in implants, including photoelastic analysis and other techniques: ((("dental implants" [MeSH Terms] OR ("dental" [All Fields] AND "implants" [All Fields]) OR "dental implants" [All Fields]) AND biomechanics [All Fields]) AND (photoelastic [All Fields] AND ("analysis" [Subheading] OR "analysis" [All Fields]))) AND ("methods" [MeSH Terms] OR "methods" [All Fields] OR "method" [All Fields]) AND ("2003/01/01" [PDAT]: "2018/12/31" [PDAT]). Articles were selected according to the presence of comparative considerations about the different methods available, being included 3 out of 10 papers.

Afterwards, the search followed different and very specific terms such as: ((dental implants) OR dental implant) AND "photoelastic analysis". Studies that applied other than the photoelastic analysis method were excluded. Based on these criteria, 23 out of 34 publications were included.

At all stages of the literature search, articles whose corresponding full-text was not possible to access were excluded. In total, from the 43 results primarily obtained, only 26 articles were selected for the current review.

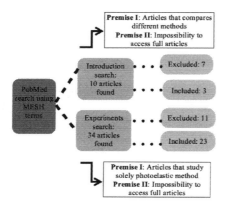

Figure 1. PubMed® search summary.

3 RESULTS AND DISCUSSION

3.1 *Types of implant-supported prosthesis retention*

Concerning the type of retention, several authors refer that there is no difference between screw— versus cemented-retained implant-supported prostheses (Aguiar et al. 2012). Some authors, however, have claimed that cemented prostheses present better stress distribution (Aguiar et al. 2012). The latter appear to provide higher levels of tolerance to poor adjustment, although exhibiting more biological issues (Lee et al. 2013) (Pimentel et al. 2015). In addition, cemented prostheses are more difficult to access in comparison to screw-retained reconstructions (Lee et al. 2013) (Pimentel et al. 2015). Implant-based rehabilitations retained by screws are technically more challenging, but a simpler solution can be found for the potential complications (Lee et al. 2013). The level of misfit and stress depends on many factors, like the type of prosthesis, loading protocol, bone quality, implant position, shape of the dental arch, diameter and length of the implant, implant surface and the prosthesis shape. Above all, the key factor for success is the precision of the connection between prosthesis and implant, with a perfectly passive fit at the implant-prosthesis interface being essential. The presence of gaps at the implant-prosthesis interface determines a delayed long-term osseointegration (Lee et al. 2013). Aiming to evaluate the consequences of the presence of gaps in three unit fixed partial dentures (FPDs), Lee et al. reported that screws retained with gaps showed more stress in the coronal portion of adjacent implants. Nevertheless, in cement-retained FDPs with gaps a transfer of non-axial stress was observed to the adjacent implants (Lee et al. 2013).

3.2 *Types of implant-supported overdentures*

To address the influence of implant-retained overdenture design on stress distribution, an O'ring and bar-clip with 2 implants (placed in the corresponding canines' region), and an association of both with 4 implants (placed in the corresponding premolars and canines' region with the O'ring at the posterior area) were used in an experimental setting, in which the axial loads simulated the protrusive and posterior contacts. The results revealed that the distribution of stress was more favorable with the bar attachment. Moreover, the bar-clip was considered the best choice because of its long-term success, providing enhanced outcomes in the posterior ridge. In fact, the bar attachment developed moderate tension levels, displaying uniform stress distribution and superior retention. On the contrary, the association group showed a non-uniform tension distribution, mostly concentrated on the posterior implants with O'ring (Machado et al. 2011).

3.3 Type of implant-prosthesis connection

In regard to implants under immediate loading, the type of prosthetic system used to manufacture frameworks does not influence the decreasing of stress around the implant, if total passivity is achieved. The type of implant-prosthesis connection, on the other hand, has been proposed to play a significant role, with the Morse taper implants presenting better stress distribution in comparison to external hexagon implants (Odo et al. 2015). This data published by Odo et al. in 2015 was corroborated by the previous findings of Pellizzer and collaborators (Pellizzer et al. 2014).

Determining the areas of higher stress in the implant-bone interface may constitute a valuable tool to predict the most appropriate type of implant system. In line with is, multiple factors as the type of connection, type of prosthesis, single or multiple implant-supported prosthesis among others, should always be considered in each particular clinical situation (Pellizzer et al. 2014).

Using the photoelastic analysis to study the performance of a 3-unit implant-supported FPD, the maximum stress distribution was found for implants with internal hexagon connections; for a single implant-supported prosthesis, however, the cone Morse taper implant demonstrated the highest stress distribution, thus minimizing the stress transmitted to the implant (Tonella et al. 2011).

The influence of implant connection modifications was recently assessed in an experimental study using external hexagon and Morse taper implants. Modified implants result from changes in the macrogeometry of conventional implants, including length, diameter, shape, prosthetic connection and thread type. In that experiment, the external geometry (threat design) was changed by extending the three preexisting grooves in the apical third towards the prosthetic platform level. When compared with conventional samples, modified implants exhibited lower stress concentration in the cervical area, a smaller bone reabsorption, but an increased stress concentration in the middle area (Valente et al. 2017).

3.4 Implant design

Attempting to verify whether the implant design has an impact on the stress transmitted to peri-implant bone, Gehrke et al. conducted a study in which implants with different length (13 and 7 mm) and two distinct designs (conical and cylindrical) were tested (Gehrke et al. 2016). Under axial loading, stress distribution was not substantially affected by the implant length. The only difference observed was imparted by the implant design, with conical implants showing the best stress distribution, contrarily to cylindrical ones, which revealed an increased stress on the crestal region for the long and short implants, and in the apical portion solely for the long cylindrical implant. Another conclusion of this study was that shorter implants tend to present lower stress concentration on the crestal bone compared to longer implants (Gehrke et al. 2016). The predictable use of short implants (<10 mm) in oral rehabilitation involving alveolar bone resorption has fueled intense discussion. Using a photoelastic experimental approach, Pimentel et al. suggested that short-wide implants may provide a biomechanical behavior comparable to longer implants with regular diameter, thus representing a valuable therapeutic alternative (Pimentel et al. 2017). Conversely, other authors have supported that short implants determine higher stress concentration at the contact bone-implant. Nonetheless, in the presence of factors that magnify stress accumulation, as increased prosthetic crown height, implant length could become not relevant (Figueirêdo et al. 2014). Besides, the design of short implants can influence the mechanical performance of the bone-implant system (Goiato et al. 2017).

3.5 Implant-abutment connection

Regarding the implant-abutment complex, Murmura et al. and Goiato et al., in independent studies, found that the design of the abutment connection area affects the functional load transfer both to the fixture and to the connection screw (Murmura et al. 2013) (Coelho et al. 2013). In the former experiment, the internal octagonal connection showed more durability than the internal hexagon after cyclic load, in conditions that simulate one year of in vivo function. It is known that the screw connection is responsible for establishing retention and mechanical continuity between abutment and fixture. To accomplish such role, an adequate preload during the tightening is mandatory, which depends on the applied torque, the geometry of the screwhead and the material that the screw and abutment are made of (Murmura et al. 2013).

3.6 Full-arch implant-supported dentures

In terms of mandibular full-arch implant-supported prostheses, the bar materials and manufacturing techniques have been also tested through photoelastic analysis. The fiber-reinforced resin bar and the titanium machined bar demonstrated the best stress distribution records. According to this study, being more lightweight than zirconium or cobalt-chromium (Co-Cr), with a similar tensile strength to zirconium, and a comparable flexural and compressive strength to Co-Cr, the fiber-reinforced resin bar emerges as a viable alternative for mandibular full-arch rehabilitations. Compared to the conventional casting technique, the use of CAD-CAM is preferred, if the rigidity of the material is adequate to adapt all the components. The advantages of this

Table 1. Summary of some findings obtained with the photoelastic method to evaluate the stress of oral rehabilitation with implants (Pesqueira *et al.* 2014; Turcio *et al.* 2009; Assunção *et al.* 2009; Pimentel *et al.* 2015; Zaparolli *et al.* 2017; Pellizzer *et al.* 2010; Galvão *et al.* 2016). *Adapted from* Pesqueira *et al.* 2014.

Author	Year	Study variable	Comments/Conclusion
Zak	1935	Types of orthodontic movements	Since this study, the application of this technique started to be used in the dentistry field (mainly related to the stress distribution)
Helldén and Derand	1998	Fit and misfit framework	The method appears to be an efficient and accurate procedure for correcting distortion in cast titanium frameworks
Nishimura *et al.*	1999	Comparison between implants and natural teeth connected with rigid or nonrigid connectors	The nonrigid connectors had less stress distribution; for a single implant-tooth connection the stress distribution were higher; for 2 implants-1 tooth, the rigid connector showed better stress distribution
Kenney and Richards Sadoswsky and Caputo Sadoswsky and Caputo Celik *et al.*	1998 2000 2004 2007	Overdenture attachment system	For vertical and inclined implant designs, the lowest stress was transferred to all implants with the bar-ball attachment system; moderate stresses were observed in implants on the loaded side with unsplinted attachment systems. The highest stress level observed with all attachment systems was moderate
Ochiai *et al.*	2003	Implants placed in the posterior edentulous jaw fabricated with photoelastic material	Stress distribution and intensity for the 2 implant conditions was similar for segmented and nonsegmented abutment designs; magnitude of stresses observed for both abutment designs was similar for the single implant condition
Ueda *et al.* Markarian *et al.*	2004 2007	Parallel and tilted implants	Stresses were generated after screw tightening of the frameworks, increasing when a load was applied and when a vertical gap was present
Barbosa *et al.*	2008	Size and location of misfit at implant—abutment interface	Great vertical misfits do not necessarily result in higher detorque values
Goiato *et al.*	2009	Attachment systems of facial prosthesis	The retention systems produced different stress distribution characteristics that, in general, were concentrated in the area around the implants; the highest concentration of fringes, in increasing order, occurred in the retention systems of the magnets, O-ring, and bar-clip
Bernardes *et al.*	2009	Connection system of cylindrical implant	Under an off-center load, the internal-hex interfaces presented the lowest stress concentrations; internal-taper interfaces presented intermediate results, and one-piece and externalhex implants resulted in high stress levels
da Silva *et al.*	2009	Different types of connectors in implant—tooth union	The internal hexagon implant established a greater depth of hexagon retention and an increase in the level of denture stability compared with the implant with the external hexagon. However, this greater stability of the internal hexagon generated greater stresses in the abutment structures
Pellizzer *et al.*	2010	Influence of platform switching on stress distribution in implants	Stress concentrations decreased in the cervical region of platform switching, and conventional/wide-diameter displayed similar stress magnitudes
Pellizzer *et al.*	2015	Stress distribution of screwed, cemented or mixed retention in implant prosthesis	The use of cemented or mixed implant prosthesis presented the worst stress distribution when submitted to compressive load, also showing lower intensity fringes when compared to screwed prosthesis
Zaparolli *et al.*	2017	Analysis of mandibular full arch implant-supported fixed dentures with different bar materials and techniques	Short implants are a reliable alternative for clinical cases with severe bone resorption

approach arise from a more precise finishing, along with less stress concentration (Zaparolli et al. 2017). Barbosa et al., intending to evaluate the passive fit of frameworks, have previously encouraged the use of CAD-CAM in future work. Both studies agree about stress distribution between titanium versus Co-Cr frameworks, with titanium showing the best results (Barbosa et al. 2016). In another investigation, three different manufacturing techniques of metal frameworks from a Co-Cr alloy (laser welding, TIG welding and monoblock) revealed no differences concerning peri-implant tensions, which exhibited identical patterns in all experimental conditions assessed (de Castro et al. 2013).

3.7 *Platform-switching on dental implants*

The platform switching is widely known and its benefits have been proven elsewhere, at least from the biological point of view. Literature has claimed that this technique prevents crestal bone loss around implants among other complications over time. In terms of biomechanical analysis, the platform switching improves stress distribution, also leading to stress reduction around the peri-implant bone of implant cervix. In fact, when compared to a conventional implant with wider diameter, the stress distribution in platform switching implants has demonstrated similar outcomes (Pellizzer et al. 2010). Also, Galvão et al. concluded that using narrower prosthetic implants (3.3–3.6 mm), prefabricated metal abutments exhibited better stress levels around the implants, with the customized metal and zirconia abutments having the lowest stress distribution (Galvão et al. 2016). On the contrary, a conventional implant with regular diameter displayed the poorer stress distribution performance (Pellizzer et al. 2010).

3.8 *Fit of prosthetic frameworks*

The photoelastic method has been employed to examine the stress transference along well-fitting and ill-fitting prosthetic frameworks. Markarian et al. observed that parallel implants generated a stress gradient that follows their axes, while angulated implants resulted in non-homogenous stress distribution, due to oblique stress patterns. The poor-fitting photoelastic model resulted in increased preload stress values, which clinically may represent a deleterious condition (Markarian et al. 2007). Many authors agree that oblique forces generate greater stress over the implant-prosthesis complex (Tonella et al. 2011) (Coelho et al. 2013) (Goiato et al. 2016). Stress resulting from oblique forces is mainly concentrated at the cervical third of implants and the surrounding bone (Pellizzer et al. 2014), which

contradicts some of Valente et al. findings (Valente et al. 2017). Also, an ill-fitting prosthesis appears to concentrate preload and occlusal load stresses around the implant laterally, rather than transferring forces along the implant axis (Markarian et al. 2007). Table 1 displays in chronological order a list of studies using photoelastic analysis to evaluate stress distribution in implant-supported oral rehabilitation.

3.9 *Cantilever length*

As regards the impact of cantilevers, photoelastic analysis has provided interesting clues as well. From a biomechanical perspective, the cantilever length negatively influences implant-supported prosthesis due to poor stress dissipation (Goiato et al. 2016). The All-on-four concept was investigated using different angulations in the maxilla (Cidade et al. 2014). Surprisingly, increasing the angulation did not necessarily result in higher stress generated around the distal implant. Under distal loading conditions (i.e., loads in the cantilever extension or in the last pillar), implants tilted with 35° displayed reduced stress values in the apical region in comparison to those tilted with 15°. Such tendency is altered when a load distributed by all pillars is applied. In these circumstances, the implant angle of 35° showed the highest levels of stress, particularly in the cervical area (Cidade et al. 2014). On the contrary, in single-element prosthesis under axial and oblique forces, increased levels of stress accumulation were found with higher implant angles. When a three-unit prosthesis was assayed, however, no differences on stress distribution were found, except for the 12° implant that showed the highest stress values (Goiato et al. 2015).

4 CONCLUSIONS

In the context of atrophic edentulous mandible or maxilla, tilted implants with or without reduced cantilever extensions, short and/or angulated implants may constitute technically easier and predictable therapeutic alternatives. Likewise, narrow implants can be feasible for short-span edentulous areas.

The presence of gaps at the implant-abutment interface represents one of the major problems in oral rehabilitation, with the type of implant connection playing a pivotal role in the implant survival rate. It should be emphasized that a passive seating at the final stages of prosthetic rehabilitation is vital to guarantee a good stress transition to the peri-implant tissues. Achieving such requirement reduces the likelihood of implant failure, also improving its long-term durability. In addition, and considering the deleterious effects of oblique loads, prosthetic structures should receive vertical loads whenever possible, since they are better tolerated.

Protocols for implant-based oral rehabilitation are multiple and should be adapted to the edentulous area of interest, taking into account the anatomy, bone resorption degree, as well as the number of prosthetic elements (single or multiple). Although there is no consensus about the ideal implant system, the use of different types of implant designs, implant lengths, methods of abutments fabrication, and overdenture systems must be assessed on a case-by-case basis, considering their particular advantages and disadvantages.

The present literature review, briefly summarized in Table 1, emphasizes the important contribution of photoelastic analysis to the oral implantology field. By investigating the biomechanical behavior of implants, it is possible to predict critical stress regions in prosthetic rehabilitations. Combined with a thorough knowledge of the stomatognathic system, understanding the mechanical properties of dental implants enable the clinician to establish an optimal customized treatment plan, thus obviating mechanical failure of biomaterials and respecting the anatomical and occlusal principles.

REFERENCES

Aguiar, F.A. de, Tiossi, R., Macedo, A.P., Mattos, M. da G.C. de, Ribeiro, R.F., Rodrigues, R.C.S. 2012. Photoelastic analysis of stresses transmitted by universal cast to long abutment on implant-supported single restorations under static occlusal loads. *The Journal of Craniofacial Surgery* 23(7 Suppl 1): 2019–23.

Assunção, W.G., Barão, V.A.R., Tabata, L.F., Gomes, E.A., Delben, J.A., dos Santos, P.H. 2009. Biomechanics studies in dentistry: bioengineering applied in oral implantology. *The Journal of Craniofacial Surgery* 20(4): 1173–7.

Barbosa, G.A.S., Bernardes, S.R., de França, D.G.B., das Neves, F.D., de Mattos, M. da GC, Ribeiro, R.F. 2016. Stress Over Implants of One-Piece Cast Frameworks Made With Different Materials. *The Journal of Craniofacial Surgery* 27(1): 238–41.

Cidade, C.P.V., Pimentel, M.J., Amaral, R.C. do, Nóbilo, M.A. de A., Barbosa, J.R. de A. 2014. Photoelastic analysis of all-on-four concept using different implants angulations for maxilla. *Brazilian Oral Research* 28.

Coelho Goiato, M., Pesqueira, A.A., Falcón-Antenucci, R.M., Dos Santos, D.M., Haddad, M.F., Bannwart, L.C., *et al.* 2013. Stress distribution in implant-supported prosthesis with external and internal implant-abutment connections. *Acta Odontologica Scandinavica* 71(2): 283–8.

de Castro, G.C., de Araújo, C.A., Mesquita, M.F., Consani, R.L.X, Nóbilo, M.A. de A. 2013. Stress distribution in Co-Cr implant frameworks after laser or TIG welding. *Brazilian Dental Journal* 24(2): 147–51.

Figueirêdo, E.P., Sigua-Rodriguez, E.A., Pimentel, M.J., Oliveira Moreira, A.R., Nóbilo, M.A. de A., de Albergaria-Barbosa, J.R. 2014. Photoelastic analysis of fixed partial prosthesis crown height and implant length on distribution of stress in two dental implant systems. *International Journal of Dentistry*: 206723.

Galvão, G.H., Grossi, J.A., Zielak, J.C., Giovanini, A.F., Furuse, A.Y., Gonzaga, C.C. 2016. Influence of Metal and Ceramic Abutments on the Stress Distribution Around Narrow Implants: A Photoelastic Stress Analysis. *Implant Dentistry* 25(4): 499–503.

Gehrke, S.A., Frugis, V.L., Shibli, J.A., Fernandez, M.P.R., Sánchez de Val, J.E.M., Girardo, J.L.C., *et al.* 2016. Influence of Implant Design (Cylindrical and Conical) in the Load Transfer Surrounding Long (13 mm) and Short (7 mm) Length Implants: A Photoelastic Analysis. *The Open Dentistry Journal* 10: 522–30.

Goiato, M.C., Arsufi, G.S., de Medeiros, R.A., Pesqueira, A.A., Guiotti, A.M., dos Santos, D.M. 2015. Stress distribution in bone simulation model with pre-angled implants. *Journal of Medical Engineering & Technology* 39(6): 322–7.

Goiato, M.C., de Medeiros, R.A., Sônego, M.V., de Lima, T.M.T., Pesqueira, A.A., Dos Santos, D.M. 2017. Stress distribution on short implants with different designs: a photoelastic analysis. *Journal of Medical Engineering & Technology* 41(2): 115–21.

Goiato, M.C., Shibayama, R., Gennari Filho, H., de Medeiros, R.A., Pesqueira, A.A., dos Santos, D.M., *et al.* 2016. Stress distribution in implant-supported prostheses using different connection systems and cantilever lengths: digital photoelasticity. *Journal of Medical Engineering & Technology* 40(2): 35–42.

Lee, J-I., Lee, Y., Kim, N-Y., Kim, Y-L., Cho, H-W. 2013. A photoelastic stress analysis of screw- and cement-retained implant prostheses with marginal gaps. *Clinical Implant Dentistry and Related Research* 15(5): 735–49.

Machado, A.C.M., Cardoso, L., Brandt, W.C., Henriques, G.E.P., de Arruda Nóbilo, M.A. 2011. Photoelastic analysis of the distribution of stress in different systems of overdentures on osseous-integrated implants. *The Journal of Craniofacial Surgery* 22(6): 2332–6.

Markarian, R.A., Ueda, C., Sendyk, C.L., Laganá, D.C., Souza, R.M. 2007. Stress distribution after installation of fixed frameworks with marginal gaps over angled and parallel implants: a photoelastic analysis. *Journal of Prosthodontics: Official Journal of the American College of Prosthodontists* 16(2): 117–22.

Murmura, G., Di Iorio, D., Cicchetti, A.R., Sinjari, B., Caputi, S. 2013. In vitro analysis of resistance to cyclic load and preload distribution of two implant/abutment screwed connections. *The Journal of Oral Implantology* 39(3): 293–301.

Odo, C.H., Pimentel, M.J., Consani, R.L.X., Mesquita, M.F., Nóbilo, M.A.A. 2015. Stress on external hexagon and Morse taper implants submitted to immediate loading. *Journal of Oral Biology and Craniofacial Research* 5(3):173–9.

Pellizzer, E.P., Carli, R.I., Falcón-Antenucci, R.M., Verri, F.R., Goiato, M.C., Villa, L.M.R. 2014. Photoelastic analysis of stress distribution with different implant systems. *The Journal of Oral Implantology* 40(2):117–22.

Pellizzer, E.P., Falcón-Antenucci, R.M., de Carvalho, P.S.P., Santiago, J.F., de Moraes, S.L.D., de Carvalho, B.M.

2010. Photoelastic analysis of the influence of platform switching on stress distribution in implants. *The Journal of Oral Implantology* 36(6): 419–24.

Pesqueira, A.A., Goiato, M.C., Filho, H.G., Monteiro, D.R., Santos, D.M.D., Haddad, M.F., *et al.* 2014. Use of stress analysis methods to evaluate the biomechanics of oral rehabilitation with implants. *The Journal of Oral Implantology* 40(2): 217–28.

Pimentel, A.C., Manzi, M.R., Polo, C.I., Sendyk, C.L., da Graça Naclério-Homem, M., Sendyk, W.R. 2015. Photoelastic Analysis on Different Retention Methods of Implant-Supported Prosthesis. *The Journal of Oral Implantology* 41(3): 258–63.

Pimentel, M.J., Silva, W.J. da, Del Bel Cury, A.A. 2017. Short implants to support mandibular complete dentures—photoelastic analysis. *Brazilian Oral Research* 31: e18.

Tonella, B.P., Pellizzer, E.P., Falcón-Antenucci, R.M., Ferraço, R., de Faria Almeida, D.A. 2011. Photoelastic analysis of biomechanical behavior of single and multiple fixed partial prostheses with different prosthetic connections. *The Journal of Craniofacial Surgery* 22(6): 2060–3.

Turcio, K.H.L., Goiato, M.C., Gennari, Filho H., dos Santos, D.M. 2009. Photoelastic analysis of stress distribution in oral rehabilitation. *The Journal of Craniofacial Surgery* 20(2): 471–4.

Valente, M.L. da C., de Castro, D.T., Macedo A.P., Shimano, AC, Dos Reis, A.C. 2017. Comparative analysis of stress in a new proposal of dental implants. *Materials Science & Engineering. C, Materials for Biological Applications* 77: 360–5.

Zaparolli, D., Peixoto, R.F., Pupim, D., Macedo, A.P., Toniollo, M.B., Mattos, M. da G.C. de 2017. Photoelastic analysis of mandibular full-arch implant-supported fixed dentures made with different bar materials and manufacturing techniques. *Materials Science & Engineering. C, Materials for Biological Applications* 81: 144–7.

Biodental Engineering V – Belinha et al. (Eds)
© 2019 Taylor & Francis Group, London, ISBN 978-0-367-21087-8

Author index

Almeida, C.F. 11, 89
Almeida, P.J. 53, 267
Alves, C. 65
Apaza-Bedoya, K. 31
Araújo, A.I. 95
Araujo, F. 61, 75
Areias, B. 101, 105
Arroyo Bote, S. 47
Azevedo, A. 89, 95
Azevedo, L. 65

Barbosa, M.I.A. 245
Barros, A. 95
Batista, R. 253, 259, 279
Belinha, J. 123, 129, 135, 141,
 147, 155, 161, 167, 171, 177,
 183, 189, 195, 201, 207, 213,
 219, 225, 231, 237, 245
Benfatti, C.A.M. 31
Borges, T. 79
Braga, A.C. 109
Brau-Aguadé, E. 47

Caldas, G.A.R. 167, 171,
 177, 183
Carvalho, A. 57
Carvalho, M.T. 89
Castro, A.T.A. 189, 195
Castro, S. 25, 113
Coelho, C.C.C. 225, 231
Correia, A. 57, 61, 65, 75, 79, 83
Côrte-Real, I. 109, 111
Costa, H. 83

da Costa, R.F.A. 119
Dantas, F. 11
de Macedo, M.G.F. 115
Diederich, H. 1
Dinis, L.M.J.S. 155, 161

Fediv, I. 57
Fernandes, B. 109, 111
Fernandes, M.G. 15
Ferrás, P. 259, 271
Ferreira, S.D. 201, 207

Figueiral, M.H. 111, 119, 253,
 267, 271, 275, 279, 285
Figueiredo, R. 79
Fonseca, E.M.M. 15, 195
Fonseca, P. 57, 75

Gehrke, S.A. 1, 43
Gentil, F. 101, 105, 129, 135
Gomes, H.I.G. 213, 219
Gomes, J.M.S. 123
Gomes, V.N. 285
Góis, F. 259, 275
Guerra, A.C. 237

Henriques, B. 31
Henriques, B.A.P.C. 115
Hernandez, P.A.G. 167,
 171

Josset, Y. 27
Juanito, G.M.P. 31

Leitão, B. 79
Lenz, J. 5
Lestriez, P. 27
Lopes, J.D. 113
Lopes, R.D. 25

Magini, R.S. 31
Manzanares Céspedes, M.C. 47
Marques, J.S. 263, 267, 271
Marques, M. 141, 147
Marques, T. 65, 75
Martinez Choy, S.E. 5
Martins, A.A. 79
Martins, D.S. 65
Martins, M. 95
Matos, S. 61
Mendes, J. 253
Mesquita, P. 89, 111
Moreira, A. 253, 259, 279
Muraille, C. 27

Naconecy, M.M. 167, 171
Natal Jorge, R.M. 15, 101, 105,

123, 129, 135, 141, 147, 155,
 161, 167, 171, 177, 183, 189,
 195, 201, 207, 213, 219, 225,
 231, 237, 245
Nogueira, R. 109

Oliveira, A. 83
Oliveira, A.F. 141, 147, 195
Oliveira, B. 83
Oliveira, S. 61
Oliveira, S. 119, 253, 259, 285
Oliveira, T. 95
Oliveira, V.C.C. 195
Özcan, C. 27
Ozkomur, A. 167, 171

Parente, M. 101, 105, 129, 135
Pereira, M. 79
Pereira, T. 89
Peyroteo, M.M.A. 155,
 161, 189
Piloto, J.F. 15, 19, 53
Piloto, P.A.G. 19
Pimenta, M. 75
Pollmann, C. 113
Ponces, M.J. 25, 113
Portela, A. 11
Prados-Frutos, J.C. 1, 43
Prados-Privado, M. 1, 43

Ramos, N. 25
Reis Campos, J.C. 11, 95, 101,
 105, 113, 119, 253, 259, 263,
 271, 275, 285
Rocha, J.M. 267, 271
Rocha, P. 53
Rojo, R. 43
Roxo, M.J. 275

Sampaio-Fernandes, J.C. 263,
 267, 279
Sampaio-Fernandes, M. 119,
 263, 275, 279
Santos, C.F. 101, 105, 129, 135
Santos, N. 65

Sarwer-Foner, S.N.D. 31
Schindler, H.J. 5
Schneider, L.E. 167, 171
Schünemann, F.H. 31
Schweizerhof, K. 5
Silva, C. 53, 263
Silva, C.F.C.L. 115
Silva, F.S. 115

Smidt, R. 167, 171
Sordi, M.B. 31
Soares, D. 263, 267, 271

Tripak, D. 285

Valente, F. 109, 111
Vargas, K.F. 167, 171

Vasconcelos, M. 11, 89, 113
Vaz, M. 25
Vaz, P. 53, 109, 111, 275, 279
Vaz, P.C. 115
Villa-Vigil, A. 47
Volpato, C.A.M. 53, 115